T0185735

SECOND EDITION

BIPOLAR DISORDER

SECOND EDITION

BIPOLAR DISORDER

A CLINICIAN'S GUIDE TO TREATMENT MANAGEMENT

EDITED BY
LAKSHMI N. YATHAM
AND
VIVEK KUSUMAKAR

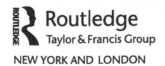

Routledge
Taylor & Francis Group

NEW YORK AND LONDON

Published 2009 by Routledge
605 Third Avenue, New York, NY 10017
4 Park Square, Milton Park, Abingdon, Oxon OX14 4RN

First issued in paperback 2014

Routledge is an imprint of the Taylor and Francis Group, an informa business

Copyright © 2009 Taylor & Francis

Library of Congress Cataloging-in-Publication Data

Bipolar disorder : a clinician's guide to treatment management / edited by Lakshmi N. Yatham, Vivek Kusumakar. -- 2nd ed.
   p. ; cm.
Includes bibliographical references and index.
ISBN 978-0-415-96136-3 (hardback : alk. paper)
  1. Manic-depressive illness. I. Yatham, Lakshmi N. II. Kusumakar, Vivek.
  [DNLM: 1. Bipolar Disorder--drug therapy. 2. Bipolar Disorder--diagnosis. 3. Tranquilizing Agents--therapeutic use. WM 207 B61575 2009]

RC516.B5246 2009
616.89'5--dc22   2008034968

ISBN 978-0-415-96136-3 (hbk)
ISBN 978-1-138-88170-9 (pbk)

In Memoriam

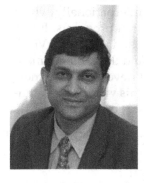

Dr. Vivek Kusumakar
1951–2009

The psychiatric community lost an outstanding colleague, clinician, scientist, educator, mentor and patient advocate, with the sudden death of Vivek Kusumakar on January 14, 2009. This book was Vivek's last major contribution to the field as he had just completed coediting this book 3 days prior to his untimely death.

Dr. Kusumakar was a professor of Psychiatry and Academic Head of Child and Adolescent Psychiatry at Dalhousie University in Halifax prior to joining Johnson & Johnson Pharmaceutical Research and Development in New Jersey in 2002. He trained and worked in India, Ireland, the UK, Canada, and the USA. His success as a clinician, researcher and educator in all of these countries was a testament to the outstanding communication skills he possessed and his vision, breadth of intellect, scientific curiosity, rigor, and generosity.

Among Dr. Kusumakar's many contributions, he was one of the founding members of the Canadian Network for Mood and Anxiety Treatments (CANMAT). It was Vivek's vision that led to a collaborative effort through the CANAMT in developing research and educational programs on bipolar disorder, which brought new treatments and information to patients, their families, physicians and other health care professionals. Vivek was the principal editor of the first Canadian Bipolar Disorder Clinical Treatment Guidelines in 1997, and these were widely adopted across Canada and in other parts of the world, and the subsequent revisions of the CANMAT guidelines are now considered the most comprehensive and up to date set of guidelines in the world. He was a coauthor of an influential consensus paper on research designs to study bipolar disorder in children and adolescents, published jointly by the American Academy of Child and Adolescent Psychiatry, the FDA, and researchers. Dr. Kusumakar's vision to help children with autism came to fruition when risperidone was the first treatment of its kind to be approved in the USA and Canada for the treatment of some of the debilitating symptoms of the disorder.

Dr. Kusumakar received many distinguished honors and awards including an award for his work on Tardive dyskinesia from the Royal College of Psychiatrists in the UK, and from the European College of Neuropsychopharmacology for his work on anticonvulsants in bipolar disorder, and Best Teacher Awards from the Universities of Glasgow and Edinburgh, as well as from the Professors of Psychiatry of the Royal College of Physicians and Surgeons of Canada.

Dr. Kusumakar's valuable contributions to science were matched by the highest of ethical standards. His commitment to volunteerism led to establishment of a variety of private foundations internationally which continue to run mental health awareness and research programs. It had been a singular privilege for me to know, collaborate, and work with Vivek for many years. His intellectual curiosity to understand the causes of mental illnesses, scientific ability to lead discovery and development of new treatments, drive for excellence, and ability to inject his vision and enthusiasm to his colleagues and those he mentored will be sorely missed.

Lakshmi N. Yatham, MBBS, FRCPC, MRCPsych (UK)

Contents

Acknowledgments ix
Preface xi
Contributors xiii

Chapter 1   Diagnosis and treatment of hypomania and mania 1
            Vivek Kusumakar, David J. Bond, and Lakshmi N. Yatham

Chapter 2   Bipolar depression: Diagnosis and treatment 19
            *David J. Muzina, David E. Kemp, Lakshmi N. Yatham, and
            Joseph R. Calabrese*

Chapter 3   Diagnosis and treatment of rapid cycling bipolar
            disorder 45
            Ralph Kupka and Mark A. Frye

Chapter 4   Bipolar II disorder: Assessment and treatment 79
            Felicity Ng, Catherine Cahill, Gin Malhi, and Michael Berk

Chapter 5   Maintenance treatment in bipolar I disorder 107
            Ryan F. Estevez and Trisha Suppes

Chapter 6   Bipolar disorders in women: Special issues 153
            Valerie H. Taylor, Meir Steiner, and Claudio N. Soares

Chapter 7   Bipolar disorder in children and adolescents 185
            Joris Berwaerts, Stanley Kutcher, and Vivek Kusumakar

Chapter 8   Bipolar disorder in the elderly 203
            Jaskaran Singh, Vivek Kusumakar, and Martha Sajatovic

Chapter 9   Comorbidity in bipolar disorder: Assessment and
            treatment 221
            Joseph F. Goldberg

Chapter 10 Lithium in the treatment of bipolar disorder 259
            Joseph Levine and K.N. Roy Chengappa

Chapter 11 Antipsychotic medications in bipolar disorder:
            A critical review of randomized controlled trials............ 295
            *David J. Bond, Eduard Vieta, Mauricio Tohen, and
            Lakshmi N. Yatham*

Chapter 12 Antidepressants for bipolar disorder: A review of
            efficacy.. 365
            Harm J. Gijsman and Willem A. Nolen

Chapter 13 Anticonvulsants in treatment of bipolar disorder:
            A review of efficacy.. 381
            Lakshmi N. Yatham and Vivek Kusumakar

Chapter 14 Somatic treatments for bipolar disorder............................ 411
            Raymond W. Lam, Peter Chan, and Andrew Howard

Chapter 15 Psychotropic medications in bipolar disorder:
            Pharmacodynamics, pharmacokinetics, drug
            interactions, adverse effects and their management....... 437
            Terence A. Ketter and Po W. Wang

Chapter 16 Practical issues in psychological approaches to
            individuals with bipolar disorders..................................... 551
            Jan Scott and Francesc Colom

Chapter 17 Psychosocial interventions for bipolar disorder:
            A critical review of evidence for efficacy......................... 575
            David J. Miklowitz

Chapter 18 Novel treatments in bipolar disorder: Future
            directions.. 591
            Jorge A. Quiroz and Robert M. Post

Index 619

Acknowledgments

We dedicate this book to patients with bipolar disorder and their families and friends, who have impressed us with their courage and perseverance in the face of adversity, and have taught us that hope comes from scientific, compassionate, and personalized treatment.

We also thank our families and colleagues for supporting us through this venture.

Lakshmi N. Yatham

Vivek Kusumakar

Preface

The previous edition of this book sold over 20,000 copies worldwide. The success of the book attests to an unmet need in this area as clinicians are clearly interested in books that provide an up-to-date synthesis of all new information in a manner that can be readily applied in clinical situations to manage patients with bipolar disorder. In keeping with this aim, the book has now been updated to include all pertinent information that will aid clinicians in the effective management of bipolar disorder.

In this revised edition, we have added a chapter on management of bipolar II disorder because of increasing recognition about its morbidity and some of the challenges in diagnosing and managing this disorder. In addition, we have devoted an entire chapter for issues related to bipolar disorder in women, while the chapter on bipolar disorder in children and elderly has been revised and updated and split into a chapter on the elderly and a chapter on children and adolescents. Evidence has accumulated over the past 10 years suggesting that psychosocial treatments as adjuncts to pharmacotherapy enhance outcome for patients with bipolar disorder. In light of this, we have added a chapter that summarizes the evidence for efficacy of psychosocial treatments and another chapter that deals with basic principles of psychosocial strategies to improve treatment adherence and outcome. Lastly, we have also added a chapter on potential new therapies for bipolar disorder to provide an overview of what is to come in terms of new treatments over the next few years.

As with the previous edition, the chapters in this revised edition fall into three main categories: the first five chapters provide diagnostic assessment and clinical guidelines for the treatment of different phases and types of bipolar disorder; the next four chapters deal with the management of bipolar disorder in women at various stages of reproductive cycle, young people, the elderly, and those with other psychiatric comorbidity. Chapters 10 through 14 review the efficacy of various psychotropic medications and somatic treatments commonly used for treatment of bipolar disorder. Chapter 15 focuses on psychotropic medication adverse effects, drug interactions and their management while Chapters 16 and 17 are devoted to psychosocial treatments. The final chapter is devoted to new and novel therapies for bipolar disorder. The division of chapters as outlined above necessitated allowing some overlap in content between the chapters.

Clinicians should be aware that the optimal treatment of bipolar disorder includes a combination of psychoeducation, life style management, psychotherapy and rehabilitative techniques with medications in the context of an empathic and longitudinal therapeutic relationship to improve symptoms, functioning and quality of life. Clinicians will need to mould their practice around the long term symptomatic and functional needs of their patients with bipolar disorder, and take a comprehensive illness management strategy, the cornerstone of which will be a collaborative multimodal approach and promotion of treatment adherence.

We sincerely hope that this book will help clinicians to provide rational evidence based treatment for patients with bipolar disorder.

This book has been made possible by numerous patients suffering from bipolar disorder whose experiences and resolve have been an inspiration to find safer and more effective treatments. We also thank all the contributing authors who have given their thought, time and energy to this book.

Lakshmi N. Yatham

Vivek Kusumakar

Contributors

Michael Berk
Department of Psychiatry
University of Melbourne
Geelong, Victoria, Australia

Joris Berwaerts
CNS, Pain and Translational
  Medicine
Johnson & Johnson
  Pharmaceutical Research and
  Development
Titusville, New Jersey, USA

David J. Bond
Division of Mood Disorders
University of British Columbia
Vancouver, British Columbia,
  Canada

Catherine Cahill
Psychological Medicine
University of Sydney
Sydney, Australia

Joseph R. Calabrese
Mood Disorders Program
Bipolar Disorder Research Center
Case Western Reserve University
Cleveland, Ohio, USA

Peter Chan
Department of Psychiatry
Vancouver General Hospital
University of British Columbia
Vancouver, British Columbia,
  Canada

K.N. Roy Chengappa
Western Psychiatric Institute
  and Clinic and Mayview State
  Hospital
University of Pittsburgh
  School of Medicine
Pittsburgh, Pennsylvania, USA

Francesc Colom
Bipolar Disorders Program
IDIBAPS Hospital Clínic
Barcelona, Spain

Ryan F. Estevez
Department of Psychiatry
University of Florida
Gainesville, Florida, USA

Mark A. Frye
Department of Psychiatry and
  Psychology
Mayo Clinic
Rochester, Minnesota, USA

Harm J. Gijsman
GGZ Nijmegen Mental
Healthcare
Trust and Department of
Psychiatry
University Medical Centre
Nijmegen
Nijmegen, The Netherlands

Joseph F. Goldberg
Mount Sinai School of Medicine
The Affective Disorders Program,
Silver Hill Hospital
New Canaan, Connecticut, USA

Andrew Howard
Department of Psychiatry
University of British Columbia
Vancouver, British Columbia,
Canada

David E. Kemp
Mood Disorders Program and
Bipolar Disorder Research Center
University Hospitals Case
Western Medical Center
Cleveland, Ohio, USA

Terence A. Ketter
Stanford University School of
Medicine
Stanford Bipolar Disorders Clinic
Stanford, California, USA

Ralph Kupka
Bipolar Disorders Program
Altrecht Institute for Mental
Health Care
Altrecht, The Netherlands

Vivek Kusumakar
Dalhousie University
Halifax, Nova Scotia, Canada
and
CNS, Pain and Translational
Medicine
Johnson & Johnson
Pharmaceutical Research and
Development
Titusville, New Jersey, USA

Stanley Kutcher
Dalhousie University and
IWK Health Centre
Halifax, Nova Scotia, Canada

Raymond W. Lam
Department of Psychiatry
University of British Columbia
Vancouver, British Columbia,
Canada

Joseph Levine
Ben Gurion University of the Negev
Beersheva Mental Health Center
Beersheva, Israel

Gin Malhi
University of Sydney
Northern Clinical School
Royal North Shore Hospital
Sydney, Australia

David J. Miklowitz
Department of Psychology
University of Colorado
Boulder, Colorado, USA
and
Department of Psychiatry
Oxford University
Oxford, England,
United Kingdom

David J. Muzina
Cleveland Clinic Neurological
 Institute/Psychiatry
Cleveland Clinic Lerner College
 of Medicine of Case Western
 University
Cleveland, Ohio, USA

Felicity Ng
Department of Clinical and
 Biomedical Sciences
Barwon Health
University of Melbourne
Geelong, Victoria, Australia

Willem A. Nolen
Department of Psychiatry
University Medical Center
 Groningen
University of Groningen
Groningen, The Netherlands

Robert M. Post
George Washington University
Washington, District of
 Columbia, USA

and

Pennsylvania State College of
 Medicine
Hershey, Pennsylvania, USA

Jorge A. Quiroz
CNS, Pain, and Translational
 Medicine
Johnson & Johnson
 Pharmaceutical Research and
 Development
Titusville, New Jersey, USA

Martha Sajatovic
School of Medicine
Case Western Reserve University
Cleveland, Ohio, USA

Jan Scott
Psychological Medicine
University of Newcastle upon Tyne
Newcastle, England,
 United Kingdom

Jaskaran Singh
University of Vermont
Burlington, Vermont, USA

and

CNS, Pain and Translational
 Medicine
Johnson & Johnson Pharmaceutical
 Research and Development
Titusville, New Jersey, USA

Claudio N. Soares
Psychiatry and Behavioral
 Neurosciences
Women's Health Concerns Clinic
McMaster University
Hamilton, Ontario, Canada

Meir Steiner
Psychiatry and Behavioural
 Neurosciences and Obstetrics
 and Gynecology
McMaster University
Hamilton, Ontario, Canada

and

Women's Health Concerns Clinic
St. Joseph's Hospital
Hamilton, Ontario, Canada

Trisha Suppes
Department of Psychiatry
VA Palo Alto Health Care System
Palo Alto, California, USA

Valerie H. Taylor
Psychiatry and Behavioral
  Neurosciences Mood Disorders
St. Joseph's Centre for Mountain
  Health Services
Hamilton, Ontario, Canada

Mauricio Tohen
Lilly Research Laboratories
Indianapolis, Indiana, USA

Eduard Vieta
University of Barcelona
Bipolar Disorders Program
Barcelona, Spain

Po W. Wang
Department of Psychiatry and
  Behavioral Sciences
Stanford University School of
  Medicine
Stanford, California, USA

Lakshmi N. Yatham
University of British Columbia
Vancouver, British Columbia,
  Canada

chapter one

Diagnosis and treatment of hypomania and mania

Vivek Kusumakar
Dalhousie University
Johnson & Johnson Pharmaceutical Research and Development

David J. Bond and Lakshmi N. Yatham
University of British Columbia

Contents

Mania: Diagnosis issues 1
Hypomania: Diagnostic issues 3
The management of mania and hypomania 5
    Assessment 5
    Initial steps, medical examination and relevant investigations 6
    Treatment strategies in mania 7
    Treatment strategies in hypomania 15
References 16

Mania: Diagnosis issues

The Diagnostic and Statistical Manual of Mental Disorders ([DSM-IV], American Psychiatric Press, 1994) defines a manic episode as a distinct period of abnormally and persistently elevated, expansive or irritable mood, lasting at least 1 week (or shorter if hospitalization is necessary), with three (four if only irritability is present) or more of the following symptoms present to a significant degree: inflated self esteem or grandiosity; decreased need for sleep; more talkative than usual; flight of ideas or a subjective experience that thoughts are racing; distractibility by unimportant and irrelevant external stimuli; increase in goal directed activity or psychomotor agitation; and an excessive involvement in pleasurable activities that have a high potential for painful or negative consequences. The mood disturbance must be sufficiently severe to cause

1

marked impairment in occupational and social functioning, sometimes requiring hospitalization to prevent harm to self or others, and may be accompanied by psychotic symptoms. Although the DSM-IV definition of mania does not include those associated with pharmacologically induced states, medical or neurological conditions, these states are important to recognize as they have significant implications for assessment, investigations and management.

In general, the severe nature of mania and the marked degree of functional impairment associated with it makes it easy to distinguish from non-pathological states such as a return to euthymia after a period of depression. However, mania and manic-like symptoms can occur in psychiatric illnesses other than Bipolar I Disorder. Differentiating bipolar disorder from schizophrenia and schizoaffective illness can be a diagnostic challenge, particularly in adolescents and young adults who are having their first or early episodes. The presence of psychotic symptoms, including bizarre or mood incongruent delusions and Schneiderian first rank symptoms, is consistent with a mania as long as there are concurrent and substantial mood symptoms as well. Cross-sectionally, acute symptoms of irritability, anger, paranoia, and catatonic-like excitement are not useful in distinguishing mania from schizophrenia, and full manias can occur in patients with schizoaffective disorder. In distinguishing between bipolar illness and psychotic disorders, the clinician should consider information about family history of psychiatric illness, premorbid functioning, nature of onset of symptoms, including presence of any prodrome, and previous history of episodes of illness, including functioning during inter-episode periods. In particular, obtaining a family history of bipolar disorder and a history of episodic illness with good interepisode functioning are helpful in confirming the diagnosis of bipolar disorder.

Mixed states, which constitute up to 30–40% of all manic episodes, can also pose diagnostic challenges. There are varied definitions of mixed mania in different diagnostic systems, and patients experiencing mixed episodes can present with a confusing mixture of manic and depressive symptoms. The lack of clear operationalized criteria can make it difficult to distinguish mixed mania from, for example, a major depressive episode with prominent psychomotor agitation or significant anxiety. As well, mixed states may represent a severe stage of mania, an intermediate or transitional state between mania and depression, or a distinct state that is a true combination of depressive and manic syndromes. The diagnostic and clinical implications of mixed states are summarized by Keck et al. (1996), and Freeman and McElroy (1999). The definitions of mixed states range from presence of full depressive episode to any depressive symptom in association with a manic episode. DSM-IV-TR defines mixed episode as patients meeting criteria for both depressive and manic episodes (except duration criteria) nearly every day for at least a 1-week period. However, it is increasingly accepted that the DSM-IV-TR definition of a mixed state is restrictive and arbitrary. The recognition of a wider spectrum of mixed states is not only important diagnostically but also has management implications, as mixed states are often associated with a turbulent course and increased suicidal risk, and a relatively poorer response to lithium and a better response to valproate and carbamazepine (The Depakote Mania Study Group, 1994; McElroy et al., 1992, Swann et al., 1997, Swann et al., 1999). McElroy and colleagues (1992) have devised operational criteria, which offer a compromise between the DSM-IV definition and other definitions that are overinclusive. They define dysphoric mania by presence of two or more specific depressive symptoms such as depressive mood, markedly diminished interest or pleasure in all or almost all activities, substantial weight gain or an increase in appetite, psychomotor retardation, hypersomnia, fatigue or loss of energy, feelings of worthlessness or excessive inappropriate guilt, feelings of helplessness or hopelessness, recurrent thought of death or suicide.

Hypomania: Diagnostic issues

Hypomania may occur as part of Bipolar II Disorder, or as a transitional state from euthymia to mania in patients with Bipolar I Disorder. A hypomanic episode, as per the DSM-IV-TR, consists of a period of elevated, expansive or irritable mood plus at least three (four, if only irritable) additional manic symptoms, lasting for a minimum of four days, and observed as a change from baseline by others. By definition, hypomania is not associated with marked impairment, hospitalization or psychotic features. Clinicians are aware that hypomania may, in fact, be associated with little or no functional impairment, or even represent a period of super-normal functioning. In addition, the criterion that symptoms should last for at least 4 days is arbitrary, and clinically relevant hypomanias may be missed with this criterion as hypomanic symptoms can often last for 1–3 days (Wicki & Angst, 1991; Yatham, 2005; Hadjipavlou et al., 2004). Clinicians should also note that many patients may simply show a decreased need for sleep and an increased energy and drive, which may all be masked within a socially or occupationally acceptable spectrum, particularly in adolescents, young adults and those in situations where a "driven" life style may be seen as acceptable or even desirable.

Bipolar II Disorder is frequently misdiagnosed as Major Depressive Disorder. The under-recognition of Bipolar II Disorder in research and clinical settings is largely attributable to the difficulty associated with obtaining a clear history of hypomania. Patients suffering from Bipolar II Disorder experience depression much more frequently than hypomania, and seek help almost exclusively during depressive episodes. Furthermore, individuals with Bipolar II Disorder may not recall previous hypomanic episodes, may not be able to distinguish them from euthymia, or even see them as desirable. Hence, it is incumbent on all physicians to retain a high index of suspicion for Bipolar II Disorder in any patient with apparent recurrent Unipolar Depression, and clinicians should carefully question all depressed patients about elevated mood states (Yatham, 2005). Careful history taking has been demonstrated to lead to a correct diagnosis of Bipolar II Disorder by experienced clinicians. Dunner and Day (1993) reported that an expert clinician using a semi-structured interview, when compared with a non-physician trained interviewer who used the Structured Clinical Interview for DSM-III-R (SCID), assigned a Bipolar II diagnosis much more often than did the less experienced interviewer. In routine clinical practice, other methods that can be used to increase the likelihood of correctly diagnosing Bipolar II Disorder include obtaining collateral information from family members, using validated questionnaires such as the Mood Disorders Questionnaire, and having patients keep a regular mood diary. Finally, clinicians should be alert for "warning signs" of bipolarity in depressed patients, including especially a family history of bipolar disorder and a history of antidepressant-associated manias or hypomanias. Additional predictors of bipolarity include early onset of depression, short (<3 months) depressive episodes, highly recurrent depressions, atypical depressive symptoms, a seasonal pattern to mood episodes, acute but not sustained response to antidepressants, and the presence of mixed depressive and hypomanic symptoms (Yatham, 2005).

Data from an ongoing genetic linkage study of Bipolar I families suggests that Bipolar II Disorder may be the most common phenotype or clinical manifestation in both Bipolar I and Bipolar II families (Simpson et al., 1993). Thus, there is some support for the clinical impression that Bipolar II Disorder may be more common than Bipolar I Disorder. Further, Bipolar II Disorder often tends to breed true to type: offspring and relatives of Bipolar II probands commonly also have Bipolar II Disorder (DePaulo et al., 1990), and genetic (Dunner, Gershon, & Goodwin, 1976), family history (Heun & Maier, 1993) and treatment studies (Calabrese et al., 2000) also suggest that Bipolar II Disorder is distinct from Bipolar I Disorder. Hence, a careful screening for a family history of Bipolar II Disorder can assist in diagnosis of a given patient. However, the clinician should also be careful not to diagnose bipolar disorder in patients, particularly those with borderline personality disorder, who often have uniphasic mood lability in the depressive to euthymic spectrum, and who may mistakenly describe euthymic states as "highs" (Akiskal, 1996). It is, however, important to bear in mind that borderline personality disorder can be comorbid with bipolar disorder in up to 30% of patients with bipolar disorder. The clinician is also well advised to be cautious in interviewing patients with Somatization

Disorder with depressive symptoms, as these patients can be highly suggestible, thus resulting in false positive assessments of hypomanic symptoms. Conversely, adolescent and young adult patients with rapid and ultra rapid biphasic mood cycling may be mistakenly diagnosed as having a primary borderline personality disorder. To safeguard against this, prospective mood charting and careful collateral histories and observations from friends and family members can be vital.

Although clear-cut mixed states are classified in the DSM-IV under mania, hypomanic patients may also suffer from dysphoric symptoms. Bipolar II Disorder, on average, has an earlier age of onset than does non-bipolar depression (Akiskal et al., 1995). This is particularly important as acts of deliberate self-harm in adolescents and young adults warrant an assessment for Bipolar II Disorder. Bipolar II patients are more likely than non-bipolar Major Depressive Disorder patients to have a history of suicide attempts (Kupfer, Carpenter, & Frank, 1988). Despite the turbulence that hypomania and recurrent depression can cause in Bipolar II patients, these patients are less likely to be hospitalized although the psychosocial impairment, risk of suicide and other functional morbidity may be significant in the Bipolar II group as well (Cook et al., 1995). Bipolar II patients also have a greater liability to rapid cycling.

The management of mania and hypomania

Assessment

The principles that guide the management of mania and hypomania include choosing a setting for treatment which will assure the safety of the patient and adherence with the treatment plan; prescribing medications which will rapidly reduce manic symptoms, protect against mania and depression during long-term treatment, and cause minimal side effects; and promoting a return to full psychosocial functioning. In the initial assessment of the patient, it is important to be aware that patients experiencing hypomania or mania often have a loss of insight fairly early in the course of the episode. Hence, obtaining collateral information from friends and relatives is vital. Clinicians should routinely screen for concurrent symptoms of depression and more complex mixed states, as well as for psychotic symptoms, suicidality, aggression, impulsive behaviors such as overspending, and dangerousness with or without homicidality. Observer rating scales have been commonly used in clinical research studies, and are increasingly being used to measure change and response to treatment in ordinary clinical settings. Rating scales that take into account patient reports, informant reports, and clinical staff observations are likely the most valid in establishing or ruling out the variety of symptoms that are present in a mania. For a review of a variety of rating scales refer to Goodwin and Jamieson (2007). Knowledge regarding the patient's psychiatric history, including severity of previous episodes and response to treatment trials, and medical history, including allergies, is also crucial. Noting the patient's mental state, particularly with respect to insight and judgment, and any evidence of psychosis, agitation, aggression, or threatening behavior, is important in assessing safety.

Initial steps, medical examination and relevant investigations

An important and necessary first step is to ascertain if the manic patient is able to give consent to treatment. If not, valid consent should be obtained as soon as possible from a person recognized in local law to be able to do so. Ensuring the safety of the acutely manic patient and those around him/her is a high priority at all stages of treatment. Hence, the initial steps may well involve screening for and managing an overt or covert attempt at suicide or other deliberate self harm, particularly by overdose. Patients who are aggressive and combative would benefit not only from being in a low stimulus, comfortable and non-challenging environment but also from rapid institution of medications to manage behavior dyscontrol and aggression. The clinician is well advised to confirm or rule out, early on in treatment, any reasonable possibility of mania secondary to an underlying medical condition, current or recent substance use and pharmacologically induced mania. Ideally, a medical evaluation and baseline investigations should be completed before the institution of biological treatment. In certain circumstances, however, because of a very acute clinical situation, treatment may have to begin prior to the completion of a full medical workup. Apart from a thorough medical examination, the following baseline investigations should be completed (Yatham et al., 2005): complete blood count including platelets; serum electrolytes; liver enzymes and serum bilirubin; urinalysis and urine toxicology for substance use; serum creatinine, and, if there is any personal or family history of renal disorder, a 24 hour creatinine clearance; TSH; ECG in patients over 40 years of age or with a previous history of cardiovascular problems; and a pregnancy test where relevant.

Serum levels of mood stabilizers should be obtained at the trough point, approximately 12 hours after the last dose of medication, at admission (as many patients are non-compliant with medications in the days or weeks leading up to an acute manic episode), and approximately 5–7 days after achieving a mood stabilizer dose titration. Two consecutive serum levels within the therapeutic range (0.8–1.2 mmols/l for lithium or 350–700 μmols/l for valproate) are sufficient during the acute phase. Any additional serum level monitoring is better guided by the clinical need and clinical state of the patient. There is no evidence that blood counts and liver enzymes need to be done more frequently than at baseline, at the end of 4 weeks and once every 6 months thereafter, unless there is a specific clinical concern. Closer monitoring is, however, required in children and the elderly, in patients being treated with multiple medications, or in any patients where there is legitimate clinical concern about hematological, hepatic, renal, endocrine, cardiovascular or neurological dysfunction.

Treatment strategies in mania

The reader is advised to refer to the chapters in this book on lithium (Chapter 10), anticonvulsants (Chapter 13), antipsychotics (Chapter 11), somatic treatments including ECT (Chapter 14), and pharmacokinetics and drug interactions (Chapter 17), for up to date reviews on the evidence of efficacy, common adverse effects and dosing strategies with various treatments. These reviews form the basis for the rationale in designing treatment strategies. However, outlined here is a summary of commonly asked questions and issues that underpin the treatment of hypomania and mania, followed by some treatment algorithms (Figure 1.1).

1. **Is the patient medically stable?** Baseline medical assessment and investigations, and medical stabilization should occur as soon as is clinically feasible. Pregnancy should be considered as a possibility and ruled out whenever clinically relevant.
2. **Is the patient competent to give consent?** If yes, record this. If not, seek the next person who can give valid consent. In most jurisdictions (check this to determine if it is the case in your city or state), patients can be treated in emergency situations without consent, but consent should be obtained as soon as possible.
3. **What treatment setting is best for the patient?** Manic patients with significant agitation, risk of gross occupational, social, financial and interpersonal misjudgments, deliberate self-harm, destructiveness, aggression, dangerousness or homicidality will commonly need the specialized observation and treatment that only a psychiatric inpatient unit can offer.
4. **What medications may be considered first-line treatments in the management of acute mania?** Mood stabilizing medications, including lithium, valproate and carbamazepine, can clearly be chosen as first line treatments for acute mania. They are all proven to be effective antimanic agents, *and* have some (valproate and carbamazepine) or good (lithium) evidence for prophylactic efficacy. Mood stabilizers can also be effective against depressive symptoms, *and* there is

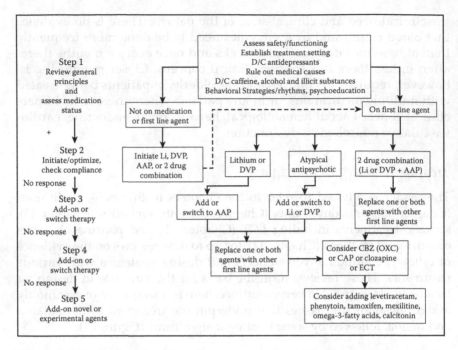

Figure 1.1 Treatment algorithm for acute mania. AAP, atypical antipsychotic; CBZ, carbamazepine; CAP, conventional antipsychotic; DVP, divalproex; ECT, electroconvulsive therapy; Li, lithium; OXC, oxcarbazepine; TOP, topiramate. (Adapted from Yatham, L.N., et al., Canadian Network for Mood and Anxiety Treatments (CANMAT) guidelines for the management of patients with bipolar disorder: Consensus and controversies. *Bipolar Disorders,* 7 (Suppl 3), 5–69, 2006.)

no evidence that they provoke depression. Although first generation antipsychotics are effective antimanic agents, they are associated with a significant risk of dystonic reactions and EPS in the short-term, and with tardive dyskinesia and exacerbation of depression in the long-term (Kukopulos et al., 1980), and are therefore not recommended as core treatments for mania except in exceptional circumstances. Recently, a great deal of evidence from randomized controlled trials (Scherk , Pajonk, & Leucht, 2007) has demonstrated that second generation antipsychotic medications, including risperidone, olanzapine, quetiapine, aripiprazole, and ziprasidone, are effective antimanic drugs, and they may be considered as initial monotherapy for mania (Yatham, 2005). However, due to their propensity to cause weight gain and metabolic disturbances (Newcomer, 2007), mood stabilizer monotherapy may be a preferred option in those with mild mania. In those with moderate to sever mania, in clinical practice, most clinicians choose a mood stabilizer and an atypical antipsychotic combination. Indeed, randomized controlled trials have demonstrated that the combination of a mood stabilizer and a second generation antipsychotic medication is superior to a mood stabilizer alone, with a more rapid onset of action and response and remission rates that are 10–20% greater than mood stabilizer monotherapy (Scherk, Pajonk, & Leucht, 2007). Current clinical practice guidelines (Yatham et al., 2005), suggest that combination therapy be used as a first line treatment for severely manic patients.

5. **Does the patient have marked behavioral dyscontrol, or is very aggressive or dangerous to self or others?** The patient may well need valid and ethical chemical or physical (i.e. low confrontation and stimulus) restraint that can be effective in minutes or at most a few hours. Treatment with benzodiazepines or first- or second-generation antipsychotics on a PRN basis should be considered in such situations. Antipsychotics should be considered especially if there is a previous history of disinhibition exacerbated by benzodiazepines. Second generation antipsychotics should be used where possible, although first generation antipsychotics may have to be used in the short term in some cases even though they may be associated with extrapyramidal side effects and have a propensity to induce depression. Consistent with clinical trial data, a recent case series suggests that intramuscular olanzapine at 10 mg is effective in reducing agitation and achieving behavioral control in mania (Bushe, Taylor, & Mathew, 2007). If the patient is not responding to optimal doses of the atypical antipsychotics or conventional antipsychotics and if the mania is escalating rapidly, then electroconvulsive therapy (ECT) needs to be considered as a treatment option.

6. **If first generation antipsychotics were used for behavioral control when patient was refusing oral medications, should the patient be switched to second generation antipsychotics and if so when and how?** As soon as the patient begins to accept treatment orally, consideration should be given to switching the patient to second-generation antipsychotics for reasons outlined above. As the dose of second-generation antipsychotic is increased, the dose of first generation antipsychotics should be cut down.

7. **Is the patient out of touch with reality due to psychotic thinking and perceptions?** There is some evidence that mood congruent psychosis will respond to mood stabilizer treatment alone. However, in the presence of persistent, severe, or chronic mood incongruent psychotic symptoms, second generation antipsychotics may be required in addition to mood stabilizers.

8. **Has the patient had a previous history of response to a particular mood stabilizer medication for mania, or was the patient ever stable**

in maintenance for bipolar disorder on a particular mood stabilizer medication or combination of medications? The previously effective medication treatment in monotherapy or combination therapy should be considered, unless newer effective medications with fewer adverse effects are available and are clinically indicated.

9. **Did the patient, historically, not respond effectively to a previous monotherapy or combination treatment or had intolerable side effects to treatment?** Consider a new option of antimanic medication.

10. **Does the patient have a recent or current history of rapid cycling or mixed state? Does the patient suffer from a bipolar disorder secondary to a medical condition or substance use?** Consider valproate or carbamazepine in a mixed state mania, or valproate in a manic episode as part of a recent rapid cycling course of illness. Second generation antipsychotics such as olanzapine can also be effective in mixed state mania (Tohen et al., 1999). Failure with lithium treatment is associated with mixed state mania and a rapid cycling course. Valproate and carbamazepine are effective in secondary mania. Also note that carbamazepine and lithium have significant interactions with other medications used in medical treatment. Prescribed substances including antidepressants that are felt to be contributing to the mania should be discontinued so long as this does not adversely impact on the patient's health.

11. **Is rapid onset of action of a medication indicated?** Loading dose treatment with valproate 20 mg per kg per day, risperidone 2–6 mg per day, olanzapine 10–30 mg per day, or zuclopenthixol acetate IM 50–150 mg every 72 hours, should be considered.

12. **How often is serum level monitoring of lithium or valproate required?** Obtain trough serum lithium or valproic acid levels after at 5–7 days after a dose increase. Titrate the dose as required. Two consecutive serum levels within the "target" range are sufficient. Serum lithium should be between 0.8 and 1.2 mmols/l and serum valproic acid between 350 and 700 μmols/l. Acutely manic and agitated patients may well need and tolerate doses producing serum levels at the higher ends of these ranges. Thereafter, the clinical picture should determine the frequency of serum medication level monitoring. Once every six months is sufficient during maintenance treatment.

13. **How often does one monitor CBC including platelets in patients being treated with valproate or carbamazepine?** After blood work proximal to the initiation of treatment, this needs to be repeated approximately 3–4 weeks into treatment, or as indicated by the clinical picture. In patients whose results are within the normal range or are clinically within normal limits, the blood work needs to be repeated only once every 6 months during continuation or maintenance treatment.

14. **In what circumstances do patients require ECG or a 24-hour creatinine clearance test?** Patients with a known risk for cardiovascular disease should have an ECG. Those with a past or family history of renal dysfunction should have a creatinine clearance test. In addition, all patients above 40 years of age and who are being considered for lithium treatment should have an ECG at baseline and as clinically indicated.

15. **If the patient has been treated for 3 weeks and does not show a trend towards improvement, and if you have optimized the medication for at least 2 weeks what are the treatment options?** Consider switching to or adding a new mood stabilizing medication or second generation antipsychotic. The best evidence currently is for the combination of a mood stabilizer and a second-generation antipsychotic, with risperidone, olanzapine, and quetiapine particularly well studied (Scherk, Pajonk, & Leucht, 2007). As well, combinations of lithium and valproate are reasonably safe, while a combination of valproate and carbamazepine should only be instituted with close serum level monitoring due to pharmacokinetic interaction. Also, if the patient has not responded to treatment up to now, it would be worthwhile, *again*, to rule out an underlying medical or neurological condition, and treat it if present. If the patient has not responded to the above strategies, combinations of three mood stabilizers or two mood stabilizers and a second generation antipsychotic might be appropriate at this stage. Experimental treatments such as levetiracetam, calcitonin nasal spray, a calcium channel blocker, or tamoxifen may be considered, if resources and clinical expertise permit. If there is no response with the above options, ECT can be considered. In patients with a history of chronic, severe refractory mania lasting over 3 months, and who do not respond to or are unable to receive ECT, clozapine treatment should be considered.

16. **Is ECT effective in bipolar disorder?** ECT is a highly effective treatment in both mania and bipolar depression. There is no clear consensus if bilateral ECT is superior to unilateral ECT. Treatment with ECT during an acute episode does not protect against recurrence of future episodes, nor does it convert medication non-responders into responders. However, the cognitive adverse effects of ECT, although clearly present—as evidenced by research—during the hours and days after a treatment, are neither long term nor permanent.

17. **Should patients with mania be treated only during the manic phase?** The lifetime risk of recurrence for a patient with Bipolar I Disorder is approximately 90%. Residual symptoms of depression or mania especially predispose patients to relapse. There is growing concern about patients who exhibit deterioration with each relapse

or recurrence. A significant number of patients who experience mania have either gone off their medications or have been under-dosed. Both these factors are associated with an increased risk for relapse and recurrence. Patients should be treated and monitored optimally, while providing timely psychoeducation and family support. Patients who have experienced a mania should be automatically considered for prophylactic mood stabilizer treatment in the majority of cases. In patients who have also received treatment with a second-generation antipsychotic, the optimal duration of maintenance treatment has not yet been determined by controlled trials, and should be a clinical decision.

18. **How can drug–drug interactions affect patients and management?** Clinicians should bear in mind that drug-drug interactions may alter the metabolism and serum levels of medications. This can result in sub therapeutic serum levels, which can be associated with treatment failure (e.g. failure of risperidone, as carbamazepine can induce hepatic enzymes to increase metabolism of risperidone resulting in low serum risperidone levels) or excessive serum levels, resulting in toxicity (e.g. lithium toxicity due to decreased clearance and increased serum level when used in conjunction with thiazide diuretics or NSAIDS). Carbamazepine in particular is known to induce the metabolism of many medications, including antipsychotics, antidepressants and oral contraceptives. Patients with developmental handicap, the elderly and those with medical or neurological problems may not only manifest exaggerated or idiosyncratic reactions to combinations of medications, but also to monotherapy.

The following treatment strategies can be effective in severely agitated or aggressive manic patients with or without psychosis:

- Admission into an intensive care psychiatric observation and treatment unit.
- Close observation for deliberate self-harm, destructiveness and aggression.
- If rapid behavioral control is required for safety, use intramuscular olanzapine 10 mg or zuclopenthixol acetate intramuscular injection 50–150 mg once every 72 hours, or haloperidol oral or IM 2–10 mg/day with or without adjunctive lorazepam oral or IM 2–12 mg/day, or a trial of first generation antipsychotic, e.g. loxapine oral or IM 20–150 mg/day can be considered. Patients who are willing to take oral medications may alternatively be prescribed olanzapine 5–30 mg daily, risperidone 2–6 mg daily, or quetiapine 400–900 mg daily, with or without concomitant lorazepam or clonazepam. Institute a mood

stabilizer and a second-generation antipsychotic as soon as patient is able to take oral medication.

- In patients where there is a need to deal with agitation and manic symptoms rapidly:
- Optimize the dose of currently prescribed mood stabilizer or initiate mood stabilizer (e.g. lithium, valproate or carbamazepine) and add a second generation antipsychotic medication, such as risperidone 1–6 mg/day, olanzapine 5–30 mg/day, or quetiapine 400–900 mg/day. Adjunctive lorazepam or clonazepam or oral or intramuscular first generation antipsychotics may be utilized on a PRN basis. Note that, to achieve efficacy, serum lithium should be at least >0.8 mmols/l, and serum valproate at least >350 μmols/l. Patients may well tolerate and need doses higher than they would tolerate when stabilized.

  Or valproate 20 mg/kg/day loading dose in combination with a second generation antipsychotic may be utilized. Adjunctive lorazepam, clonazepam or a first generation antipsychotic may be used on a PRN basis. Or ECT if the patient worsens rapidly or is excessively aggressive or does not respond to other strategies within a reasonable period or has a previous history of response to only ECT in a severely manic situation.

- In manic patients with a history of only a partial or a non-response to a combination of a mood stabilizer and antipsychotic, or a combination of two mood stabilizers, a switch to a different atypical antipsychotic or a mood stabilizer should be considered. We recommend following the CANMAT treatment algorithm in these cases (Yatham, 2005; Yatham et al., 2006).

- In patients who have a history of non-response to optimal use of the above strategies, or there is severe chronic mania that is persistent, Clozapine 50–900 mg/day (serum level 200–350 ng/ml) should be considered.

In manic patients with significant psychotic symptoms without significant aggression or behavior dyscontrol the following strategies:

- Restart or optimize previous treatment, or initiate a mood stabilizer (e.g. lithium, valproate or carbamazepine) and a second-generation antipsychotic medication. Adjunctive lorazepam, clonazepam, or a first-generation antipsychotic medication may be used on a PRN basis.
- If a patient does not respond to the above treatment within 3 weeks, consider combining valproate and lithium (safer than a valproate–carbamazepine combination), with or without a second generation antipsychotic.

- If a patient does not respond to the above regime within 4 weeks of optimal dosing, switch to a different second generation antipsychotic should be considered. These steps should be repeated a few times as per CANMAT algorithm before ECT can be considered.
- If there is a history of non-response to the above regimes, or if the psychotic mania does not respond to any of the above strategies in a timely manner, then clozapine 50–900 mg/day (serum level 200–350 ng/ml) should be considered.

In patients with pure mania without psychotic symptoms and with no significant behavioral dyscontrol the following strategy should be considered:

- Monotherapy with lithium (0.8–1.2 mmols/l), valproate (350–700 μmols/l) or carbamazepine in monotherapy may be sufficient for the core manic symptoms. However, in order to regulate sleep, lorazepam 1–4 mg/day, clonazepam 0.5–2 mg/day, zopiclone 7.5–15 mg/day, or quetiapine 12.5–50 mg/day over the first 7–10 days may be necessary.
- If there is poor or no response to the above regime within 3 weeks, consider the following: Switching to a different mood stabilizer or to a second generation antipsychotic; Adding a second generation antipsychotic to the mood stabilizing medication; or combining lithium and valproate (safer than a valproate–carbamazepine combination) can be considered.
- Those that fail to respond to the above strategies, consider the CANMAT treatment algorithm for further options.

In patients in a mixed state the following strategy should be considered:

- Valproate (serum level >350 mmols/l) or olanzapine 5–30 mg/day would be the first medications of choice. Mixed states are associated with failure to respond to lithium.
- If patient fails to respond to the above, adding or switching to a second generation antipsychotic would be appropriate especially in the presence of severe symptoms, excessive agitation, hostility or psychotic symptoms.
- Lorazepam 1–12 mg/day can be used for mild, moderate or severe behavior dyscontrol without a history of benzodiazepine induced disinhibition.
- ECT should be considered if the above strategies, even when optimized, are ineffective.
- Clozapine 50–900 mg/day (serum level 200–350 ng/ml) should be considered if the above strategies fail after an adequate trial.

Treatment strategies in hypomania

Hypomania is rarely the presenting complaint in a patient with Bipolar II Disorder. Bipolar II patients experience depressive symptoms anywhere from three- to thirty-fold more frequently than hypomania, and hypomania rarely causes sufficient distress or functional impairment to lead patients to seek treatment. However, patients with Bipolar II Disorder may present with hypomania during long-term follow-up, or give a history of frequent hypomanias associated with some degree of impaired functioning. Clinicians should bear in mind that, given the frequency and severity of depression relative to hypomania, the main goals of treatment for most patients with Bipolar II Disorder are to treat acute depression and to prevent depression and hypomania during maintenance therapy. To date, no randomized controlled trials have assessed any pharmacologic treatment in the management of hypomania. Nonetheless, clinical experience suggests that hypomania can be managed with the following strategies.

- Hypomania can commonly be managed in an ambulatory setting, and, in special circumstances, in a day hospital or day treatment setting.
- A trial of a mood stabilizing medication should be initiated, or optimized if the patient is already taking one. There is some evidence for lithium, lamotrigine, carbamazepine, and quetiapine in preventing episodes of hypomania and depression during the long-term management of Bipolar II Disorder, and for quetiapine in the treatment of acute Bipolar II depression. Lithium, lamotrigine, or quetiapine can be considered for initial pharmacotherapy, while carbamazepine should be reserved for non-responders due to its numerous pharmacokinetic interactions.
- Good sleep hygiene should be encouraged. If needed, a bedtime sedative such as lorazepam 1–2 mg, zopiclone 7.5–15 mg, clonazepam 0.5–1 mg, or quetiapine 12.5–50 mg may be prescribed.
- As a general rule, antidepressants should be discontinued. However, clinical judgment should be exercised in this situation. The evidence as to whether antidepressants increase the frequency of hypomania in Bipolar II Disorder is mixed, and patients with a clear history of antidepressant response and, historically, no increased frequency of hypomania and no severe mood elevations may in some cases continue antidepressant medications under close clinical observation.
- Where there is a previous history of rapid escalation into mania, and this hypomania is clinically deemed to be a transitional phase into mania, treatment with second generation antipsychotics may have to commenced or recommenced. Consideration should be given to in-patient admission for such patients.

References

Akiskal HS, Maser JE, Zeller PF, Endicott J, Coryell W, Keller M, Warshaw M, Clayton P, & Goodwin F. (1995). Switching from unipolar to bipolar II: An eleven year prospective study of clinical and temperamental predictors in 559 patients. *Archives of General Psychiatry, 52*,114–123.

Akiskal HS. (1996). The prevalent clinical spectrum of bipolar disorders: Beyond DSM IV. *Journal of Clinical Psychopharmacology, 16*, 2S–14S.

Bushe CJ, Taylor M, & Mathew M. (2007). Intramuscular olanzapine—a UK case series of early cases. *Annals of General Psychiatry, 6*, 11.

Calabrese JR, Suppes T, Bowden CL, Sachs GS, Swann AC, McElroy SL, Kusumakar V, Ascher JA, Earl NL, Greene PL, Monaghan ET. (2000). A double-blind, placebo-controlled, prophylaxis study of lamotrigine in rapid-cycling bipolar disorder. *Journal of Clinical Psychiatry, 61*, 841–850.

Cooke RG, Young LT, Levitt AJ, Pearce MM, & Joffe RT. (1995). Bipolar II: Not so different when co-morbidity is excluded. *Depression, 3*, 154–156.

DePaulo DR, Simpson SG, Gayle JO, & Folstein SE. (1990). Bipolar II disorder in six sisters. *Journal of Affective Disorders, 19*, 259–264.

Dunner DL, Gershon ES, & Goodwin FK. (1976). Heritable factors in the severity of affective illness. *Biological Psychiatry, 11*, 31–42.

Dunner DL, & Day LK. (1993). Diagnostic reliability of the history of hypomania in bipolar II patients and patients with major depression. *Comprehensive Psychiatry, 34*, 303–307.

Freeman MP, & McElroy SL. (1999). Clinical picture and etiologic models of mixed states. In: Akiskal HS. (Ed.), *The Psychiatric Clinics of North America. Bipolarity: Beyond Classic Mania, 22* (3), 535–546.

Goodwin FK, & Jamieson KR. (2007). Assessment. In: Goodwin FK & Jamieson KR (Eds.), *Manic Depressive Illness: Bipolar Disorders and Recurrent Depression* (pp. 355–378). Oxford University Press, New York, NY.

Hadjipavlou G, Mok H, & Yatham LN. (2004). Bipolar II disorder: An overview of recent developments. *Canadian Journal of Psychiatry, 49* (12), 802–812.

Heun R, & Maier W. (1993). The distinction of bipolar II disorder from bipolar I and recurrent unipolar depression: Results of a controlled family study. *Acta Psychiatrica Scandinavica, 87*, 279–284.

Keck PE, McElroy SL, Smetz GF, & Sax KW. (1996). Clinical features of mania in adulthood. In Shulman KI, Tohen M, Kutcher SP. (Eds.), *Mood Disorders Across the Life Span* (pp. 272–274). Wiley-Liss, New York, NY.

Kukopulos A, Reginaldi D, Laddomada P, Floris G, Serra G, & Tondo L (1980). Course of manic depressive cycle and changes caused by treatments. *Pharmokopsychiatr Neuropsychopharmacology, 13*, 156–167.

Kupfer, DJ, Carpenter, LL, & Frank, E. (1988). Is bipolar II a unique disorder? *Comprehensive Psychiatry, 29*, 228–236.

McElroy SL, Keck PE Jr, Pope HG Jr, Hudson JI, Faedda GL, & Swann AC. (1992). Clinical and research implications of the diagnosis of dysphoric or mixed mania or hypomania. *American Journal of Psychiatry, 149*, 1633–1644.

Newcomer JW. (2007). Metabolic considerations in the use of antipsychotic medications: A review of recent evidence. *Journal of Clinical Psychiatry, 68* (Suppl 1), 20–27.

Scherk H, Pajonk FG, & Leucht S. (2007). Second-generation antipsychotic agents in the treatment of acute mania: A systematic review and meta-analysis of randomized controlled trials. *Archives of General Psychiatry, 64,* 442–455.

Simpson SG, Folstein SE, Meyers DA, McMahon FJ, Brusco DM, & DePaulo JR Jr. (1993): Bipolar II. The most common phenotype? *American Journal of Psychiatry, 150,* 901–903.

Swann A, Bowden C, Morris D, Calabrese JR, Petty F, Small J, Dilsaver SC, & Davis JM. (1997). Depression during mania. Treatment response to lithium or divalproex. *Arch Gen Psychiatry, 54,* 37–42.

Swann A, Bowden C, Calabrese J, Dilsaver S, & Morris D. (1999). Differential effect of number of previous episodes of affective disorder on response to lithium or divalproex in acute mania. *American Journal of Psychiatry, 156,* 1264–1266.

The Depakote Mania Study Group (1994). Efficacy of divalproex vs lithium and placebo in the treatment of mania. *JAMA, 271,* 918–924.

Thomas A. Widiger, Allen J. Frances, Harold Alan Pincus, Michael B. First, Ruth Ross, and Wendy Davis (1994). *The Diagnostic and Statistical Manual of Mental Disorders* (4th ed). American Psychiatric Press, Washington, D.C.

Tohen M, Sanger TM, McElroy SL, Tollefson GD, Chengappa KN, Daniel DG, Petty F, Centorrino F, Wang R, Grundy SL, Greaney MG, Jacobs TG, David SR, & Toma V. (1999). Olanzapine versus placebo in the treatment of acute mania. *American Journal of Psychiatry, 156,* 702–709.

Wicki W, & Angst J. (1991). The Zurich Study: Hypomania in a 28–30 year old cohort. *European Archives of Psychiatry and Clinical Neurosciences, 240,* 339–348.

Yatham LN. (2005). Diagnosis and management of patients with bipolar II disorder. *Journal of Clinical Psychiatry, 66* (Suppl 1), 13–17.

Yatham LN, Kennedy SH, O'Donovan C, Parikh S, MacQueen G, McIntyre R, Sharma V, Silverstone P, Alda M, Baruch P, Beaulieu S, Daigneault A, Milev R, Young LT, Ravindran A, Schaffer A, Connolly M, Gorman CP, & Canadian Network for Mood and Anxiety Treatments. (2005). Canadian Network for Mood and Anxiety Treatments (CANMAT) guidelines for the management of patients with bipolar disorder: Consensus and controversies. *Bipolar Disorders, 7* (Suppl 3), 5–69.

Yatham LN, Kennedy SH, O'Donovan C, Parikh SV, McIntyre R, Sharma V, & Beaulieu S. (2006). CANMAT guidelines for management of patients with bipolar disorder: An update for 2007. *Bipolar Disorders, 8* (6), 721–739.

chapter two

Bipolar depression: Diagnosis and treatment

David J. Muzina
Cleveland Clinic Lerner College of Medicine of Case Western University

David E. Kemp
University Hospitals Case Western Medical Center

Lakshmi N. Yatham
University of British Columbia

Joseph R. Calabrese
Case Western Reserve University

Contents

Early and accurate diagnosis of bipolar depression 20
    A family history of bipolar disorder has
       positive predictive value 21
    Depression is the hallmark of bipolar disorder 22
    Any failed antidepressant treatment is cause for
       diagnostic review 23
    The presence of comorbidities should heighten suspicion of
       bipolar depression 24
Pharmacological treatment of bipolar depression 25
    What are the first line treatment options for
       bipolar depression? 26
    When should combination or add-on
       therapies be considered? 30
       (1) Switching agents 31
       (2) Combining or adding alternate agents 31
       (3) Augmenting 32

What other somatic therapies should be considered
for refractory bipolar depression? 33
Clinical recommendations 34
References 37

Clinicians are increasingly aware of the challenges associated with making an early and accurate diagnosis of bipolar disorder. Absent a current or past history of obvious mania, the recognition of bipolarity is often late. The key distinction to be made principally is the differentiation of unipolar major depression from bipolar depression.

Our current diagnostic conceptualization of bipolar disorder revolves around the identified historical presence of at least one prior manic, mixed, or hypomanic episode. The occurrence of a major depressive episode or episodes itself does not allow for diagnosing bipolar disorder; in fact, DSM-IV criteria for a major depressive episode for major depressive disorder and bipolar disorder are identical. A history of a previous manic or mixed episode suggests a diagnosis of bipolar disorder, type I, whereas a past hypomania would indicate bipolar disorder, type II. Although these "above-baseline" poles of bipolar disorder can cause considerable distress, negative consequences, and disability, most individuals with bipolar disorder suffer more frequent and more extended periods of mood disturbance that are depressive in nature. Therefore, it is imperative that a diagnosis of bipolar depression be considered in any patient presenting with a major depressive episode.

The importance of accurate diagnosis is intuitively obvious. Proper treatment planning and success hinge on diagnostic certainty, particularly in bipolar depression. More systematic reviews of the efficacy of lithium, anticonvulsants, antipsychotics, and antidepressants may be found elsewhere in this book. The focus of this chapter will be a clinical and practical approach to the early and accurate diagnosis of bipolar depression and the general strategies employed to deal with acute bipolar depression.

Early and accurate diagnosis of bipolar depression

There is no better substitute for a thorough and confirmed history obtained from clinical interview of the patient and collateral sources, such as family and medical records, when attempting to accurately diagnose bipolar disorder. Taking a DSM-IV directed approach to diagnosis via informal or structured clinical interview augmented by collateral information should lead to accurate diagnosis. Simply asking depressed patients about any history of manic or hypomanic episodes using a symptom-based approach or screening instrument may be all that is needed in many cases. However, patients sometimes cannot recall or are embarrassed to admit to past manic episodes or behaviors. Furthermore, hypomanic episodes may often go undetected. The use of some "data-based clues" might afford the clinician with an index of suspicion regarding the possibility of bipolar disorder as the cause for a major depressive episode and thus improve the rate and accuracy of diagnosis. The following clues encourage the clinician to "think bipolar" based on family history, the depression history itself, the overall course of the mood disorder, response to past treatments, and the presence of comorbidities.

A family history of bipolar disorder has positive predictive value

The depressed patient presenting for evaluation and treatment should always be asked about a family history of bipolar disorder or manic-depressive illness. It is worthwhile to make a more detailed inquiry about any relative reported to have had a depressive episode, "nervous breakdown", psychiatric hospitalization or institutionalization, or suicide attempt since many times an exact diagnosis in these affected family members is not known by the patient. There are several lines of evidence supporting the belief that a family history of bipolar disorder may have positive predictive value in diagnosing bipolar depression in depressed individuals.

Some investigators have interpreted the work of Emil Kraepelin and others and stated that family history is the most important external diagnostic validator in psychiatry (Akiskal & Benazzi, 2006). A family history of bipolar disorder increases the likelihood that a patient's major depressive episode is bipolar in nature or that a bipolar course will follow in time (Akiskal & Benazzi, 2006; Akiskal et al., 1983; Coryell et al., 1995). In terms of the more difficult to diagnose bipolar II depression, Akiskal and Benazzi (2006) reported that not only was a family history of bipolar disorder much more common in bipolar II disorder than in major depressive disorder (odds ratio 4.4), but that with higher bipolar family loading there are more hypomanic symptoms seen during a major depressive episode ("depressive-mixed states"). Beyond clinical validation of bipolar II disorder and its inclusion in the Diagnostic and Statistical Manual (DSM) of Mental Disorders, there is support that bipolar II disorder is a genetically valid subtype that may be distinguishable from bipolar I disorder. Whereas linkage on chromosome 6q is strongly associated with bipolar I disorder, a broader phenotype, which includes bipolar II and bipolar spectrum disorders, appears to be linked to chromosome 8q (McQueen et al., 2005).

Numerous studies continue to strengthen the genetic and familial basis for bipolar disorder. A complex genetic etiology involving multiple susceptibility genes and an environmental component is suggested by family, twin, and adoption studies while pedigree studies using high-density genome scans have identified several potential bipolar-disorder susceptibility loci (Detera-Wadleigh et al., 1999). It is postulated that rather than one specific gene defect causing bipolar disorder, multiple genes are likely linked and have smaller effects that interact with each other to modulate susceptibility and/or disease phenotype (Kennedy et al., 2003). Imaging studies have found various potential abnormalities in families with bipolar disorder, perhaps implicating the anterior cingulate and medial frontal regions in mediating resiliency and vulnerability in these affected families (Kruger et al., 2006). Episode frequency and some clinical features have been found to be significantly correlated among relatives (Fisfalen et al., 2005). Numerous indicators of severity have also been reported to be familial, including earlier age of onset, hallucinations or delusions, alcoholism, and suicidal behavior (Fisfalen et al., 2005).

Routine and in-depth questioning about family history is warranted in the evaluation of any depressed patient, potentially leading to improved recognition of bipolar disorder or heightened clinical awareness of susceptibility and future risk of bipolarity.

Depression is the hallmark of bipolar disorder

Although a manic, mixed, or hypomanic episode is required by DSM-IV criteria to make a diagnosis of bipolar disorder, depression is the greatest burden of bipolar disorder. Depression often strikes early, recurs frequently, and leads to considerable distress and disability for those patients afflicted with bipolar disorder.

The majority of patients with bipolar disorder first demonstrate symptoms during childhood or adolescence (Lish et al., 1994). Depression, not mania, is typically the first episode at onset of bipolar disorder (Suppes et al., 2001). Overall time spent depressed is significantly greater than time spent manic (3:1) or hypomanic (37:1) emphasizing the predominantly depressive nature of bipolar disorder (Judd et al., 2002; Judd et al., 2003). Simply screening positive for the possible presence of bipolar disorder has been associated with significantly increased difficulties with work, social or leisure interactions, and extended family interactions (Calabrese et al., 2003). Furthermore, when questioned about the impact of bipolar disorder on occupational and psychosocial functioning, patients repeatedly attribute greater impairment in their work and family life to depressive symptoms rather than to mania (Calabrese et al., 2004). Suicide during bipolar depression is a well-known risk, with suicide attempts observed at rates 20 times higher than in the general population (Tondo Isacsson & Baldessarini, 2003).

Several studies suggest that bipolar depression is more commonly associated with certain attributes than unipolar major depression, including reverse vegetative symptoms (e.g. hypersomnia and hyperphagia), chronicity of the index episode, extraversion, novelty-seeking, and being less judgmental (Akiskal et al., 1983; Coryell et al., 1995; Bowden, 2005). The presence of psychotic features may also be a harbinger of bipolarity. Delusions that develop during an episode of major depression have been found to be predictive of bipolar disorder (Solomon et al., 2006) and longitudinal studies of post-partum psychosis most often reveal the underlying disorder to fall within the bipolar spectrum (Chaudron & Pies, 2003). Although these features might increase clinical suspicion of bipolarity in an individual depressed patient, they are not reliably present in all bipolar depressed patients. Indeed, current diagnostic classifications do not distinguish major depressive episodes of the bipolar versus unipolar variety.

Any failed antidepressant treatment is cause for diagnostic review

When patients presumed to have unipolar major depression do not respond, or even worsen upon receiving conventional antidepressant treatment, clinicians should be observant for signs of activation or agitation that may signal a "pseudo-unipolar" state (Akiskal et al., 2005). Such agitated depressions have been associated with suicidality when treated with antidepressant monotherapy and emphasize the fact that a diagnosis of bipolar disorder should be revisited in the setting of antidepressant treatment failure. Pharmacologic induction of hypomania or mania, sometimes referred to as "switching", is a phenomenon more commonly observed in the patient with bipolar disorder. Although debated as to its frequency, various antidepressant and other medications may confer some risk for switching or increasing cycles of abnormal mood states in some individuals with bipolar disorder. More important may be the recognition that a failed treatment should lead the clinician to revisit the diagnosis of bipolar disorder in any depressed patient.

In examining the predictors of bipolar disorder risk among patients being treated for major depression with standard antidepressant medications and at least one antidepressant failure, Calabrese and colleagues (2006) examined patient self-reports and medical records from 602 outpatients being treated by 60 psychiatrists across the United States. The Mood Disorders Questionnaire (MDQ) was used to screen for bipolar disorder. In this cohort, five variables were found to be associated with bipolar disorder risk (MDQ positive): family history of bipolar disorder, comorbid anxiety, depression diagnosis within five years, legal problems, and the subjective feeling of the patient that "people were unfriendly" toward them. Of interest, nearly one in five (18.6%) of these patients who were thought to have unipolar major depression screened positively for bipolar disorder and this rate was not impacted by the number of prior antidepressant failures. Whether the patient failed just one antidepressant or five or more did not change the likelihood of screening positive for bipolar disorder. Extending these data to the clinical practice of differentiating bipolar disorder from unipolar, clinicians should be aware that nearly 20% of their antidepressant failures may be related to potential misdiagnosis. Failure to respond to a conventional antidepressant treatment should prompt re-examination of the initial diagnosis to exclude bipolar disorder as the cause of the depressive episode prior to proceeding with the next antidepressant trial.

The presence of comorbidities should heighten suspicion of bipolar depression

Upon review of the literature, it becomes apparent that a strong association exists between substance use disorders, anxiety disorders, impulse control disorders, eating disorders and attention-deficit hyperactivity disorder (Singh & Zarate, 2006). Over a decade ago, substance abuse and dependence were recognized as comorbidities more likely to be present in patients with bipolar disorder than major depressive disorder (Regier et al., 1990). More recently, the 2001–2002 National Epidemiologic Survey on Alcohol and Related Conditions surveyed 43,093 respondents and similarly found the absolute rates of comorbid substance use disorders to be higher in subjects with bipolar disorder as compared with unipolar major depressive disorder (Hasin et al., 2005; Grant et al., 2005). Among the 883 respondents found to have bipolar disorder, the 12-month prevalence rate for any alcohol use disorder and any drug use disorder was 23.6% and 12.9%, respectively (Grant et al., 2005). This contrasts with the lower 12-month prevalence rates for respondents with unipolar disorder, where any alcohol use disorder was present in 14.1% and any drug use disorder was present in 4.6% of respondents (Hasin et al., 2005). Absolute lifetime rates for generalized anxiety disorder, social phobia, and personality disorders were also found to be higher among the individuals diagnosed with bipolar disorder. The results of this large epidemiological study are consistent with anxiety disorder research that shows specific anxiety disorders, such as panic disorder and generalized anxiety disorder, are more common in bipolar than unipolar disorder, even after controlling for potential confounding variables such as age and gender (Simon et al., 2003).

Not all reports suggest a greater prevalence of co-occurring psychiatric disorders in patients with bipolar disorder. Mantere and colleagues (1996) found that patients with unipolar major depressive disorder had significantly more Axis I comorbidity than those with bipolar disorder (69% vs 57%, respectively) in a Finnish population. However, patients with bipolar disorder had more cluster B personality disorders, while cluster A and

C personality disorders were more commonly found to be comorbid with major depression (Mantere et al., 2006). In summary, the presence of comorbid substance use disorders and/or cluster B personality disorders in a patient with a depressive episode should heighten suspicion of bipolarity. Other impulse control problems, such as pathologic gambling, may also differentially affect individuals with bipolar disorder (McIntyre et al., 2007).

Perhaps more significant is the observation that medical comorbidities are quite commonly associated with bipolar disorder. Patients with bipolar disorder have been reported to suffer with higher rates of chronic fatigue syndrome, migraine, asthma, chronic bronchitis, multiple chemical sensitivities, hypertension, and gastric ulcer (McIntyre et al., 2006). Early onset depression, characteristic of bipolar disorder, may lead to negative health behaviors that result in the development of comorbid medical conditions. The role of medications used in the treatment of bipolar disorder to the development of cardiovascular disease should also not be overlooked. Obesity not only results in adverse medical outcomes, but is correlated with greater lifetime numbers of depressive episodes and depressive recurrence (Fagiolini et al., 2003). Comorbid medical disorders are associated with a more severe course of bipolar disorder, including psychosocial difficulties, unemployment, disability, and more frequent medical service utilization (McIntyre et al., 2006). Additionally, patients with bipolar disorder are vulnerable to developing key modifiable risk factors for cardiovascular disease, such as obesity, smoking, hypertension, dyslipidemia, and type 2 diabetes mellitus (Newcomer, 2006).

Although certainly not definitive in differentiating unipolar from bipolar depression, a pattern of psychiatric and/or medical comorbidities as described above should alert the clinician to the possible presence of an undiagnosed bipolar disorder in the depressed patient.

Pharmacological treatment of bipolar depression

A more detailed review of the efficacy of lithium, anticonvulsants, antidepressants, and atypical antipsychotics in the treatment of bipolar depression can be found elsewhere in this book. This section of the chapter aims to provide clinicians with rational and pragmatic approaches for treating patients with bipolar depression.

The majority of clinical trials using antidepressant drugs for depression have systematically excluded bipolar depressed patients due to fears about inducing manic switches or because the use of concomitant mood stabilizers might confound the interpretation of clinical efficacy of antidepressants. Interestingly, between 1968 and 2001 only 10 randomized trials (total $n = 533$) were reported on the use of traditional marketed antidepressants for acute bipolar depression (Muzina et al., 2006). Given the limitations in sample sizes, study designs, and interpretability one might conclude that to date there has yet to be demonstration via a large scale, randomized controlled trial that traditional antidepressant medication as monotherapy is both safe and efficacious. Nor is it clear whether antidepressants contribute any long-term benefit in bipolar disorder, as there are no controlled trials of maintenance phase treatment comparing the selective serotonin reuptake inhibitors or the second-generation antidepressants to placebo. This lack of supportive evidence for standard antidepressants along with concerns of destabilizing mood in the patient with bipolar depression are major factors contributing to the lower ranking of these agents as therapeutic options in most evidence-based practice guidelines and algorithms. When recommended, it is almost always in conjunction with known mood stabilizers or anti-manic agents.

Only recently have rigorous and methodical evaluations of pharmacological treatments for acute bipolar depression emerged. The recommendations formulated in this chapter for treatment of bipolar depression will be based mainly on these more recent treatment studies that have led to US-FDA approval or that have replicated, double-blind, placebo-controlled monotherapy trials. The questions that will be addressed here include: What is the first line treatment for bipolar depression? When should combination or add-on therapies be considered? What other somatic therapies should be considered for refractory bipolar depression? Finally, we will provide clinical guidelines for treating patients with bipolar depression.

What are the first line treatment options for bipolar depression?

An individual patient history of past response (efficacy and tolerability) should guide initial treatment decisions, if available. A family history of response to pharmacological treatment of bipolar depression may also prompt an informed first-step therapy choice. In terms of evidence-based first line treatments, lithium, lamotrigine, olanzapine–fluoxetine combination, and quetiapine take priority.

Although methodological problems limit the interpretability of data from early bipolar depression trials of lithium for bipolar depression, most suggest at least moderate efficacy (see Yatham et al., 1997; Muzina & Calabrese, 2003 for review). More recent study of lithium suggests that higher blood levels may be more effective, as no additional antidepressant benefit was achieved by the co-administration of paroxetine or imipramine when blood levels of lithium were maintained above 0.8 mEq/L (Nemeroff et al., 2001). Lithium's reported ability to protect patients from suicide with long-term use also confers some advantage when considering initial treatment strategies for this chronic, relapsing mood disorder (Baldessarini et al., 2006).

The only anticonvulsant that has been rigorously examined for its efficacy in bipolar depression to date is lamotrigine. Other anticonvulsants have not been extensively studied, have shown no significant efficacy, or have demonstrated only modest beneficial effects (see Muzina et al., 2006 for review). In the first double-blinded, placebo-controlled study of lamotrigine in the acute treatment of bipolar I depression, patients receiving lamotrigine 200 mg/day had significant improvement in depressive symptomatology compared to placebo as measured by several standardized rating scales (Calabrese et al., 1999). Lamotrigine has also been reported as a beneficial treatment for patients with rapid cycling bipolar disorder, particularly type II, as well as in a smaller cohort of treatment refractory subjects using a 6-week randomized and placebo controlled crossover design (Calabrese et al., 2001; Frye et al., 2000). It must be noted that lamotrigine failed to separate from placebo in the treatment of acute bipolar depression in four out of the five double-blind, placebo controlled trials completed to date (Calabrese et al., 2008), casting some doubt on the hope that robust antidepressant effects would be found consistently in acutely depressed bipolar patients. However, lamotrigine's proven efficacy as maintenance treatment in bipolar I disorder with more robust protection against depressive relapse and recurrence place it among leading first line options for acute bipolar depression as part of a regimen to potentially alleviate acute symptomatology as well as to delay or prevent future depressive episodes.

A recent report comparing lamotrigine to placebo add-on to lithium attempted to address the question of whether or not lamotrigine had any additional effect to lithium in patients with bipolar depression breaking through on lithium therapy (van der Loos et al., 2007). This study randomized 124 patients experiencing a depressive episode associated with bipolar I or II disorder to receive either lamotrigine ($n = 64$) or placebo ($n = 60$) added to prior lithium (0.6–1.2 mmol/L). Lamotrigine was dosed according to approved prescribing information guidelines starting with 25 mg/day and titrating to 200 mg/day. During the course of this 8-week double-blind study, a statistically significant reduction in Montgomery-Asberg Depression Rating Scores (MADRS) with lamotrigine use compared to placebo emerged at week 6 ($p = 0.031$) and was observed again at week 8 ($p = 0.006$). Lamotrigine add-on was also statistically superior to placebo add-on in response rates ($\geq 50\%$ MADRS reduction), with more than half of the lamotrigine-treated patients responding compared to less than one-third in the placebo group ($p = 0.030$). Lamotrigine add-on was well tolerated with no significant increase in observed switch rates or adverse events, including rash, as compared with placebo.

There is some historical foundation supporting the utility of antipsychotics to treat mood states acutely, with recent explorations of atypical antipsychotics for bipolar disorder—including the depressed phase—appearing in the literature (see Muzina et al., 2006 for review). The first placebo-controlled trial with an atypical antipsychotic for the treatment of bipolar depression was completed by Tohen and colleagues (2003). In this study, both olanzapine and the olanzapine–fluoxetine combination demonstrated significantly greater and sustained mean improvements in total depression scores over placebo. The olanzapine–fluoxetine combination was significantly better on all efficacy measures of depression in comparison to both olanzapine and placebo, including higher rates of response, remission, study completion, and faster times to response and remission. In addition, only the olanzapine–fluoxetine combination was able to significantly improve core mood symptoms such as apparent and reported sadness, lassitude, inability to feel, and pessimistic thoughts. Only bipolar I subjects were included in this acute bipolar depression trial. In 2003, olanzapine–fluoxetine combination became the first pharmacological treatment approved by the US-FDA for acute depressive episodes associated with bipolar disorder. An adequate trial of olanzapine–fluoxetine combination would encompass dosing with a minimum of 6/25 per day (olanzapine 6 mg plus fluoxetine 25 mg) for 6–8 weeks, increasing up to 12/50 per day as needed based on response.

The second agent, and only monotherapy, to receive US-FDA approval for acute bipolar depression was quetiapine. Two monotherapy trials of quetiapine for bipolar depression have been conducted. In the first, which represents the largest double-blinded, placebo controlled trial of bipolar depression to date ($n=542$) (Calabrese et al., 2005), quetiapine-treated subjects experienced higher response and remission rates than placebo-treated subjects as well as greater improvement on the core symptoms of depression. The second study (Thase et al., 2006) confirmed the findings of this initial trial with combined data for efficacy and tolerability of quetiapine monotherapy leading to an approved indication for the treatment of depressive episodes in bipolar disorder. Quetiapine monotherapy showed a broad effect against all core depression items, including suicidal thoughts. An adequate trial with quetiapine for bipolar depression would employ a minimum dose of 300 mg/day for 6–8 weeks, increasing up to 600 mg/day as suggested by clinical response while noting that 300 mg/day is the US-FDA recommended dose.

Quetiapine monotherapy has also been investigated beyond the acute phase of bipolar depression management and up to 52-weeks of continuation therapy in two similarly designed multicenter, randomized, double-blind, placebo-controlled studies referred to as EMBOLDEN (Efficacy of Monotherapy in BipOLar DEpressioN). In EMBOLDEN-I, quetiapine monotherapy (300 or 600 mg daily) was more effective than placebo for the treatment of acute depression episodes in bipolar I and bipolar II disorder; subjects randomized to a lithium monotherapy-treatment arm in this study did not demonstrate significant reduction in depression compared with placebo (lithium dosed to maintain serum level of 0.6–1.2 mEq/L). The acute antidepressant efficacy of quetiapine was maintained during long-term treatment up to 52 weeks (Young et al., 2008a). Similarly, in EMBOLDEN-II, quetiapine monotherapy (300 or 600 mg daily) was more significantly more effective than placebo in reducing depression acutely and maintaining this therapeutic effect over up to 52 weeks of continuation treatment. In this study, subjects randomized to paroxetine monotherapy (20 mg daily) fared no better than placebo with respect to reduction in depression (Young et al., 2008b). In the EMBOLDEN studies, long term quetiapine was generally well tolerated with treatment emergent adverse events similar to those observed with acute therapy.

However, it does not appear that a class antidepressant effect exists for the atypical antipsychotics in bipolar depression. Two identical, multi-center, double-blind trials comparing aripiprazole with placebo have been conducted in subjects with bipolar I disorder experiencing non-psychotic major depressive episodes (Thase et al., 2008). Subjects received aripiprazole starting with 10 mg daily with subsequent flexible dosing between 5 and 30 mg/day. Despite early statistical separation from placebo, by end of study (8 weeks) no significant differences were found in either of the two trials on primary or secondary efficacy measures. In addition, in a pooled analysis of the two studies a large proportion of aripiprazole-treated subjects developed akathisia as compared with placebo (24.4% vs 3.8%).

There is less strength of evidence for treatment of acute bipolar depression with all other available medications, including carbamazepine, divalproex, other atypical antipsychotics, or adjunctive antidepressants (see Kemp et al., 2006 for review).

However, in the recent largest randomized controlled trial of divalproex ER versus placebo in acute bipolar depression reported to date ($n=54$), divalproex ER monotherapy was associated with significantly greater reduction in depressive symptomatology than placebo beginning at week 3 and throughout the remainder of the 6 week study (Muzina et al., 2008). Subjects enrolled in this two-site study were mood stabilizer naïve and newly diagnosed with either bipolar I or II disorder in depressed phase. The therapeutic effect size was moderately large (0.68) with a mean dose of divalproex ER of 1,606 mg daily and mean blood level of 82 ug/ml. Subjects with bipolar I disorder, but not those with bipolar II disorder, experienced statistically significant improvement. Response rates to divalproex ER were significantly greater than with placebo; remission rates did not significantly differ. Follow-up study of divalproex in a larger sample size of patients with acute bipolar depression is warranted.

Although double blind controlled data are lacking, electroconvulsive therapy has consistently been shown to have efficacy in bipolar depression (Bratfos & Haug, 1965; Stromgren, 1973; Abrams & Taylor, 1974; Homan et al., 1982). In fact, electroconvulsive therapy appears to have comparable efficacy for both unipolar and bipolar depression, with bipolar depressives experiencing more rapid clinical improvement and requiring fewer treatments than their unipolar counterparts (Daly et al., 2001). Clinical consensus indicates that electroconvulsive therapy may be particularly effective for severe depressions complicated by marked suicidality or psychosis, supporting its use as first line treatment for acute bipolar depression in certain cases demanding urgent amelioration of symptoms.

First line treatment of bipolar depression typically calls for selection of quetiapine, olanzapine–fluoxetine combination, lamotrigine, or lithium based on available evidence and strength of data. Taking into account individual and family variables, as well as clinical experience, allows for a customized treatment strategy for bipolar depression. Electroconvulsive therapy should be considered for extremely depressed patients with bipolar disorder, especially if psychosis or severe suicidality is present.

The use of combined mood stabilizer plus a traditional antidepressant (most notably a selective serotonin reuptake inhibitor (SSRI) or bupropion) is common practice in clinical psychiatry. Scant controlled evidence supports such practice. Indeed, the recent report showing no difference in sustained remission rates between mood stabilizer alone and mood stabilizer plus SSRI or bupropion over 6 months suggests that combining mood stabilizer with antidepressants confers no great benefit in bipolar disorder and perhaps should not be considered a first-line treatment option (Sachs et al., 2007).

When should combination or add-on therapies be considered?

Combining two or more medications to treat bipolar depression is common practice. Expert consensus guidelines often support the use of two mood stabilizers in combination to treat bipolar depression, especially for refractory cases. Yet, the clinical trial evidence to support this practice remains lacking. Young and colleagues (2000) evaluated whether a second mood stabilizer (lithium or divalproex) or an antidepressant would be beneficial when administered to patients who experienced a major depressive episode while taking either lithium or divalproex. Results showed that both treatments were equally effective at reducing depression severity, though the trial was limited by a small sample size ($n=27$) and it is not known whether the administration of placebo would have resulted in similar levels of mood improvement. Among patients refractory to at least one trial of a mood stabilizer in combination with an antidepressant, there is open-label support for adding lamotrigine to the pharmacologic regimen, though this option is expected to result in recovery for about only one-fourth of patients (Nierenberg et al., 2006). Typically, patients with bipolar depression are treated with combinations of medications due to severity of the episode or lack of complete response to a monotherapy. Rapid cycling bipolar disorder is often associated with treatment refractoriness, perhaps to any treatment modality, and frequently requires multiple medications to achieve symptomatic recovery (Calabrese & Delucchi, 1989; Calabrese et al., 2005).

Prior to the emergence of evidence supporting the atypical antipsychotics for bipolar depression, refractory bipolar depression has been defined as "depression that failed to respond to a trial with lithium at serum levels of 0.8 mEq/L and above for six weeks" (Yatham et al., 2002). There is no consensus definition—Sachs (1996) initially defined refractory bipolar depression as depression without remission despite two adequate trials (6 weeks each) of standard classes of antidepressant agents with or without augmentation strategies. More recently, Nierenberg and colleagues (2006) utilized a definition of treatment resistance based on not responding to two trials of antidepressants or an antidepressant plus mood stabilizer regimen. Based on more recent studies noted above and the historical role of lithium, an alternate definition for refractory bipolar depression would be "depression that failed to fully respond to an adequate trial of at least two of the four first line options (olanzapine–fluoxetine combination, quetiapine, lithium, lamotrigine)".

Treatment strategies that should be considered for patients with refractory bipolar depression thus defined include: (1) switching agents, (2) combining or adding alternate agents, and (3) augmenting.

(1) Switching agents

The decision as to whether switch or combination is more appropriate hinges on whether a patient has shown no response or partial response to the current treatment. If adequate dosing of initial treatment with first line agents has been met with treatment failure, then switching agents among this group of four medications should be considered first if there is minimal or no response to the agent tried. As an example, a patient with bipolar depression who has failed to respond to quetiapine may be tried on OFC or lithium or lamotrigine. Given the prominence of data to support these four agents over all others, it is our view that this approach should be utilized during initial management of the refractory bipolar depressed patient. Based on the lack of replicated studies supporting lamotrigine monotherapy in bipolar depression, and its limited efficacy in preventing mania, lamotrigine monotherapy may be only appropriate for those patients with bipolar depression with a history of no recent or only mild manias.

(2) Combining or adding alternate agents

Another approach to managing the refractory patient would be a combination strategy, particularly if a patient had a partial response to previous agent. Combining mood stabilizers, such as adding valproate to lithium or combining carbamazepine with lithium may be effective for some patients as outlined above (Young et al., 2000; Kramlinger & Post, 1989). Combining alternate atypical antipsychotics with mood stabilizers may be helpful in some cases, although a class antidepressant effect for atypical antipsychotics has not been demonstrated thus far.

The addition of an antidepressant may be effective in treating some patients with bipolar depression with reports supporting tranylcypromine (Himmelhoch, Fuchs, & Symons, 1982; Himmelhoch et al., 1991; Thase et al., 1992), fluoxetine (Cohn et al., 1989), imipramine (Baumhackl et al., 1989; Cohn et al., 1989; Himmelhoch et al., 1991; Thase et al., 1992), moclobemide (Baumhackl et al., 1989), paroxetine (Young et al., 2000; Vieta et al., 2002), citalopram (Kupfer et al., 2001), bupropion (Sachs et al., 1994; McIntyre et al., 2002; Leverich et al., 2006), venlafaxine (Vieta et al., 2002; Leverich et al., 2006), sertraline (Leverich et al., 2006) and escitalopram (Fonseca et al., 2006). Similar effectiveness with other antidepressants might be likely although systematic studies have not been completed. The issue of antidepressant induced switching or cycling is covered in detail elsewhere in this book. Tricyclic and monoamine oxidase inhibitor antidepressants are thought to carry higher risk for mood destabilization in bipolar disorder (Peet, 1994; Calabrese et al., 1999; Boerlin et al., 1998). Although still under debate, the use of antidepressants in any patient with bipolar disorder must be approached with caution—even when prescribed with a known mood stabilizer. One study observed that although patients with bipolar disorder on antidepressants plus a mood stabilizer did not experience more switches to mania or cycling compared to those not taking an antidepressant, they more frequently remained in subsyndromal depressive states (Bauer et al., 2006). Another study reported significant rates of switching to full duration hypomania or mania in both acute and long-term continuation treatment with adjunctive antidepressants (venlafaxine>sertraline>bupropion) (Leverich et al., 2006). If antidepressants are used and depressive symptoms remit, controversy surrounds the issue of duration of antidepressant exposure and potential risk, with some recommending tapering off the antidepressant within 4–6 weeks of remission (Yatham et al., 1997; Yatham et al., 2006).

(3) Augmenting
Augmentation strategies involve adding an agent without known antidepressant properties but which may have the potential to augment the antidepressant properties of another drug. Several augmentation agents have been reported beneficial in unipolar major depression, including pindolol, tryptophan, methyphenidate, thyroid hormone, modafinil, gabapentin, pramipexole, and ropinirole (Perez et al.,

1997; Tome et al., 1997; Coppen, Shaw, & Farrell, 1963; Aronson et al., 1996; Wharton et al., 1971; Fawcett et al., 1991; Stoll et al., 1996; Menza, Kaufman, & Castellanos, 2000; Cassano et al., 2004; Cassano et al., 2005; Wang et al., 2002). These agents may be considered for use as augmentation in refractory bipolar depression with caution, particularly due to potential switching with stimulant use.

Recent reports have noted promise for the dopamine agonist pramipexole as augmentation to mood stabilizers in acute bipolar depression (Sporn et al., 2000; Zarate et al., 2004; Goldberg, Burdick, & Endick, 2004). Inositol, a sugar derivative with a role in intracellular signaling, has had modest and variable benefit to date as an augmenting agent (Nierenberg et al., 2006; Eden Evins et al., 2006). Riluzole, a glutamate-modulating agent used to treat amyotrophic lateral sclerosis, has shown antidepressant effects in an open-label trial in combination with lithium (Zarate et al., 2005). Omega-3 eicosapentaenoic acid (also known as fatty acids or "fish oils") have demonstrated some encouraging results as augmenting agents in bipolar depression (Osher, Bersudsky, & Belmaker, 2005; Frangou, Lewis, & McCrone, 2006), although no benefit was detected in a recent double-blind randomized controlled trial by Keck and colleagues (2006). However, a meta-analysis demonstrated statistically significant benefit for both unipolar and bipolar depression for omega-3 fatty acids and pointed out other health benefits associated with their use (Freeman et al., 2006). Most recently, Frye and colleagues reported significant benefit with modafinil add-on for acute bipolar depression that was inadequately responsive to therapeutic doses of a mood stabilizer, with some patients also failing adjunctive antidepressants (Frye et al., 2007).

What other somatic therapies should be considered for refractory bipolar depression?

Chronotherapeutic interventions, including the combination of light therapy and total sleep deprivation, are other biological treatments that have been tested for the relief of acute bipolar depression (Benedetti et al., 2005). Although the short-term efficacy associated with such interventions is intriguing from a mechanistic standpoint, the inability to provide sustained relief for more than a few weeks is a substantial limitation.

Variant forms of brain stimulation are also worthy of consideration in the treatment of refractory bipolar depression. As described previously in this chapter, electroconvulsive therapy is a particularly effective treatment for bipolar depression with efficacy rates reported to be at least 50% and as high as 100% (see Srisurapanont, Yatham, & Zis, 1995 for review).

Electroconvulsive therapy may be the preferred treatment for severe depression late in life although very little data exists regarding this treatment in geriatric bipolar depression (Dombrovski & Mulsant, 2007; Aziz, Lorberg, & Tampi, 2006). Similarly, although this treatment has been suggested as a non-teratogenic option for pregnant women with depression, it has not been sufficiently studied in terms of efficacy and safety in women with bipolar depression. Nonetheless electroconvulsive therapy remains a clinically effective treatment for refractory bipolar depression.

Vagus nerve stimulation (VNS) has been used for treatment refractory depression. Although acute beneficial effects have been observed to be marginally better than sham treatments, 1 and 2-year outcomes suggest a more gradual antidepressant benefit (Rush et al., 2000; Rush et al., 2005a; Rush et al., 2005b; Nahas et al., 2005). Only a very small number of these treatment refractory depressive patients were known to have bipolar disorder. Acute and long-term outcomes for bipolar depression are not well studied.

Repetitive transcranial magnetic stimulation (rTMS) has gained attention as a potential tool to treat depression although the optimum methodologies have not yet been defined (stimulus frequency, intensity, coil placement). Preliminary evidence suggests that this form of non-invasive brain stimulation may have a role in treating bipolar depression (Dolberg et al., 2002; Su, Huang, & Wei, 2005).

Deep brain stimulation (DBS) of the white matter tracts adjacent to the subgenual cingulate gyrus has been associated with a striking and sustained remission in a small number of patients with treatment resistant depression (Mayberg et al., 2005). Further investigation of this non-destructive form of neuromodulation for psychiatric disorders, including treatment refractory bipolar depression, is warranted.

Clinical recommendations

Recent and emerging data regarding the acute treatment of bipolar depression continue to reshape the hierarchy of clinical management strategies. Evidence-based practice guidelines change, with algorithmic approaches commonly updated in an effort to provide clinicians with additional information and tools to better manage bipolar depression (see updated CANMAT guidelines, Yatham et al., 2006). Until recently, initial treatment with lithium targeting blood levels of ≥ 0.8 mEq/L—either alone or in combination with an antidepressant or second mood stabilizer—may have been a common first line recommendation. Large studies have led to indications in acute bipolar depression for an atypical antipsychotic (quetiapine) and an atypical antipsychotic/SSRI medication combination (olanzapine–fluoxetine), thus altering the treatment landscape as have newer adjunctive therapy trials. Additional controlled trials validating a monotherapy role for lamotrigine acutely in the depressed phase have not been favorable and have surfaced in opposition to prior findings supporting its use in this manner, although its use as an adjunctive agent is better supported by the evidence.

As previously discussed, the treatment of acute bipolar depression should initially be undertaken with one of the first-line, evidence-favored options: OFC, quetiapine, lithium, or lamotrigine. In many cases, a combination of these agents may be the first step although monotherapy trials should be considered along with close follow-up and readiness to adjust the regimen based on treatment response. If the patient fails to respond to initial monotherapy with one of these four medications, the best next treatment strategy will depend on whether the patient experienced partial or no response. If no response, switch to an alternate first-line agent is recommended. If partial response, the addition of a second drug is advised—with the choice of added agent depending on which medication the patient was already taking and partially responding to. For example, if the patient was on lithium and had only a partial response, lamotrigine could be added based on the van der Loos study (2007) or antidepressant added based on the studies referenced above. If the initial approach to bipolar depression utilized quetiapine and only partial response occurs, SSRI's could be added based on open label data. If OFC initially led to only partial response, next steps might include substituting for olanzapine with quetiapine or lithium, or fluoxetine switched to bupropion.

For the newly diagnosed patient with bipolar disorder in the depressed phase who is not receiving a mood stabilizer, we recommend that treatment with one of the four first line agents (OFC, quetiapine, lithium, lamotrigine) be initiated after appropriate medical screening and blood work. This would include a thorough systems review and physical examination (to include height, weight, and waist circumference). Blood work including routine chemistries and blood count, thyroid stimulating hormone, and fasting blood sugar and lipid profile should be obtained at baseline. Discussions regarding most common concerns with these four agents, such as metabolic issues associated with atypical antipsychotics, lithium toxicities, and rash with lamotrigine can be found elsewhere in this book. Quetiapine should be dosed to 300 mg at bedtime, starting with 50 mg the first night, and increasing to 300 mg on day 4. Olanzapine–fluoxetine combination can be started at 6/25 once daily and titrated up later if clinically appropriate. Adequate trial duration should be a minimum of 6 weeks. A preference for quetiapine over olanzapine-fluoxetine is noted for those patients with bipolar II depression, with a history of antidepressant induced mania or cycling, or in clinical situations where weight gain or an increase in cardiometabolic risk may be particularly problematic. We recommend always following dosing guidelines for lamotrigine found in its prescribing information in order to minimize rash risk, paying particular attention to any co-prescribed medications that may inhibit or accelerate its clearance. When lithium is used to treat acute bipolar depression, starting divided daily doses totaling 600–900 mg with subsequent blood level determinations to target at least 0.8 mEq/L is advised.

Usual precautions when starting lithium (creatinine, thyroid panel, toxicity) or lamotrigine (risk for rash, dosing guidelines) should be observed (covered elsewhere in this book). For those patients with a recent or severe history of mania or hypomania, or for whom suicide risk may be elevated or chronic, the addition of lithium is preferred. Lamotrigine added to quetiapine or olanzapine–fluoxetine combination should be considered ahead of lithium in those who have a more prominent depressive course of bipolar disorder, those with bipolar II depression or rapid cycling, or those who may not be able to tolerate lithium.

If bipolar depression is more severe, particularly if hospitalization is necessary, ECT should strongly be considered. In cases where the patient with bipolar depression is already on a mood stabilizer, has failed the above initial treatments or is otherwise determined to be treatment refractory, the above reviewed strategies of switching, combining alternative agents or augmentation with novel compounds should be employed. Switching to another medication with a good evidence base or a closely related drug should be considered particularly if very limited or no response was obtained with the most recent regimen. Combining or adding on additional medication is also a viable next step, especially if some partial response has been obtained with the first drug or if additional symptomatology has emerged that requires attention. Examples include adding another mood stabilizer such as valproate if irritability or impulsivity is noted, or combining the ongoing mood stabilizer with an atypical antipsychotic if agitation or psychosis is present. The introduction of a standard antidepressant medication may be necessary for some patients, particularly in those with more severe or anergic depression, those with comorbid anxiety disorders or bulimia, those with chronic dysphoria and impulsive aggression stemming from a personality disorder, and those failing to respond to mood stabilizers alone. In these cases, SSRI's or bupropion should be the first choices with careful attention paid to the possibility that any antidepressant might carry a risk of manic or hypomanic switches or cycling of mood.

Augmentation with T3, pramipexole, modafinil, riluzole, inositol, or omega-3 fatty acids should be reserved for those patients with persistent resistance to the better studied treatments discussed above who either do not consent to or who are not eligible for electroconvulsive therapy. Electroconvulsive therapy is a very effective treatment for bipolar depression and should not be ignored or unduly delayed when initial treatment sequences fail to address depression, particularly when symptoms are severe, suicidal ideation is intense, or psychosis is present. Electroconvulsive therapy should also be considered for bipolar depression in the elderly and during pregnancy.

Developing somatic treatments, such as light therapy, VNS, rTMS, and DBS, offer hope for non-pharmacological interventions for refractory mood disorders. However, until larger studies that include a focus on refractory bipolar depression are done, their use should not be routinely considered.

References

Abrams, R., & Taylor, M. A. (1974). Unipolar and bipolar depressive illness. Phenomenology and response to electroconvulsive therapy. *Arch. Gen. Psychiatry, 30* (3), 320–321.

Akiskal, H. S., & Benazzi, F. (2006). The DSM-IV and ICD-10 categories of recurrent [major] depressive and bipolar II disorders: evidence that they lie on a dimensional spectrum. *J. Affect. Disord., 92* (1), 45–54.

Akiskal, H. S., Benazzi, F., Perugi, G., & Rihmer, Z. (2005). Agitated "unipolar" depression re-conceptualized as a depressive mixed state: implications for the antidepressant-suicide controversy. *J. Affect. Disord., 85* (3), 245–258.

Akiskal, H. S., Walker, P., Puzantian, V. R., King, D., Rosenthal, T. L., & Dranon, M. (1983). Bipolar outcome in the course of depressive illness. Phenomenologic, familial, and pharmacologic predictors. *J. Affect. Disord., 5* (2), 115–128.

Aronson, R., Offman, H. J., Joffe, R. T., & Naylor, C. D. (1996). Triiodothyronine augmentation in the treatment of refractory depression. A meta-analysis. *Arch. Gen. Psychiatry, 53* (9), 842–848.

Aziz, R., Lorberg, B., & Tampi, R. R. (2006). Treatments for late-life bipolar disorder. *Am. J. Geriatr. Pharmacother., 4* (4), 347–364.

Baldessarini, R. J., Tondo, L., Davis, P., Pompili, M., Goodwin, F. K., & Hennen, J. (2006). Decreased risk of suicides and attempts during long-term lithium treatment: a meta-analytic review. *Bipolar Disord., 8* (5 Pt 2), 625–639.

Bauer, M., Rasgon, N., Grof, P., Glenn, T., Lapp, M., Marsh, W., Munoz, R., Suwalska, A., Baethge, C., Bschor, T., Alda, M., & Whybrow, P. C. (2006). Do antidepressants influence mood patterns? A naturalistic study in bipolar disorder. *Eur. Psychiatry, 21* (4), 262–269.

Baumhackl, U., Biziere, K., Fischbach, R., Geretsegger, C., Hebenstreit, G., Radmayr, E., & Stabl, M. (1989). Efficacy and tolerability of moclobemide compared with imipramine in depressive disorder (DSM-III): an Austrian double-blind, multicentre study. *Br. J. Psychiatry, 6* (Suppl), 78–83.

Benedetti, F., Barbini, B., Fulgosi, M. C., Colombo, C., Dallaspezia, S., Pontiggia, A., & Smeraldi, E. (2005). Combined total sleep deprivation and light therapy in the treatment of drug-resistant bipolar depression: acute response and long-term remission rates. *J. Clin. Psychiatry, 66* (12), 1535–1540.

Boerlin, H. L., Gitlin, M. J., Zoellner, L. A., & Hammen, C. L. (1998). Bipolar depression and antidepressant-induced mania: a naturalistic study. *J. Clin. Psychiatry, 59* (7), 374–379.

Bowden, C. L. (2005). A different depression: clinical distinctions between bipolar and unipolar depression. *J. Affect. Disord., 84* (2–3), 117–125.

Bratfos, O., & Haug, J. O. (1965). Electroconvulsive therapy and antidepressant drugs in manic-depressive disease. Treatment results at discharge and 3 months later. *Acta Psychiatr. Scand.*, *41* (4), 588–596.

Calabrese, J. R., Bowden, C. L., Sachs, G. S., Ascher, J. A., Monaghan, E., & Rudd, G. D. (1999). A double-blind placebo-controlled study of lamotrigine monotherapy in outpatients with bipolar I depression. Lamictal 602 Study Group. *J. Clin. Psychiatry*, *60* (2), 79–88.

Calabrese, J. R., & Delucchi, G. A. (1989). Phenomenology of rapid cycling manic depression and its treatment with valproate. *J. Clin. Psychiatry*, *50* (Suppl), 30–34.

Calabrese, J. R., Hirschfeld, R. M., Frye, M. A., & Reed, M. L. (2004). Impact of depressive symptoms compared with manic symptoms in bipolar disorder: results of a U.S. community-based sample. *J. Clin. Psychiatry*, *65* (11), 1499–1504.

Calabrese, J. R., Hirschfeld, R. M., Reed, M., Davies, M. A., Frye, M. A., Keck, P. E., Lewis, L., McElroy, S. L., McNulty, J. P., & Wagner, K. D. (2003). Impact of bipolar disorder on a U.S. community sample. *J. Clin. Psychiatry*, *64* (4), 425–432.

Calabrese, J. R., Huffman, R. F., White, R. L., Edwards, S., Thompson, T. R., Ascher, J. A., Monaghan, E. T., & Leadbetter, R. A. (2008). Lamotrigine in the acute treatment of bipolar depression: results of five double blind, placebo-controlled clinical trials. *Bipolar Disord.*, *10* (2), 323–333.

Calabrese, J. R., Keck, P. E., Jr., Macfadden, W., Minkwitz, M., Ketter, T. A., Weisler, R. H., Cutler, A. J., McCoy, R., Wilson, E., & Mullen, J. (2005). A randomized, double-blind, placebo-controlled trial of quetiapine in the treatment of bipolar I or II depression. *Am. J. Psychiatry*, *162* (7), 1351–1360.

Calabrese, J. R., Muzina, D. J., Kemp, D. E., Sachs, G. S., Frye, M. A., Thompson, T. R., Klingman, D., Reed, M. L., & Hirschfeld, R. M. (2006). Predictors of bipolar disorder among patients currently treated for major depression. *MedGenMed.*, *15*, *8* (3), 38.

Calabrese, J. R., Rapport, D. J., Kimmel, S. E., & Shelton, M. D. (1999). Controlled trials in bipolar I depression: focus on switch rates and efficacy. *Eur. Neuropsychopharmacol.*, *9* (Suppl 4), S109–S112.

Calabrese, J. R., Shelton, M. D., Bowden, C. L., Rapport, D. J., Suppes, T., Shirley, E. R., Kimmel, S. E., & Caban, S. J. (2001). Bipolar rapid cycling: focus on depression as its hallmark. *J. Clin. Psychiatry*, *62* (Suppl 14), 34–41.

Calabrese, J. R., Shelton, M. D., Rapport, D. J., Youngstrom, E. A., Jackson, K., Bilali, S., Ganocy, S. J., & Findling, R. L. (2005). A 20-month, double-blind, maintenance trial of lithium versus divalproex in rapid-cycling bipolar disorder. *Am. J. Psychiatry*, *162* (11), 2152–2161.

Cassano, P., Lattanzi, L., Fava, M., Navari, S., Battistini, G., Abelli, M., & Cassano, G. B. (2005). Ropinirole in treatment-resistant depression: a 16-week pilot study. *Can. J. Psychiatry*, *50* (6), 357–360.

Cassano, P., Lattanzi, L., Soldani, F., Navari, S., Battistini, G., Gemignani, A., & Cassano, G. B. (2004). Pramipexole in treatment-resistant depression: an extended follow-up. *Depress Anxiety*, *20* (3), 131–138.

Chaudron, L. H., & Pies, R. W. (2003). The relationship between postpartum psychosis and bipolar disorder: a review. *J. Clin. Psychiatry*, *64* (11), 1284–1292.

Cohn, J. B., Collins, G., Ashbrook, E., & Wernicke, J. F. (1989). A comparison of fluoxetine imipramine and placebo in patients with bipolar depressive disorder. *Int. Clin. Psychopharmacol.*, *4* (4), 313–322.

Coppen, A., Shaw, D. M., & Farrell, J. P. (1963). Potentiation of the antidepressive effect of a monoamine-oxidase inhibitor by tryptophan. *Lancet*, *1*, 79–81.

Coryell, W., Endicott, J., Maser, J. D., Keller, M. B., Leon, A. C., & Akiskal, H. S. (1995). Long-term stability of polarity distinctions in the affective disorders. *Am. J. Psychiatry, 152* (3), 385–390.

Daly, J. J., Prudic, J., Devanand, D. P., Nobler, M. S., Lisanby, S. H., Peyser, S., Roose, S. P., & Sackeim, H. A. (2001). ECT in bipolar and unipolar depression: differences in speed of response. *Bipolar Disord., 3* (2), 95–104.

Detera-Wadleigh, S. D., Badner, J. A., Berrettini, W. H., Yoshikawa, T., Goldin, L. R., Turner, G., Rollins, D. Y., Moses, T., Sanders, A. R., Karkera, J. D., Esterling, L. E., Zeng, J., Ferraro, T. N., Guroff, J. J., Kazuba, D., Maxwell, M. E., Nurnberger, J. I., Jr., & Gershon, E. S. (1999). A high-density genome scan detects evidence for a bipolar-disorder susceptibility locus on 13q32 and other potential loci on 1q32 and 18p11.2. *Proc. Natl. Acad. Sci. USA, 96* (10), 5604–5609.

Dolberg, O. T., Dannon, P. N., Schreiber, S., & Grunhaus, L. (2002). Transcranial magnetic stimulation in patients with bipolar depression: a double blind, controlled study. *Bipolar Disord., 4* (Suppl 1), 94–95.

Dombrovski, A. Y., & Mulsant, B. H. (2007). ECT: the preferred treatment for severe depression in late life. *Int. Psychogeriatr., 19* (1), 10–14.

Eden Evins, A., Demopulos, C., Yovel, I., Culhane, M., Ogutha, J., Grandin, L. D., Nierenberg, A. A., & Sachs, G. S. (2006). Inositol augmentation of lithium or valproate for bipolar depression. *Bipolar Disord., 8* (2), 168–174.

Fagiolini, A., Kupfer, D. J., Houck, P. R., Novick, D. M., & Frank, E. (2003). Obesity as a correlate of outcome in patients with bipolar I disorder. *Am. J. Psychiatry, 160* (1), 112–117.

Fawcett, J., Kravitz, H. M., Zajecka, J. M., & Schaff, M. R. (1991). CNS stimulant potentiation of monoamine oxidase inhibitors in treatment-refractory depression. *J. Clin. Psychopharmacol., 11* (2), 127–132.

Fisfalen, M. E., Schulze, T. G., DePaulo, J. R., Jr., DeGroot, L. J., Badner, J. A., & McMahon, F. J. (2005). Familial variation in episode frequency in bipolar affective disorder. *Am. J. Psychiatry, 162* (7), 1266–1272.

Fonseca, M., Soares, J. C., Hatch, J. P., Santin, A. P., & Kapczinski, F. (2006). An open trial of adjunctive escitalopram in bipolar depression. *J. Clin. Psychiatry, 67* (1), 81–86.

Frangou, S., Lewis, M., & McCrone, P. (2006). Efficacy of ethyl-eicosapentaenoic acid in bipolar depression: randomised double-blind placebo-controlled study. *Br. J. Psychiatry, 188*, 46–50.

Freeman, M. P., Hibbeln, J. R., Wisner, K. L., Davis, J. M. & Mischoulon, D., Peet, M., Keck, P. E., Jr., Marangell, L. B., Richardson, A. J., Lake, J., & Stoll, A. L. (2006). Omega-3 fatty acids: evidence basis for treatment and future research in psychiatry. *J. Clin. Psychiatry, 67* (12), 1954–1967.

Frye, M. A., Grunze, H., & Suppes, T. (2007). A placebo-controlled evaluation of adjunctive modafinil in the treatment of bipolar depression. *Am. J. Psychiatry., 164* (8), 1242–1249.

Frye, M. A., Ketter, T. A., Kimbrell, T. A., Dunn, R. T., Speer, A. M., Osuch, E. A., Luckenbaugh, D. A., Cora-Ocatelli, G., Leverich, G. S., & Post, R. M. (2000). A placebo-controlled study of lamotrigine and gabapentin monotherapy in refractory mood disorders. *J. Clin. Psychopharmacol., 20* (6), 607–614.

Goldberg, J. F., Burdick, K. E., & Endick, C. J. (2004). Preliminary randomized, double-blind, placebo-controlled trial of pramipexole added to mood stabilizers for treatment-resistant bipolar depression. *Am. J. Psychiatry, 161* (3), 564–566.

Grant, B. F., Stinson, F. S., Hasin, D. S., Dawson, D. A., Chou, S. P., Ruan, W. J., & Huang, B. (2005). Prevalence, correlates, and comorbidity of bipolar I disorder and axis I and II disorders: results from the National Epidemiologic Survey on Alcohol and Related Conditions. *J. Clin. Psychiatry, 66* (10), 1205–1215.

Hasin, D. S., Goodwin, R. D., Stinson, F. S., & Grant, B. F. (2005). Epidemiology of major depressive disorder: results from the National Epidemiologic Survey on Alcoholism and Related Conditions. *Arch. Gen. Psychiatry, 62* (10), 1097–1106.

Himmelhoch, J. M., Fuchs, C. Z., & Symons, B. J. (1982). A double-blind study of tranylcypromine treatment of major anergic depression. *J. Nerv. Ment. Dis., 170* (10), 628–634.

Himmelhoch, J. M., Thase, M. E., Mallinger, A. G., & Houck, P. (1991). Tranylcypromine versus imipramine in anergic bipolar depression. *Am. J. Psychiatry, 148* (7), 910–916.

Homan, S., Lachenbruch, P. A., Winokur, G., & Clayton, P. (1982). An efficacy study of electroconvulsive therapy and antidepressants in the treatment of primary depression. *Psychol. Med., 12* (3), 615–624.

Judd, L. L., Akiskal, H. S., Schettler, P. J., Coryell, W., Endicott, J., Maser, J. D., Solomon D. A., Leon, A. C., & Keller, M. B. (2003). A prospective investigation of the natural history of the long-term weekly symptomatic status of bipolar II disorder. *Arch. Gen. Psychiatry, 60 (3)*, 261–269.

Judd, L. L., Akiskal, H. S., Schettler, P. J., Endicott, J., Maser, J., Solomon, D. A., Leon, A. C., Rice, J. A., & Keller, M. B. (2002). The long-term natural history of the weekly symptomatic status of bipolar I disorder. *Arch. Gen. Psychiatry, 59* (6), 530–537.

Keck, P. E., Jr., Mintz, J., McElroy, S. L., Freeman, M. P., Suppes, T., Frye, M. A., Altshuler, L. L., Kupka, R., Nolen, W. A., Leverich, G. S., Denicoff, K. D., Grunze, H., Duan, N., & Post, R. M. (2006). Double-blind, randomized, placebo-controlled trials of ethyl-eicosapentanoate in the treatment of bipolar depression and rapid cycling bipolar disorder. *Biol. Psychiatry, 60* (9), 1020–1022.

Kemp, D. E., Gao, K., Muzina, D. J., & Calabrese, J. R. (2006). Progress in the treatment of bipolar depression: advances and challenges. *Psychiatric Times, 23* (9), 39.

Kennedy, J. L., Farrer, L. A., Andreasen, N. C., Mayeux, R., & St George-Hyslop, P. (2003). The genetics of adult-onset neuropsychiatric disease: complexities and conundra? *Science, 302* (5646), 822–826.

Kramlinger, K. G., & Post, R. M. (1989). The addition of lithium to carbamazepine. Antidepressant efficacy in treatment-resistant depression. *Arch. Gen. Psychiatry, 46* (9), 794–800.

Kruger, S., Alda, M., Young, L. T., Goldapple, K., Parikh, S., & Mayberg, H. S. (2006). Risk and resilience markers in bipolar disorder: brain responses to emotional challenge in bipolar patients and their healthy siblings. *Am. J. Psychiatry, 163 (2)*, 257–264.

Kupfer, D. J., Chengappa, K. N., Gelenberg, A. J., Hirschfeld, R. M., Goldberg, J. F., Sachs, G. S., Grochocinski, V. J., Houck, P. R., & Kolar, A. B. (2001). Citalopram as adjunctive therapy in bipolar depression. *J. Clin. Psychiatry, 62* (12), 985–990.

Leverich, G. S., Altshuler, L. L., Frye, M. A., Suppes, T., McElroy, S. L., Keck, P. E., Jr., Kupka, R. W., Denicoff, K. D., Nolen, W. A., Grunze, H., Martinez, M. I., & Post, R. M. (2006). Risk of switch in mood polarity to hypomania or mania in patients with bipolar depression during acute and continuation trials of venlafaxine, sertraline, and bupropion as adjuncts to mood stabilizers. *Am. J. Psychiatry, 163* (2), 232–239.

Lish, J. D., Dime-Meenan, S., Whybrow, P. C., Price, R. A., & Hirschfeld, R. M. (1994). The National Depressive and Manic-depressive Association (DMDA) survey of bipolar members. *J. Affect. Disord.*, *31* (4), 281–294.

Mantere, O., Melartin, T. K., Suominen, K., Rytsälä, H. J., Valtonen, H. M., Arvilommi, P., Leppämäki, S., & Isometsä, E. T. (2006). Differences in Axis I and II comorbidity between bipolar I and II disorders and major depressive disorder. *J. Clin. Psychiatry*, *67* (4), 584–593.

Mayberg, H. S., Lozano, A. M., Voon, V., McNeely, H. E., Seminowicz, D., Hamani, C., Schwalb, J. M., & Kennedy, S. H. (2005). Deep brain stimulation for treatment-resistant depression. *Neuron*, *45* (5), 651–660.

McIntyre, R. S., Konarski, J. Z., Soczynska, J. K., Wilkins, K., Panjwani, G., Bouffard, B., Bottas, A., & Kennedy, S. H. (2006). Medical comorbidity in bipolar disorder: implications for functional outcomes and health service utilization. *Psychiatr. Serv.*, *57* (8), 1140–1144.

McIntyre, R. S., Mancini, D. A., McCann, S., Srinivasan, J., Sagman, D., & Kennedy, S. H. (2002). Topiramate versus bupropion SR when added to mood stabilizer therapy for the depressive phase of bipolar disorder: a preliminary single-blind study. *Bipolar Disord.*, *4* (3), 207–213.

McIntyre, R. S., McElroy, S. L., Konarski, J. Z., Soczynska, J. K., Wilkins, K., & Kennedy, S. H. (2007). Problem gambling in bipolar disorder: Results from the Canadian Community Health Survey. *J. Affect. Disord.*, *102* (1–3), 27–34.

McQueen, M. B., Devlin, B., Faraone, S. V., Nimgaonkar, V. L., Sklar, P., Smoller, J. W., Abou Jamra, R., Albus, M., Bacanu, S. A., Baron, M., Barrett, T. B., Berrettini, W., Blacker, D., Byerley, W., Cichon, S., Coryell, W., Craddock, N., Daly, M. J., Depaulo, J. R., Edenberg, H. J., Foroud, T., Gill, M., Gilliam, T. C., Hamshere, M., Jones, I., Jones, L., Juo, S. H., Kelsoe, J. R., Lambert, D., Lange, C., Lerer, B., Liu, J., Maier, W., Mackinnon, J. D., McInnis, M. G., McMahon, F. J., Murphy, D. L., Nothen, M. M., Nurnberger, J. I., Pato, C. N., Pato, M. T., Potash, J. B., Propping, P., Pulver, A. E., Rice, J. P., Rietschel, M., Scheftner, W., Schumacher, J., Segurado, R., Van Steen, K., Xie, W., Zandi, P. P., & Laird, N. M. (2005). Combined analysis from eleven linkage studies of bipolar disorder provides strong evidence of susceptibility loci on chromosomes 6q and 8q. *Am. J. Hum. Genet.*, *77* (4), 582–595.

Menza, M. A., Kaufman, K. R., & Castellanos, A. (2000). Modafinil augmentation of antidepressant treatment in depression. *J. Clin. Psychiatry*, *61* (5), 378–381.

Muzina, D. J., & Calabrese, J. R. (2003). Recent placebo-controlled acute trials in bipolar depression: focus on methodology. *Int. J. Neuropsychopharmacol.*, *6* (3), 285–291.

Muzina, D. J., Gajwani, P., Kemp, D. E., Gao, K., & Calabrese, J. R. (2006). Antiepileptic drugs for acute bipolar depression: applying data to clinical practice. *Psych. Annals*, *36* (9), 637–644.

Muzina, D. J., Ganocy, S., Khalife, S., Gao, K., Kemp, D., & Bachtel, M.B. (2008). A Double-Blind, Placebo-Controlled Study of Divalproex Extended-Release in Newly Diagnosed Mood Stabilizer Naïve Patients with Acute Bipolar I or II Depression. Presented at American Psychiatric Association Annual Meeting, Washington, DC.

Muzina, D. J., Kemp, D. E., Gao, K., Gajwani, P., & Calabrese, J. R. (2006). Atypical antipsychotics in bipolar *depression:* applying emerging evidence to clinical practice. *Psych. Annals*, *36* (9), 646–652.

Nahas, Z., Marangell, L. B., Husain, M. M., Rush, A. J., Sackeim, H. A., Lisanby, S. H., Martinez, J. M., & George, M. S. (2005). Two-year outcome of vagus nerve stimulation (VNS) for treatment of major depressive episodes. *J. Clin. Psychiatry*, 66 (9), 1097–1104.

Nemeroff, C. B., Evans, D. L., Gyulai, L., Sachs, G. S., Bowden, C. L., Gergel, I. P., Oakes, R., & Pitts, C. D. (2001). Double-blind, placebo-controlled comparison of imipramine and paroxetine in the treatment of bipolar depression. *Am. J. Psychiatry*, 158 (6), 906–912.

Newcomer, J. W. (2006). Medical risk in patients with bipolar disorder and schizophrenia. *J. Clin. Psychiatry*, 67 (11), e16.

Nierenberg, A. A., Ostacher, M. J., Calabrese, J. R., Ketter, T. A., Marangell, L. B., Miklowitz, D. J., Miyahara, S., Bauer, M. S., Thase, M. E., Wisniewski, S. R., & Sachs, G. S. (2006). Treatment-resistant bipolar depression: a STEP-BD equipoise randomized effectiveness trial of antidepressant augmentation with lamotrigine, inositol, or risperidone. *Am. J. Psychiatry*, 163 (2), 210–216.

Osher, Y., Bersudsky, Y., & Belmaker, R. H. (2005). Omega-3 eicosapentaenoic acid in bipolar depression: report of a small open-label study. *J. Clin. Psychiatry*, 66 (6), 726–729.

Peet, M. (1994). Induction of mania with selective serotonin re-uptake inhibitors and tricyclic antidepressants. *Br. J. Psychiatry*, 164 (4), 549–550.

Perez, V., Gilaberte, I., Faries, D., Alvarez, E., & Artigas, F. (1997). Randomised, double-blind, placebo-controlled trial of pindolol in combination with fluoxetine antidepressant treatment. *Lancet*, 349 (9065), 1594–1597.

Regier, D. A., Farmer, M. E., Rae, D. S., Locke, B. Z., Keith, S. J., Judd, L. L., & Goodwin, F. K. (1990). Comorbidity of mental disorders with alcohol and other drug abuse. Results from the Epidemiologic Catchment Area (ECA) Study. *JAMA*, 264 (19), 2511–2518.

Rush, A. J., George, M. S., Sackeim, H. A., Marangell, L. B., Husain, M. M., Giller, C., Nahas, Z., Haines, S., Simpson, R. K., Jr., & Goodman, R. (2000). Vagus nerve stimulation (VNS) for treatment-resistant depressions: a multicenter study. *Biol. Psychiatry*, 47 (4), 276–286.

Rush, A. J., Marangell, L. B., Sackeim, H. A., George, M. S., Brannan, S. K., Davis, S. M., Howland, R., Kling, M. A., Rittberg, B. R., Burke, W. J., Rapaport, M. H., Zajecka, J., Nierenberg, A. A., Husain, M. M., Ginsberg, D., & Cooke, R. G. (2005). Vagus nerve stimulation for treatment-resistant depression: a randomized, controlled acute phase trial. *Biol. Psychiatry*, 58 (5), 347–354.

Rush, A. J., Sackeim, H. A., Marangell, L. B., George, M. S., Brannan, S. K., Davis, S. M., Lavori, P., Howland, R., Kling, M. A., Rittberg, B., Carpenter, L., Ninan, P., Moreno, F., Schwartz, T., Conway, C., Burke, M., Barry, J. J. (2005). Effects of 12 months of vagus nerve stimulation in treatment-resistant depression: a naturalistic study. *Biol. Psychiatry*, 58 (5), 355–363.

Sachs, G. S. (1996). Treatment-resistant bipolar depression. *Psychiatr. Clin. North Am.*, 19 (2), 215–236.

Sachs, G. S., Lafer, B., Stoll, A. L., Banov, M., Thibault, A. B., Tohen, M., & Rosenbaum, J. F. (1994). A double-blind trial of bupropion versus desipramine for bipolar depression. *J. Clin. Psychiatry*, 55 (9), 391–393.

Sachs, G. S., Nierenberg, A. A., Calabrese, J. R., Marangell, L. B., Wisniewski, S. R., Gyulai, L., Friedman, E. S., Bowden, C. L., Fossey, M. D., Ostacher, M. J., Ketter, T. A., Patel, J., Hauser, P., Rapport, D., Martinez, J. M., Allen, M. H., Miklowitz, D. J., Otto, M. W., Dennehy, E. B., & Thase, M. E. (2007).

Effectiveness of adjunctive antidepressant treatment for bipolar depression. *N. Engl. J. Med., 356* (17), 1711–1722.

Simon, N. M., Smoller, J. W., Fava, M., Sachs, G., Racette, S. R., Perlis, R., Sonawalla, S., & Rosenbaum, J. F. (2003). Comparing anxiety disorders and anxiety-related traits in bipolar disorder and unipolar depression. *J. Psychiatr. Res., 37* (3), 187–192.

Singh, J. B., & Zarate, C. A., Jr. (2006). Pharmacological treatment of psychiatric comorbidity in bipolar disorder: a review of controlled trials. *Bipolar Disord., 8* (6), 696–709.

Solomon, D. A., Leon, A. C., Maser, J. D., Truman, C. J., Coryell, W., Endicott, J., Teres, J. J., & Keller, M. B. (2006). Distinguishing bipolar major depression from unipolar major depression with the screening assessment of depression-polarity (SAD-P). *J. Clin. Psychiatry, 67* (3), 434–442.

Sporn, J., Ghaemi, S. N., Sambur, M. R., Rankin, M. A., Recht, J., Sachs, G. S., Rosenbaum, J. F., & Fava, M. (2000). Pramipexole augmentation in the treatment of unipolar and bipolar depression: a retrospective chart review. *Ann. Clin. Psychiatry, 12* (3), 137–140.

Srisurapanont, M., Yatham, L. N., & Zis, A. P. (1995). Treatment of acute bipolar depression: a review of the literature. *Can. J. Psychiatry, 40* (9), 533–544.

Stoll, A. L., Pillay, S. S., Diamond, L., Workum, S. B., & Cole, J. O. (1996). Methylphenidate augmentation of serotonin selective reuptake inhibitors: a case series. *J. Clin. Psychiatry, 57* (2), 72–76.

Stromgren, L. S. (1973). Unilateral versus bilateral electroconvulsive therapy. Investigations into the therapeutic effect in endogenous depression. *Acta Psychiatr. Scand. Suppl., 240,* 8–65.

Su, T. P., Huang, C. C., & Wei, I. H. (2005). Add-on rTMS for medication-resistant depression: a randomized, double-blind, sham-controlled trial in Chinese patients. *J. Clin. Psychiatry, 66* (7), 930–937.

Suppes, T., Leverich, G. S., Keck, P. E., Nolen, W. A., Denicoff, K. D., Altshuler, L. L., McElroy, S. L., Rush, A. J., Kupka, R., Frye, M. A., Bickel, M., Post, R. M. (2001). The Stanley Foundation Bipolar Treatment Outcome Network. II. Demographics and illness characteristics of the first 261 patients. *J. Affect. Disord., 67* (1–3), 45–59.

Thase, M. E., Mallinger, A. G., McKnight, D., & Himmelhoch, J. M. (1992). Treatment of imipramine-resistant recurrent depression, IV: a double-blind crossover study of tranylcypromine for anergic bipolar depression. *Am. J. Psychiatry, 149* (2), 195–198.

Thase, M. E., Macfadden, W., Weisler, R. H., Chang, W., Paulsson, B., Khan, A., Calabrese, J. R. (2006). Efficacy of quetiapine monotherapy in bipolar I and II depression: a double-blind, placebo-controlled study (the BOLDER II study). *J Clin Psychopharmacol, 26,* 600–609.

Thase, M. E., Jonas, A., Khan, A., Bowden, C. L., Wu, X., McQuade, R. D., Carson, W. H., Marcus, R. N., & Owen, R. (2008). Aripiprazole monotherapy in non-psychotic bipolar I depression: results of 2 randomized, placebo-controlled studies. *J Clin Psychopharmacol, 28,* 13–20.

Tohen, M., Vieta, E., Calabrese, J., Ketter, T. A., Sachs, G., Bowden, C., Mitchell, P. B., Centorrino, F., Risser, R., Baker, R. W., Evans, A. R., Beymer, K., Dube, S., Tollefson, G. D., & Breier, A. (2003). Efficacy of olanzapine and olanzapine-fluoxetine combination in the treatment of bipolar I depression. *Arch. Gen. Psychiatry, 60* (11), 1079–1088.

Tome, M. B., Isaac, M. T., Harte, R., & Holland, C. (1997). Paroxetine and pindolol: a randomized trial of serotonergic autoreceptor blockade in the reduction of antidepressant latency. *Int. Clin. Psychopharmacol., 12* (2), 81–89.

Tondo, L., Isacsson, G., & Baldessarini, R. (2003). Suicidal behaviour in bipolar disorder: risk and prevention. *CNS Drugs, 17* (7), 491–511.

van der Loos, M. L. M., Zwolle, I. K., Vieta, E., & Nolen, W. A. (2007, June 7–9). Lamotrigine as Add-on to Lithium in Bipolar Depression. Paper presented at the Seventh International Conference on Bipolar Disorder, Pittsburgh, PA.

Vieta, E., Martinez-Arán, A., Goikolea, J. M., Torrent, C., Colom, F., Benabarre, A., & Reinares, M. (2002). A randomized trial comparing paroxetine and venlafaxine in the treatment of bipolar depressed patients taking mood stabilizers. *J. Clin. Psychiatry, 63* (6), 508–512.

Wang, P. W., Santosa, C., Schumacher, M., Winsberg, M. E., Strong, C., & Ketter, T. A. (2002). Gabapentin augmentation therapy in bipolar depression. *Bipolar Disord., 4* (5), 296–301.

Wharton, R. N., Perel, J. M., Dayton, P. G., & Malitz, S. (1971). A potential clinical use for methylphenidate with tricyclic antidepressants. *Am. J. Psychiatry, 127* (12), 1619–1625.

Yatham, L., Kusumakar, V., & Kutcher, S. (2002). Treatment of bipolardepression. In L. Yatham, V. Kusumakar & S. Kutcher (Eds.), Bipolar Disorder: A Clinician's Guide to Biological Treatments (pp. 17–32). New York, NY: Brunner-Routledge.

Yatham, L. N., Kennedy, S. H., O'Donovan, C., Parikh, S. V., MacQueen, G., McIntyre, R. S., Sharma, V., & Beaulieu, S. (2006). Canadian Network for Mood and Anxiety Treatments (CANMAT) guidelines for the management of patients with bipolar disorder: update 2007. *Bipolar Disord., 8* (6), 721–739.

Yatham, L. N., Kusumakar, V., Parikh, S. V., Haslam, D. R., Matte, R., Sharma, V., & Kennedy, S. (1997). Bipolar depression: treatment options. *Can. J. Psychiatry, 42* (Suppl 2), 87S–91S.

Young A. H., McElroy, S., Chang, W., Paulsson, B., Brecher, M. (2008a). Placebo-controlled study with acute and continuation phase of quetiapine in adults with bipolar depression (EMBOLDEN I). Presented at 21st European College of Neuropsychopharmacology Congress, Sept 1, 2008. *Eur. Neuropsychopharmacology, 18* (Suppl 4), S371.

Young A. H., McElroy, S., Chang, W., Paulsson, B., Brecher, M. (2008b). Placebo-controlled study with acute and continuation phase of quetiapine in adults with bipolar depression (EMBOLDEN II). Presented at 21st European College of Neuropsychopharmacology Congress, Sept 1, 2008. *Eur. Neuropsychopharmacology, 18* (Suppl 4), S371.

Young, L. T., Joffe, R. T., Robb, J. C., MacQueen, G. M., Marriott, M., & Patelis-Siotis, I. (2000). Double-blind comparison of addition of a second mood stabilizer versus an antidepressant to an initial mood stabilizer for treatment of patients with bipolar depression. *Am. J. Psychiatry, 157* (1), 124–126.

Zarate, C. A., Jr., Payne, J. L., Singh, J., Quiroz, J. A., Luckenbaugh, D. A., Denicoff, K. D., Charney, D. S., & Manji, H. K. (2004). Pramipexole for bipolar II depression: a placebo-controlled proof of concept study. *Biol. Psychiatry, 56* (1), 54–60.

Zarate, C. A. Jr., Quiroz, J. A., Singh, J. B., Denicoff, K. D., De Jesus, G., Luckenbaugh, D. A., Charney, D. S., & Manji, H. K. (2005). An open-label trial of the glutamate-modulating agent riluzole in combination with lithium for the treatment of bipolar depression. *Biol. Psychiatry, 57* (4), 430–432.

chapter three

Diagnosis and treatment of rapid cycling bipolar disorder

Ralph Kupka
Altrecht Institute for Mental Health Care

Mark A. Frye
Mayo Clinic

Contents

Introduction 46
Clinical features 47
Prevalence of rapid cycling 54
Persistence of rapid cycling 54
Genetics 56
Associated features and possible risk factors 57
Induction of rapid cycling by antidepressants 58
Treatment 59
    Lithium 60
    Valproate 62
    Lamotrigine 63
    Other anticonvulsants 64
    Atypical antipsychotics 64
    Other pharmacological treatment options 65
    The use of antidepressants in rapid cyclers 66
    Combination treatment 67
    Non-pharmacological treatment 67
Conclusions and clinical management recommendations 68
References 70

Introduction

Cyclicity is the hallmark of bipolar disorder, and is especially prominent in patients with a rapid cycling course (Goodwin & Jamison, 2007). Among patients with bipolar disorder, manic, hypomanic, depressive, and mixed episodes may occur in any given sequence and frequency. As early as in 1809, an English physician John Haslam, described the frequent alternation of mania and depression as a bad prognostic sign: *"When the furious state is succeeded by melancholy, and after this shall have continued a short time, the violent paroxysm returns, the chance of recovery is very slight. Indeed, whenever these states of the disease frequently change, such alterations may be considered as very unfavorable."*

In 1854, Baillarger described *"La folie à double forme"*, and Falret *"La folie circulaire"*, both indicating the alternation of manic and depressive phases, whether they were followed by lucid intervals or not. Kraepelin (1913) and Bleuler (1949) both maintained that regularity in what they called circular insanity was the exception rather than the rule. These and other observations from the pre-pharmacological era are of great importance for understanding the natural course of bipolar disorder, since most patients in more contemporary longitudinal studies have received both acute and prophylactic treatment, which may have modified the course of illness for the better or the worse. It is estimated from these early studies that "circular" or "chronic" manic-depressive illness was present in 4–20% of bipolar patients (Alarcon, 1985).

The term rapid cycling, that is the occurrence of four or more separate mood episodes within a year, was introduced in 1974 by Dunner and Fieve (1974) to describe a variant of bipolar disorder that was relatively unresponsive to lithium prophylaxis. They defined rapid cycling as a course of illness in which four or more mood episodes had occurred in the year preceding treatment. Rapid cycling patient would typically have at least two episodes of mania and two depressions per year, often in a biphasic pattern. The minimum of four episodes per year was chosen arbitrarily to obtain a study population of sufficient size. Lithium prophylaxis was effective in only 18% of the rapid cyclers, although it did attenuate the further course of illness in many others. In contrast, lithium prophylaxis was effective in 59% of the non-rapid cyclers. Over the past three decades, it has become clear that rapid cyclers are relatively resistant to most pharmacological treatment, and that lithium is far from being the least effective (Tondo, Hennen, & Baldessarini, 2003).

Based on a multisite data reanalysis that gave some support for the original cut-off of four episodes per year (Bauer et al., 1994), rapid cycling was included in DSM-IV (American Psychiatric Association [APA], 1994) as a course specifier for bipolar I and II disorder using the original definition

(Dunner, 1998). The concept of rapid cycling has been widely studied, and over the past decades excellent reviews of rapid-cycling bipolar disorder have been published (e.g. Alarcon, 1985; Kilzieh & Akiskal, 1999; Mackin & Young, 2004; Coryell, 2005; Bauer et al., 2008). Studies that have made direct comparisons between rapid and non-rapid cyclers to shed light on the differential characteristics of both conditions, are reviewed by Kupka et al. (2003) and summarized in Table 3.1.

Clinical features

As defined in DSM-IV and DSM-IV-TR, the specifier "with rapid cycling" can be applied to bipolar I disorder or bipolar II disorder. The essential feature of rapid cycling is the occurrence of four or more mood episodes during the preceding 12 months, occurring in any combination and order. The episodes must meet both the duration and symptom criteria for a major depressive, manic, mixed, or hypomanic episode, and must be demarcated by a partial or full remission for at least two months or by a switch to an episode of opposite polarity. Manic, hypomanic, and mixed episodes are counted as being of the same pole (e.g. a hypomanic episode immediately followed by a manic or mixed episode counts as only one episode in considering the specifier with rapid cycling). Apart from the fact that they occur more frequently, episodes that occur in a rapid-cycling pattern are assumed to be no different from those that occur in a non-rapid-cycling pattern. Mood episodes that count toward defining a rapid-cycling pattern exclude those episodes directly caused by a substance (e.g. cocaine or corticosteroids), antidepressants, or a general medical condition.

The definition of rapid cycling of at least four episodes per year has not changed since its introduction in 1974. Studies that specifically addressed the issue of rapid cycling as a course modifier in DSM-IV endorsed the definition of rapid cycling as having at least four episodes per year. Bauer et al. (1994) suggested that the reliability of the definition would be enhanced by a more valid definition of remission and its minimum duration than the arbitrary DSM-IV requirement of a rather lengthy two months, especially when consecutive episodes are of the same polarity. Since the presence of subsyndromal symptoms is generally associated with an increased risk of relapse, partial remission rather than complete recovery will be the rule in rapid cyclers.

Maj et al. (1994, 1999) found that the occurrence of a pole-switching pattern (direct switching from depression to mania or vice versa within 24 hours) predicted rapid cycling and treatment resistance at follow-up, and suggested that the requirement of a pole-switching pattern would enhance the predictive validity of rapid cycling. The criterion of switch is relatively underappreciated in DSM-IV-TR criteria, which has focused

Table 3.1 Overview of 25 Studies Comparing Rapid Cycling (RC) and Non-Rapid Cycling (N-RC) Bipolar Disorder

Study	Primary focus	Subjects	n RC (%) n N-RC	n (%) Females	n (%) Bipolar II	Mean age onset (SD)
Dunner, Patrick, & Fieve (1977)	Descriptive and effects of lithium	N=306 lithium outpatients followed up to 7 years	40 RC (13) 266 N-RC	RC: 28 (70) N-RC: 123 (46) (p<.01)	RC: 16 (40) N-RC: 87 (33)	RC: 29.9 (12.0) N-RC: 31.3 (10.9)
Koukopulos et al. (1980)	Course of illness and influence of treatments	N=434 in/outpatients follow-up 4.5 years	87 RC (20) 347 N-RC	RC: 61 (70) N-RC: 195 (56) (p=.02)	RC: 71 (82) N-RC: 156 (45) (p<.0000)	n/r
Cowdry et al. (1983)	Thyroid dysfunction	N=43 NIMH in/outpatients on lithium; follow-up 1 year	24 RC (56) 19 N-RC	RC: 20 (83) N-RC: 10 (53) (p<.05)	n/r	n/r
Wehr et al. (1988)	Descriptive and treatment response	N=66 NIMH inpatients follow-up 1–12 years	47 RC (71) 19 N-RC	RC: 47 (100) N-RC: 19 (100)	RC: 22 (47) N-RC: 6 (32)	RC: 30 (11) N-RC: 27 (12)
Nurnberger et al. (1988)	Family history	N=195 NIMH in/outpatients	29 RC (15) 166 N-RC	RC: 25 (86) N-RC: 88 (53) (p<.001)	n/r	n/r
Joffe, Kutcher, & MacDonald (1988)	Thyroid dysfunction	N=42 outpatients	17 RC (40) 25 N-RC	RC: 7 (41) N-RC: 20 (80) (p<.01)	n/r	n/r

Maj, Pirozzi, & Starace (1989)	Course of illness and treatment response	N=118 outpatients follow-up ≥2 years	14 RC (12) 104 N-RC	RC: 9 (64) N-RC: 59 (57)	n/r	RC: 32. (6.0) N-RC: 31.3 (4.6)
Bartalena et al. (1990)	Thyroid dysfunction	N=22 outpatients	11 RC (50) 11 N-RC (*matched*)	RC: 11 (100) N-RC: 11 (100)	n/r	n/r
Kusalic (1992)	Thyroid dysfunction	N=20 in/outpatients	10 RC (50) 10 N-RC (*matched*)	RC: 7 (70) N-RC: 7 (70) (*matched*)	n/r	RC: 29 (6) N-RC: 28 (8)
Coryell, Endicott, & Keller (1992)	Descriptive (NIMH-CDS)	N=243 in/outpatients follow-up 1–5 years	45 RC (19) 198 N-RC	RC: 32 (71) N-RC: 98 (50) (p=.009)	RC: 16 (36) N-RC: 35 (18) (p=.008)	RC: 25.4 (8.4)
Lish et al. (1993)	Family history	N=89 outpatients from three specialized clinics	45 RC (51) 44 N-RC	RC: 37 (82) N-RC: 28 (64) (p<.05)	n/r	n/r
Wu & Dunner (1993)	History of suicide attempts	N=220 outpatients	100 RC (45) 120 N-RC	RC: 60 (60) N-RC: 64 (53)	RC: 78 (78) N-RC: 78 (65) (p<.003)	RC: 21 (12) N-RC: 23 (12)
Bauer et al. (1994)	Validity of RC as course specifier	N=239 outpatients Reanalysis of existing studies	120 RC (50) 119 N-RC (*matched*)	RC: 84 (70) N-RC: 60 (50) (p=.003)	RC: 54 (45) N-RC: 45 (38)	RC: 22.9 (0.1) N-RC: 22.9 (0.1)
Maj et al. (1994)	Validity of RC as course specifier	N=111 in/outpatients follow-up 2–5 years	37 RC (33) 74 N-RC (*matched*)	RC: 24 (65) N-RC: 38 (51)	RC: 15 (41) N-RC: 18 (24)	RC: 29.9 (4.7) N-RC: 29.3 (5.2)

(continued)

Table 3.1 Overview of 25 Studies Comparing Rapid Cycling (RC) and Non-Rapid Cycling (N-RC) Bipolar Disorder (*Continued*)

Study	Primary focus	Subjects	n RC (%) n N-RC	n (%) Females	n (%) Bipolar II	Mean age onset (SD)
Post et al. (1997)	Thyroid dysfunction	N=67 NIMH inpatients all medication-free	31 RC (46) 36 N-RC	n/r all: 38 (58)	n/r	n/r
Kirov et al. (1998)	Genetic (COMT-gene)	N=165 outpatients from a genetic study	55 RC (33) 110 N-RC	RC: 34 (62) N-RC: 58 (53)	RC: 10 (18) N-RC: 6 (5)	n/r
Avasthi et al. (1999)	Descriptive	N=270 in/outpatients follow-up ≥1 year	33 RC (12) 237 N-RC	RC: 14 (42) N-RC: 88 (37)	RC: 8 (24) N-RC: n/r	RC: 30.2 (7.1) N-RC: 27.7 (11.2)
Bowden et al. (1999)	Efficacy of Lamotrigine	N=75 open treatment trial follow-up 48 weeks	41 RC (55) 34 N-RC	RC: 25 (61) N-RC: 20 (59)	n/r	RC: 19.4 (8.8) N-RC: 29.6 (11.2) ($p<.00001$)
Maj et al. (1999)	Validity of RC as course specifier	N=210 outpatients follow-up ≥1year	31 RC(24) 97 N-RC	RC: 21 (68) N-RC: 51 (53) ($p<.05$)	RC: 13 (42) N-RC: 28 (29) ($p<.05$)	n/r
Baldessarini et al. (2000)	Response to lithium prophylaxis	N=360 outpatients follow-up 4.5 years	56 RC (16) 304 N-RC	RC: 41 (73) N-RC: 188 (62)	RC: 43 (77) N-RC: 99 (33) ($p=.0001$)	RC: 33.6 (12.5) N-RC: 28.7 (11.9) ($p=.005$)
Serretti et al. (2002)	Descriptive	N=595 inpatients from various studies pooled	275 RC (46) 320 N-RC	RC: 175 (63) N-RC: 176 (55) ($p=.03$)	RC: 49 (18) N-RC: 63 (20)	RC: 32.1 (11.8) N-RC: 29.4 (10.9) ($p=.004$)

Vo & Dunner (2003)	Treatment response	*N*=152 treatment-resistant outpatients	102 RC (67) 50 N-RC	RC: 63 (62) N-RC: 28 (56)	RC: 55 (54) N-RC: 30 (60)	n/r
Coryell et al. (2003)	Descriptive (NIMH-CDS)	*N*=345 outpatients long-term follow-up 14 years	89 RC (26) 256 N-RC	RC: 62 (70) N-RC: 137 (54) (*p*=.008)	RC: 29 (33) N-RC: 89 (35)	RC: 21.6 (8.9) N-RC: 24.4 (10.6) (*p*=.03)
Yildiz & Sachs (2003)	Descriptive	*N*=197 outpatients (BP-I only)	84 RC (43) 113 N-RC	RC: 55 (65) N-RC: 58 (51)	n/a n/a	RC: 18.9 (8.7) N-RC: 21.8 (9.3) (*p*=.02)
Schneck et al. (2004)	Descriptive (STEP-BD)	*N*=456 outpatients	91 RC (20) 365 N-RC	RC: 61 (67) N-RC: 210 (58)	RC: 22 (24) N-RC: 89 (24)	RC: 16.7 (8.7) N-RC: 20.0 (8.5) (*p*=.01)
Kupka et al. (2005)	Descriptive (SFBN)	*N*=539 outpatients Follow-up 1 year	206 RC (38) 333 N-RC	RC: 129 (63) N-RC: 173 (52) (*p*=.02)	RC: 29 (14) N-RC: 75 (23) (*p*=.03)	RC: 17.6 (9.1) N-RC: 23.1 (10.0) (*p*=<.0001)

Source: Adapted and expanded from Kupka et al. (2003).

RC=rapid cyclers; N-RC = non-rapid cyclers.
Percentages are rounded off to whole numbers.
n/r=not reported in original study.
n/a=not applicable.
Statistical significant differences between rapid cyclers and non-rapid cyclers reported in original studies are indicated by *p*-values in italics.

more on illness burden quantified as episode frequency; the switch criterion would likely enhance validity by obviating the challenges encountered identifying partial remission and minimal duration criteria for
rapid cycling.

Bauer et al. (1994) distinguished between two ways of conceptualizing rapid cycling: counting separate episodes, and looking at the temporal
linkage of episodes of opposite polarity. The simple approach is to count
individual episodes according to explicit duration and severity criteria,
and then define a cut-off point to separate rapid from non-rapid cycling.
This is the way that rapid cycling was operationalized by Dunner and
Fieve (1974) and currently in DSM-IV-TR, and it requires no particular pattern or sequence of episodes. Most modern studies of rapid cycling used
definitions based on episode counting. In contrast, the "classic" approach
focused more on (continuous) cyclicity, and included particularly those
patients with rapid alternations of polarity. These two approaches
may result in overlapping but different patient groups. Maj et al. (2002)
addressed the confusion that may result when one is not fully aware of
these two concepts of rapid cycling.

Beyond the DSM-IV definition, faster cycle frequencies have been
described in case reports as "ultra-rapid cycling" (cycles of 48 hours) and
"ultradian cycling" (mood shifts within a day) (Alarcon, 1985; Kramlinger
& Post, 1996). It is clear that formal duration criteria are not met in these
patients, and therefore they would be classified as "Bipolar Disorder Not
Otherwise Specified" or "Bipolar I Disorder, Mixed Episode", without the
additional course specifier "rapid cycling". Even when cycle frequency is
less extreme, brief episodes, that is not meeting DSM-IV duration criteria,
are abundant in patients with rapid cycling (Bauer et al., 1994; Kupka et
al., 2005). If these "truncated episodes" are taken into account in addition to full-duration episodes, considerably more patients would be classified as rapid cyclers, as is probably the case in everyday clinical practice.
Moreover, brief mood episodes may be abundant in bipolar spectrum
disorder like recurrent brief depression and recurrent brief hypomania
(Angst et al., 2003).

It is obvious that the distinction between (ultra-) rapid cycling and true
mixed episodes may be difficult, given their complex relationship. Rapid
cyclers may have true mixed episodes (dysphoric manias) in the course
of their illness, alternating with depressions. Mixed states may form the
transition between manic and depressive episodes, and cycling may be so
frequent that it is conceived as one single protracted mixed episode.

All in all, rapid cycling has a considerable variability among patients:
the occasional occurrence of four mood episodes within one year, a more
regular and continuous cycling pattern, or a longer period of chaotic mood
alternations. Examples of these patterns are shown in Figure 3.1.

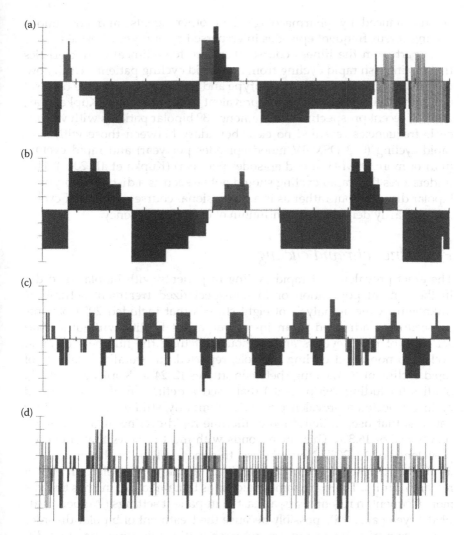

Figure 3.1 Examples of one-year prospective illness course in four patients with rapid cycling bipolar I disorder. Mania/hypomania above baseline, depression below baseline: (a) alternation of manic, depressive, and mixed episodes; (b) regular alternation of euphoric manias and depressions; (c) continuous cycling with full-duration and brief episodes; (d) ultra-rapid and ultradian cycling. (NIMH-LifeChart™ data from the Stanley Foundation Bipolar Treatment Network naturalistic follow-up study, Kupka et al., 2005.)

Although not mentioned in DSM-IV-TR, rapid cycling could be further specified as: early onset (from the very onset of bipolar illness, estimated at 20% of cases) (Goodwin & Jamison, 2007) versus late onset; spontaneous versus induced by pharmacological or other agents; and continuous cycling versus frequent episodes interspersed by euthymic periods.

Apart from the illness course, there are few clinical characteristics that distinguish rapid cycling from non-rapid cycling patients. Until now, only female gender, bipolar II subtype and possibly an early age of onset are found to be somewhat more prevalent in rapid cyclers (Kupka et al., 2003). A recent prospective study among 539 bipolar patients with various cycle frequencies revealed no clear boundary between those with non-rapid cycling (0–3 DSM-IV mood episodes per year) and rapid cycling (four or more DSM-IV mood episodes per year) (Kupka et al., 2005). This underscores that rapid cycling should not be seen as a distinct subtype of bipolar disorder, but rather as is a dimensional course specifier of cyclicity, arbitrarily defined on a continuum of episode frequency.

Prevalence of rapid cycling

The exact prevalence of rapid cycling in patients with bipolar disorder in the general population or in non-specialized treatment settings is unknown. A meta-analysis of eight studies that included 2054 patients consecutively admitted to an in- or outpatient facility without *a priori* selection of rapid cyclers and without matching the numbers of rapid cyclers to non-rapid cycling controls, reported an overall prevalence of rapid cycling of 16.3% (range between studies 12–24%) (Kupka et al., 2003). Studies (including 795 patients) that used a definition of current rapid cycling reported a prevalence of 16.4%. Similarly, studies (including 1259 patients) that used a definition of lifetime rapid cycling also reported a prevalence of 16.3%. This corresponds with most reviews that suggest a prevalence of 13–20%. Nevertheless, this may still be at the upper limits of the true prevalence in bipolar disorder due to the selection bias of research clinics. There are some indications that rapid cycling has become more frequent in recent years, at least in in-patient settings (Wolpert et al., 1990; Frye et al., 2000), possibly because the treatment of bipolar disorder is now common practice in non-research settings, leaving the more difficult cases for treatment in specialized centers. However, it may also be that widespread treatment with antidepressants has increased the incidence of rapid cycling (Wehr & Goodwin, 1979). Increased awareness after the inclusion of rapid cycling in DSM-IV may also have contributed to an apparent increased prevalence.

Persistence of rapid cycling

Most follow-up studies have suggested that rapid cycling is a transient phenomenon in most patients (Table 3.2), although some found particular

Table 3.2 Prospective Follow-Up Studies of Rapid Cycling Bipolar Disorder

Study	n	Years follow-up (mean ±SD)	Persistent RC course	Converted to non-RC course	Complete or nearly complete remission
Wehr et al. (1988)	51	1–12 (4.9 ± 3.5)	21 (41%)	8 (16%)	19 (37%)
Coryell, Endicott, & Keller (1992)	39	5	1 (3%) in all 5 years	25 (64%) after first year 7 (18%) after second year	10 (25%)
Bauer et al. (1994)	58	1–3 (2.9 ± 0.4)	27 (47%)	26 (45%)	5 (9%)
Maj et al. (1994)	37	5	22/37 (59%) in first year 16/36 (44%) in second year 8/23 (35%) after 5 years 7/37 (19%) throughout follow-up	15/37 (41%) in first year 20/36 (56%) in second year 15/23 (65%) after 5 years	n/r
Maj et al. (1999)	31	1	18 (58%) in first year	13 (42%) in first year	n/r
Coryell et al. (2003)	89	(15.2 ± 4.9)	20 (22%) for ≥2 years	69 (78%) within 2 years	n/r
Koukopoulos et al. (2003)	109	2–36 years (12.6 ± 7.5)	55 (54%) throughout follow-up	17 (16%)	36 (33%)

high rates of persistent rapid cycling throughout follow-up (Maj et al., 1999; Koukopoulos et al., 2003). Close clinical follow-up is critical in these assessments as ongoing use of alcohol, drugs, and possibly continuous or pulsatile use of antidepressants may contribute to misattribution of "true" rapid cyclers. There is evidence that persistence of rapid cycling is associated with the occurrence of brief mood episodes and a pole-switching pattern, especially a switch from depression to (hypo-) mania as seen in patients with a DMI or DmI course (Koukopoulos et al., 1980; Maj et al., 1999; Maj et al., 2002). Other features associated with persistent rapid cycling were agitated depression and the pre-existence of a hyper-thymic or cyclothymic temperament (Koukopoulos et al., 1980). It has been suggested that transient rapid cycling may result from intermit-tent treatment with antidepressants (Koukopoulos et al., 1980), although another study gave no evidence for this association (Coryell et al., 2003). Koukopoulos et al. (2003) suggested that the persistence of rapid cycling beyond the first year of adequate treatment, that is a duration of at least 2 years, would identify "true" rapid cyclers. This is supported by the fact that most studies reported the largest reduction of rapid cycling after the first year of follow-up (Table 3.2). Still, even if rapid cycling as such resolves, in the short and the long term these patients will have more subsequent affective morbidity than non-rapid cyclers (Coryell et al., 2003).

Genetics

There is strong evidence that bipolar disorder has a significant genetic background (Goodwin & Jamison, 2007), but consistent evidence for rapid cycling as a specific endophenotype is lacking. A meta-analysis of studies that investigated the impact of a family history of mood disorders on the prevalence of rapid cycling reported that only one of six studies found a significantly increased prevalence of mood disorders among first-degree relatives of patients with rapid cycling when compared to patients without rapid cycling (Kupka et al., 2003). Moreover, three studies with rigorous methodology that were specifically designed to assess the morbidity risk among first-degree relatives also found no differences. Although Fisfalen et al. (2005) determined that episode frequency was a highly familial trait after investigating 407 subjects with affective disorder from 86 families of probands with bipolar disorder, they also reported that there was no evidence that DSM-IV rapid cycling a was familial trait. These results suggest that a family history of mood disorders does not substantially increase the risk for rapid cycling.

Using molecular genetic techniques to study candidate genes that may be related to the development of rapid cycling, one study found an association with low COMT activity allele (chromosome 22q11.2) (Kirov et al., 1998). A similar association was found in six patients with ultra-rapid cycling (Papolos et al., 1998), but not in prepubertal and adolescent subjects with ultradian cycling (Geller & Cook, 2000).

The long allele polymorphism of the serotonin transporter gene-linked functional polymorphic region (5-HTTLPR) was found to be more prevalent in patients with rapid cycling as compared to controls and patients with other forms of bipolar and remitting mood disorders (Cusin et al., 2001). In contrast, another group found an association between a lifetime history of rapid cycling and the short form of the 5-HTTLPR (Rousseva et al., 2003). Two recent studies (Green et al., 2006; Muller et al., 2006) reported that variations at the Val66Met polymorphism of the BDNF gene were associated with the susceptibility for rapid cycling but not with bipolar disorder in general.

Associated features and possible risk factors

Several features have been associated with rapid cycling, of which female gender, clinical or subclinical hypothyroidism, and treatment with antidepressants are most often mentioned. These factors could point towards underlying etiological or pathophysiological mechanisms (Papadimitriou et al., 2005).

A modest overrepresentation of women among rapid cyclers is a relatively consistent finding across studies and contrasts with the even sex distribution in bipolar disorder in general (Tondo & Baldessarini, 1998; Kupka et al., 2003). The possible endocrine or other factors that may account for this gender difference have not been delineated. Although many bipolar women exhibited mood fluctuations across the menstrual cycle (Rasgon et al., 2005), no consistent association between menstrual cycle and rapid cycling has been found (Wehr et al., 1988; Leibenluft et al., 1999). Moreover, rapid cycling also exists in men and in postmenopausal women. This does not, however, exclude either the possible role of gonadal steroids in the modulation of brain mechanisms involved in mood regulation, or their potential, indirect, contribution to mood cycling through their effects on circadian rhythms and activity levels (Leibenluft, 1996). Female gender has been associated with other potential concomitants of rapid cycling such as bipolar II pattern, hypothyroidism, preponderance of depression, and hence exposure to antidepressants. In addition, the occurrence of faster cycle frequencies has been reported in bipolar patients with a history of early physical and sexual abuse, and such early traumas are more prevalent in women (Leverich et al., 2002). Nonetheless, female preponderance among rapid cyclers tends to be somewhat overstated, and it is obvious that men are also at a substantial risk of developing a rapid cycling course. Mood disorders have long been associated with clinical or subclinical thyroid dysfunction, and vice versa. However, there is ongoing controversy about whether there is an association of rapid cycling with hypothyroidism. If so, there are two hypotheses: (1) Patients with rapid cycling are predisposed to the development of clinical or subclinical hypothyroidism, especially when treated with lithium (Cho et al., 1979); (2) Patients with (impending) thyroid failure become more susceptible to a rapid cycling course (Bauer, Whybrow, & Winokur, 1990).

When compared with healthy controls, rapid cycling bipolar patients showed a significant decrease in serum thyroxine, an increase in serum thyroid stimulating hormone, and a disturbed thyrotropin-releasing hormone stimulation test after 4 weeks' lithium treatment (Gyulai et al., 2003). Although there was no control group of non-rapid cycling patients, these findings suggest that rapid cycling bipolar disorder is associated with a latent hypofunction of the hypothalamic-pituitary-thyroid axis, which may become manifest with short-term lithium challenge. An increased prevalence of thyroperoxidase (TPO) antibodies has been reported in rapid cycling bipolar patients (Oomen, Schipperijn, & Drexhage, 1996). Another study confirmed a high prevalence of TPO-antibodies in bipolar patients, but found no association with a prospectively assessed rapid cycling course (Kupka et al., 2002).

In a meta-analysis of clinical studies published between 1974 and 2002 that compared rapid cycling and non-rapid cycling patients, female gender (P=.000) and bipolar II subtype (P=.001) were significant differentiating features, although the effect sizes of these differences were small (Kupka et al., 2003). In addition, a family history of mood disorder, onset of bipolar illness with a depressive episode, a lifetime history of suicide attempts, and lithium non-responsiveness were more prevalent in rapid cyclers but these differences did not reach statistical significance. Studies investigating the association between rapid cycling and hypothyroidism reported very inconsistent results, thus lacking overall significance.

Subsequent studies of large naturalistic samples could not confirm an overrepresentation of rapid cyclers among patients with bipolar II subtype. Schneck et al. (2004) found an equal 20% rapid cycling among bipolar I and bipolar II patients, while Kupka et al. (2005) reported 41.3% rapid cycling among bipolar I and 27.9% among bipolar II patients. Interestingly, these and other recently published studies (Coryell et al., 2003; Yildiz & Sachs, 2003) consistently reported a younger age of onset of bipolar disorder in rapid cyclers (see Table 3.1).

Induction of rapid cycling by antidepressants

The induction of rapid cycling by antidepressants was originally addressed by Wehr and Goodwin (1979) and is still a subject of controversy (Wehr & Goodwin, 1987; Coryell et al., 1992; Wehr, with reply by Coryell, 1993; Coryell et al., 2003). Wehr and Goodwin (1979) found a pattern of increased cycling in a small study using an on-off-on design adding tricyclics or placebo to lithium prophylaxis. They, as well as Koukopoulos et al. (1975; 1980; 1983) hypothesized that antidepressants induce remission of depressive symptoms by accelerating the natural course of the illness, that is by shortening the cycle length. This implies that, after remission, the symptom-free interval would be shorter and the next episode would occur earlier than expected, sometimes following immediately after recovery, leading to a continuous cycling course. If so, then, paradoxically, the short-term therapeutic effect would not prevent but rather favour the subsequent evolution of the illness. Women and bipolar II patients may be more at risk for antidepressant-induced rapid cycling, as well as those who typically have manias or hypomanias following depression, and/ or premorbid hyperthymic or cyclothymic temperament (Koukopoulos et al., 1975, 1980; Altshuler et al., 1995). In a retrospective review of life charts of 51 treatment-refractory bipolar patients, Altshuler et al. (1995) found an antidepressant-induced manic episode in 35% of the patients, and antidepressant-induced cycle acceleration in 26%, with a strong association between the two phenomena. It has been suggested that antidepressant-induced rapid cycling is not different from and fully explained by antidepressant-induced (hypo-) mania (Mattes, 2006).

Alternatively, the association between rapid cycling and antidepressants may be related to the frequent occurrence of depression or to a natural course of mania following depression, and not to the antidepressant itself (Coryell, Endicott, & Keller., 1992; Coryell et al., 1993). In other words, in that case, rapid cycling increases the likelihood of the use of antidepressants rather than vice versa. It is difficult to differentiate the natural course of illness from switches into mania and cycle acceleration attributable to use of antidepressants as prospective randomized control trials to address this specific question are lacking. In a recent long-term follow-up study of 89 rapid cycling and 254 non-rapid cycling patients over a period of on average 14 years, the use of tricyclic antidepressants in combination with lithium was not associated with an increased risk for switching from depression to (hypo-) mania, nor was the cessation of a rapid cycling course associated with decrease in the use of antidepressants (Coryell et al., 2003).

Treatment

As with bipolar disorder in general the main objective of the treatment of rapid cycling is remission of acute episodes as well as prevention of future episodes. However, given the inherent nature of rapid cycling and the likelihood of spontaneous remission of individual episodes within a relatively short time, prevention of episodes should be the main focus. In fact, it may even be counterproductive to focus on the treatment of individual episodes. While treatment of manic episodes is in general congruent with prophylaxis, the treatment of depression is often more difficult and may lead to further destabilization of a patient as some treatments such as antidepressants may induce mania or faster cycling. Hence, before reviewing the efficacy of various treatments, some general treatment strategies are discussed.

The first step is to identify any factor that may promote cycling (e.g. antidepressants, substance abuse, hormonal treatments, endocrine disorders) (Sachs, 2004). If present, those should be addressed. Those on antidepressant, the antidepressant should be tapered and a mood stabilizer added. If after 4 months the cycle frequency is significantly reduced, this treatment should be continued. Otherwise, a second mood stabilizer or psychotherapy is added. If this remains ineffective after a trial of 16 weeks, a third mood stabilizer or a more experimental treatment option is added. Key features in an algorithm are refraining from antidepressants and allowing every new treatment or treatment combination sufficient time to exhibit its efficacy.

Since spontaneous remission and early recurrence is the rule rather than the exception in rapid cycling, acute short-term clinical trials have only limited relevance to its overall treatment. Until now, there are only two published studies of continuation treatment in patients with rapid cycling bipolar disorder using a formal double-blind, parallel-group design (Calabrese et al., 2000; Calabrese et al., 2005a) (Table 3.3). These will be discussed below, together with open studies in rapid cyclers and studies comparing the efficacy of various treatments in rapid cyclers and non-rapid cyclers.

Tondo, Hennen, & Baldessarini (2003) compared the responses to long-term treatments of rapid cycling versus non-rapid cycling patients in a meta-analysis of 16 studies that included lithium, valproate, carbamazepine, lamotrigine, and topiramate, alone or in combination with other agents. These studies involved 905 rapid cycling and 951 non-rapid cycling patients who were treated over an average of 47.5 months. Rapid cyclers had a 2.9-fold greater risk of recurrence or non-improvement, and a pooled risk-ratio for inferior treatment response of 1.40 (CI 1.26–1.56; $p < .0001$). All treatment modalities were associated with lower effectiveness in rapid cycling, with no evidence of superiority of one particular treatment. These authors state that total long-term protection from recurrences is an unrealistic expectation in bipolar disorder in general and particularly in rapid cycling, and that one should aim at symptomatic and functional improvement.

Lithium

Failure of lithium prophylaxis was one of the key features of rapid cycling when the term was introduced (Dunner & Fieve, 1974). However, in later

Table 3.3 Studies Comparing the Effects of Lithium Treatment in
Rapid-Cycling (RC) and Non-Rapid-Cycling (N-RC) Bipolar Disorder

Study	Subjects (n)[a]	Follow-up (years)	% Rapid cyclers	Lithium responders[b,c] n (%)
Dunner & Fieve (1974)	55	0.5–5.5	20	RC: 2/11 (18)[b,d] ; N-RC: 26/44 (59)[b,d]
Kukopulos et al. (1980)	434	4.5	20	RC: 36/65 (55)[b]; N-RC: 157/244 (64)[b]
Wehr et al. (1988)	66	1–12	71	RC: 12/51 (24)[b,d]; N-RC: 11/12 (92)[b,d]
Maj et al. (1989)	118	≥2	12	RC: 3/12 (25)[c]; N-RC: 53/87 (61)[c]
Okuma (1993)	108	2	56	RC: 1/60 (2)[b,d]; N-RC: 16/48 (33)[b,d]
Okuma (1993)	108	2	56	RC: 18/60 (30)[c,d]; N-RC: 31/48(65)[c,d]
Maj et al. (1999)	128	≥1	24	RC: 13/22 (59)[c]; N-RC: 74/89 (83)[c]
Baldessarini et al. (2000)	360	4.5	16	RC: 10/56 (18)[b]; N-RC: 96/304 (32)[b]
Baldessarini et al. (2000)	360	4.5	16	RC: 37/56 (66)[c]; N-RC: 184/304 (61)[c]

[a] Total numbers in the study may differ from numbers in fifth column since not all participants had been treated with lithium.

[b] Lithium response defined as complete or near complete prevention of recurrences on lithium prophylaxis: overall in five studies: 61/243 (25.1%) in RC and 306/667 (45.9%) in N-RC (x^2=31.1, df=1, P<.000).

[c] Lithium response defined as at least 50% improvement on lithium prophylaxis: overall in four studies: 71/150 (47.3%) in RC and 342/528 (64.8%) in N-RC (x^2=14.2, df=1, P<.000).

[d] Significant difference between lithium response among rapid cyclers and non-rapid cyclers.

reports the same authors concluded that lithium is still recommended
in rapid cyclers since many of these patients have a reduction of the frequency and/or the severity and duration of both depressive and manic
episodes (Dunner, Patrick, & Fieve, 1977; Dunner, 1979). Interestingly,
the notion that lithium is of little use in rapid cyclers remains widespread. This may be true if complete remission and the prevention of
further recurrences are the criteria of response. If one aims at significant reduction of symptoms, a more favorable picture emerges. Table 3.4
shows all studies comparing the efficacy of lithium in rapid cyclers and
non-rapid cyclers.

Overall, 47% of rapid cyclers compared with 65% of non-rapid cyclers
had at least 50% symptomatic improvement. In contrast, only 25% of rapid

Table 3.4 Published Double-Blind, Parallel-Group Studies of
Continuation Treatment in Patients with Rapid-Cycling Bipolar Disorder

Study	Study drugs (n)	Duration	Outcome measures	Result	Comments
Calabrese et al. (2000)	LMT (92) PBO (88)	6 months after 12-week open-stabilization phase	Time to additional treatment for emerging symptoms	BP-I: LMT = PBO BP-II: LMT > PBO	Relapse with LMT: 59% Relapse with PBO: 74% Difference only in BP-II group
Calabrese et al. (2005a)	Li (32) VPA (28)	20 months after open-stabilization phase	Time to any episode	Li=VPA;	Relapse with Li: 56% Relapse with VPA: 50%

LMT, lamotrigine; PBO, placebo; Li, lithium; VPA, valproate; BP-I, bipolar I disorder; BP-II, bipolar II disorder.

cyclers and 46% of non-rapid cyclers had no further recurrences during lithium prophylaxis. However, pooling of these data must be interpreted with caution given the considerable differences in study designs. In particular, the duration of follow-up in these seven studies varied widely from 6 months to 12 years. In two of these studies (Koukopoulos et al., 1980; Baldessarini et al., 2000), the authors suggest that a relative favorable response to lithium maybe partly due to the limited use of antidepressants. In a 5-year follow-up of 247 patients who remained on lithium prophylaxis, 94 (38%; all non-rapid cyclers) had no recurrences, 115 (47%; including 31 rapid cyclers) had at least one recurrence but also a reduction of at least 50% of the time spent in hospital, and 38 (15%; including ten rapid cyclers) were not significantly improved (Maj et al., 1998). In the meta-analysis cited above, Tondo, Hennen, & Baldessarini (2003) concluded that lithium is no less effective than valproate, carbamazepine, lamotrigine, or topiramate, and that all these agents are relatively ineffective when total protection from episodes is the treatment goal. In conclusion, patients with rapid cycling bipolar disorder may indeed benefit from long-term lithium treatment, alone or in combination with other mood stabilizers.

Valproate

Initial open studies reported a favorable response to valproate in rapid cyclers, with marked prophylactic antimanic and antimixed effects, but only minimal to moderate prophylactic antidepressant effects (Calabrese &

Delucchi, 1990; Calabrese et al., 1992; Calabrese et al., 1993). These observations have given valproate a reputation of treatment of choice for any clinical presentation of rapid cycling (Sachs et al., 2000). However, a recent 20-month double-blind comparison of valproate and lithium in 60 rapid cycling bipolar patients found no significant difference between the treatment groups in terms of overall rates of relapse (51% on valproate, level ≥50 µg/ml, versus 56% on lithium, level ≥0.8 mEq/l), median time to the initiation of additional pharmacotherapy to treat emerging symptoms (45 vs 18 weeks), and median survival (26 vs 14 weeks) (Calabrese et al., 2005a). In the open-stabilization phase of this study all patients received a combination of lithium and valproate. Only 60 of 254 patients (24%) responded in the acute phase, while 76% discontinued the study prematurely due to poor adherence (28%), intolerable side effects (19%), or non-response (26%). Of the patients who did not discontinue in the open phase and remained symptomatic after 6 months, 73% had refractory depression and 27% had refractory mania, hypomania or mixed states, confirming that depressive symptoms are the least responsive to treatment.

Lamotrigine

An open study gave some evidence for the efficacy of lamotrigine in rapid cycling patients with depressive and mild-to-moderate but not severe manic symptoms (Bowden et al., 1999). In a double-blind crossover study comparing lamotrigine, gabapentine, and placebo in patients with refractory mood disorders, mainly bipolar rapid cyclers, only lamotrigine was significantly more effective than placebo (Frye et al., 2000). In a large double-blind, placebo-controlled 6-months maintenance trial, 182 of 324 patients with rapid cycling bipolar disorder who were stabilized on lamotrigine with or without other moodstabilizing agents, were subsequently randomized to lamotrigine monotherapy (100–500 mg/day) or placebo (Calabrese et al., 2000). A majority of patients (71%) had bipolar I disorder. Median time to intervention for emerging mood symptoms was statistically different between lamotrigine and placebo groups in bipolar II but not bipolar I patients. Overall, 41% of lamotrigine-treated patients remained stable without relapse into hypomania, mania, or depression for the entire 6 months, compared with 26% receiving placebo (*P*=.03). It is of interest, as in the lithium-divalproex maintenance study cited above, that only a relatively small proportion (56%) was stabilized during the acute treatment phase, underlining the difficulties in the treatment of rapid cycling patients. Efficacy in bipolar II but not bipolar I patients with rapid cycling, although fairly modest, is consistent with findings that lamotrigine is effective in the acute treatment of bipolar depression (Calabrese et al., 1999) and has prophylactic efficacy against depression but not against mania (Calabrese et al., 2003; Bowden et al., 2003). Although severe rash is often mentioned as a side-effect of lamotrigine, increasing the dose slowly and careful monitoring should reduce this risk substantially (Calabrese et al., 2002).

Other anticonvulsants

Like valproate, carbamazepine has no advantage over lithium in the treatment of rapid cycling (Okuma, 1993; Tondo, Hennen, & Baldessarini, 2003), and evidence for it's overall long-term efficacy from controlled studies is limited. In a 3-year cross-over study comparing the efficacy of lithium, carbamazepine , and in the third year the combination in treatment-refractory bipolar patients with a history of rapid cycling, 28% responded to lithium, 19% to carbamazepine, and 56% to the combination (Denicoff et al., 1997). However, the effect of time on overall response cannot be ruled out. If carbamazepine is given in combination with other treatments, one should consider the possibility of interactions through enzyme induction.

Although in a recent case report two patients with rapid cycling responded to levetiracepam (Braunig & Kruger, 2003), this agent was not clearly effective in an open-case series including rapid cyclers (Post et al., 2005). Augmentation of an ongoing moodstabilizing regime with tiagabine has shown some efficacy in a small number of rapid cyclers, but treatment with this anticonvulsant has been associated with frequent and severe adverse effects (Schaffer, Schaffer, & Howe, 2002; Suppes et al., 2002). Small studies with gabapentin add-on treatment reported unconvincing results in patients with rapid cycling (Altshuler et al., 1999; Wang et al., 2002), while gabapentin monotherapy was ineffective (Frye et al., 2000).

Atypical antipsychotics

Atypical antipsychotics have shown antimanic efficacy (Hirschfeld, 2003). Quetiapine reduced manic symptoms in a small case-series of rapid cyclers (Vieta et al., 2002). These short-term studies give evidence that atypical antipsychotics are primarily indicated in the manic phase of rapid cycling. In a small open study, clozapine add-on treatment up to one year proved to be more effective in non-rapid cyclers than in rapid cyclers (Suppes, Ozcan, & Carmody, 2004). A *post-hoc* analysis of 1-year open-label maintenance treatment with olanzapine in bipolar I patients with a rapid cycling and non-rapid cycling course reported less favorable long-term outcomes in rapid cyclers (Vieta et al., 2004). Although rapid cyclers had slightly better antimanic responses in the preceding double-blind acute treatment phase, they showed less overall symptomatic remission (i.e. remission of both manic and depressive symptoms), and more recurrences, especially depressive episodes. This study clearly reveals the caveat of short-term studies in rapid cyclers: relatively quick remission of symptoms of the index-episode is almost inherent to this illness course, as is the likelihood of recurrences.

Although there is less evidence for the efficacy of atypical antipsychotics in bipolar depression (McIntyre & Katzman, 2003), in a recently published study quetiapine was more efficacious than placebo for depression in bipolar I and II disorder (Calabrese et al., 2005b). This difference remained present in an *post-hoc* analysis of a subgroup of 108 patients with rapid cycling bipolar I and II disorder (Vieta et al., 2007). This suggests that quetiapine would be an interesting treatment option in rapid cycling, but there are currently no studies available to give evidence for such a recommendation.

In a recent, as yet unpublished multicenter, international trial (Alphs et al., 2008), patients with bipolar I and II disorder with a frequently relapsing course, defined as having had four or more mood episodes that required treatment intervention in the previous 12 months, were included. These patients continued to receive their treatment-as-usual (TAU), which most commonly consisted of mood stabilizers, like lithium and valproate. In addition to TAU, these patients were initially treated in an open-label manner with adjunctive risperidone long-acting injectable (LAI) for 12 weeks. Subjects who were in symptom remission were randomized to TAU only or TAU with adjunctive risperidone LAI treatment in a double-blind, placebo controlled phase of the trial. Patients treated with risperidone LAI adjunctive to TAU showed significantly fewer relapses into a mood episode when compared to those treated with TAU alone. The majority of subjects received risperidone LAI 25 mg once every two weeks in addition to their treatment-as-usual. It should be noted that the definition of "frequently relapsing bipolar disorder" in these subjects was wider than the category of "rapid cycling" in DSM IV. It is noteworthy that risperidone LAI demonstrated efficacy and safety in this population.

Other pharmacological treatment options

Given an association of rapid cycling with clinical and subclinical hypothyroidism, however controversial, there has been considerable interest in using the thyroid hormone thyroxin (L-T4) in treatment-refractory mood disorders (Bauer et al., 2003). Until now, evidence of the efficacy of thyroxin in patients with rapid cycling is restricted to single-case studies and three small open case series (Stancer & Persad, 1982; Bauer, Whybrow, & Winokur, 1990; Afflelou et al., 1997). In these studies overall 27 patients (22 women) were treated, who received 50–500 mcg of thyroxin daily over a period of 1–108 months. Among these patients were 16 (59%) responders, six (22%) partial responders, and five (19%) non-responders. Although most of these patients had thyroid indexes in the normal range, there is some evidence that during lithium maintenance treatment, a relatively low free T4 (although within normal limits) is associated with more affective episodes and greater severity of depression as shown by the Beck Depression Inventory (Frye et al., 1999). This could be a potential rationale for thyroxin add-on treatment in rapid cycling. In general, patients tolerated these supraphysiological doses of thyroxin very well (Bauer et al., 2001). Taken together, these observations suggest that some euthyroid rapid cyclers, especially women, may respond when supraphysiological doses of thyroxin are added to an ongoing mood stabilizer. Given the limited evidence, such treatment should be reserved for treatment-resistant cases.

Several other options have been recommended as add-on treatments to a mood-stabilizer regime (Post et al., 2000) particularly clozapine, topiramate, nimodipine, buspirone, inositol and omega-3 fatty acids. A recent double-blind placebo-controlled study of add-on omega-3 fatty acids reported no significant efficacy in patients with rapid cycling bipolar disorder after 6 months of treatment (Keck et al., 2006).

The use of antidepressants in rapid cyclers

Although antidepressants clearly induce hypomania or mania in some patients with bipolar disorder, the evidence that antidepressants destabilize mood, increase cycle frequency, and induce rapid cycling is still open to debate (see earlier). Still, their use in rapid cyclers is in general best avoided, and limited to severe depressive episodes that last long enough to benefit from the delayed-onset antidepressant effect. There is some evidence that one should be especially hesitant to use antidepressants in patients whose depressions are usually followed by (hypo-) manias, or who previously had a manic switch after starting an antidepressant. If antidepressants are used during acute depression, they should be tapered after remission and avoided in the maintenance phase. Selective serotonin re-uptake inhibitors may have somewhat less cycling-inducing properties than tricyclic antidepressants, although evidence from controlled studies is lacking.

Combination treatment

Few available treatments for bipolar disorder can be regarded as true long-term mood stabilizers with acute and prophylactic efficacy for both manic and depressive episodes. The current evidence for lithium comes closest to this ideal, which may be in part due to the large number of studies that have involved lithium over the years (Bauer & Mitchner, 2004; Muzina & Calbrese, 2005). Still, long-term stabilization preventing "break-through" episodes is rarely achieved with any monotherapy. By definition, the need for a bimodal action is most pressing in patients with rapid cycling. It is therefore useful to distinguish agents with mood-stabilizing properties "from above", that is predominantly effective for mania (lithium, carbamazepine, valproate, atypical antipsychotics, electroconvulsive therapy [ECT]), and mood-stabilizers "from below", that is predominantly effective for depression (lithium, lamotrigine, ECT) (Ketter & Calabrese, 2002). Combining agents from these two classes is a rational approach in the treatment of rapid cycling. Starting agents sequentially, rather than simultaneously, allows for the evaluation of the relative efficacy of each drug (Sachs, 2004). Lithium should be considered in combination treatments, with the addition of lamotrigine in predominant depression, and valproate, carbamazepine or olanzapine in predominant mania (Bowden, 2004). When combining lamotrigine and valproate one should reduce the dose of the former and be even more alert for signs of rash (Calabrese et al., 2002).

Non-pharmacological treatment

Psychotherapeutic interventions (psychoeducation [PE], cognitive-behavioral therapy [CBT], interpersonal social rhythm therapy [IP/SRT], and family-focused treatment [FFT]) are effective in the long-term treatment of bipolar disorder by improving environmental risk factors, coping behavior, life style and adherence to medication treatment (Bauer, 2002). Although some form of psychoeducational therapy is indicated in any treatment regime for bipolar disorder, there is no evidence for specific efficacy in rapid cycling. Theoretically it might be expected that rapid cycling patients would specifically benefit from IP/SRT, since there is some indication they have less adherence to social rhythms than controls (Ashman et al., 1999). However, studies of psychotherapeutic interventions in rapid cyclers are lacking.

There are some case reports of the application of sleep deprivation in the depressive phase of rapid cycling bipolar disorder (Papadimitriou et al., 1993; Koukopoulos et al., 2003), which suggest a temporary improvement but also the risk of switching to hypomania.

Bright light therapy has been established an effective treatment for seasonal depression, and there are a few case reports of its application in rapid cycling (reviewed by Papadimitriou et al., 2007). In a study of nine rapid cycling patients, Leibenluft et al. (1995) found that light therapy in the afternoon improved mood during the depressive phase, in contrast to morning or evening applications.

Electroconvulsive therapy (ECT) is a safe and effective treatment for depression as well as for mania, suggesting that it would have mood stabilizing potential, and successful treatment of rapid cycling patients have been reported. However, there is only equivocal evidence of the efficacy of ECT in rapid cycling, coming from case-reports and small case-series indicating that the overall response is low and not sustained in most cases (Papadimitriou et al., 2007).

Conclusions and clinical management recommendations

Rapid cycling is relatively common in clinical populations of patients with bipolar disorder and is generally associated with unfavorable results with currently available pharmacologic treatment. These patients need careful assessment of previous illness course, elimination of potentially cycling-inducing factors, and systematic step-wise treatment planning with a focus on long-term stabilization rather than short-term remission. Combining all currently available evidence, expert opinion, and our own clinical experience, we provide a treatment algorithm as presented in Figure 3.2.

Combining mood-stabilizing agents which have predominantly antimanic and antidepressant properties appears to be the most promising approach if initial mood stabilizer monotherapy (lithium or valproate for bipolar I, and lamotrigine for bipolar II rapid cycling) is not successful. When evaluating treatment, significant reduction of symptoms (i.e. milder, briefer, and fewer episodes) is a more realistic goal than complete prevention of further episodes. Agents that show partial efficacy in a given patient should not be abandoned too soon but rather be part of a subsequent combination treatment. This strategy should be discussed with the patient to enhance treatment adherence. Rapid cycling is a transient phase of illness in many, if not most patients, but there are a substantial number of patients in whom it takes a protracted course of years or even decades. Despite a growing therapeutic armamentarium, patients with rapid cycling remain one of the great challenges in the treatment of bipolar illness.

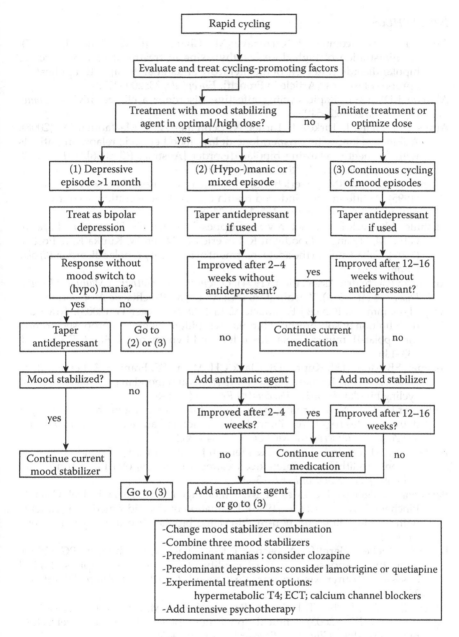

Figure **3.2** A suggested algorithm for the treatment of rapid cycling bipolar disorder.

References

Afflelou S, Auriacombe M, Cazenave M, Chartres JP, & Tignol J. (1997). Administration of high dose levothyroxine in treatment of rapid cycling bipolar disorders. Review of the literature and initial therapeutic application apropos of 6 cases. [Article in French]. *Encephale, 23*: 209–217.

Alarcon RD. (1985). Rapid cycling affective disorders: a clinical review. *Comp. Psychiatry, 26*: 522–540.

Alphs L, Haskins J, Turkoz I, Turner N, Schreiner A, & Macfadden W. (2008). Adjunctive long-acting risperidone delays mood episode relapse in patients with frequently relapsing bipolar disorder [Abstract P.3.c.066]. *J. Eur. Coll. Neuropsychopharmacol., 18* (Suppl 4): S441.

Altshuler LL, Post RM, Leverich GS, Mikalauskas K, Rosoff A, & Ackerman L. (1995). Antidepressant-induced mania and cycle acceleration: a controversy revisited. *Am. J. Psychiatry, 152*: 1130–1138.

Altshuler LL, Keck PE Jr, McElroy SL, Suppes T, Brown ES, Denicoff K, Frye M, Gitlin M, Hwang S, Goodman R, Leverich G, Nolen W, Kupka R, & Post R. (1999). Gabapentin in the acute treatment of refractory bipolar disorder. *Bipolar Disord., 1*: 61–65.

American Psychiatric Association. (1994). *Diagnostic and Statistical Manual of Mental Disorders* (4th Edn). Washington, DC: American Psychiatric Association.

Angst J, Gamma A, Benazzi F, Ajdacic V, Eich D, & Rässler W. (2003). Toward a re-definition of subthreshold bipolarity: epidemiology and proposed criteria for bipolar-II, minor bipolar disorders and hypomania. *J. Affect. Disord., 73*: 133–146.

Ashman SB, Monk TH, Kupfer DJ, Clark CH, Myers FS, Frank E, & Leibenluft E. (1999). Relationship between social rhythms and mood in patients with rapid cycling bipolar disorder. *Psychiatry Res., 86* (1): 1–8.

Baillarger J. (1854). Note sur un genre de folie dont les accès sont characterises par deux périodes régulières, l'une de dépression et l'autre d'excitation. *Bulletin de l'Académie Impériale de Médecine, 19*: 340–352.

Baldessarini RJ, Tondo L, Floris G, & Hennen J. (2000). Effects of rapid cycling on response to lithium maintenance treatment in 360 bipolar I and II disorder patients. *J. Affect. Disord., 61*: 13–22.

Bartalena L, Pellegrini L, Meschi M, Antonangeli L, Bogazzi F, Dell'Osso L, Pinchera A, & Placidi GF. (1990). Evaluation of thyroid function in patients with rapid-cycling and non-rapid-cycling bipolar disorder. *Psychiatry Res., 34*: 13–17.

Bauer M, Priebe S, Berghfer A, Bschor T, Kiesslinger U, & Whybrow PC. (2001). Subjective response to and tolerability of long-term supraphysiological doses of levothyroxine in refractory mood disorders. *J. Affect. Disord., 64*: 35–42.

Bauer M, Adli A, Bschor T, Heinz A, Rasgon N, Frye M, Grunze H, Kupka R, & Whybrow PC. (2003). Clinical applications of levothyroxine in refractory mood disorders. *Clin. App. Bipolar Disord., 2*: 49–56.

Bauer M, Beaulieu S, Dunner DL, Lafer B, & Kupka R. (2008). Rapid cycling bioplar—diognostic conceptsl. *Bipolar Disorders, 10*: 153–162.

Bauer MS, Whybrow PC, & Winokur A. (1990). Rapid cycling bipolar affective disorder. I. Association with grade I hypothyroidism. *Arch. Gen. Psychiatry,* 47: 427–432.

Bauer MS, Calabrese JR, Dunner DL, Post R, Whybrow PC, Gyulai L, Tay LK, Younkin SR, Bynum D, Lavori P, & Price RA. (1994). Multisite data reanalysis of the validity of rapid cycling as a course modifier for bipolar disorder in DSM-IV. *Am. J. Psychiatry,* 151: 506–515.

Bauer MS. (2002). Psychosocial interventions for bipolar disorder: a review. In: Maj M, Akiskal HS, Lopez-Ibor JJ, Sartorius N (Eds.), *Bipolar Disorder.* New York: John Wiley & Sons.

Bauer MS, & Mitchner L. (2004). What is a "mood stabilizer"? An evidence-based response. *Am. J. Psychiatry,* 161: 3–18.

Bleuler E. (1949). *Lehrbuch der Psychiatrie. Achte Auflage.* Berlin: Springer Verlag.

Bowden CL, Calabrese JR, McElroy SL, Rhodes LJ, Keck PE Jr., Cookson J, Anderson J, Bolden-Watson C, Asher J, Monaghan E, & Zhou J. (1999). The efficacy of lamotrigine in rapid cycling and non-rapid cycling patients with bipolar disorder. *Biol. Psychiatry,* 45: 953–958.

Bowden CL, Calabrese JR, Sachs G, Yatham LN, Asghar SA, Hompland M, Montgomery P, Earl N, Smoot TM, DeVeaugh-Geiss J, & Lamictal 606 Study Group. (2003). A placebo-controlled 18-month trial of lamotrigine and lithium maintenance treatment in recently manic or hypo manic patients with bipolar I disorder. *Arch. Gen. Psychiatry,* 60: 392–400.

Bowden CL. (2004). Making optimal use of combination pharmacotherapy in bipolar disorder. *J. Clin. Psychiatry,* 65 (Suppl 15): 21–24.

Braunig P, & Kruger S. (2003). Levetiracepam in the treatment of rapid cycling bipolar disorder. *J. Psychopharmacol.,* 17: 239–241.

Calabrese JR, Suppes T, Bowden CL, Sachs GS, Swann AC, McElroy SL, Kusumakar V, Ascher JA, Earl NL, Greene PL, & Monaghan ET, Lamictal 614 Study Group. (2000). A double-blind, placebo-controlled, prophylaxis study of lamotrigine in rapid-cycling bipolar disorder. *J. Clin. Psychiatry,* 61: 841–850.

Calabrese JR, & Delucchi GA. (1990). Spectrum of efficacy of valproate in 55 patients with rapid-cycling bipolar disorder. *Am. J. Psychiatry,* 147: 431–434.

Calabrese JR, Markovitz PJ, Kimmel SE, & Wagner SC. (1992). Spectrum of efficacy of valproate in 78 rapid-cycling bipolar patients. *J. Clin. Psychopharmacol.,* 12 (Suppl): 53S–56S.

Calabrese JR, Rapport DJ, Kimmel SE, Reece B, & Woyshville MJ. (1993). Rapid cycling bipolar disorder and its treatment with valproate. *Can. J. Psychiatry,* 38 (Suppl 2): S57–61.

Calabrese JR, Bowden CL, Sachs GS, Ascher JA, Monaghan E, Rudd GD, & Lamictal 602 Study Group. (1999). A double-blind placebo-controlled study of lamotrigine monotherapy in outpatients with bipolar I depression. *J. Clin. Psychiatry,* 60: 79–88.

Calabrese JR, Suppes T, Bowden CL, Sachs GS, Swann AC, McElroy SL, & Lamictal 614 Study Group. (2000). A double-blind, placebo-controlled, prophylaxis study of lamotrigine in rapid-cycling bipolar disorder. *J. Clin. Psychiatry,* 61: 841–850.

Calabrese JR, Bowden CL, Sachs G, Yatham LN, Behnke K, Mehtonen OP, Montgomery P, Ascher J, Paska W, Earl N, DeVeaugh-Geiss J, & Lamictal 605 Study Group. (2003). A placebo-controlled 18-month trial of lamotrigine and lithium maintenance treatment in recently depressed patients with bipolar I disorder. *J. Clin. Psychiatry, 64*: 1013–1024.

Calabrese JR, Sullivan JR, Bowden CL, Suppes T, Goldberg JF, Sachs GS, Shelton MD, Goodwin FK, Frye MA, & Kusumakar V. (2002). Rash in multicenter trials of lamotrigine in mood disorders: clinical relevance and management. *J. Clin. Psychiatry, 63*: 1012–1019.

Calabrese JR, Shelton MD, Rapport DJ, Youngstrom EA, Jackson K, Bilali S, Ganocy SJ, & Findling RL. (2005a). A 20-month, double-blind, maintenance trial of lithium versus divalproex in rapid-cycling bipolar disorder. *Am. J. Psychiatry, 162*: 2152–2161.

Calabrese JR, Keck PE, Macfadden W, Minkwitz M, Ketter TA, Weisler RH, Cutler AJ, McCoy R, Wilson E, & Mullen J. (2005b). A randomized, double-blind, placebo-controlled trial of quetiapine in the treatment of bipolar I or II depression. *Am. J. Psychiatry, 162*: 1351–1360.

Cho JJ, Bone S, Dunner DL, Colt E, & Fieve RR. (1979). The effect of lithium treatment on thyroid function in patients with primary affective disorder. *Am. J. Psychiatry, 136*: 115–116.

Coryell W, Endicott J, & Keller M. (1992). Rapidly cycling affective disorder. Demographics, diagnosis, family history and course. *Arch. Gen. Psychiatry, 49*: 126–131.

Coryell W, Solomon D, Turvey C, Keller M, Leon AC, Endicott, Schettler P, Judd L, & Mueller T. (2003). The long-term course of rapid-cycling bipolar disorder. *Arch. Gen. Psychiatry, 60*: 914–920.

Cowdry RW, Wehr TA, Zis A, & Goodwin FK. (1983). Thyroid abnormalities associated with rapid cycling bipolar illness. *Arch. Gen. Psychiatry, 40*: 414–420.

Coryell W. (2005). Rapid cycling bipolar disorder. Clinical characteristics and treatment options. *CNS Drugs, 19*: 557–569.

Cusin C, Serretti A, Lattuada E, Lilli R, Lorenzi C, Mandelli L, Pisati E, & Smeraldi E. (2001). Influence of 5-HTTLPR and TPH variants on illness time course in mood disorders. *J. Psychiatric Res., 35*: 217–223.

Denicoff KD, Smith-Jackson EE, Disney Er, Ali SO, Leverich GS, & Post RM. (1997). Comparative prophylactic efficacy of lithium, carbamazepine and the combination in bipolar disorder. *J. Clin. Psychiatry, 158*: 470–478.

Dunner DL, & Fieve RR. (1974). Clinical factors in lithium carbonate prophylaxis failure. *Arch. Gen. Psychiatry, 30*: 229–233.

Dunner DL. (1979). Rapid cycling bipolar manic depressive illness. *Psych. Clin. North Am., 2*: 461–467.

Dunner DL. (1998). Bipolar Disorders in DSM–IV: Impact of rapid cycling as a course modifier. *Neuropsychopharmacology, 19*: 189–193.

Dunner DL, Patrick V, & Fieve RR. (1977). Rapid cycling manic depressive patients. *Compr. Psychiatry, 18*: 561–566.

Falret JP. (1854). Mémoire sur la folie circulaire, forme de maladie mentale caractérisée par la reproduction successive et régulière de l'état maniaque, de l'état mélancolique, et d'un intervalle lucide plus ou moins prolongé. *Bulletin de l'Académie de Médecine, 19*: 382–415.

Fisfalen ME, Schulze TG, DePaulo JR Jr, DeGroot LJ, Badner JA, & McMahon FJ. (2005). Familial variation in episode frequency in bipolar affective disorder. *Am. J. Psychiatry, 162*: 1266–1272.

Frye MA, Ketter TA, Leverich GS, Huggins T, Lantz C, Denicoff KD, & Post RM. (2000). The increasing use of polypharmacotherapy for refractory mood disorders: 22 years of study. *J. Clin. Psychiatry, 61*: 9–15.

Frye MA, Ketter TA, Kimbrell TA, Dunn RT, Speer AM, Osuch EA, Luckenbaugh DA, Cora-Ocatelli G, Leverich GS, & Post RM. (2000). A placebo-controlled study of lamotrigine and gabapentin monotherapy in refractory mood disorders. *J. Clin. Psychopharmacol., 20*: 607–614.

Frye MA, Denicoff KD, Bryan AL, Smith-Jackson EE, Ali SO, Luckenbaugh D, Leverich GS, & Post RM. (1999). Association between lower serum free T4 and greater mood instability and depression in lithium-maintained bipolar patients. *Am. J. Psychiatry, 156*: 1909–1914.

Geller B, & Cook EH Jr. (2000). Ultradian rapid cycling in prepubertal and early adolescent bipolarity is not in transmission disequilibrium with val/met COMT alleles. *Biol. Psychiatry, 47*: 605–609.

Goodwin FK, & Jamison KR. (2007). Manic-depressive illness. *Bipolar disorders and recurrent depression* (2nd Edn). Oxford: Oxford University Press.

Green EK, Raybould R, Macgregor S, Hyde S, Young AH, O'Donovan MC, Owen MJ, Kirov G, Jones L, Jones I, & Craddock N. (2006). Genetic variation of brain-derived neurotrophic factor (BDNF) in bipolar disorder: case-control study of over 3000 individuals from the UK. *Br. J. Psychiatry, 188*: 21–25.

Gyulai L, Bauer M, Bauer MS, García-España F, Cnaan A, & Whybrow PC. (2003). Thyroid hypofunction in patients with rapid cycling bipolar disorder after lithium challenge. *Biol. Psychiatr, 53*: 899–905.

Haslam J. (1809). *Observations on madness and melancholy.* London: Callow.

Hirschfeld RM. (2003). The efficacy of atypical antipsychotics in bipolar disorders. *Clin. Psychiatry, 64* (Suppl 8): 15–21.

Joffe RT, Kutcher S, & MacDonald C. (1988). Thyroid function and bipolar affective disorder. *Psychiatry Res., 25*: 117–121.

Keck PE, Mintz J, McElroy SL, Freeman MP, Suppes T, Frye MA, Altshuler LL, Kupka R, Nolen WA, Leverich GS, Denicoff KD, Grunze H, Duan N, & Post RM. (2006). Double-blind, randomized, placebo-controlled trials of ethyl-eicosapentanoate in the treatment of bipolar depression and rapid cycling bipolar disorder. *Biol. Psychiatry, 60*: 1020–1022.

Ketter TA, & Calabrese JR. (2002). Stabilization of mood from below versus above baseline in bipolar disorder: a new nomenclature. *J. Clin. Psychiatry, 63*: 146–151.

Kilzieh N, & Akiskal H. (1999). Rapid cycling bipolar disorder. An overview of research and clinical experience. *Psych. Clin. North Am., 22*: 585–607.

Kirov G, Murphy KC, Arranz MJ, Jones I, McCandles F, Cunugi H, Murray RM, McGuffin P, Collier DA, Owen MJ, & Craddock N. (1998). Low activity allele of catecholamine-O-methyltransferase gene associated with rapid cycling bipolar disorder. *Mol. Psychiatry, 3*: 342–345.

Koukopoulos A, Sani G, Koukopoulos AE, Minnai GP, Girardi P, Pani L, Albert MJ, & Reginaldi D. (2003). Duration and stability of the rapid-cycling course: a long-term personal follow-up of 109 patients. *J. Affect. Disord., 73*: 75–85.

Koupopoulos A, Reginaldi D, Laddomada P, Floris G, Serra G, & Tondo L. (1980). Course of the manic-depressive cycle and changes caused by treatment. *Pharmakopsychiatr Neuropsychopharmakol, 13*: 156–167.

Koukopoulos A, Caliari B, Tundo A, Minnai G, Floris G, Reginaldi D, & Tondo L. (1983). Rapid cyclers, temperament and antidepressants. *Comp. Psychiatry, 24*: 249–258.

Koukopoulos A, Reginaldi D, Girardi P, & Tondo L. (1975). Course of manic-depressive recurrences under lithium. *Comp. Psychiatry, 16*: 517–524.

Kraepelin E. (1913). Psychiatrie. *Ein Lehrbuch für Studirende und Aerzte. III. Band.* Achte Auflage. Leipzig: Verlag Barth.

Kramlinger KG, & Post RM. (1996). Ultra-rapid and ultradian cycling in bipolar affective illness. *Br. J. Psychiatry, 168*: 314–323.

Kupka RW, Luckenbaugh DA, Post RM, Leverich GS, & Nolen WA. (2003). Rapid and non-rapid cycling bipolar disorder: a meta–analysis of clinical studies. *J. Clin. Psychiatry, 64*: 1483–1494.

Kupka RW, Luckenbaugh DA, Post RM, Suppes T, Altshuler LL, Keck PE Jr, Frye MA, Denicoff KD, Grunze H, Leverich GS, McElroy SL, Walder J, & Nolen WA. (2005). A comparative study of rapid and non-rapid cycling bipolar disorder using daily prospective mood ratings in 539 out-patients. *Am. J. Psychiatry, 162*: 1273–1280.

Kupka RW, Nolen WA, Post RM, McElroy SL, Altshuler LL, Denicoff KD, Frye MA, Keck PE Jr, Leverich GS, Rush AJ, Suppes T, Pollio C, & Drexhage HA. (2001). High rate of autoimmune thyroiditis in bipolar disorder: lack of association with lithium exposure. *Biol. Psychiatry, 51*: 305–311.

Kusalic M. (1992). Grade II and grade III hypothyroidism in rapid-cycling bipolar patients. *Neuropsychobiology, 25*: 177–181.

Leibenluft E, Ashman SB, Feldman-Naim S, Feldman-Naim S, & Yonkers KA. (1999). Lack of relationship between menstrual cycle phase and mood in a sample of women with rapid cycling bipolar disorder. *Biol. Psychiatry, 46*: 577–580.

Leibenluft E. (1996). Women with bipolar illness: clinical and research issues. *Am. J. Psychiatry, 153*: 163–173.

Leibenluft E, Turner EH, Feldman-Naim S, Schwartz PJ, Wehr TA, & Rosenthal NE. (1995). Light therapy in patients with rapid cycling bipolar disorder: preliminary results. *Psychopharmacol Bull., 31*: 705–710.

Leverich GS, McElroy SL, Suppes T, Keck PE, Denicoff KD, Nolen WA, Altshuler LL, Rush AJ, Kupka R, Frye MA, Autio KA, & Post RM. (2002). Early physical and sexual abuse associated with an adverse course of bipolar illness. *Biol. Psychiatry, 51*: 288–297.

Lish JD, Gyulai L, Resnick SM, Kirtland A, Amsterdam JD, Whybrow PC, & Arlen Price R. (1993). A family history study of rapid-cycling bipolar disorder. *Psychiatry Res., 48*: 37–46.

Mackin P, & Young AH. (2004). Rapid cycling bipolar disorder: historical overview and focus on emerging treatments. *Bipolar Disord., 6*: 523–529.

Maj M, Pirozzi R, Formicola AM, & Tortorella A. (1999). Reliability and validity of four alternative definitions of rapid-cycling bipolar disorder. *Am. J. Psychiatry, 156*: 1421–1424.

Maj M, Pirozzi R, Magliano L, & Bartoli L. (2002). The prognositic significance of "switching" in patients with bipolar disorder: a 10-year prospective follow-up study. *Am. J. Psychiatry, 159*: 1711–1717.

Maj M, Magliano L, Pirozzi R, Marasco C, & Guarneri M. (1994). Validity of rapid cycling as a course specifier for bipolar disorder. *Am. J. Psychiatry, 151*: 1015–1019.

Maj M, Pirozzi R, & Starace F. (1989). Previous pattern of course of the illness as a predictor of response to lithium prophylaxis in bipolar patients. *J. Affect. Disord., 17*: 237–241.

Maj M, Pirozzi R, Magliano L, & Bartoli L. (1998). Long-term outcome of lithium prophylaxis in bipolar disorder: a 5-year prospective study of 402 patients at a lithium clinic. *Am. J. Psychiatry, 155*: 30–35.

Mattes JA. (2006). Antidepressant-induced rapid cycling: another perspective. *Ann. Clin. Psychiatry, 18*: 195–199.

McIntyre R, & Katzman M. (2003). The role of atypical antipsychotics in bipolar depression and anxiety disorders. *Bipolar Disord., 5* (Suppl 2): 20–35.

Muzina DJ, & Calabrese JR. (2005). Maintenance therapies in bipolar disorder: focus on randomized controlled trials. *Aust N Z J Psychiatry, 39* (8): 652–61.

Muller DJ, de Luca V, Sicard T, King N, Strauss J, & Kennedy JL. (2006). Brain-derived neurotrophic factor (BDNF) gene and rapid-cycling bipolar disorder: family-based association study. *Br. J. Psychiatry, 189*: 317–323.

Nurnberger Jr J, Guroff JJ, Hamovit J, Berrettini W, & Gershon E. (1988). A family study of rapid-cycling bipolar illness. *J. Affect. Disord., 15*: 87–91.

Okuma T. (1993). Effects of carbamazepine and lithium on affective disorders. *Neuropsychobiology, 27*: 138–145.

Oomen HAPC, Schipperijn AJM, & Drexhage HA. (1996). The prevalence of affective disorder and in particular of a rapid cycling of bipolar disorder in patients with abnormal thyroid function tests. *Clin. Endocrinol., 45*: 215–223.

Papolos DS, Veit S, Faedda GL, Saito T, & Lachman HM. (1998). Ultra-ulta rapid cycling bipolar disorder is associated with the low activity catecholamine-O-methyltransferase allele. *Mol. Psychiatry, 3*: 346–349.

Papadimitriou GN, Christodoulou GN, Katsouyanni K, & Stefanis CN. (1993). Therapy and prevention of affective illness by total sleep deprivation. *J. Affect. Disord., 27* (2): 107–116.

Papadimitrou GN, Calabrese JR, Dikeos DG, & Christodoulou GN. (2005). Rapid cycling bipolar disorder: biology and pathogenesis. *Int. J. Neuropsychopharmacol., 8*, 281–292.

Papadimitriou GN, Dikeos DG, Soldatos CR, & Calabrese JR. (2007). Non-pharmacological treatments in the management of rapid cycling bipolar disorder. *J. Affect. Disord., 98*: 1–10.

Post RM, Kramlinger KG, Joffe RT, Roy-Byrne PP, Rosiff A, Frye MA, & Huggins T. (1997). Rapid cycling bipolar disorder: lack of relation to hypothyroidism. *Psychiatry Res., 72*: 1–7.

Post RM, Altshuler LL, Frye MA, Suppes T, McElroy SL, Keck PE Jr, Leverich GS, Kupka R, Nolen WA, Luckenbaugh DA, Walden J, & Grunze H. (2005). Preliminary observations on the effectiveness of levetiracetam in the open adjunctive treatment of refractory bipolar disorder. *J. Clin. Psychiatry, 66*: 370–374.

Rasgon N, Bauer M, Grof P, Gyulai L, Elman S, Glenn T, & Whybrow PC. (2005). Sex-specific self-reported mood changes by patients with bipolar disorder. *J. Psychiatr. Res., 39*: 77–83.

Rousseva A, Henry C, van den Bulke D, Fournier G, Laplanche JL, Leboyer M, Bellivier F, Aubry JM, Baud P, Boucherie M, Buresi C, Ferrero F, & Malafosse A. (2003). Antidepressant-induced mania, rapid cycling and the serotonin transporter gene polymorphism. *Pharmacogenomics J.*, *3*: 101–104.

Sachs GS, Printz DJ, Kahn DA, Carpenter D, & Docherty JP. (2000). The expert consensus guideline series: medication treatment of bipolar disorder 2000. *Postgrad Med.*, 1–104.

Sachs G. (2004). Managing bipolar affective disorder. London: Science Press.

Schaffer LC, Schaffer CB, & Howe J. (2002). An open case series on the utility of tiagabine as an augmentation in refractory bipolar outpatients. *J. Affect. Disord.*, *71*: 259–263.

Schneck CD, Miklowitz DJ, Calabrese JR, Allen MH, Thomas MR, Wisniewski SR, Miyahara S, Shelton MD, Ketter TA, Goldberg JF, Bowden CL, & Sachs GS. (2004). Phenomenology of rapid cycling bipolar disorder: data from the first 500 participants in the Systematic Treatment Enhancement Program. *Am. J. Psychiatry*, *161*: 1902–1908.

Serretti A, Mandelli L, Lattuada E, & Smeraldi E. (2002). Rapid cycling mood disorder: clinical and demographic feature. *Comp. Psychiatry*, *43*: 336–343.

Stancer HC, & Persad E. (1982). Treatment of intractable rapid-cycling manic-depressive disorder with levothyroxine. Clinical observations. *Arch. Gen. Psychiatry*, *39*: 311–312.

Suppes T, Chisholm KA, Dhavale D, Frye MA, Altshuler LL, McElroy SL, Keck PE, Nolen WA, Kupka R, Denicoff KD, Leverich GS, Rush AJ, & Post RM. (2002). Tiagabine in treatment refractory bipolar disorder: a clinical case series. *Bipolar Disord.*, *4*: 283–289.

Suppes T, Ozcan ME, & Carmody T. (2004). Response to clozapine of rapid cycling versus non-cycling patients with a history of mania. *Bipolar Disord.*, *6*: 329–332.

Tondo L, & Baldessarini LU. (1998). Rapid cycling in women and men with bipolar manic-depressive disorders. *Am. J. Psychiatry*, *155*: 1434–1436.

Tondo, L., Hennen, J., & Baldessarini, R.J. (2003). Rapid cycling bipolar disorder: effects of long-term treatment. *Acta Psychiatrica Scand.*, *108*: 4–14.

Vieta E, Parramon G, Padrell E, Nieto E, Martinez-Aràn A, Corbella B, Colom F, Reinares M, Goikolea JM, & Torrent C. (2002). Quetiapine in the treatment of rapid cycling bipolar disorder. *Bipolar Disord.*, *4*: 335–340.

Vieta E, Calabrese JR, Hennen J, Colom F, Martinez-Aran A, Sanchez-Moreno J, Yatham LN, Tohen M, & Baldessarini RJ. (2004). Comparison of rapid-cycling and non-rapid-cycling bipolar I manic patients during treatment with olanzapine: analysis of pooled data. *J. Clin. Psychiatry*, *65*: 1420–1428.

Vieta E, Calabrese J, Goikolea J, Raines S, & Macfadden W; for the BOLDER Study Group. (2007). Quetiapine monotherapy in the treatment of patients with bipolar I or II depression and a rapid-cycling disease course: a randomized, double-blind, placebo-controlled study. *Bipolar Disord.*, *9*: 413–425.

Vo D, & Dunner DL. (2003). Treatment-resistant bipolar disorder: a comparison of rapid cyclers and nonrapid cyclers. *CNS Spectrums*, *8*: 948–952.

Wang PW, Santosa C, Schumacher M, Winsberg ME, Strong C, & Ketter TA. (2002). Gabapentin augmentation therapy in bipolar depression. *Bipolar Disord.*, *4*: 296–301.

Wehr TA, & Goodwin FK. (1979). Rapid cycling in manic–depressives induced by tricyclic antidepressants. *Arch. Gen. Psychiatry, 36*: 555–559.

Wehr TA, & Goodwin FK. (1987). Can antidepressants cause mania and worsen the course of affective illness? *Am. J. Psychiatry, 144*: 1403–1411.

Wehr TA, Sack DA, Rosenthal NE, & Cowdry RW. (1988). Rapid cycling affective disorder: contributing factors and treatment responses in 51 patients. *Am. J. Psychiatry, 145*: 179–184.

Wehr TA. (1993). Can antidepressants induce rapid cycling? (with reply by Coryell). *Arch. Gen. Psychiatry, 50*: 495–498.

Wolpert EA, Goldberg JF, & Harrow M. (1990). Rapid cycling in unipolar and bipolar affective disorders. *Am. J. Psychiatry, 147*: 725–728.

Wu LH, & Dunner DL. (1993). Suicide attempts in rapid cycling bipolar disorder patients. *J. Affect. Disord., 29*: 57–61.

Yildiz A, & Sachs GS. (2003). Do antidepressants induce rapid cycling? A gender-specific association. *J. Clin. Psychiatry, 64*: 814–818.

chapter four

Bipolar II disorder: Assessment and treatment

Felicity Ng
University of Melbourne

Catherine Cahill and Gin Malhi
University of Sydney

Michael Berk
University of Melbourne

Contents

Introduction 80
Epidemiology 80
Diagnosis 81
    Conceptualisation and diagnostic validity 83
Clinical features 84
Treatment 87
    Hypomania 87
    Depression 88
        Antidepressants 88
        Mood stabilizers 91
        Atypical antipsychotics 91
        Others 92
    Maintenance 93
    Rapid-cycling 94
    Psychological therapies 95
Clinical recommendations for management 95
Conclusions 96
References 97

Introduction

The longitudinal association of depression with hypomania was proposed as a distinct bipolar subtype over three decades ago (Dunner et al., 1976a), and was subsequently formally defined as a diagnostic entity called bipolar II disorder in the fourth edition of the Diagnostic and Statistical Manual of Mental Disorders (DSM-IV) in 1994 (American Psychiatric Association [APA], 1994). However, controversies regarding its diagnostic criteria, validity, boundaries with other disorders, and treatment still exist. The meaningful application of a diagnosis of bipolar II disorder requires an understanding of its core features, heterogeneous aetiology, diagnostic boundaries and treatment options.

Epidemiology

The precise prevalence rate of bipolar II disorder is not available, but its magnitude may be inferred from epidemiological data on bipolar disorder as a whole. Conservative lifetime prevalence estimates for bipolar disorder derived from large epidemiological studies have been in the vicinity of 1%. The most influential of these have included the Epidemiologic Catchment Area (ECA) study (Regier et al., 1988) and the National Comorbidity Survey (Kessler et al., 1994) conducted in the United States, which reported lifetime prevalences of 1.2 and 1.6%, respectively. Weissman et al. (1996) reported rates of 0.3–1.5% based on their epidemiological survey across 10 countries. However, these figures were based on interview schedules with narrow and ill-defined criteria for hypomania, and can reasonably be expected to underestimate the prevalence of the full bipolar spectrum.

More recent lifetime prevalence estimates of bipolar disorder have tended to be greater in magnitude. A Hungarian sample estimated a lifetime prevalence of 5.1%, using DSM-III-R criteria (Szadoczky et al., 1998). In a secondary analysis of the ECA data that included the category of subsyndromal manic symptoms, lifetime prevalence rates of 0.8, 0.5 and 5.1% were obtained for mania, hypomania and subsyndromal manic symptoms, respectively, thus yielding an overall rate of 6.4% for the bipolar spectrum (Judd & Akiskal, 2003). A Zurich cohort study reported a prevalence rate of 5.5% for DSM-IV mania/hypomania up to the age of 35 years, and a further rate of 2.8% for recurrent, brief (of 1–3 days' duration) hypomania in the same population (Angst, 1998). In a subsequent analysis of this study using broader definitions of bipolarity, the lifetime prevalence rate was reported to be as high as 10.9%, compared to 11.4% for broadly-defined major depression (Angst et al., 2003). Some of these studies can be criticised for their inconsistent definitions of bipolarity and for sacrificing diagnostic specificity by encompassing subsyndromal symptoms. Due to the lack of methodological consensus, the lifetime prevalence of the bipolar II subtype is unknown, but could be deduced from the above studies to lie between 1 and 5%.

Bipolar disorder is a common diagnosis among the psychiatric patient population. Cassano et al. (1989) reported that one in three primary depressed patients had a bipolar spectrum disorder, while Ghaemi, Boiman, and Goodwin (2000) cited that 60% of outpatients with affective disorders had a diagnosis of bipolar disorder (30% for bipolar I, 12% for bipolar II and 18% for bipolar not otherwise specified). Benazzi (1997, 1999a) reported prevalence rates of 43.4–45% for bipolar II disorder among private practice outpatients with a major depressive episode. The diagnosis may be over-represented in clinical cohorts of individuals with depression that is refractory to treatment (Sharma, Khan, & Smith, 2005).

Diagnosis

The DSM-IV-TR diagnostic criteria for bipolar II disorder requires a history of at least one major depressive episode and one hypomanic episode, in the absence of any manic or mixed episodes (APA, 2000). Although bipolar II disorder has shown robust diagnostic validity, the diagnostic criteria for hypomania has been under some debate. A hypomanic episode is stipulated by DSM-IV-TR to consist of persistently elevated, expansive or irritable mood lasting for at least 4 days, during which the patient must have at least three (four if mood is irritable) of the following symptoms: inflated self-esteem or grandiosity, decreased need for sleep, talkativeness or pressure to keep talking, flight of ideas or subjective experience of racing thoughts, distractibility, increase in goal-directed activity or psychomotor activation, and excessive involvement in pleasurable activities (APA, 2000). Shorter durations of hypomania have been demonstrated to be common in both bipolar I and II subtypes (Bauer et al., 2006), and hypomanic episodes of 1–3 days' duration have been found to be of comparable clinical significance to those lasting 4 days or more, as measured by illness characteristics such as age of onset, family history, depressive duration, suicide attempts and conduct problems (Angst et al., 2003). The shortening of the duration criterion for diagnosis from 4 to 2 days has been proposed (Akiskal & Pinto, 1999), while others have proposed the abandonment of temporal criteria altogether (Angst et al., 2003). Additionally, there have been data supporting overactivity as the most common and most strongly correlated hypomanic symptom in bipolar II disorder, and its inclusion as a stem criterion for hypomania has been suggested (Benazzi, 2006b).

As a syndromal phenomenon, bipolar II disorder can be difficult to diagnose, as suggested by its lengthy mean lag time to diagnosis, which has been estimated to be longer by several years than bipolar I disorder (Ghaemi, Boiman, & Goodwin, 2000; Mantere et al., 2004). This diagnostic elusiveness may have a number of explanations pertaining to characteristics of the disorder, the patient and the clinician. Diagnostic uncertainty is likely to occur because the disorder has a typical depressive onset (Berk et al., 2007) and predominance of depressive episodes over its longitudinal course, which may present initially as unipolar depression. The misleading nature of initial bipolar presentations is illustrated by longitudinal follow up studies that have shown a steady transition rate of unipolar to bipolar diagnoses over time. In one study conducted over a mean duration of 23.4 years, 50% of individuals initially diagnosed with unipolar disorder have switched to a bipolar diagnosis (32.1% bipolar I, 17.9% bipolar II) (Angst et al., 2005), while another study reported that 27% of patients with unipolar depression developed hypomania over a period of 15 years (Goldberg, Harrow, & Whiteside, 2001). Both studies showed a steady linear conversion pattern that was age independent, suggesting ongoing risk for conversion with time.

This is further compounded by the vastly greater likelihood of patients seeking treatment for depression than hypomania, and under-reporting of hypomanic symptoms. Under-reporting may relate to impaired insight into the presence of hypomania, due to their typically brief durations, subtle quality and the often distorted affective reference point of patients with mood disorders, or to a conscious preference of hypomania as reprieve from depression. An additional confound is that hypomania is frequently not impairing or distressing, increasing the likelihood that it may be seen as not abnormal, and even desirable, thus complicating recognition. For a variety of reasons that include time limitation, educational background, psychiatric expertise and availability of collateral historical accounts, clinicians may fail to specifically inquire about hypomania or recognize its presence. Personality factors, anxiety and substance use commonly coexist with mood disorders, which may further obscure diagnostic clarity. Lastly, hypomania associated with substance use and antidepressants is frequently dysphoric, resulting in overlap and confusion with depressive phenotypes. DSM-IV does not recognize drug- or antidepressant-induced hypomania. The nosological differences between major diagnostic classification systems, such as the International Classification of Diseases (ICD-10) (WHO, 1992) and the text revision edition of DSM-IV (DSM-IV-TR) (APA, 2000), may also contribute to the lack of conceptual unity for bipolar disorders, although conceptual diversity extends to other psychiatric disorders and may be a more general reflection of the nebulous quality and multi-dimensional aetiologies of psychiatric complaints.

To assist in the diagnosis of latent bipolar spectrum disorders, Ghaemi et al. have suggested a number of clinical clues of bipolarity in a patient's history (Ghaemi, Ko, & Goodwin, 2001). These include: early age of onset of major depressive episode (<25); recurrent major depressive episodes (>3); atypical depressive features; psychotic major depressive episodes; postpartum depression, brief major depressive episodes (<3 months); antidepressant-induced hypomania or mania; antidepressant "wear-off" effect; lack of response to three or more adequate antidepressant treatment trials; family history of bipolarity in first degree relatives; and hyperthymic personality. However, these are most useful as indicators for suspicion of bipolarity, and are not criteria for a specific diagnosis of bipolar II disorder.

Conceptualisation and diagnostic validity

The conceptualisation of bipolar disorders, in particular their scope and relationship to unipolar depression, is contentious and has been so since the time of Kraepelin (1913). In the contemporary literature for affective disorders, there has been support for the concept of both bipolar spectrum disorders and the affective spectrum (Akiskal, 1996; Ghaemi, Ko, & Goodwin, 2001), while others have cautioned against such expansive diagnostic boundaries and advocated for the preservation of a more narrow definition of bipolar disorder (Baldessarini, 2000).

The bipolar spectrum has been proposed by Akiskal to capture the range of affective clinical presentations between unipolar depression and bipolar I disorder, including bipolar II, iatrogenic (commonly antidepressant-induced) mania, cyclothymia, hyperthymic personality and unipolar depression in the presence of bipolarity in the family history (Akiskal, 1996). In a similarly broad paradigm, the majority of affective disorders have been suggested to exist on a spectrum of overlapping manifestations from dysthymia at one end, through the unipolar and bipolar spectrums, to bipolar I disorder at the other end (Ghaemi, Ko, & Goodwin, 2001). In an echo of the Kraepelian notion of "manic-depressive insanity", the import of cycling has been emphasised as an expression of bipolarity, which argues for continuity between recurrent unipolar depression and bipolar disorder. This has received some support from data illustrating the continual distribution of symptoms between these two conditions (Benazzi, 2002; 2003b), and the presence of substantial hypomanic symptoms in those with recurrent unipolar depression (Cassano et al., 2004).

In spite of the disputed boundaries among affective disorders, various lines of research support the validity of bipolar II disorder as a distinct diagnosis. Familial bipolar II patterns suggest a genetic basis, and have been documented in the form of case reports (Kuyler, 1988) and family studies (Dunner, Gershon, & Goodwin, 1976b; Coryell et al., 1984). In one study, probands with bipolar II disorder were more likely to have similarly afflicted first-degree relatives than bipolar I or non-bipolar probands, and were more likely than non-bipolar probands but less likely than bipolar I probands to have first-degree relatives with bipolar I disorder (Coryell et al., 1984). Other studies support genetic heterogeneity in bipolar II disorder, but suggest that a subgroup may "breed true" (Coryell et al., 1984). Preliminary findings linking bipolar II disorder to chromosome 18q provides additional genetic support for its validity as a bipolar subtype (McMahon et al., 2001). More recently, distinction among bipolar II disorder and the "soft" bipolar subtypes was demonstrated in the French National EPIDEP Study, where, using Akiskal's classification, bipolar subtypes II–IV showed significant differences on several clinical dimensions including clinical features, treatment responses and familial affective patterns (Akiskal, Akiskal, & Lancrenon, 2006). The diagnostic stability of bipolar I and II disorders, as illustrated by a 10-year follow-up study (Coryell et al., 1995), as well as the high inter-rater reliability of bipolar II disorder (Simpson et al., 2002), also lend strength to its diagnostic validity.

Clinical features

Bipolar II disorder appears to have a gender distribution that is either equal or has a slight female preponderance (Hendrick et al., 2000; Arnold, 2003), although a female predominance as high as 67.3% has been reported in a private practice outpatient bipolar II cohort. This study also found that females had a younger age of onset of the disorder and greater psychiatric comorbidity, atypical depression, mixed depression and suicidal ideation. However, the symptom structure of hypomania was similar for both sexes (Benazzi, 2006a). An earlier study of bipolar II and unipolar depressed outpatients likewise found atypical features to be more common in female bipolar II patients compared with male bipolar II patients and female unipolar patients, but found no gender differences in age of onset or various markers of severity and chronicity of illness (Benazzi, 1999b).

Age of onset for bipolar II disorder tends to be earlier than that for unipolar depression by several years, and approximates that for bipolar I disorder (Peselow et al., 1982; Angst, 1986). Symptoms usually start in adolescence, although the time gap between onset of symptoms and diagnosis of bipolar disorder is often over 10 years, with the disorder commonly having first been misdiagnosed as unipolar depression (Hirschfeld, Lewis, & Vornik, 2003). The delay in diagnosis for bipolar II has been reported to be longer than for bipolar I disorder (Mantere et al., 2004). Young age of onset has been proposed as a clinical marker of a bipolar subtype that is associated with greater genetic loading (Taylor & Abrams, 1981; Strober et al., 1988; Somanath, Jain, & Reddy, 2002) and illness severity (Geller et al., 2002).

In a large study of bipolar disorder, including the bipolar II subtype, the mean age of illness onset was 17.37 years, with the majority having experienced either very early onset before the age of 13 (27.7%) or early onset between the ages of 13 and 18 (37.6%), while the remainder (34.7%) were classified as adult onset after the age of 18 (Perlis et al., 2004). The two earlier onset groups had significantly higher rates of comorbid anxiety disorders and substance abuse, a more severe illness course marked by more recurrences and shorter periods of euthymia, and a greater likelihood of suicide attempts and violence. The association of earlier onset with greater comorbidity and more severe illness course has also been reported by a subsequent epidemiologically-based study (Goldstein & Levitt, 2006) and is well substantiated in the literature (Carlson & Meyer, 2000; Hollander et al., 2001; Wozniak et al., 2005). Despite evidence in the literature and clinical experience indicating that bipolar disorder is largely a condition with an adolescent onset, it is interesting to observe that bipolar II disorder is not recognized as a diagnostic entity in children and adolescents under some guidelines (The National Institute for Health and Clinical Excellence [NICE], 2006), but is accepted under others (National Institute of Mental Health [NIMH], 2000; 2001). This diagnostic discrepancy highlights the need to bridge the different conceptualisations of the disorder, to enable better diagnosis and intervention (Cahill et al., 2007).

The course of bipolar II disorder is characterized by a predominance of depressive symptoms. Its chronicity and illness burden are illustrated by naturalistic prospective data over 13.4 years from Judd et al. (2003a), which show the presence of symptoms during 53.9% of follow-up time, primarily comprising of depressive symptoms (50.3% of follow-up time), in contrast to infrequent hypomanic and cycling/mixed symptoms (1.3% and 2.3% of follow-up time, respectively). Additionally, the combined duration of sub-syndromal, minor depressive and hypomanic symptoms was three times longer than the total duration of major depressive symptoms. In comparison, a similar naturalistic study of bipolar I patients detected mood symptoms over 47.3% of follow-up time, with 31.9% of follow-up time marked by the presence of depressive symptoms (Judd et al., 2002). Compared with bipolar I disorder, the bipolar II variant may have more major and minor depressive episodes and shorter inter-episode intervals (Judd et al., 2003b). In a shorter study that followed up patients with bipolar I and II disorder over 3 years, both bipolar patient groups were found to be symptomatic approximately half of the time, during which subsyndromal and moderate depressive symptoms predominate (Joffe et al., 2004). The importance of subsyndromal symptoms lies in their predictive power for pole-specific relapse (Goodnick et al., 1987; Tohen, Waternaux, & Tsuang, 1990; Keller et al., 1992), and the functional impact of subsyndromal depressive symptoms (Altshuler et al., 2002; Judd et al., 2005).

The most distinctive cross-sectional clinical marker of bipolar II disorder is perhaps the presence of atypical depression, the recognition of which should prompt careful inquiry into a history of hypomania. Atypical features, as defined by DSM-IV-TR criteria, include hypersomnia, increase in appetite or significant weight gain, leaden paralysis, mood reactivity, and a longstanding pattern of interpersonal rejection sensitivity (APA, 2000). These symptoms have been demonstrated to be more common in bipolar II than in unipolar disorder (Benazzi, 2000). Since the DSM-IV-TR diagnosis of a mixed state requires the full criteria for major depression and mania to be concurrently satisfied, by definition, mixed states are not recognized for bipolar II disorder, as threshold mania can only be met in bipolar I disorder. In this context, alternative criteria for subthreshold mixed states may be more applicable to bipolar II disorder, such as the criteria for mixed depression that have been proposed and validated by Akiskal and Benazzi, which require the presence of three or more symptoms of hypomania in conjunction with a major depressive episode (Benazzi, 2003a; 2005). A softer criteria of two or more hypomanic symptoms in combination with threshold major depression has also been suggested to be useful (Benazzi, 2004; Benazzi, Koukopoulos, & Akiskal, 2004). The detection of subthreshold mixed states, and their differentiation from depressive phenotypes, particularly agitated depression, is of critical salience (Benazzi, 2007). The former requires mood stabilizer treatment akin to those used in mania, where antidepressants may be a risk factor and a contraindication, while in the latter antidepressants may have a therapeutic role.

Comorbidities, both physical and psychiatric, are exceedingly common in bipolar II disorder, although the direction of causality and the nature of the relationship are not usually clear. Borderline personality disorder, anxiety disorders (especially panic disorder, obsessive-compulsive disorder and post-traumatic stress disorder, simple and social phobia), substance use disorder (especially alcohol abuse and dependence) and eating disorders are among the commonest psychiatric comorbid conditions (McElroy et al., 2001; Mantere et al., 2006). In one study, 76% of bipolar II disorder patients had at least one DSM Axis I comorbidity, the presence of which was associated with an earlier age of bipolar disorder onset, a history of cycle acceleration and more severe mood episodes over time (McElroy et al., 2001). Another study reported comorbid psychiatric conditions in half of their bipolar II disorder patients, and the only clinical difference was significantly more prevalent suicidal ideation and suicide attempts among the comorbid bipolar group (Vieta et al., 2000).

The clinical and functional sequelae of bipolar II disorder are numerous and cause considerable impact on patients' lives. The lifetime risk of suicide attempts has been estimated to be higher in bipolar II than in both bipolar I disorder and unipolar depression, and bipolar II disorder has been reported to be an over-represented diagnosis in completed suicides (Rihmer, Rutz, & Pihlgren, 1995; Rihmer & Pestality, 1999). This over-representation may in part relate to the prominence of mixed depression and comorbid substance use (Tondo, Baldessarini, & Floris, 1999), and raises additional concerns regarding the therapeutic use of agents that may induce mixed states. In a long-term naturalistic study, psychosocial disability was found to increase with symptomatic severity for depressive episodes and subsyndromal depressive symptoms for both bipolar I and II disorder patients. Interestingly, hypomanic and manic episodes, but not subsyndromal hypomanic symptoms, have been associated with stepwise functional impairment in bipolar I patients, whereas neither subsyndromal nor syndromal hypomania were associated with functional impairment in a bipolar II comparison group. During euthymia, both bipolar I and II groups showed a small but significant functional decrease in comparison with controls (Judd et al., 2005). Such functional disability may partly ensue from cognitive impairment, especially in executive functions. There is evidence for cognitive impairment in both bipolar I and II disorders that is independent of mood status, but their reported profiles of impairment have thus far shown inconsistencies (Summers et al., 2006; Torrent et al., 2006). In view of its early onset, delayed diagnosis, chronicity, comorbidities and functional disability, it is not difficult to appreciate the burden of bipolar II disorder, at an individual and societal level (Stimmel, 2004).

Treatment

There is a dearth of high quality trials for both pharmacological and psychological treatments of bipolar II disorder. The existing data is often derived from studies that combine bipolar I and II disorder, and occasionally bipolar not otherwise specified (NOS) and unipolar depression, in their designs. Pharmacotherapy trials typically focus on the effect of one agent, as monotherapy or adjunctive therapy, on one affective pole (mania/hypomania or depression) in either the acute or maintenance setting.

Hypomania

The treatment of hypomania has virtually been unexplored in research, a situation that possibly reflects the presumed equivalence of mania and hypomania treatments (Vieta, et al., 2001) and the often brief durations of hypomania that may not cause significant distress or impairment, and do not necessitate clinical intervention.

   Nevertheless, a small open-labelled trial has specifically investigated the efficacy of risperidone in the acute treatment and short-term prophylaxis of hypomania in bipolar II disorder (Vieta et al., 2001). In this study, 44 bipolar II disorder patients with scores above 7 on the Young Mania Rating Scale (YMRS) were treated with open-labelled risperidone, at a mean dose of 2.8 mg per day, as monotherapy or adjunctive treatment over 6 months. The majority (73%) met response criteria, and 60% were rated as asymptomatic on the Clinical Global Impressions Scale (CGI) at end-point. At follow-up, 12% had experienced a depressive episode, compared with 2% for hypomania relapse and 2% for both depressive and hypomanic break-through episodes. The interpretation of these results, however, is difficult in view of the lack of randomization or control group and inadequate power of the study.

A second open-labelled study examined the use of adjunctive topiramate for bipolar II patients in hypomania ($N=15$) or depression ($N=4$), who were not candidates for conventional mood stabilizers due to previous poor response or intolerance. At the end of the 12-week trial, the group showed highly significant improvements in YMRS, CGI for bipolar disorder and Hamilton Rating Scale for Depression (HAM-D$_{17}$). Of those who had index hypomania, eight responded and five remitted, compared with two and one, respectively, among those with index depression (Vieta et al., 2003). Again, interpretation is difficult given the low number of patients in each group, and the fact that topiramate has failed to show efficacy in unpublished registration trials.

More recently, a pilot randomized study compared oxcarbazepine ($N=15$) and divalproex ($N=15$) as either adjunctive treatment or monotherapy for hypomania. Improvement over the course of 8 weeks was comparable between the two groups, as measured with the YMRS, suggesting potential utility of oxcarbazepine in this setting (Suppes et al., 2007).

Depression

This predominant pole of bipolar disorder is challenging to treat, as the effects of the available pharmacotherapeutic options can be inadequate and concerns about antidepressant-induced mania and aggravation of mood cycling impinge on their use. Furthermore, clinical trials are limited in both number and methodological rigour, and often produce inconsistent results. The main groups of medications used in bipolar depression are the antidepressants, mood stabilizers and atypical antipsychotics.

Antidepressants

Amsterdam et al. have published a small collection of studies that specifically investigated antidepressant monotherapy in bipolar II major depression (Amsterdam, 1998; Amsterdam et al., 1998; Amsterdam & Garcia-Espana, 2000; Amsterdam & Shults, 2005b). The largest of these studies used retrospective data from a prospective, placebo-controlled trial of fluoxetine monotherapy in major depression to examine the efficacy and safety of this treatment in the bipolar II subgroup (Amsterdam et al., 1998). Bipolar II patients (N=89) were compared against age- and gender-matched unipolar patients (N=89) and unmatched unipolar patients (N=661). All were treated with fluoxetine at a daily dose of 20 mg for 12 weeks, after which those in remission were randomized to receive placebo or fluoxetine continuation for 14, 38 or 50 weeks. Both the short-term efficacy of fluoxetine, as measured by mean reductions in HAM-D$_{17}$ scores, and its prophylactic efficacy, as measured by depressive relapse rates, were comparable for bipolar II and unipolar patients. Manic switch was determined retrospectively without a specific instrument such as mood charting, and was reported at a rate of 3.8% for bipolar II patients, 0% for matched unipolar patients and 0.3% for unmatched unipolar patients in the acute treatment phase. Manic switch occurred at a rate of 3.6% for bipolar II patients and 0.8% for unmatched unipolar patients in the prophylactic phase.

In a subsequent study, 37 bipolar II patients in a major depressive episode were treated with open-labelled fluoxetine monotherapy at a daily dose of 20 mg for 8 weeks, and those who achieved HAM-D$_{17}$ scores below nine were randomized to either placebo (N=4) or fluoxetine continuation (N=8) for 6 months. Major depressive relapse occurred in 43% of fluoxetine-treated patients compared with 100% of placebo-treated patients, although this difference did not achieve statistical significance. Five patients scored at or above 12 on the YMRS at some point during the acute treatment phase, and fluoxetine-treated patients had a significantly higher mean increment on YMRS than the placebo-treated group (3.0 ± 1.8 vs 0.2 ± 0.45, $p = 0.01$) in the prophylaxis phase. However, none met DSM-IV criteria for hypomania, or was considered to have clinically meaningful hypomania (Amsterdam & Shults, 2005b).

In a trial of venlafaxine monotherapy in bipolar II (N=16) and unipolar (N=30) patients in a major depressive episode, efficacy was similar for both groups as measured by HAM-D$_{21}$ and Montgomery–Åsberg Depression Rating Scale (MADRS) score reductions, and no manic switch was observed over the 6-week study period (Amsterdam, 1998). A post-hoc analysis of this study that only examined female patients likewise found no significant difference in antidepressant efficacy between the bipolar II and unipolar subgroups (Amsterdam & Garcia-Espana, 2000).

A further study compared fluoxetine monotherapy, olanzapine monotherapy, combination fluoxetine and olanzapine, and placebo for bipolar major depression over an 8-week period, although bipolar I patients comprised almost the entirety of the sample (N=34, bipolar I N=32, bipolar II N=2). Significant reductions in HAM-D$_{17}$ and MADRS scores were found for all treatment groups, with no differentiation among groups. No significant increase in YMRS scores were observed, although a significant reduction in YMRS score was found in the fluoxetine monotherapy group (Amsterdam & Shults, 2005a).

Among other studies involving antidepressants in bipolar II depression, a double-blind trial found significantly superior efficacy of tranylcypromine over imipramine in the treatment of bipolar I and II anergic depression (Himmelhoch et al., 1991), an open-labelled study reported efficacy of adjunctive citalopram for bipolar I and II depression (Kupfer et al., 2001), and a case series documented good response to fluoxetine in chronically depressed bipolar II patients who had not previously responded to tricyclic antidepressants, monoamine oxidase inhibitors and lithium (Simpson & DePaulo, 1991).

Taken as a whole, these studies have inconclusive results that are limited by methodological weaknesses. As no placebo-control data is available for acute antidepressant efficacy, these study findings can only support comparable acute efficacy of fluoxetine and venlafaxine for bipolar II and unipolar major depression. For depressive relapse prevention, only one study contained placebo-controlled data that suggested prophylactic benefits from fluoxetine, but the sample size was small and the difference non-significant. The determination of both illness relapse and manic switch were disadvantaged by the absence of prospective measures of switch such as mood charting, limits of the study durations and small sample sizes, although a greater risk of switching appears to exist for bipolar II patients relative to their unipolar counterparts. Considerations of power further confound interpretation of those trials.

The debate surrounding the risks and benefits of antidepressant use in bipolar disorder is far from resolution. The induction of hypomania, mania, mixed states and rapid cycling by antidepressants have been recognized for all classes of antidepressants (El-Mallakh & Karippot, 2002), although greater risk has been reported with tricyclic antidepressants than selective serotonin reuptake inhibitors (SSRIs) (Peet, 1994). A recent study has investigated the comparative hypomanic and manic switch rates for three second-generation antidepressants (sertraline, venlafaxine and bupropion) when used adjunctively to mood stabilizers in bipolar I and II disorders. A total of 174 patients with bipolar I (N=126), II (N=46) and NOS (N=2) subtypes who were in a depressive episode were randomized to 10-week trials of the three agents. Approximately two thirds completed the trial, and showed similar response (49–53%) and remission (34–41%) rates for all three antidepressants. Venlafaxine was associated with a significantly higher switch rate than sertraline or bupropion, with no significant differences between the latter two. Furthermore, the switch rate differences for the three medications were only significant for rapid-cycling patients (Post et al., 2006). The bipolar II subtype was also significantly less likely than the bipolar I subtype to undergo hypomanic or manic switching (Altshuler et al., 2006).

Mood stabilizers

Despite the established practice of treating bipolar II disorder with mood stabilizers, there is scarce high-level clinical trial data, especially of its efficacy in acute bipolar II depression.

In a 12-week, open-labelled trial of divalproex sodium monotherapy in bipolar II depression ($N=19$), 63% met the criteria for response, but the predominance of medication-naïve patients among the responders was notable and likely skewed the results (Winsberg et al., 2001). A double-blind, placebo-controlled trial of divalproex sodium was conducted in 30 women with comorbid bipolar II disorder and borderline personality disorder over 6 months. Although divalproex sodium was associated with significantly better outcomes in the domains of interpersonal sensitivity, anger/hostility and aggression, no significant difference was found in the depression measure (Frankenburg & Zanarini, 2002).

There is open-labelled data supporting the efficacy of lamotrigine as monotherapy and adjunctive therapy in the acute treatment of bipolar I and II depression (Calabrese et al., 1999a; Nierenberg et al., 2006). Double-blind, placebo-controlled evidence also exists for the efficacy of lamotrigine monotherapy in bipolar I major depression (Calabrese et al., 1999b), but there is no similar trial specifically devoted to bipolar II depression. In a small study ($N=31$) with a double-blind, randomized, cross-over design, lamotrigine monotherapy was compared with gabapentin and placebo for refractory unipolar and bipolar disorder that included a bipolar II subset. The results suggested efficacy of lamotrigine in refractory affective illness, but was unable to differentiate between the index illness pole (Frye et al., 2000). Another small study ($N=23$) demonstrated an advantage of lamotrigine adjunctive to fluoxetine over fluoxetine monotherapy in a group with treatment-resistant major depression that contained a bipolar II subset (Barbosa, Berk, & Vorster, 2003).

Atypical antipsychotics

Of studies that included bipolar II disorder, there is open-labelled data in support of the usefulness of adjunctive olanzapine, risperidone, quetiapine and zonisamide in the treatment of acute bipolar depression (McIntyre et al., 2004; Ghaemi et al., 2006; Milev, Abraham, & Zaheer, 2006), although these findings are restricted by small sample sizes and methodological weaknesses.

Two large placebo-controlled trials have been conducted with quetiapine monotherapy for acute bipolar major depression in bipolar I and II disorder patients. Named the BOLDER I and II studies, these trials randomized patients to receive quetiapine at 300 mg and 600 mg per day, or placebo over 8 weeks. The results were significantly in favor of quetiapine for bipolar II depression in BOLDER II trial but not in BOLDER I trial. Of interest, the effect sizes for the bipolar II subgroup were lower (0.39 for quetiapine at 600 mg per day and 0.28 at 300 mg per day) than the bipolar I subgroup (1.09 for quetiapine at 600 mg per day and 0.91 at 300 mg per day), which may reflect different characteristics of major depression in the two subtypes (Calabrese et al., 2005a; Thase et al., 2006).

A small (N=30), 8-week study compared olanzapine, fluoxetine, combination olanzapine/fluoxetine and placebo in bipolar I and II major depression, and reported significant reductions in depression severity as measured by HAM-D$_{28}$ and MADRS, for all treatment groups (Amsterdam & Shults, 2005a). There have also been small studies of adjunctive atypical antipsychotics in bipolar I and II major depression. In one such study, 30 patients were randomly allocated to receive risperidone, paroxetine or both, adjunctive to an established mood stabilizer. All groups showed modest but significant improvement but did not differentiate from one another (Shelton & Stahl, 2004). Another study compared adjunctive risperidone with lamotrigine and inositol in a sample of 66 bipolar patients with treatment-resistant depression. Over the 16-week, open-labelled trial, recovery rates were not different between comparator groups, but lamotrigine was superior on selected depression severity and functional ratings (Nierenberg et al., 2006). These results are of ancillary relevance, but are too limited in power and methodology to serve as convincing evidence of efficacy.

Others

The impact of a dopamine agonist on bipolar II depression was investigated in two small preliminary studies. In one study, 21 patients in depressive phase of bipolar II disorder were randomized to pramipexole or placebo for 6 weeks, in addition to their established lithium or valproate. Significantly more patients responded to pramipexole (60%) than placebo (9%) (p=0.02) (Zarate et al., 2004). The second study included 22 patients with treatment-resistant bipolar depression, but only a minority were diagnosed with the bipolar II subtype. Compared with placebo, pramiprexole adjunctive to mood stabilizers over 6 weeks led to a significantly higher response rate (67% vs 20%) and greater magnitude of improvement, as measured by HAM-D$_{17}$ and the CGI Severity Scale (Goldberg, Burdick, & Endick, 2004).

Maintenance

Among the early literature, some researchers have found superior prophy-lactic outcomes with lithium over placebo for bipolar II disorder patients, in terms of reducing both the frequency and severity of depressive relapses (Dunner, Stallone, & Fieve, 1976c; Fieve, Kumbaraci, & Dunner, 1976). A placebo-controlled trial comparing lithium, imipramine, and lithium plus imipramine as prophylaxis for unipolar ($N=27$) and bipolar II ($N=22$) dis-order found no benefits from imipramine over placebo or in addition to lithium, but lithium was associated with a significantly reduced risk of relapse in the unipolar group and a trend of reducing bipolar relapses of any type (Kane et al., 1982).

Further evidence for the prophylactic efficacy of lithium in bipolar II disorder was provided by a long-term, observational study of lithium monotherapy in 317 patients with bipolar I and II disorder. Lithium was associated with reduced morbidity in both bipolar subtypes, but showed comparatively superior outcomes in bipolar II patients, in terms of reduced hospitalizations, reduction in illness episodes and time spent ill, and longer interepisodic intervals (Tondo et al., 1998). A subsequent study of the same population confirmed these findings, and found no increase in morbidity with long-term (up to 30 years) continuation of lithium. Minor and statisti-cally non-significant increase in recurrences was observed with lithium re-treatment following discontinuation (Tondo, Baldessarini, & Floris, 2001). A reduction of suicide risk to the magnitude of 8.3-fold has been estimated with long-term lithium maintenance for bipolar disorder, but a sharp risk reversal was observed in the first year upon discontinuation of lithium (Baldessarini, Tondo, & Hennen, 1999), although this has been suggested to be less marked in bipolar II than in bipolar I disorder (Faedda et al., 1993).

A prophylactic trial conducted over 2.5 years compared lithium with carbamazepine in classical (bipolar I) ($N=67$) and non-classical (including a subset of bipolar II disorder) ($N=104$) patients. Whilst reduced rehospitaliza-tion was associated with lithium in the classical group, there was a trend in favor of carbamazepine for the non-classical group (Greil et al., 1998; Greil & Kleindienst 1999). However, the aggregation of various bipolar subtypes in a single non-classical group may have diluted the specificity of these findings.

For the novel anticonvulsants, there are randomized, controlled pro-phylaxis trials of lamotrigine with favorable results, but these were con-ducted on bipolar I disorder samples only. A small ($N=25$) randomized, placebo-controlled prophylaxis trial of adjunctive gabapentin reported no emergent manic or depressive symptoms in either the gabapentin or pla-cebo group, but overall improvement over the 12-month period was sig-nificantly greater for gabapentin as measured by CGI for bipolar disorder (Vieta et al., 2006).

The dilemma surrounding antidepressant use in bipolar depression extends to bipolar maintenance treatment. The previously-cited randomized, controlled study of adjunctive antidepressants in acute bipolar depression (Post et al., 2006) had a 1-year continuation phase, which involved more detailed mood charting and a different measure for switching. For the combined bipolar I and II sample, switch rates for brief hypomania, recurrent brief hypomania, full-duration hypomania and mania in the acute trial phase were estimated to be 4.8%, 7.0%, 11.4% and 7.9%, respectively. Corresponding switch rates during the continuation phase were, respectively, 4.6%, 13.8%, 21.8% and 14.9%. The overall switch rates did not significantly differ among the individual antidepressants, although venlafaxine had the highest ratio of threshold to subthreshold switches. Interestingly, the switch rate was unrelated to the number or type of baseline mood stabilizers (Leverich et al., 2006).

Balancing against the risk of mood switching and rapid cycling is the risk of depressive relapse. In a prospective study, bipolar disorder patients who had remitted from a depressive episode with antidepressants adjunctive to mood stabilizers were followed up over a 1-year period. The diagnostic distribution included bipolar I ($N=53$) and II ($N=24$) disorders, bipolar disorder NOS ($N=5$), and schizoaffective disorder ($N=2$). At the end of 1 year, 70% of those who had discontinued their antidepressants within 6 months of remission had relapsed with a depressive episode, compared with 36% of those who had continued their antidepressants beyond 6 months. Those who had discontinued antidepressant treatment within 6 months also experienced significantly earlier relapses (Altshuler et al., 2003). It is important to note that this sample was a subset of a far larger sample ($N=1078$) within the Stanley Bipolar Network, and only those individuals who had settled on an antidepressant ($N=84$) were eligible for the trial. These results may not be generalizable beyond that subgroup. A controversial viewpoint has more recently been presented in a proof of concept study suggesting that SSRIs may have potential mood stabilizing effects in bipolar II disorder (Parker et al., 2006). However, this limited data from a cross-over study with a small sample size ($N=10$) must be interpreted with caution in the face of comparatively more established evidence to the contrary.

Rapid-cycling

For the rapid-cycling subtype, the efficacy of lamotrigine was investigated in a double-blind, placebo-controlled trial of bipolar I and II disorder patients, in which 182 stabilized subjects were randomized to 6-month maintenance with lamotrigine monotherapy or placebo. The lamotrigine group was superior in terms of survival in study and illness relapse, which on subtype analysis, was only significant for the bipolar II subset (Calabrese et al., 2000).

With regards to other agents, low-dose sodium valproate (daily dose range of 125–500 mg) was found to be associated with sustained partial or complete mood stabilization in the majority (79%) of patients in an open-labelled study of rapid-cycling cyclothymic ($N=15$) and bipolar II ($N=11$) patients conducted over 3 years (Jacobsen, 1993). The utility of sodium valproate in rapid-cycling was also supported by an open-labelled trial in 63 refractory affective disorder patients, including a bipolar II subgroup (Schaff, Fawcett, & Zajecka, 1993). However, when divalproex was compared with lithium in a double-blind, maintenance trial of rapid-cycling bipolar disorder over 20 months that included both bipolar I and II subtypes ($N=60$), no significant differences in relapse were found between the two agents, although the majority of patients were ineligible to enter the randomization phase (Calabrese et al., 2005b). A small case series of six treatment-resistant, rapid-cycling bipolar II patients suggested that the addition of bupropion to established lithium and/or levothyroxine was efficacious and was not associated with mood switching over a period of 2 years (Haykal & Akiskal, 1990), but these results are awaiting confirmatory studies.

Psychological therapies

Psychotherapy trials are uncommon in bipolar disorder, especially for bipolar II and bipolar spectrum disorders, and the variable form that psychotherapy takes complicates this area of research. Nevertheless, studies on bipolar I or unspecified bipolar disorder patients have shown that adjunctive psychotherapy, in the forms of cognitive-behavioral therapy, interpersonal social rhythms therapy, family therapy and psychoeducation, may be useful in relapse prevention (Scott & Gutierrez, 2004). A minor bipolar II subset was included in a randomized controlled trial of adjunctive group psychoeducation ($N=120$), delivered over 21 sessions with a 2-year follow-up period. The intervention group demonstrated significantly superior outcome as measured by total number of relapses, time to all types of affective relapse and time of subsequent hospitalizations (Colom et al., 2003). A smaller ($N=52$) randomized trial of 6 months of cognitive therapy in bipolar I and II disorder patients also reported better global outcome and trends of reduced symptoms and longer time to depressive relapse among the intervention group (Ball et al., 2006).

Clinical recommendations for management

Given the limited quantity and quality of efficacy studies in bipolar II disorder, extrapolation of findings from bipolar I disorder trials and clinical experience may serve as reasonable substitutes in guiding clinical management.

In the treatment of hypomania, lithium, valproate, carbamazepine and the atypical antipsychotics are all appropriate options. As lithium has the most solid evidence base for all aspects of mood stabilization, it would seem to be the most logical first-line treatment. The use of valproate, carbamazepine and atypical antipsychotics are recommended as post-first-line treatments, either alone or in combination.

The treatment of acute bipolar depression is a contentious issue. Existing concerns over antidepressant-induced manic switch or rapid cycling illness require further clarification through high-quality research. At present, a cautious approach would entail first-line treatment with mood stabilizers, and the combined use of an antidepressant and mood stabilizer(s) as second-line treatment. Of the mood stabilizers, lithium, valproate and lamotrigine are options. There is no good evidence to suggest that antidepressant efficacies differ in bipolar II patients from those with unipolar major depression. It is recommended that antidepressant therapy be time-limited, and avoided where possible in those with a rapid-cycling course. The atypical antipsychotics may have a role, but the current evidence for bipolar depression treatment is preliminary. Electroconvulsive therapy (ECT) remains an efficacious option, and should be kept in mind, especially in those with severe or refractory bipolar depression.

In maintenance, lithium retains the best evidence for efficacy in preventing both poles of the disorder. Valproate and lamotrigine are also long-term maintenance options, albeit with lesser evidence behind their overall efficacies.

Conclusions

Bipolar II disorder is still evolving as a diagnostic entity, but evidence implies that it is a valid diagnosis, which is prevalent in the psychiatric population and common in the general community. Current diagnostic classifications have acknowledged limitations in bipolar II disorder, complicating recognition and management. The current literature on bipolar II disorder is at its infancy, and much remains to be learnt in the areas of aetiology, optimal diagnostic criteria and treatment. From a practical viewpoint, there is strong evidence that certain clinical features such as young age of onset, atypical or mixed depression, though not pathognomonic, can serve as indicators of the disorder. In treatment, there is a dearth of clinical trial data of adequate quality to guide clinical practice, a situation that is made more complex by the risks of iatrogenic aggravation of the illness. Extrapolation from the evidence base for bipolar I disorder treatments may provide the best available, albeit suboptimal, guidance. Until more specific and higher quality data emerges, an open-minded and vigilant approach to clinical management of bipolar II disorder patients may be the most realistic option.

References

The National Institute for Health and Clinical Excellence [NICE] (2006). *Bipolar Disorder: The Managment of Bipolar Disorder in Adults, Children and Adolescents in Primary and Secondary Care* (pp. 57–60). London: National Collaborating Centre for Mental Health.

Akiskal, H. S. (1996). The prevalent clinical spectrum of bipolar disorders: beyond DSM-IV. *J. Clin. Psychopharmacol., 16*, 4S–14S.

Akiskal, H. S., Akiskal, K. K. & Lancrenon, S. (2006). Validating the soft bipolar spectrum in the French National EPIDEP Study: The prominence of BP-II 1/2. *J. Affect. Disord., 96*(3), 207–213.

Akiskal, H. S. & Pinto, O. (1999). The evolving bipolar spectrum. Prototypes I, II, III, and IV. *Psychiatr. Clin. North Am., 22*, 517–534.

Altshuler, L., Suppes, T., Black, D., Nolen, W. A., Keck, P. E., Jr., Frye, M. A. et al. (2003). Impact of antidepressant discontinuation after acute bipolar depression remission on rates of depressive relapse at 1-year follow-up. *Am. J. Psychiatry, 160*, 1252–1262.

Altshuler, L. L., Gitlin, M. J., Mintz, J., Leight, K. L. & Frye, M. A. (2002). Subsyndromal depression is associated with functional impairment in patients with bipolar disorder. *J. Clin. Psychiatry, 63*, 807–811.

Altshuler, L. L., Suppes, T., Black, D. O., Nolen, W. A., Leverich, G., Keck, P. E., Jr. et al. (2006). Lower switch rate in depressed patients with bipolar II than bipolar I disorder treated adjunctively with second-generation antidepressants. *Am. J. Psychiatry, 163*, 313–315.

Amsterdam, J. (1998). Efficacy and safety of venlafaxine in the treatment of bipolar II major depressive episode. *J. Clin. Psychopharmacol., 18*, 414–417.

Amsterdam, J. D. & Garcia-Espana, F. (2000). Venlafaxine monotherapy in women with bipolar II and unipolar major depression. *J. Affect. Disord., 59*, 225–229.

Amsterdam, J. D., Garcia-Espana, F., Fawcett, J., Quitkin, F. M., Reimherr, F. W., Rosenbaum, J. F. et al. (1998). Efficacy and safety of fluoxetine in treating bipolar II major depressive episode. *J. Clin. Psychopharmacol., 18*, 435–440.

Amsterdam, J. D. & Shults, J. (2005a). Comparison of fluoxetine, olanzapine, and combined fluoxetine plus olanzapine initial therapy of bipolar type I and type II major depression--lack of manic induction. *J. Affect. Disord., 87*, 121–130.

Amsterdam, J. D. & Shults, J. (2005b). Fluoxetine monotherapy of bipolar type II and bipolar NOS major depression: a double-blind, placebo-substitution, continuation study. *Int. Clin. Psychopharmacol., 20*, 257–264.

Angst, J. (1986). The course of affective disorders. *Psychopathology, 19*(Suppl 2), 47–52.

Angst, J. (1998). The emerging epidemiology of hypomania and bipolar II disorder. *J. Affect. Disord., 50*, 143–151.

Angst, J., Gamma, A., Benazzi, F., Ajdacic, V., Eich, D. & Rossler, W. (2003). Toward a re-definition of subthreshold bipolarity: epidemiology and proposed criteria for bipolar-II, minor bipolar disorders and hypomania. *J. Affect. Disord.*, 73, 133–146.

Angst, J., Sellaro, R., Stassen, H. H. & Gamma, A. (2005). Diagnostic conversion from depression to bipolar disorders: results of a long-term prospective study of hospital admissions. *J. Affect. Disord.*, 84, 149–157.

APA (1994). *Diagnostic and Statistical Manual of Mental Disorders (4th edition)*. Washington, DC: American Psychiatric Association.

APA (2000). *Diagnostic and Statistical Manual of Mental Disorders (4th edition text revision)*. Washington, DC: American Psychiatric Association.

Arnold, L. M. (2003). Gender differences in bipolar disorder. *Psychiatr. Clin. North Am.*, 26, 595–620.

Baldessarini, R. J. (2000). A plea for integrity of the bipolar disorder concept. *Bipolar Disord.*, 2, 3–7.

Baldessarini, R. J., Tondo, L. & Hennen, J. (1999). Effects of lithium treatment and its discontinuation on suicidal behavior in bipolar manic-depressive disorders. *J. Clin. Psychiatry*, 60(Suppl 2), 77–84; discussion 111–116.

Ball, J. R., Mitchell, P. B., Corry, J. C., Skillecorn, A., Smith, M. & Malhi, G. S. (2006). A randomized controlled trial of cognitive therapy for bipolar disorder: focus on long-term change. *J. Clin. Psychiatry*, 67, 277–286.

Barbosa, L., Berk, M. & Vorster, M. (2003). A double-blind, randomized, placebo-controlled trial of augmentation with lamotrigine or placebo in patients concomitantly treated with fluoxetine for resistant major depressive episodes. *J. Clin. Psychiatry*, 64, 403–407.

Bauer, M., Grof, P., Rasgon, N. L., Marsh, W., Munoz, R. A., Sagduyu, K. et al. (2006). Self-reported data from patients with bipolar disorder: Impact on minimum episode length for hypomania. *J. Affect. Disord.*, 96, 101–105.

Benazzi, F. (1997). Prevalence of bipolar II disorder in outpatient depression: a 203-case study in private practice. *J. Affect. Disord.*, 43, 163–166.

Benazzi, F. (1999a). Bipolar II disorder is common among depressed outpatients. *Psychiatry Clin. Neurosci.*, 53, 607–609.

Benazzi, F. (1999b). Gender differences in bipolar II and unipolar depressed outpatients: a 557-case study. *Ann. Clin. Psychiatry*, 11, 55–59.

Benazzi, F. (2000). Depression with DSM-IV atypical features: a marker for bipolar II disorder. *Eur. Arch. Psychiatry Clin. Neurosci.*, 250, 53–55.

Benazzi, F. (2002). Highly recurrent unipolar may be related to bipolar II. *Compr Psychiatry*, 43, 263–268.

Benazzi, F. (2003a). Bipolar II depressive mixed state: finding a useful definition. *Compr Psychiatry*, 44, 21–27.

Benazzi, F. (2003b). Bipolar II disorder and major depressive disorder: continuity or discontinuity? *World J. Biol. Psychiatry*, 4, 166–171.

Benazzi, F. (2004). Mixed states in bipolar II disorder: should full hypomania always be required? *Psychiatry Res.*, 127, 247–257.

Benazzi, F. (2005). Mixed depression: a clinical marker of bipolar-II disorder. *Prog. Neuropsychopharmacol. Biol. Psychiatry*, 29, 267–274.

Benazzi, F. (2006a). Gender differences in bipolar-II disorder. *Eur. Arch. Psychiatry Clin. Neurosci.*, 256, 67–71.

Benazzi, F. (2006b). Is overactivity the core feature of hypomania in bipolar II disorder? *Psychopathology*, 40, 54–60.

Benazzi, F. (2007). Bipolar disorder—focus on bipolar II disorder and mixed depression. *Lancet, 369,* 935–945.

Benazzi, F., Koukopoulos, A. & Akiskal, H. S. (2004). Toward a validation of a new definition of agitated depression as a bipolar mixed state (mixed depression). *Eur. Psychiatry, 19,* 85–90.

Berk, M., Dodd, S., Callaly, P., Berk, L., Fitzgerald, P., de Castella, A. R. et al. (2007). History of illness prior to a diagnosis of bipolar disorder or schizoaffective disorder. *J. Affect. Disord., 103*(1–3), 181–186.

Cahill, C., Hanstock, T., Jairam, R., Hazell, P., Walter, G. & Malhi, G. S. (2007). Comparison of diagnostic guidelines for juvenile bipolar disorder. *Aust. N Z J. Psychiatry, 41,* 479–484.

Calabrese, J. R., Bowden, C. L., McElroy, S. L., Cookson, J., Andersen, J., Keck, P. E., Jr. et al. (1999a). Spectrum of activity of lamotrigine in treatment-refractory bipolar disorder. *Am. J. Psychiatry, 156,* 1019–1023.

Calabrese, J. R., Bowden, C. L., Sachs, G. S., Ascher, J. A., Monaghan, E. & Rudd, G. D. (1999b). A double-blind placebo-controlled study of lamotrigine monotherapy in outpatients with bipolar I depression. Lamictal 602 Study Group. *J. Clin. Psychiatry, 60,* 79–88.

Calabrese, J. R., Keck, P. E., Jr., Macfadden, W., Minkwitz, M., Ketter, T. A., Weisler, R. H. et al. (2005a). A randomized, double-blind, placebo-controlled trial of quetiapine in the treatment of bipolar I or II depression. *Am. J. Psychiatry, 162,* 1351–1360.

Calabrese, J. R., Shelton, M. D., Rapport, D. J., Youngstrom, E. A., Jackson, K., Bilali, S. et al. (2005b). A 20-month, double-blind, maintenance trial of lithium versus divalproex in rapid-cycling bipolar disorder. *Am. J. Psychiatry, 162,* 2152–2161.

Calabrese, J. R., Suppes, T., Bowden, C. L., Sachs, G. S., Swann, A. C., McElroy, S. L. et al. (2000). A double-blind, placebo-controlled, prophylaxis study of lamotrigine in rapid-cycling bipolar disorder. Lamictal 614 Study Group. *J. Clin. Psychiatry, 61,* 841–850.

Carlson, G. A. & Meyer, S. E. (2000). Bipolar disorder in youth. *Current Psychiatry Reports, 2,* 90–94.

Cassano, G. B., Akiskal, H. S., Musetti, L., Perugi, G., Soriani, A. & Mignani, V. (1989). Psychopathology, temperament, and past course in primary major depressions. 2. Toward a redefinition of bipolarity with a new semistructured interview for depression. *Psychopathology, 22,* 278–288.

Cassano, G. B., Rucci, P., Frank, E., Fagiolini, A., Dell'Osso, L., Shear, M. K. et al. (2004). The mood spectrum in unipolar and bipolar disorder: arguments for a unitary approach. *Am. J. Psychiatry, 161,* 1264–1269.

Colom, F., Vieta, E., Martinez-Aran, A., Reinares, M., Goikolea, J. M., Benabarre, A. et al. (2003). A randomized trial on the efficacy of group psychoeducation in the prophylaxis of recurrences in bipolar patients whose disease is in remission. *Arch. Gen. Psychiatry, 60,* 402–407.

Coryell, W., Endicott, J., Maser, J. D., Keller, M. B., Leon, A. C. & Akiskal, H. S. (1995). Long-term stability of polarity distinctions in the affective disorders. *Am. J. Psychiatry, 152,* 385–390.

Coryell, W., Endicott, J., Reich, T., Andreasen, N. & Keller, M. (1984). A family study of bipolar II disorder. *Br. J. Psychiatry, 145,* 49–54.

Dunner, D. L., Fleiss, J. L. & Fieve, R. R. (1976a). The course of development of mania in patients with recurrent depression. *Am. J. Psychiatry, 133,* 905–908.

Dunner, D. L., Gershon, E. S. & Goodwin, F. K. (1976b). Heritable factors in the severity of affective illness. *Biol. Psychiatry, 11,* 31–42.

Dunner, D. L., Stallone, F. & Fieve, R. R. (1976c). Lithium carbonate and affective disorders. V: A double-blind study of prophylaxis of depression in bipolar illness. *Arch. Gen. Psychiatry, 33,* 117–120.

El-Mallakh, R. S. & Karippot, A. (2002). Use of antidepressants to treat depression in bipolar disorder. *Psychiatr. Serv., 53,* 580–584.

Faedda, G. L., Tondo, L., Baldessarini, R. J., Suppes, T. & Tohen, M. (1993). Outcome after rapid vs gradual discontinuation of lithium treatment in bipolar disorders. *Arch. Gen. Psychiatry, 50,* 448–455.

Fieve, R. R., Kumbaraci, T. & Dunner, D. L. (1976). Lithium prophylaxis of depression in bipolar I, bipolar II, and unipolar patients. *Am. J. Psychiatry, 133,* 925–929.

Frankenburg, F. R. & Zanarini, M. C. (2002). Divalproex sodium treatment of women with borderline personality disorder and bipolar II disorder: a double-blind placebo-controlled pilot study. *J. Clin. Psychiatry, 63,* 442–446.

Frye, M. A., Ketter, T. A., Kimbrell, T. A., Dunn, R. T., Speer, A. M., Osuch, E. A. et al. (2000). A placebo-controlled study of lamotrigine and gabapentin monotherapy in refractory mood disorders. *J. Clin. Psychopharmacol, 20,* 607–614.

Geller, B., Craney, J. L., Bolhofner, K., Nickelsburg, M. J., Williams, M. & Zimerman, B. (2002). Two-year prospective follow-up of children with a prepubertal and early adolescent bipolar disorder phenotype. *Am. J. Psychiatry, 159,* 927–933.

Ghaemi, S. N., Boiman, E. E. & Goodwin, F. K. (2000). Diagnosing bipolar disorder and the effect of antidepressants: a naturalistic study. *J. Clin. Psychiatry, 61,* 804–808; quiz 809.

Ghaemi, S. N., Ko, Y. J. & Goodwin, F. (2001). The bipolar spectrum and the antidepressant view of the world. *J. Psychiatric Practice, 7,* 287–297.

Ghaemi, S. N., Zablotsky, B., Filkowski, M. M., Dunn, R. T., Pardo, T. B., Isenstein, E. et al. (2006). An open prospective study of zonisamide in acute bipolar depression. *J. Clin. Psychopharmacol., 26,* 385–388.

Goldberg, J. F., Burdick, K. E. & Endick, C. J. (2004). Preliminary randomized, double-blind, placebo-controlled trial of pramipexole added to mood stabilizers for treatment-resistant bipolar depression. *Am. J. Psychiatry, 161,* 564–566.

Goldberg, J. F., Harrow, M. & Whiteside, J. E. (2001). Risk for bipolar illness in patients initially hospitalized for unipolar depression. *Am. J. Psychiatry, 158,* 1265–1270.

Goldstein, B. I. & Levitt, A. J. (2006). Further evidence for a developmental subtype of bipolar disorder defined by age at onset: results from the national epidemiologic survey on alcohol and related conditions. *Am. J. Psychiatry, 163,* 1633–1636.

Goodnick, P. J., Fieve, R. R., Schlegel, A. & Baxter, N. (1987). Predictors of interepisode symptoms and relapse in affective disorder patients treated with lithium carbonate. *Am. J. Psychiatry, 144,* 367–369.

Greil, W. & Kleindienst, N. (1999). Lithium versus carbamazepine in the maintenance treatment of bipolar II disorder and bipolar disorder not otherwise specified. *Int. Clin. Psychopharmacol., 14,* 283–285.

Greil, W., Kleindienst, N., Erazo, N. & Muller-Oerlinghausen, B. (1998). Differential response to lithium and carbamazepine in the prophylaxis of bipolar disorder. *J. Clin. Psychopharmacol., 18*, 455–460.

Haykal, R. F. & Akiskal, H. S. (1990). Bupropion as a promising approach to rapid cycling bipolar II patients. *J. Clin. Psychiatry, 51*, 450–455.

Hendrick, V., Altshuler, L. L., Gitlin, M. J., Delrahim, S. & Hammen, C. (2000). Gender and bipolar illness. *J. Clin. Psychiatry, 61*, 393–396; quiz 397.

Himmelhoch, J. M., Thase, M. E., Mallinger, A. G. & Houck, P. (1991). Tranylcypromine versus imipramine in anergic bipolar depression. *Am. J. Psychiatry, 148*, 910–916.

Hirschfeld, R. M., Lewis, L. & Vornik, L. A. (2003). Perceptions and impact of bipolar disorder: how far have we really come? Results of the national depressive and manic-depressive association 2000 survey of individuals with bipolar disorder. *J. Clin. Psychiatry, 64*, 161–174.

Hollander, E., Allen, A., Lopez, R. P., Bienstock, C. A., Grossman, R., Siever, L. J. et al. (2001). A preliminary double-blind, placebo-controlled trial of divalproex sodium in borderline personality disorder. *J. Clin. Psychiatry, 62*, 199–203.

Jacobsen, F. M. (1993). Low-dose valproate: a new treatment for cyclothymia, mild rapid cycling disorders, and premenstrual syndrome. *J. Clin. Psychiatry, 54*, 229–234.

Joffe, R. T., MacQueen, G. M., Marriott, M. & Young T. L. (2004). A prospective, longitudinal study of percentage of time spent ill in patients with bipolar I or bipolar II disorders. *Bipolar Disord., 6*, 62–66.

Judd, L. L. & Akiskal, H. S. (2003). The prevalence and disability of bipolar spectrum disorders in the US population: re-analysis of the ECA database taking into account subthreshold cases. *J. Affect. Disord., 73*, 123–131.

Judd, L. L., Akiskal, H. S., Schettler, P. J., Coryell, W., Endicott, J., Maser, J. D. et al. (2003a). A prospective investigation of the natural history of the long-term weekly symptomatic status of bipolar II disorder. *Arch. Gen. Psychiatry, 60*, 261–269.

Judd, L. L., Akiskal, H. S., Schettler, P. J., Coryell, W., Maser, J., Rice, J. A. et al. (2003b). The comparative clinical phenotype and long term longitudinal episode course of bipolar I and II: a clinical spectrum or distinct disorders? *J. Affect. Disord., 73*, 19–32.

Judd, L. L., Akiskal, H. S., Schettler, P. J., Endicott, J., Leon, A. C., Solomon, D. A. et al. (2005). Psychosocial disability in the course of bipolar I and II disorders: a prospective, comparative, longitudinal study. *Arch. Gen. Psychiatry, 62*, 1322–1330.

Judd, L. L., Akiskal, H. S., Schettler, P. J., Endicott, J., Maser, J., Solomon, D. A. et al. (2002). The long-term natural history of the weekly symptomatic status of bipolar I disorder. *Arch. Gen. Psychiatry, 59*, 530–537.

Kane, J. M., Quitkin, F. M., Rifkin, A., Ramos-Lorenzi, J. R., Nayak, D. D. & Howard, A. (1982). Lithium carbonate and imipramine in the prophylaxis of unipolar and bipolar II illness: a prospective, placebo-controlled comparison. *Arch. Gen. Psychiatry, 39*, 1065–1069.

Keller, M. B., Lavori, P. W., Kane, J. M., Gelenberg, A. J., Rosenbaum, J. F., Walzer, E. A. et al. (1992). Subsyndromal symptoms in bipolar disorder. A comparison of standard and low serum levels of lithium. *Arch. Gen. Psychiatry, 49*, 371–376.

Kessler, R. C., McGonagle, K. A., Zhao, S., Nelson, C. B., Hughes, M., Eshleman, S. et al. (1994). Lifetime and 12-month prevalence of DSM-III-R psychiatric disorders in the United States. Results from the National Comorbidity Survey. *Arch. Gen. Psychiatry, 51,* 8–19.

Kraepelin, E. (1913). *Manic-Depressive Insanity and Paranoia.* Edinburgh: E and S Livingstone.

Kupfer, D. J., Chengappa, K. N., Gelenberg, A. J., Hirschfeld, R. M., Goldberg, J. F., Sachs, G. S. et al. (2001). Citalopram as adjunctive therapy in bipolar depression. *J. Clin. Psychiatry, 62,* 985–990.

Kuyler, P. L. (1988). Rapid cycling bipolar II illness in three closely related individuals. *Am. J. Psychiatry, 145,* 114–115.

Leverich, G. S., Altshuler, L. L., Frye, M. A., Suppes, T., McElroy, S. L., Keck, P. E., Jr. et al. (2006). Risk of switch in mood polarity to hypomania or mania in patients with bipolar depression during acute and continuation trials of venlafaxine, sertraline, and bupropion as adjuncts to mood stabilizers. *Am. J. Psychiatry, 163,* 232–239.

Mantere, O., Melartin, T. K., Suominen, K., Rytsala, H. J., Valtonen, H. M., Arvilommi, P. et al. (2006). Differences in Axis I and II comorbidity between bipolar I and II disorders and major depressive disorder. *J. Clin. Psychiatry, 67,* 584–593.

Mantere, O., Suominen, K., Leppamaki, S., Valtonen, H., Arvilommi, P. & Isometsa, E. (2004). The clinical characteristics of DSM-IV bipolar I and II disorders: baseline findings from the Jorvi Bipolar Study (JoBS). *Bipolar Disord., 6,* 395–405.

McElroy, S. L., Altshuler, L. L., Suppes, T., Keck, P. E., Jr., Frye, M. A., Denicoff, K. D. et al. (2001). Axis I psychiatric comorbidity and its relationship to historical illness variables in 288 patients with bipolar disorder. *Am. J. Psychiatry, 158,* 420–426.

McIntyre, R. S., Mancini, D. A., Srinivasan, J., McCann, S., Konarski, J. Z. & Kennedy, S. H. (2004). The antidepressant effects of risperidone and olanzapine in bipolar disorder. *Can. J. Clin. Pharmacol., 11,* e218–e226.

McMahon, F. J., Simpson, S. G., McInnis, M. G., Badner, J. A., MacKinnon, D. F. & DePaulo, J. R. (2001). Linkage of bipolar disorder to chromosome 18q and the validity of bipolar II disorder. *Arch. Gen. Psychiatry, 58,* 1025–1031.

Milev, R., Abraham, G. & Zaheer, J. (2006). Add-on quetiapine for bipolar depression: a 12–month open-label trial. *Can. J. Psychiatry, 51,* 523–530.

Nierenberg, A. A., Ostacher, M. J., Calabrese, J. R., Ketter, T. A., Marangell, L. B., Miklowitz, D. J. et al. (2006). Treatment-resistant bipolar depression: A STEP–BD equipoise randomized effectiveness trial of antidepressant augmentation with lamotrigine, inositol, or risperidone. *Am. J. Psychiatry, 163,* 210–216.

NIMH (2000). *Child and adolescent bipolar disorder: An update from the National Institute of Mental Health.* Bethesda, MD: National Institute of Mental Health.

NIMH. (2001). Research roundtable on prepubertal bipolar disorder *J. Am. Acad. Child. Adolesc. Psychiatry, 40,* 871–878.

Parker, G., Tully, L., Olley, A. & Hadzi-Pavlovic, D. (2006). SSRIs as mood stabilizers for Bipolar II Disorder? A proof of concept study. *J. Affect. Disord., 92,* 205–214.

Peet, M. (1994). Induction of mania with selective serotonin re-uptake inhibitors and tricyclic antidepressants. *Br. J. Psychiatry, 164,* 549–550.

Perlis, R. H., Miyahara, S., Marangell, L. B., Wisniewski, S. R., Ostacher, M., DelBello, M. P. et al. (2004). Long-Term implications of early onset in bipolar disorder: data from the first 1000 participants in the systematic treatment enhancement program for bipolar disorder (STEP-BD). *Biol. Psychiatry, 55,* 875–881.

Peselow, E. D., Dunner, D. L., Fieve, R. R., Deutsch, S. I. & Rubinstein, M. E. (1982). Age of onset of affective illness. *Psychiatr. Clin. (Basel), 15,* 124–132.

Post, R. M., Altshuler, L. L., Leverich, G. S., Frye, M. A., Nolen, W. A., Kupka, R. W. et al. (2006). Mood switch in bipolar depression: comparison of adjunctive venlafaxine, bupropion and sertraline. *Br. J. Psychiatry, 189,* 124–131.

Regier, D. A., Boyd, J. H., Burke, J. D., Jr., Rae, D. S., Myers, J. K., Kramer, M. et al. (1988). One-month prevalence of mental disorders in the United States. Based on five epidemiologic catchment area sites. *Arch. Gen. Psychiatry, 45,* 977–986.

Rihmer, Z. & Pestality, P. (1999). Bipolar II disorder and suicidal behavior. *Psychiatr. Clin. North Am., 22,* 667–673.

Rihmer, Z., Rutz, W. & Pihlgren, H. (1995). Depression and suicide on Gotland. An intensive study of all suicides before and after a depression-training programme for general practitioners. *J. Affect. Disord., 35,* 147–152.

Schaff, M. R., Fawcett, J. & Zajecka, J. M. (1993). Divalproex sodium in the treatment of refractory affective disorders. *J. Clin. Psychiatry, 54,* 380–384.

Scott, J. & Gutierrez, M. J. (2004). The current status of psychological treatments in bipolar disorders: a systematic review of relapse prevention. *Bipolar Disord., 6,* 498–503.

Sharma, V., Khan, M. & Smith, A. (2005). A closer look at treatment resistant depression: is it due to a bipolar diathesis? *J. Affect. Disord., 84,* 251–257.

Shelton, R. C. & Stahl, S. M. (2004). Risperidone and paroxetine given singly and in combination for bipolar depression. *J. Clin. Psychiatry, 65,* 1715–1719.

Simpson, S. G. & DePaulo, J. R. (1991). Fluoxetine treatment of bipolar II depression. *J. Clin. Psychopharmacol., 11,* 52–54.

Simpson, S. G., McMahon, F. J., McInnis, M. G., MacKinnon, D. F., Edwin, D., Folstein, S. E. et al. (2002). Diagnostic reliability of bipolar II disorder. *Arch. Gen. Psychiatry, 59,* 736–740.

Somanath, C. P., Jain, S. & Reddy, Y. C. (2002). A family study of early-onset bipolar I disorder. *J. Affect. Disord., 70,* 91–94.

Stimmel, G. L. (2004). Economic grand rounds: the economic burden of bipolar disorder. *Psychiatr. Serv., 55,* 117–118.

Strober, M., Morrell, W., Burroughs, J., Lampert, C., Danforth, H. & Freeman, R. (1988). A family study of bipolar I disorder in adolescence. Early onset of symptoms linked to increased familial loading and lithium resistance. *J. Affect. Disord., 15,* 255–268.

Summers, M., Papadopoulou, K., Bruno, S., Cipolotti, L. & Ron, M. A. (2006). Bipolar I and bipolar II disorder: Cognition and emotion processing. *Psychol. Med.,* 1–11.

Suppes, T., Kelly, D. I., Hynan, L. S., Snow, D. E., Sureddi, S., Foster, B. et al. (2007). Comparison of two anticonvulsants in a randomized, single-blind treatment of hypomanic symptoms in patients with bipolar disorder. *Aust. N Z J. Psychiatry, 41*, 397–402.

Szadoczky, E., Papp, Z., Vitrai, J., Rihmer, Z. & Furedi, J. (1998). The prevalence of major depressive and bipolar disorders in Hungary. Results from a national epidemiologic survey. *J. Affect. Disord., 50*, 153–162.

Taylor, M. A. & Abrams, R. (1981). Early- and late-onset bipolar illness. *Arch. Gen. Psychiatry, 38*, 58–61.

Thase, M. E., Macfadden, W., Weisler, R. H., Chang, W., Paulsson, B., Khan, A. et al. (2006). Efficacy of quetiapine monotherapy in bipolar I and II depression: A double-blind, placebo-controlled study (the BOLDER II study). *J. Clin. Psychopharmacol., 26*, 600–609.

Tohen, M., Waternaux, C. M. & Tsuang, M. T. (1990). Outcome in Mania. A 4-year prospective follow-up of 75 patients utilizing survival analysis. *Arch. Gen. Psychiatry, 47*, 1106–1111.

Tondo, L., Baldessarini, R. J. & Floris, G. (2001). Long-term clinical effectiveness of lithium maintenance treatment in types I and II bipolar disorders. *Br. J. Psychiatry, 178*, S184–S190.

Tondo, L., Baldessarini, R. J., Hennen, J. & Floris, G. (1998). Lithium maintenance treatment of depression and mania in bipolar I and bipolar II disorders. *Am. J. Psychiatry, 155*, 638–645.

Tondo, L., Baldessarini, R. J., Hennen, J., Minnai, G. P., Salis, P., Scamonatti, L. et al. (1999). Suicide attempts in major affective disorder patients with comorbid substance use disorders. *J. Clin. Psychiatry, 60*(Suppl 2), 63–69; discussion 75–66, 113–116.

Torrent, C., Martinez-Aran, A., Daban, C., Sanchez-Moreno, J., Comes, M., Goikolea, J. M. et al. (2006). Cognitive impairment in bipolar II disorder. *Br. J. Psychiatry, 189*, 254–259.

Vieta, E., Colom, F., Martinez-Aran, A., Benabarre, A., Reinares, M. & Gasto, C. (2000). Bipolar II disorder and comorbidity. *Comp. Psychiatry, 41*, 339–343.

Vieta, E., Gasto, C., Colom, F., Reinares, M., Martinez-Aran, A., Benabarre, A. et al. (2001). Role of risperidone in bipolar II: an open 6-month study. *J. Affect. Disord., 67*, 213–219.

Vieta, E., Manuel Goikolea, J., Martinez-Aran, A., Comes, M., Verger, K., Masramon, X. et al. (2006). A double-blind, randomized, placebo-controlled, prophylaxis study of adjunctive gabapentin for bipolar disorder. *J. Clin. Psychiatry, 67*, 473–477.

Vieta, E., Sanchez-Moreno, J., Goikolea, J. M., Torrent, C., Benabarre, A., Colom, F. et al. (2003). Adjunctive topiramate in bipolar II disorder. *World J. Biol. Psychiatry, 4*, 172–176.

Weissman, M. M., Bland, R. C., Canino, G. J., Faravelli, C., Greenwald, S., Hwu, H. G. et al. (1996). Cross-national epidemiology of major depression and bipolar disorder. *JAMA, 276*, 293–299.

WHO. (1992). *International Statistical Classification of Diseases and Related Health Problems (ICD-10)*. Geneva: World Health Organization.

Winsberg, M. E., DeGolia, S. G., Strong, C. M. & Ketter, T. A. (2001). Divalproex therapy in medication-naive and mood-stabilizer-naive bipolar II depression. *J. Affect. Disord., 67*, 207–212.

Wozniak, J., Biederman, J., Kwon, A., Mick, E., Faraone, S., Orlovsky, K. et al. (2005). How cardinal are cardinal symptoms in pediatric bipolar disorder? An examination of clinical correlates. *Biol. Psychiatry, 58*, 583–588.

Zarate, C. A., Jr., Payne, J. L., Singh, J., Quiroz, J. A., Luckenbaugh, D. A., Denicoff, K. D. et al. (2004). Pramipexole for bipolar II depression: a placebo-controlled proof of concept study. *Biol. Psychiatry, 56*, 54–60.

chapter five

Maintenance treatment in bipolar I disorder

Ryan F. Estevez
University of Florida

Trisha Suppes
VA Palo Alto Health Care System

Contents

Introduction 108
The importance of maintenance treatment 108
    When should maintenance treatment be started? 110
    Choosing the right maintenance treatment 110
    Lithium 112
Anticonvulsants 115
    Valproate 115
    Carbamazepine 116
    Lamotrigine 117
    Topiramate 118
Anticonvulsants—other 118
Antipsychotics 119
    Clozapine 119
    Olanzapine 120
    Quetiapine 121
    Risperidone 122
    Aripiprazole 123
    Ziprasidone 124
    Side effects of atypical antipsychotics 124
    Antidepressants 125
    Summary of maintenance pharmacotherapy 127

Refractory patients... 127
    Importance of monitoring 128
    Psychosocial and other therapies 129
Conclusion 131
References 131

Introduction

There has been a recent shift among clinicians in the focus of treatment for bipolar disorder from simply treating a manic or depressed phase acutely, to more long term approaches that incorporate psychopharmaco-logical, psychosocial, familial, and the consideration of comorbid medical conditions. This chapter will focus on the treatment of bipolar disorder in the maintenance phase of the illness.

According to DSM-IV, 2 months of sustained recovery is considered sufficient for remission, and this is where the maintenance therapy phase begins (Calabrese et al., 2006). Choosing the best maintenance treatment based on the available research to date presents a formidable challenge to clinicians (Sachs & Thase, 2000). There have only been a handful of studies that have even attempted to address this important phase of treatment (Tohen et al., 2003b), and the studies that have been performed have not been conducted in a manner that has produced an adequately large data set conducive for meta-analyses with externally valid clinical implications.

The importance of maintenance treatment

When treating any patient who has been diagnosed with bipolar disorder, it is important that the clinician recognize the chronic relapsing nature of the disorder. As many as 50% of both bipolar I and bipolar II patients remain symptomatic over the long-term (Judd et al., 2003) while as many as 60% of patients will experience a relapse within 4 years of an episode of illness (Tohen et al., 2003b). This high risk of relapse remains even if a patient has not had an episode in several years if treatment is discontinued (Angst et al., 2003a). These patients suffer a significant amount of functional impairment (Ferrier et al., 1999) and even when euthymic, neurocognitive deficits that negatively impact (Thompson et al., 2005). Untreated bipolar patients are 2.5 times more likely to die in the next 12 months than individuals of the same sex and age without bipolar disorder (Angst et al., 2002). The incredibly high morbidity and mortality of bipolar patients largely depends on how many episodes an individual experiences (Begley et al., 2001). It has been suggested that relapse prevention may lead to a more benign course of illness (Goodwin, 2003).

Maintenance treatment is also important as it has been shown that frequent episodes of illness alter the response to subsequent acute episodes (Swann et al., 2000) and to maintenance treatment (Gelenberg et al., 1989). It seems that episodes beget episodes (Kessing et al., 2004). It is clear that the long term prevention of acute bipolar episodes is as vital as the amelioration of acute episodes.

The depressed phase of bipolar disorder accounts for a substantial portion of the illness's mortality and morbidity, including increased medical costs, occupational impairment, family disruption, and reduced quality of life, all leading to substantial costs to society (Svarstad et al., 2001; Li et al., 2002; Endicott et al., 2007). Even in the absence of full blown episodes, patients may experience substantial impairment (Gelenberg et al., 1989) and reduced quality of life as the result of residual symptoms going untreated (Altshuler et al., 2006; Frye et al., 2006). These residual or subsyndromal symptoms are not trivial, as their presence has been shown to be extremely common among patients as well as a strong predictor for relapse (Revicki et al., 2005; Perlis et al., 2006a; Tohen et al., 2006a).

Controlled clinical trials in maintenance can be divided into two categories: prophylaxis trials involving patients considered to be euthymic, and relapse prevention trials involving patients who have recently recovered from an acute episode and are then randomized to continue active treatment or switch to placebo (Ghaemi et al., 2004). The majority of studies fall into the relapse prevention category. In addition to typically including only bipolar I patients, those with substantial medical, psychiatric, or substance abuse comorbidities are almost always excluded. Most studies also only involve monotherapy, and do not allow adjunctive psychosocial therapies (Perlis et al., 2006a) despite evidence demonstrating the utility of such additional treatments in reducing the risk of recurrence (Colom et al., 2003). Further complicating matters is the fact that that most maintenance trials have primarily studied recently manic (as opposed to depressed) patients using responder enriched subjects (excluding those who are known to be intolerable or refractory to the study drug). Selection bias is an unavoidable consequence as patients who continue into the maintenance phase have already been stabilized acutely, making the chances of finding a difference from the drug and placebo statistically more probable (Chou & Fazzio, 2006).

Despite the limited available treatment data and increasing amount of evidence supporting the need for additional maintenance trials (Suppes et al., 1991), having a good strategy for maintenance therapy is an essential aspect of a comprehensive treatment plan. Episode prevention and treatment of sub-syndromal residual symptoms should be the primary goals of long-term treatment as it has been estimated that 25% of bipolar patients are rehospitalized within 11 months of their first episode, and 50% within 4 years (Kessing et al., 2004).

When should maintenance treatment be started?

Bipolar disorder, like most psychiatric illnesses, can be manifested in a number of different and unique ways depending on the patient. Treatment decisions must be tailored to the unique needs and clinical presentation of each patient, taking into account a number of medical, physical, and socio-economic factors. To date, there are several published guidelines for the management of bipolar disorder (McAllister-Williams, 2006) including the British Association of Psychopharmacology (BAP) guidelines (Goodwin, 2003), the American Psychiatric Association (APA) guidelines (APA, 2002), the Canadian Network for Mood and Anxiety Treatment (CANMAT) guidelines (Yatham et al., 2005), the Australian and New Zealand clinical practice guidelines for the treatment of bipolar disorder, the Texas Implementation of Medication Algorithms (TIMA) for bipolar I disorder (Suppes et al., 2005), and the World Federation of Societies of Biological Psychiatry (WFSBP) guidelines (Grunze et al., 2004). The BAP and APA recommend that maintenance treatment be started after a single manic episode. The CANMAT guidelines suggest that if patients refuse maintenance treatment, they should be continued on acute treatment for 3–6 months (antidepressants for 1–3 months) and provided with psychoeducation. The TIMA guideline endorse a collaborative approach, suggesting that clinicians and patients discuss maintenance treatment options after stabilization of an acute episode. Suggest discussing maintenance treatment for all patients stabilized on an acute treatment. Although the data regarding the long term treatment of bipolar depression is less robust, it is recommended that treatment continue indefinitely due to the high risk of relapse (McAllister-Williams, 2006).

Choosing the right maintenance treatment

Although the utility of alternative and adjunctive treatments is becoming apparent, pharmacotherapy remains the mainstay of treatment in the both the acute and maintenance phase of bipolar disorder. Choosing medications that have the largest probability of being both effective and well tolerated are especially important in bipolar disorder. Bipolar patients are commonly non-adherent to their treatment regimens, with reported rates as high as 66% (Lingam & Scott, 2002). This carries enormous consequences as it is well recognized that compliance with treatment greatly improves long term outcome (Revicki et al., 2005). Some studies of bipolar patients have found that the percentage of time not spent in euthymia during maintenance treatment is as high as 30–50%, a majority of which (as much as three times) is spent in the depressive phase of the illness (Judd et al., 2002; Judd & Akiskal, 2003; Post et al., 2003; Baldessarini et al., 2004; Suppes et al., 2005). It may be that such residual morbidity is in part the result of incomplete treatment adherence (Gonzalez-Pinto et al., 2006), as long term treatment non-adherence has been shown to be particularly prevalent among psychiatric patients with increasingly of complex treatment regimens. (Colom et al., 2000; Scott & Pope, 2002; Vieta, 2005a). As well, ongoing subsyndromal symptoms reflect the complexities of the illness and limitations of available treatments.

Physicians should make a concerted effort to keep dosing regimens simple, establish clear and realistic goals for treatment, and to educate patients about the drug(s) they are taking with their accompanying side effects. Involving family and friends in treatment whenever possible has also been shown to be helpful in reinforcing adherence (Keller, 2004). This is especially important for patients who have recovered from an initial presentation of dysphoric mania, as there is evidence to suggest that this subgroup of recently manic patients are particularly prone to experience adverse side effects (Bowden et al., 2005a). Similarly, recent placebo-controlled studies have suggested that depressed patients with a bipolar II diagnosis experience more side effects on the same medications than bipolar I patients (Suppes et al., 2007).

There is growing amount of data to guide selection of individual treatments, given a particular set of conditions or circumstances. For example, knowing the predominant mood states of patients have important implications for which mood stabilizer(s) will produce the best outcome.

There is a general consensus that the polarity of the index (or presenting) episode tends to predict the polarity of relapse into a subsequent episode in a ratio of about 2:1 to 3:1 (Calabrese et al., 2004). In other words, a patient who presents in a manic state is more likely to subsequently relapse to a manic state, whereas a patient presenting in a depressed mood is more likely to have depressive relapse.

It is essential that any maintenance regimen include a mood stabilizer, however there is currently no consensus on what criteria define a "mood stabilizer". The Food and Drug Administration (FDA) has not recognized this term and there is no medication approved by the FDA as a "mood stabilizer" (Chou & Fazzio, 2006). The most stringent definition, as articulated by Bauer and Mitchner (2004) is a drug or treatment that has shown both acute and maintenance efficacy for both depression and mania in placebo-controlled studies, without causing an exacerbation or destabilization of the opposite polar mood. For the purposes of this chapter, we will utilize the broader definition of a mood stabilizer (Suppes et al., 1991; Bowden,

1998), defined as a pharmacotherapy that has demonstrated efficacy in either mania or depression. Because of the cycling nature of bipolar disorder, a vital component to a copasetic long term treatment plan is one that addresses both phases of the illness, without neglecting or exacerbating one phase for the sake of managing the other (Calabrese et al., 2002). These long term considerations must be made during all phases of the illness in choosing the most appropriate pharmacological treatment (Table 5.1).

Lithium

Lithium, the earliest archetypal treatment for bipolar disorder (Carney & Goodwin, 2005) is perhaps one of the only currently utilized medication in bipolar disorder that meets the more stringent criteria for a mood stabilizer (Bauer & Mitchner, 2004). It was the first drug approved by the FDA (in 1974) for the maintenance treatment of bipolar disorder. While the evidence for lithium's effectiveness in acute mania is well established (Geddes et al., 2004; Baldessarini et al., 2006), its value in maintenance treatment is receiving renewed attention.

Double-blind, placebo controlled studies performed in the 1970s first demonstrated superior efficacy in preventing relapse compared to placebo (Baastrup et al., 1970; Melia, 1970; Cundall et al., 1972; Coppen et al., 1973;

Table 5.1 Medications with FDA Indications for Treatment of Bipolar Disorder as of April 1, 2007

Generic name	Trade name	Acute bipolar mania	Mixed	Maintenance treatment of bipolar I	Acute bipolar depression
Lithium	Eskalith	X		X	
Valproate	Depakote and Depakote ER	X			
Lamotrigine	Lamictal			X	
Carbamazepine extended release	Equetro	X	X		
Aripiprazole	Abilify	X	X	X	
Olanzapine	Zyprexa	X	X	X	
Quetiapine	Seroquel	X			X
Ziprasidone	Geodon	X	X		
Risperidone	Risperdal	X	X		
Olanzapine/ fluoxetine Combination	Symbyax				X
Chlorpromazine	Thorazine	X			

Prien et al., 1973). More recent studies have confirmed the efficacy of lithium in maintenance treatment (Maj et al., 1998; Geddes et al., 2004), particularly in certain subgroups of bipolar patients. In two large, well designed maintenance studies comparing lithium to lamotrigine (LTG), lithium was shown to be effective in the prevention of new mood episodes, and was more effective than LTG in the prevention of mania (Bowden et al., 2003; Calabrese et al., 2003). Many factors have been shown to be predictive of prophylactic response to lithium treatment, including high social status, good compliance, social support, and dominance (Kleindienst et al., 2005).

Other factors that have been shown to predict a good therapeutic response include having an episodic pattern of mania-depressed-euthymia, an older age of illness onset, and the presence of euphoric or "classic" manic. symptoms (Schurhoff et al., 2000; Swann et al., 2002; Goodwin & Goldstein, 2003). Conversely, stress, high expressed emotions, neurotic personality traits, unemployment, multiple previous hospitalizations, illness severity, an episodic pattern of depressed-mania-euthymia, or having a pattern of continuous cycling have all shown to predict a poor response to lithium although one recent study suggests the equal limited effectiveness of monotherapy lithium or valproate (VPA) in rapid cycling patients. (Bowden et al., 2005a; Calabrese et al., 2005a; Calabrese et al., 2005b; Kleindienst et al., 2005). It could be the case that rapid cycling patients are more likely to respond to lithium if they are not concurrently prescribed antidepressants (Kukopulos et al., 1980).

Lithium has enjoyed a reputation of being an effective antidepressant in maintenance treatment in spite of limited empirical support (Frye et al., 2006). This widely held belief has recently been challenged (Denicoff et al., 1997; Bowden, 2000; Bowden et al., 2003; Calabrese et al., 2003; Goodwin et al., 2004; Coryell et al., 1997; Moncrieff, 1997; Geddes et al., 2004). It has been hypothesized that the higher depression scores reported in many of these studies are a result of lithium induced motor slowing in patients who are no longer in a manic episode (Swann et al., 2002).

The totality of the evidence to date suggests that lithium has a moderate beneficial effect and at worst, an equivocal effect in preventing depressive episodes (Fawcett, 2003; Bauer & Mitchner, 2004; Geddes et al., 2004; Calabrese et al., 2006). One factor that has been shown to be a good predictor for lithium's efficacy against depressive relapse/recurrence is whether a response during the preceding acute episode was achieved by lithium (Severus et al., 2006). The proper use of lithium in the depressed phase of bipolar disorder remains an area of controversy. The continued examination of this issue will provide much needed clarification and consensus to guide clinical treatment selections.

One important feature that distinguishes lithium among other pharmacological treatments for bipolar disorder is that it is the one agent that has consistently demonstrated intrinsic anti-suicidal properties (Tondo et al., 1997; Baldessarini et al., 2006). Long term maintenance treatment with lithium has repeatedly shown to reduce the risk of suicide and suicide attempts, (Muller-Oerlinghausen et al., 1992; Tondo et al., 2001; Rucci et al., 2002; Baldessarini et al., 2003a; Muller-Oerlinghausen et al., 2003; Dunner, 2004; Angst et al., 2005; Kessing et al., 2005; Muller-Oerlinghausen et al., 2005; Gonzalez-Pinto, Mosquera et al., 2006) with the most recent comprehensive meta-analysis showing reduced rates of suicide and suicidal behaviors (including completed and attempted suicides) six to eight times that of untreated patients (Cipriani et al., 2005; Baldessarini et al., 2006). Although it is not known why lithium possesses this unique property, it has been suggested that it is a result of lithium's ability to limit impulsivity and aggressiveness(Baldessarini et al., 2006).

Lithium appears to be most effective when used in combination with VPA (Sharma et al., 1993; Solomon et al., 1997), LTG (Goodwin & Goldstein, 2003), carbamazepine (CBZ) (Denicoff et al., 1997), and for patients with a history of psychosis or treatment resistance, olanzapine (Tohen et al., 2002b) or risperidone (Vieta et al., 2001a; 2001b; Yatham et al., 2003). In fact, combination treatments have been shown to increase compliance (Keck et al., 1997) perhaps because combination treatments can be given at lower doses than monotherapy requires, reducing the likelihood of experiencing adverse effects (Goodwin, 2003). Controlled studies have not yet been conducted establishing the veracity of this assertion.

The side effects of lithium include tremor, drowsiness, nausea/ vomiting, increased urine output, muscle weakness, thirst, dry mouth, cognitive impairment, toxicity above 2.0 µEq/L, dermatological effects including acne, and weight gain. Patients should be encouraged to exercise, to restrict fluid intake to non-sugary liquids, and to avoid the intake of simple carbohydrates, particularly early in the day (Goodwin, 2003). Physicians should monitor electrolytes, thyroid and renal function at treatment initiation and annually. A recommended serum level between 0.5 and 0.9 µEq/L is adequate for some people, although levels between 0.8 and 1.2 µEq/L have been shown to be the most effective in the prevention of manic relapses/recurrences (Severus et al., 2006). If side effects are prominent, a trial at lower levels is recommended in lieu of immediate discontinuation or switching to another medication as there is good evidence that the abrupt discontinuation of lithium carries a significant risk of relapse (Suppes et al., 1991; Goodwin, 1994; Burgess et al., 2001).

There are many clinicians, who are not as familiar with using lithium and thus fear prescribing it because of its potential lethality. The available evidence does not support this fear in clinical practice as the choice of lithium as a toxin for suicide attempts seems to be uncommon (Waddington & McKenzie, 1994). Even more assuring is that the fatality risk of overdoses has been shown to be moderate, and very similar to those of modern antidepressants and second-generation antipsychotics (Watson, Litovitz et al., 2004) which are considered to be much safer than lithium.

Available data support the use of lithium monotherapy or combination treatment as a first line treatment for the maintenance phase of bipolar disorder (Baldessarini et al., 2002; Goodwin et al., 2003; Cipriani et al., 2005). As the evidence suggests that lithium is most effective in prevention of manic episodes, it may be an important part of a maintenance treatment regimen for bipolar patients likely to relapse into mania or to experience suicidal ideation.

Anticonvulsants

Valproate

VPA is one of the most commonly prescribed mood-stabilizing drugs in the United States (Goodwin, 2003). There is an abundance of evidence supporting the efficacy of VPA monotherapy in acute bipolar mania both before and since its FDA approval for acute bipolar mania in 1995 (Bowden et al., 1994; 2006) However, its use in maintenance therapy, although widespread in clinical practice, has limited empirical support (Calabrese et al., 1992; Lambert & Venaud, 1992; Gyulai et al., 2003; Tohen et al., 2003; Keck et al., 2005). There is some evidence to suggest that patients with rapid cycling, mixed, or dysphoric manic states respond better to long term treatment with VPA (Calabrese & Delucchi, 1990; Calabrese et al., 1992; Swann et al., 1997; Davis et al., 2004) although more recent data is equivocal (Calabrese et al., 2005b; Bowden et al., 2005a). VPA has been shown to be better tolerated than lithium (Bowden et al., 2000; Bowden et al., 2005a). It has also been shown to be a more cost effective treatment than olanzapine (Revicki et al., 2003) as well as lithium (for all bipolar patients except those presenting with "classic mania" [Keck et al., 1996]).

The evidence supporting the use of VPA in the treatment of bipolar depression is limited. There are a few small placebo controlled studies that have shown promising results (Calabrese & Delucchi, 1990; Bowden et al., 2000; Winsberg et al., 2001; Gyulai et al., 2003; Bowden et al., 2005a; Davis, Bartolucci et al., 2005), including demonstrated effectiveness in reducing subsyndromal depressive in comparison to lithium (Bowden, 2003; Gyulai et al., 2003) but other studies have not (Calabrese & Delucchi, 1990; Calabrese et al., 2005b) Unlike lithium, VPA has not been shown to reduce risk of suicide (Goodwin et al., 2003) although it has been shown to be helpful in decreasing irritability, anger, and impulsive aggressiveness in women with bipolar II disorder and comorbid borderline personality disorder (Jacobsen, 1993; Frankenburg & Zanarini, 2002). It is perhaps a good choice for patients with comorbid disorders such as alcoholism, cluster B personality disorders, dementia, and patients with impulusivity, irritability, aggression (Davis et al., 2000), or hyperactivity (Bowden, 2007).

VPA is perhaps most efficacious when used in combination with olanzapine (Solomon et al., 1997; Tohen et al., 2003), a selective serotonin reuptake inhibitor (Gyulai et al., 2003), or with lithium (Solomon et al., 1997). Along with the state that the patient is experiencing, their individual susceptibility to certain side effects should help clinicians determine whether or not VPA is an appropriate choice. For example, if a patient's renal function is compromised, lithium is not a viable option but VPA might be. However, unlike lithium, VPA is highly protein bound so caution must be used when giving it with other medications as it can easily displace other drugs (a common example being warfarin) and result in toxicity. Serum levels between 75 and 99 µEq/L have been shown to be maximally protective against relapse/recurrence of any mood episode (Keck et al., 2005) while serum levels above 100 µEq/L have been highly correlated with the development of gastrointestinal side effects.

In addition to dose related gastrointestinal side effects, nausea and vomiting are common (Bowden, 2007). This is often alleviated over time or by taking the medication with food. Additional side effects include increased appetite, weight gain, sedation, hair loss, reversible increases in liver function tests, thrombocytopenia, and rarely pancreatitis or liver failure. Polycystic ovary syndrome has been associated with long-term VPA therapy (Joffe et al., 2006) although the pathophysiological causality has not been well established.

Carbamazepine

CBZ has been studied in at least 19 controlled trials (McElroy & Keck, 2000; Weisler et al., 2006) and has demonstrated anti-manic activity, even in some patients who are refractory to lithium. CBZ extended release was recently approved by the FDA for acute manic and mixed episodes, although the prophylactic use of CBZ versus lithium has produced mixed results (Denicoff et al., 1997). The most consistently shown difference in efficacy between CBZ and lithium seems to be related to whether or not a patient has a diagnosis of "classic" bipolar I disorder (i.e. lacking mood-incongruent features, mixed states, or comorbid psychiatric illness) (Kleindienst & Greil, 2000; Kleindienst et al., 2005). CBZ is perhaps more effective than lithium for patients with non-classical bipolar disorder, those with a head injury, or other neurological problems. There is some early evidence that CBZ is an effective maintenance treatment for rapid cycling disorder (Calabrese et al., 1992) although this finding has not been universal (Denicoff et al., 1997; Muzina et al., 2005).

The evidence for use of CBZ in bipolar depression remains equivocal although promising (Ballenger & Post, 1980; Post et al., 1986), particularly for bipolar I mixed patients. Unlike lithium, CBZ has not been shown to reduce the risk for suicide (Thies-Flechtner et al., 1996; Weisler et al., 2005; 2006). Similar to other mood stabilizers, the weight of the evidence suggests that CBZ achieves its highest efficacy when used in conjunction with another mood stabilizer or antipsychotic (Keck & Mc Elroy, 2002), particularly lithium (Denicoff et al., 1997; Goodwin, 2003; Baethge et al., 2005).

Side effects include dizziness, drowsiness, double vision, fatigue, nausea, vomiting, ataxia, tremor, discomfort due to indigestion, abnormal gait, hyponatremia, rash, agranulocytosis and rarely Stevens–Johnson syndrome. Although VPA appears to be more tolerable than CBZ for short-term use, CBZ might be a better choice than VPA for long term use in terms of risk for weight gain, polycystic ovary syndrome, bone loss, and teratogenicity (Nasrallah et al., 2006). For these reasons, current consensus supports the use of CBZ as a second choice mood-stabilizing agent that is appropriate to consider for certain patients, such as those intolerant or non-responsive to lithium or VPA (Suppes et al., 2005; Yatham et al., 2005).

Lamotrigine

LTG is approved by the FDA for the maintenance treatment of bipolar disorder (2003). This indication was described as prevention of new mood episodes, reflecting the study design leading to LTG approval. It is an effective monotherapy option for use in maintenance treatment of bipolar depression (Calabrese et al., 1999; Frye et al., 2000; Calabrese et al., 2003; McElroy et al., 2004), including treatment refractory patients (Calabrese et al., 1999; Frye et al., 2000). It isn't recommended in acute treatment, however (Calabrese et al., 2008). Unlike antidepressants, LTG does not appear to place patients at risk for switching into mania or cycle acceleration (Calabrese et al., 2002b).

Recent evidence suggests that LTG has similar overall efficacy to lithium, but that it may be more effective in certain subgroups of patients including those with prominent anxiety and substance use comorbidity (Grof, 2003), as well as rapid cycling bipolar II disorder (Calabrese et al., 2000; Calabrese et al., 2005a). While lithium is still considered to be a more effective agent for prophylaxis against mania (Bowden et al., 2003; Calabrese et al., 2003), LTG has emerged as the preferred agent for protection against depressive episodes. The combination of lithium and LTG has been shown to be an effective treatment for refractory patients (Ghaemi et al., 2006).

Side effects include headache, dizziness, diplopia, ataxia, fatigue, nausea, dry mouth, hypersensitivity reactions, and most importantly, rash (with the subsequently rare although medically serious development of Stevens–Johnson syndrome). An additional advantage to LTG is that it appears to be weight neutral (Sachs et al., 2006). Caution should be exercised when combining LTG and VPA as VPA doubles the serum levels of lamotrigine (Kanner & Frey, 2000). LTG should be very gradually titrated to minimize the risk of rash and Stevens-Johnson syndrome (Messenheimer et al., 1998; Guberman et al., 1999; Wong et al., 1999; Grasela et al., 1999).

Topiramate

There is not a sufficient amount of evidence to support the use of topiramate in bipolar disorder. A recent combined analysis of four studies treating patients with an acute manic or mixed episode showed topiramate to be an ineffective treatment (Kushner et al., 2006) with another recent study supporting these findings (Chengappa et al., 2006). Several open label trials have suggested that it may be effective as an adjunctive treatment for bipolar disorder (McElroy et al., 2000; Ghaemi et al., 2001; McIntyre et al., 2002; McIntyre et al., 2005; Chengappa et al., 2006) although in most recent published randomized double blind study,did not show any difference in outcomes between placebo and topiramate-adjunctive treatment to a mood stabilizer (Chengappa et al., 2006). As in other studies, patients taking topiramate experienced a significant decrease in body weight (mean 2.5 kg) (Chengappa et al., 2006).

This positive effect could explain its continued widespread use in bipolar disorder despite the lack of evidence to support its effectiveness in treating the symptoms of bipolar disorder. While clinicians may utilize topirimate for the adjunctive benefit of weight loss, topiramate is not recommended as a core option for maintenance treatment in bipolar disorder.

It is worthy to note the publication of several reports of topiramate induced metabolic acidosis in both adults and children (Wilner et al., 1999; Stowe et al., 2000; Ko & Kong 2001; Takeoka et al., 2001; Philippi et al., 2002; Groeper & McCann, 2005).

Anticonvulsants—other

Many other anticonvulsants have been studied as potential mood stabilizing agents including gabapentin (Altshuler et al., 1999; Vieta et al., 2006), phenytoin (Mishory et al., 2000; 2003), oxcarbazepine (Benedetti et al., 2004; Conway et al., 2006, Suppes et al., 2007), zonisamide (McElroy et al., 2005; Ghaemi et al., 2006), levetiracetam (Post et al., 2005), tiagabine (Kaufman, 1998; Schaffer et al., 2002; Suppes et al., 2002), as have modafinil (Post et al., 2006a), stimulants (Carlson et al., 2004), omega-3 fatty acids (Stoll et al., 1999; Keck et al., 2002; Keck et al., 2006), and riluzole (Zarate et al., 2005). Only four of these studies (two for zonisamide, one each for phenytoin, and gabapentin) even attempted to measure the long term effectiveness of these treatments (Mishory et al., 2003; McElroy et al., 2005; Ghaemi et al., 2006; Vieta et al., 2006). These studies have also been limited by small sample sizes and methodological problems making definitive conclusions on efficacy limited and at this time speculative (Evins, 2003; Yatham, 2004).

Antipsychotics

Typical antipsychotics such as haloperidol, chlorpromazine, thioridazine, and perphenazine have all been shown to possess antimanic efficacy. However side effects such as increased risk of depression, dystonias, akathisia, tardive dyskinesia, prolactin elevation and sexual side effects have all limited their long term use. Atypical antipsychotics have demonstrated equal and at times better (particularly in regards to depressive symptoms) efficacy with an improved overall side-effect profile when compared to typical antipsychotics (Hirschfeld, 2003; Hirschfeld et al., 2003).

The most recent data suggests that atypical antipsychotics are similarly effective when used in combination with lithium or VPA (Vieta & Goikolea, 2005). Although the evidence suggests that there are no statistically significant differences between the atypical antipsychotics in their effectiveness in acute mania (Perlis et al., 2006b), they do perform differently for treatment of bipolar depression. Quetiapine has demonstrated the most robust efficacy followed by olanzapine-fluoxetine combination (Yatham, 2005).

Similar to other medications used for bipolar maintenance, the available research data supporting the use of atypicals in maintenance treatment is limited. To date only olanzapine, aripiprazole, and quetiapine have been studied in placebo-controlled monotherapy studies with olanzapine having the most published data to suggest its effectiveness in this phase of the illness (Yatham, 2002; Hellewell, 2006). Some reports suggest that patients who have been stabilized from acute episodes on antipsychotics can have them tapered without increasing the risk of an episode relapse (Saksa et al., 2004). The relative long term benefit of lithium plus an anticonvulsant versus lithium or an anticonvulsant plus an atypical antipsychotic has yet to be determined. The section on side effects management, later in this chapter, will detail recommended monitoring when atypical antipsychotics are prescribed.

Clozapine

Numerous studies have shown the effectiveness of clozapine in difficult to treat patients, such as those experiencing lithium-resistant rapid cycling or dysphoric mania, as well as others not responding to conventional treatments like lithium or anticonvulsants (Calabrese et al., 1991; Suppes et al., 1994; Zarate et al., 1995; Suppes et al., 2004; Fehr et al., 2005). Its use in maintenance treatment of bipolar disorder should be reserved for difficult to treat patients, particularly if they are prone to mania or mood lability, and for those who have failed other atypical antipsychotics (Suppes et al., 1992; Calabrese et al., 1996; Suppes et al., 1999). Side effects include the possibility of blood dyscrasias, including life-threatening agranulocytosis, seizures, sedation, and weight gain. Clozapine also carries a black-box warning regarding cardiac toxicity that can lead to fatal myocarditis.

Olanzapine

Olanzapine is the most widely studied atypical antipsychotic in bipolar disorder and was the first atypical antipsychotic to receive FDA approval for the treatment of acute mania. It has demonstrated a broad range of efficacy across several subgroups of patients (Baldessarini et al., 2003a). Olanzapine has been shown to reduce symptoms of acute mania alone or in combination with a mood stabilizer (Tohen et al., 1999; Tohen et al., 2000; Baldessarini et al., 2003a; Sanger et al., 2003). The intramuscular formulation has been shown to be effective in the management of agitated manic patients. It has also been shown by some measures to be superior to VPA in the treatment of acute mania (Tohen et al., 2002a) although side effects including weight gain and metabolic abnormalities are more common with olanzapine.

The olanzapine–fluoxetine combination has demonstrated efficacy in reducing symptoms of bipolar depression (Tohen et al., 2003), although often at the cost of weight gain, elevation of hemoglobin A1c, prolactin, total cholesterol, LDL cholesterol, and triglycerides (Tohen et al., 2004). The combination of olanzapine with VPA or lithium has shown superior efficacy in the treatment of manic and mixed episodes to that of either mood stabilizer plus placebo (Tohen et al., 2002b).

Olanzapine has demonstrated effectiveness in the maintenance phase of the illness and received FDA approval for maintenance treatment in 2004 (Tohen, Bowden et al ., 2006a.; Vieta et al., 2001d; Sanger et al., 2003; Tohen et al., 2005; Ketter et al., 2006). It is important to note that the wording of this indication is for maintenance therapy after achieving a responder status for an average duration of 2 weeks. This verbiage is a reflection of how these studies were methodologically structured. A recent study suggested olanzapine monotherapy was effective for relapse prevention of mood episodes in patients who responded to olanzapine in an acute manic or mixed episode (Tohen et al., 2006b) while other studies have shown it to be superior to VPA (Tohen et al., 2003) or lithium monotherapy in preventing recurrence of manic and mixed episodes (Tohen et al., 2004; Tohen et al., 2005) and suicidal ideation (Houston et al., 2006). Its effectiveness appears to be especially robust in patients with bipolar I disorder with a recent onset of illness (Ketter et al., 2006).

Side effects include weight gain, movement disorders, and metabolic changes, with some suggestion that olanzapine causes the most egregious metabolic changes among all of the atypicals approved for bipolar disorder (Newcomer, 2005; 2007).

Quetiapine

The FDA has approved quetiapine for treatment of acute depressive and manic episodes in bipolar I disorder, and for maintenance treatment of bipolar I disorder in combination with either lithium or divalproex. This is due to several randomized controlled trials demonstrating theeffi cacy of quetiapine in bipolar mania as either monotherapy (Bowden et al., 2005b; McIntyre et al., 2005) or in combination with lithium or VPA (Zarate et al., 2000; Vieta et al., 2002; Sachs et al., 2004). Recent studies have shown strong evidence to support the use of quetiapine monotherapy (Calabrese et al., 2005c; Thase et al., 2006) or add on therapy (Milev et al., 2006) in bipolar I and II depression (Suppes et al., 2005; Dando & Keating, 2006; Suppes et al., 2007). It has also been shown to reduce depression associated anxiety symptoms in patients with bipolar I depression (Hirschfeld et al., 2006b) and increase quality of life and improve sleep (Endicott et al., 2007).

There is some evidence from open-label trials that quetiapine is effective for patients with poorly controlled bipolar and schizoaffective mood disorders (Zarate et al., 2000) as well as those with comorbidities such as substance dependence (Brown et al., 2002; Brown et al., 2003), psychosis (Zarate et al., 2000), and rapid-cycling (Vieta et al., 2002).

Recently placebo-controlled maintenance phase trials have been completed with quetiapine. In two recently completed placebo-controlled maintenance phase trials, quetiapine plus mood stabilizer was significantly more effective than placebo plus mood stabilizer in delaying time to new mood symptoms (Suppes et al., 2008; Vieta et al., 2008). These two studies used the trial design currently being required by the FDA for a maintenance indication: open treatment for a period of time following an acute episode, a clinically stabilized open period (12 weeks) on lithium or VPA plus atypical agent, then randomization to continue open lithium or VPA with blind atypical or placebo. Both studies showed that quetiapine plus mood stabilizer was more effective than placebo plus mood stabilizer in delaying both manic and depressive episodes, leading to FDA indication for this approach. This newer design reflects a more true maintenance effect of a medication, although the sample is enriched by those being randomized who have responded to the medication. Side effects included weight gain and also increase in the incidence of elevated glucose levels in the quetiapine group.

Side effects include weight gain, somnolence, dizziness, dry mouth, and metabolic changes (Calabrese, Keck et al., 2005; Newcomer, 2005; Newcomer & Haupt, 2006; Newcomer, 2007). The incidence of EPS-related adverse events including akathisia has been shown to be similar to placebo (McIntyre et al., 2005; Pini et al., 2006). Quetiapine has been shown to be better tolerated than risperidone (Chi-Un et al., 2004), olanzapine (Sussman, 2003), aripiprazole (Ghaemi et al., 2006), and haloperidol (McIntyre et al., 2005). The available evidence to date suggests that quetiapine is emerging as a viable bimodal mood stabilizer, with the combined effectiveness and safety profile to justify it as a preferred option among the currently available atypical antipsychotics (Vieta, 2005). Furthermore, the combined data from acute treatment trials and the recent maintenance studies suggests that quetiapine may be the first agent to meet the strictest definition of mood stabilizer (Bauer & Mitchner, 2004).

Risperidone

Many trials have demonstrated the efficacy of risperidone as monotherapy (Hirschfeld et al,. 2004; Gopal et al., 2005; Khanna et al., 2005) and when combined with lithium, VPA, or CBZ in the treatment of acute mania (Rendell et al., 2006). There is only sparse evidence to support the use of risperidone in the treatment of bipolar depression (Shelton & Stahl, 2004). No randomized controlled trials of oral risperidone in long-term maintenance therapy have been published to date (Rendell et al., 2006; Rendell & Geddes, 2007).

One small study showed promise for treatment of breakthrough episodes (Ghaemi & Sachs, 1997) and another large open label trial showed promising results for use as maintenance (Hirschfeld et al., 2006a). Data analyzed from the largest naturalistic study ever conducted with risperidone as an open add-on to mood stabilizers suggests efficacy for many symptoms on the bipolar spectrum (Vieta et al., 2001c).

However, two recent double blind trials assessed the efficacy of Risperdal Consta, the long-acting injectable formulation of risperidone, in relapse prevention of mood episodes in bipolar disorder (Alphs et al., 2008, Yatham, 2008). In the first double blind controlled study with a placebo withdrawal design (Alphs et al., 2008), patients with bipolar I and II disorders with a frequently relapsing course (≥4 mood episodes requiring intervention in the previous 12 months) were stabilized on treatment as usual (usually mood stabilizers) and Risperdal Consta LAI. During long term follow up, the augmentation of treatment as usual with the atypical antipsychotic LAI was superior to treatment as usual alone in preventing mood episodes. In a second double blind study of patients with bipolar I disorder, also using placebo withdrawal design, monotherapy with Risperdal Consta LAI was superior to placebo in preventing relapse into a mood episode (Yatham, 2008). Risperdal Consta long-acting injectable treatment was well tolerated in both studies. These data suggest a new paradigm of maintenance treatment for patients accepting of a long-acting injectable therapy.

Aripiprazole

Aripiprazole has demonstrated efficacy in the treatment of acute manic and mixed episodes (Keck et al., 2003; Vieta et al., 2005; Sachs et al., 2006) as well as in maintenance treatment (Keck et al., 2003; Keck et al., 2006). It received FDA approval for the treatment of bipolar mania and maintenance in 2004. The seminal trial that led to approval included acutely manic or mixed patients who were stabilized for 6–18 weeks and then randomly assigned to double-blind maintenance treatment with aripiprazole or placebo for 26 weeks, provided they met criteria for stabilization. Time to relapse of a mood episode was significantly longer for the aripiprazole group than for the placebo group. There have been preliminary reports describing that aripiprazole augmentation may be useful for treatment resistant bipolar depression (Worthington et al., 2005; Keck et al., 2006; Kemp et al., 2006; Ketter et al., 2006; Sokolski, 2007) although its use may be limited by extrapyramidal side-effects including akathisia (Worthington et al., 2005; Kemp et al., 2006).

The potential development of EPS is a deterrant to the consideration of aripiprazole among some clinicians. Vieta et al. (2005) showed a low dropout rate due to side effects such as weight gain, hyperprolactinemia and EPS in aripiprazole compared to placebo, suggesting a potential for greater adherence in the maintenance phase (Vieta et al., 2005). A more recent trial replicated the absence of significant weight gain or the development of prolactinemia, however the incidence of akathisia and tremor were significantly higher for patients taking aripiprazole than placebo (Keck et al., 2006).

Although it seems that aripiprazole does not contribute to the development of weight gain and other metabolic abnormalities to the same extent as other atypical antipsychotics, this benefit might come at the cost of a slightly increased risk of extra-pyramidal symptoms. The potential of this medication to contribute to metabolic disturbances in the absence of weight gain is still being assessed.

Ziprasidone

Two randomized controlled studies of ziprasidone monotherapy in acute mania have shown efficacy in symptom reduction with tolerability similar to placebo (Keck et al., 2003; Potkin et al., 2005). However, there is no evidence showing its effectiveness in bipolar depression or in maintenance at this time.

Side effects include an increased risk of extra-pyramidal symptoms, nausea or other gastrointestinal distress, and dizziness. The FDA has included a black box warning for QT prolongation risk with ziprasidone, although the clinical implications for this in practice are minimal for patients without cardiovascular comorbidities (Harrigan et al., 2004; Levy et al., 2004; Kudla et al., 2006).

Side effects of atypical antipsychotics

As the use of atypical antipsychotics has steadily risen over the past 10 years, and expanded to treatment of diverse psychiatric diagnoses, unanticipated side effects such as weight gain, hyperlipidemia, hypertension, and type 2 diabetes mellitus have been well documented (Fagiolini et al., 2002; Atmaca et al., 2003; Keck & McElroy, 2003; Kilbourne et al., 2004; McElroy et al., 2004; Fagiolini et al., 2005; Newcomer, 2005; Yumru et al., 2007). This led to the FDA mandated black-box warnings for all atypical antipsychotics for the possibility of developing life threatening diabetes mellitus in 2003 and a subsequent black-box warning for an increased risk of death related to psychosis and behavioral problems in elderly patients with dementia in 2005 (Rosack, 2005). Olanzapine, risperidone, and aripiprazole also carry warnings against an increased risk of cerebrovascular events including stroke and an increased risk of death from stroke.

Having a diagnosis of bipolar disorder has been shown to double the mortality from cardiovascular disease and pulmonary embolism compared to the general population (Morriss & Mohammed, 2005). In fact, the rate of metabolic syndrome in bipolar patients taking either olanzapine, risperidone, or quetiapine has been shown to be as high as 30% (Fagiolini et al., 2005; Yumru et al., 2007).

Atypical antipsychotics are not the only medications used in bipolar disorder that cause weight gain. However, the weight gain associated with atypicals is often seen with other serious metabolic abnormalities not commonly seen or at least recognized in patients who gain weight from agents such as lithium or VPA.

This increase in weight seems to be the genesis of subsequent risk factors, as adiposity is related to increased plasma glucose and lipids as well as decrease insulin sensitivity (Newcomer & Haupt, 2006). Weight gain has also been associated with a decrease in functioning and well-being (Revicki et al., 2003), and has been considered to be the factor most commonly related to medication discontinuation (Sachs, 2003). Although a difference between clozapine, risperidone, olanzapine, and quetiapine in the development of diabetes has not been demonstrated (Sumiyoshi et al., 2004), ziprasidone and aripiprazole appear to be the atypicals that are least likely to cause many of the precursors (such as obesity) implicated in the development of significant medical corporeal morbidity. In addition to considering the medical consequences of weight gain and metabolic anomalies, clinicians should consider the psychological impact of adverse effects such as weight gain on adherence, as it has a tremendous impact in long term effectiveness (Vieta & Goikolea, 2005).

The American Diabetes association together with the American Psychiatric Association, the American Association of Clinical Endocrinologists, and the North American Association for the Study of Obesity issued a consensus statement which includes a monitoring protocol for patients on atypical antipsychotics (Barrett et al., 2004). Table 5.2 lists these recommendations.

Antidepressants

The FDA has recently issued a warning that "a major depressive episode may be the initial presentation of bipolar disorder … and that treating such an episode with an antidepressant alone may increase the likelihood of precipitation of a mixed/manic episode in patients at risk for bipolar disorder" (US FDA. http://www.fda.gov/cder/drug/antidepressants/default.htm, issued 6/30/2005). The appropriate use of antidepressants in persons with bipolar disorders continues to remain controversial, with concerns about suicidality, relapse, chronic depressive symptoms, and lack of demonstrated effectiveness (McElroy et al., 2006; Altshuler et al., 2003; Sachs et al., 2007).

Selective serotonin reuptake inhibitors (SSRIs) are often prescribed for patients with both unipolar and bipolar depression. Of the SSRIs, fluoxetine, paroxetine, and citalopram, have shown some efficacy for the treatment of acute bipolar depression when combined with a mood stabilizer (Cohn et al., 1989; Kupfer et al., 2001; Nemeroff et al., 2001). However, a recent placebo-controlled study of add-on antidepressants for acute depression found no benefit for the addition of antidepressants (Sachs et al., 2007).

Table 5.2 ADA, APA, AACE, and the NAASO Recommendations for
Monitoring Patients Taking Atypical Antipsychotics

- Before starting therapy, personal and family **history** should be evaluated for obesity, diabetes, dyslipidemia, hypertension, or cardiovascular disease.
- **Weight** (BMI) should be checked at baseline, then at 4, 8, and 12 weeks after initiating or changing atypical therapy. To be followed by quarterly checks thereafter. If a patient gains ≥5% of their initial weight, consider switching to a different agent.
- **Waist circumference** should be measured at baseline and then annually.
- **Blood pressure** should be checked at baseline, 12 weeks, and then annually. More frequent checks are recommended for patients with a higher baseline risk for development of hypertension.
- **Fasting plasma glucose** should be checked at baseline, 12 weeks, and then annually. Check more frequently in patients with a higher baseline risk for diabetes. (Note: some clinicians recommend a fasting blood glucose every three to six months, with more frequent initial checks for high risk patients.[a,b]
- **Fasting lipid profile** should be checked at baseline, 12 weeks, then every 5 years if normal. Check more frequently if clinically indicated. (Note: some clinicians recommend checking lipid panels from every three months[b] to yearly[a].

Source: Barrett, E., et al., Consensus development conference on antipsychotic drugs and obesity and diabetes. *Diabetes Care, 27*: 596–601, 2004.
[a] Lebovitz, H. E. (2003). Metabolic consequences of atypical antipsychotic drugs. *Psychiatr. Q., 74*: 277–290.
[b] Wirshing, D. A., et al. (2003). Understanding the new and evolving profile of adverse drug effects in schizophrenia. *Psychiatr. Clin. North Am., 26*: 165–190.

Because of their inferior side effect profile and their tendency to switch patients into hypomania/mania in comparison to SSRIs, TCAs such as imipramine and amitriptyline, and MAOIs such as tranylcypromine, have largely been relegated to second choice agents although they still might be preferred in individual cases (Zornberg & Pope, 1993). Of all of the antidepressants, buproprion may be associated with the smallest risk of hypo/manic switch (Sachs et al., 1994; Leverich et al., 2006), while tricyclics and MAOI antidepressants have been shown to induce switching in as many as 25% and 21% of patients, respectively (Himmelhoch et al., 1991).The serotonin-norepinephrine reuptake inhibitor venlafaxine, may also pose a greater risk of manic/hypomanic switching in comparison to other new generation antidepressants (Nemeroff et al., 2001; Leverich et al. 2006), particularly among patients with a prior history of rapid cycling (Post et al., 2006b). In a meta-analysis, Peet (1994) confirmed that tricyclics induce switching at a higher rate than SSRIs, which had switch rates that were statistically equal to placebo.

There is some evidence to suggest caution when prescribing antidepressants to women with a history of bipolar disorder as the chances of inducing a rapid cycling switch are enhanced (Yildiz & Sachs, 2003). Additional predictors of antidepressant induced mania include patients with a family history of bipolar disorder (Howland, 1996), number of past manic episodes (Boerlin et al., 1998), comorbid alcohol or other drug abuse (Goldberg & Whiteside, 2002), history of rapid cycling (Ghaemi et al., 2003), and in the absence of lithium (Henry et al., 2001). These findings emphasize the importance of recognizing individual risk factors for susceptibility of antidepressant induced switching and tailoring treatment decisions accordingly (Goldberg & Truman, 2003).

Summary of maintenance pharmacotherapy

The evidence to date suggests that lithium monotherapy remains the gold standard of treatment because it protects against both manic and depressive relapses (although it is more effective in protecting against manic relapse) and has also been shown to reduce the risk of suicide. VPA, olanzapine, or quetiapine should be utilized if lithium is ineffective or poorly tolerated. CBZ should be considered an alternative option that may be effective in non-classic presentations of illness. LTG is an option that can be considered when the depressive phase of the illness is predominant.

For patients who fail monotherapy, choosing an effective combination therapy should begin with determining what the main burden of illness is within a particular patient. If it is mania, lithium or VPA (with CBZ and oxcarbazepine being second line options) in combination with an antipsychotic such as olanzapine, quetiapine, risperidone, or aripiprazole are reasonable choices. If the main burden of illness is depression, then the combination of lithium, VPA, or quetiapine (with CBZ and oxcarbazepine as second line options) with LTG, a SSRI, or buproprion is a viable options.

Risperidone long-acting injectable can be helpful in preventing relapse, particularly of mania, in monotherapy in bipolar I disorder, or as adjunctive treatment to mood stabilizers in frequently relapsing bipolar I and II disorder. This treatment option is particularly relevant to patient with poor treatment adherence or poor response to mood stabilizers.

Refractory patients

Unfortunately, there are many bipolar patients who remain symptomatic despite conventional mono and combination pharmacotherapies. It is essential to re-evaluate these patients for any underlying medical comorbidities (such as hypothyroidism) or substance abuse that may be contributing to their morbidity. For rapid cycling patients, discontinuing antidepressants may be helpful in stabilization. The use of clozapine or ECT are also considerations for refractory patients. The data regarding the efficacy of other pharmacotherapies such as gabapentin, topiramate, omega-3-fatty acids, phenytoin and others, while in widespread clinical use and likely effective in certain patients, are too sparse to warrant specific recommendations.

Importance of monitoring

In order to maximize the effectiveness of any long term treatment regimen, individual clinicians must be vigilant in the monitoring of their patients. This includes, but is not limited to, providing patients with options for psychotherapy and other psychosocial therapies, routine psychoeduction, the constant emphasis on the importance of treatment adherence, and when possible the incorporation of family members into the treatment plan. Clinicians should routinely monitor for suicidality and subsyndromal symptoms through the use of standardized mood scales, such as the Young Mania Rating Scale (YMRS) (Young et al., 1978) and the Hamilton Rating Scale for Depression (HAM-D) (Hamilton, 1959). Patients should be monitored for weight gain and any other medication side effects such as tardive dyskinesia if taking antipsychotics. Women should be assessed for polycystic ovary syndrome.

At the initiation of any drug treatment, baseline laboratory investigations should include CBC, fasting glucose, fasting lipid levels (TC, vLDL, HDL, LDL, TG), platelets, electrolytes, liver enzymes, serum bilirubin, prothrombin time, partial thromboplastin time, urinalysis, urine toxicology, serum creatinine, 24 hour creatinine clearance (if positive for a history of renal disease), thyroid stimulating hormone, prolactin, pregnancy test, and electrocardiogram (for those above the age of 40) (Yatham et al., 2005). These tests should be repeated 4 weeks after treatment and then every 3–6 months afterwards or sooner at the appearance of any new clinical symptoms or signs of medical illness. For patients taking lithium, thyroid and renal function tests should be assessed annually.

For patient taking lithium or VPA, regular monitoring of serum medication levels should be performed, particularly with patients with a history of non-compliance. Lithium levels should be targeted at 0.8–1.1 mmol/L while an ideal VPA level is between 70 and 120 micrograms/ml (Allen et al., 2006). Tegretol levels should be targeted between 4 and 12 micrograms/ml. Serum levels should be drawn at 12 hours after the last dose (trough level) approximately 5 days after the most recent dose titration and every 3–6 months afterwards. Any dose increases should be performed slowly and if a decision is made to switch medication, a smooth cross tapering regimen should be employed, particularly with lithium as rapid discontinuation has been shown to increase the likelihood of relapse (Strober, Morrell et al. 1990).

For patient taking atypical antipsychotics, a personal and family history of diabetes, obesity, hypertension, cardiovascular disease, and dyslipidemia should be assessed at baseline. Weight and BMI should be measured at baseline, and then every 4, 8, and 12 weeks thereafter. An alternative medication should be considered for any patient that gains >5% of their initial body weight, particularly if dietary interventions and/ or lifestyle changes have failed. Waist circumference should be measured at baseline and then annually. Blood pressure should be taken at baseline, 12 weeks, and then annually, with more frequent monitoring for patients with an increased risk for the development of hypertension. Fasting plasma glucose should be assessed at baseline, 12 weeks, and then every 6–12 months depending on each patient's unique risk for developing diabetes. Fasting lipid profile should be checked at baseline, 12 weeks, and then every 5 years if normal or more frequently if clinically indicated. Some clinicians have recommended checking total triglycerides and cholesterol every 3 months during the first year of treatment with atypicals.

Psychosocial and other therapies

Non-adherence to psychotropic medications is often associated with illness recurrence (Colom et al., 2000). A number of factors affect patient adherence (Sajatovic et al., 2004) (see Tables 5.3 and 5.4). When choosing a particular drug, clinicians must consider the impact of each pharmacotherapy beyond their efficacy, taking into account tolerability and potential for side effects. The combination of effective drug treatment and psychoeducation may be the optimal approach for a successful long-term outcome of bipolar disorder (Vieta & Colom, 2004).

While pharmacotherapy is essential for effective treatment of bipolar disorder, there is an increasing amount of evidence suggesting the utility of adjunctive psychosocial treatments that reduce morbidity, decrease residual symptoms, enhance drug compliance, and help to prevent relapses. High levels of critical, hostile, or emotionally overinvolved attitudes (high expressed emotion, or EE) in parents or spouses are associated with high rates of relapse, poor symptomatic outcomes, or both (Miklowitz et al., 1988; Priebe et al., 1989; O'Connell et al., 1991; Honig et al., 1997). Family-focused treatment that includes education, communication training, and problem-solving skills training, added to pharmacotherapy, has been shown to be more effective at preventing relapses and reducing suicidality than pharmacotherapy alone (Miklowitz et al., 2000; Miklowitz & Taylor, 2006). Psychotherapy, especially cognitive-behavioral techniques that focus on compliance, education about the illness, and

Table 5.3 Characteristics of Effective Therapies
that Maximize Adherence

Education
Self-monitoring
Recurrence prevention
Managing side effects
Identifying and managing stressors
Addressing belief system and attitudes to illness

Source: Sajatovic, M., M. Davies, & Hrouda, D. R., Enhancement of treatment adherence among patients with bipolar disorder. *Psychiatr. Serv., 55*(3): 264–269, 2004.

Table 5.4 Factors Associated with Poor
Treatment Adherence

Side effects of medications
Poor attitudes towards treatment
Poor insight
Denial of illness or symptoms
Comorbid substance abuse
Comorbid personality disorders
Lack of psychosocial support
Low education level
Younger age, single, and male

Source: Sajatovic, M., M. Davies, & Hrouda, D. R., Enhancement of treatment adherence among patients with bipolar disorder. *Psychiatr. Serv., 55*(3): 264–269, 2004.

maintaining circadian integrity, has been shown to improve the effectiveness of medication (Goodwin, 2003). In fact, medication alone versus medication plus psychotherapy has been shown to be greater than the difference between medication alone versus placebo (Feighner et al., 1998). In a recently published large, randomized-controlled study where psychosocial treatments were added to pharmacotherapy, intensive psychosocial treatments were more beneficial than brief treatment in enhancing stabilization for patients with bipolar depression (Miklowitz et al., 2007). Finally, continuation and maintenance electroconvulsive shock treatment, while seldom employed, remains a viable treatment option for chronic, severe, medication-refractory or intolerant, or non-adherent patients, (Vaidya et al., 2003).

Conclusion

Studies in the last 10 years have greatly added to our knowledge base of how to approach maintenance therapy for patients with bipolar disorder. Recent studies have reaffirmed the efficacy of lithium, particularly in the prevention of new manic episodes, and introduced new therapies such as LTG, which has been shown to be effective in the prevention of new depressive episodes. The second generation atypical agents, such as olanzapine and aripiprazole, have shown effectiveness at maintaining efficacy and preventing relapse in recently stabilized patients and more recent studies provide evidence for the use of quetiapine and risperidone long-acting injectable in preventing relapse into a mood episode.

This recent body of work supports the importance of ongoing maintenance treatments and the need for future studies to guide treatment. We do not know if lithium plus an anticonvulsant will out-perform an atypical antipsychotic used in combination. The best strategy to prevent depression has only been studied in monotherapy. There is a critical need for more combination treatment maintenance studies to explore this issue.

Finally, the relative benefit and risk ratio of the use of antidepressants in maintenance phase treatment needs to be explored in placebo controlled prospective studies.

References

Allen, M. H., Hirschfeld, R. M., Wozniak, P. J., Baker J. D., & Bowden, C. L. (2006). Linear relationship of valproate serum concentration to response and optimal serum levels for acute mania. *Am. J. Psychiatry, 163*(2): 272–275.

Alphs, L., Haskins, J., Turkoz, I., et al. (2008). Adjunctive long-acting risperidone delays mood episode relapse in patients with frequently relapsing bipolar disorder [Abstract P.3.c.066]. *J. Eur. Coll. Neuropsychopharmacol, 18*(Suppl 4): S441.

Altamura, A. C., Salvadori, D., Madaro, D., Santini, A., & Mundo E. (2003). Efficacy and tolerability of quetiapine in the treatment of bipolar disorder: preliminary evidence from a 12-month open-label study. *J. Affect. Disord., 76*(1–3): 267–271.

Altshuler, L., Suppes, t., Black, D., Nolen, W. A., Keck, P. E., Frye, M. A., McElroy, S., Kupka, S., Grunze, H., Walden, J., Leverich, G., Denicoff, K., Luckenbaugh, D., & Post, R. (2003). Impact of antidepressant discontinuation after acute bipolar depression remission on rates of depressive relapse at 1-year follow-up. *Am. J. Psychiatry, 160*(7): 1252.

Altshuler, L. L, Keck, P. E. Jr., McElroy, S. L., Suppes, T., Brown, E. S., Denicoff, K., Frye, M., Gitlin, M., Hwang, S., Goodman, R., Leverich, G., Nolen, W., Kupka, R., & Post, R. (1999). Gabapentin in the acute treatment of refractory bipolar disorder. *Bipolar Disord., 1*(1): 61–65.

Altshuler, L. L., Post, R. M., Black, D. O., Keck, P. E. Jr., Nolen, W. A., Frye, M. A., Suppes, T., Grunze, H., Kupka, R. W., Leverich, G. S., McElroy, S. L., Walden, J., & Mintz, J. (2006). Subsyndromal depressive symptoms are associated with functional impairment in patients with bipolar disorder: results of a large, multisite study. *J. Clin. Psychiatry, 67*(10): 1551–1560.

American Psychiatric Association (2002). Practice guideline for the treatment of patients with bipolar disorder (revision). *Am. J. Psychiatry, 159*: 1–50.

Angst, F., Stassen, H. H., Clayton, P. J., & Angst, J. (2002). Mortality of patients with mood disorders: follow-up over 34-38 years. *J. Affect. Disord., 68*: 167–181.

Angst, J., F. Angst, F., Gerber-Werder R., & Gamma, A. (2005). Suicide in 406 mood-disorder patients with and without long-term medication: a 40 to 44 years follow-up. *Arch. Suicide Res., 9*: 279–300.

Angst, J., Gamma, A., Sellaro, R., Lavori, P. W., & Zhang, H. (2003a). Recurrence of bipolar disorders and major depression. A life-long perspective. *Eur. Arch. Psychiatry Clin. Neurosci., 253*(5): 236–240.

Atmaca, M., Kuloglu, M., Tezcan, E., & Ustundag, B. (2003b). Serum leptin and triglyceride levels in patients on treatment with atypical antipsychotics. *J. Clin. Psychiatry, 64*: 598–604.

Baastrup, P. C., Poulsen, J. C., Schou, M., Thomsen, K., & Amdisen, A. (1970). Prophylactic lithium: double blind discontinuation in manic-depressive and recurrent-depressive disorders. *Lancet, 2*(7668): 326–330.

Baethge, C., Baldessarini, R. J, Mathiske-Schmidt, K., Hennen, J., Berghöfer, A., Muller-Oerlinghausen, B., Bschor, T., Adli, M., & Bauer, M. (2005). Long-term combination therapy versus monotherapy with lithium and carbamazepine in 46 bipolar I patients. *J. Clin. Psychiatry, 66*(2): 174–182.

Baldessarini, R., Salvatore, P., Tohen, M., Khalsa, H. K., Hennen, J., Gonzalez-Pinto, A., & Baethge C. (2004). Morbidity from onset in first-episode bipolar I disorder patients: the International-300 study. *Neuropsychopharmacology, 29* (Suppl 1): S88.

Baldessarini, R. J., Hennen, J., Wilson, M., Calabrese, J., Chengappa, R., Keck, P. E. Jr., McElroy, S., Sachs, G., Vieta, E., Welge, J., Yatham, L. N., Zarate, C., Baker, R. W., & Tohen, M. (2003a). Olanzapine vs. placebo in acute mania: treatment responses in subgroups. *J. Clin. Psychopharmacol., 23*: 370–376.

Baldessarini, R. J., Tondo L., & Hennen J. (2003b). Lithium treatment and suicide risk in major affective disorders: update and new findings. *J. Clin. Psychiatry, 64*(Suppl 5): 44–52.

Baldessarini, R. J., Tondo, L., Davis, P., Pompili, M., Goodwin, F. K., & Hennen, J. (2006). Decreased risk of suicides and attempts during long-term lithium treatment: a meta-analytic review. *Bipolar Disord., 8*(5 Pt 2): 625–639.

Baldessarini, R. J., Tondo L., Hennen J., & Viguera A. C. (2002). Is lithium still worth using? An update of selected recent research. *Harv. Rev. Psychiatry, 10*(2): 59–75.

Ballenger, J. C., & Post, R. M. (1980). Carbamazepine in manic-depressive illness: a new treatment. *Am. J. Psychiatry, 137*: 782–790.

Barrett, E., Blonde, L., Clement, S., Davis, J., Devlin, J., Kane, J., Klein, S., & Torrey, W., (2004). Consensus development conference on antipsychotic drugs and obesity and diabetes. *Diabetes Care, 27*: 596–601.

Bauer, M. S., & Mitchner, L. (2004). What is a mood stabilizer? An evidence-based response. *Am. J. Psychiatry, 161*: 3–18.

Begley, C. E., Annegers, J. F., Swann, A. C., Lewis, C., Coan, S., Schnapp, W. B., & Bryant-Comstock, L. (2001). The lifetime cost of bipolar disorder in the US: An estimate for new cases in 1998. *Pharmacoeconomics, 19*: 483–495.

Benedetti, A., Lattanzi, L., Pini, S., Musetto, L., Dell'Osso l., & Cassano, G. B. (2004). Oxcarbazepine as add-on treatment in patients with bipolar manic, mixed or depressive episode. *J. Affect. Disord., 79*: 273–277.

Boerlin, H., Gitlin, M. J., Zoellner, L. A., & Hammen, C. L. (1998). Bipolar depression and antidepressant-induced mania: a naturalistic study. *J. Clin. Psychiatry, 59*: 374–379.

Bowden, C. (1998). New concepts in mood stabilization: Evidence for the effectiveness of valproate and lamotrigine. *Neuropsychopharmacology, 19*: 194–199.

Bowden, C. (2003). Acute and maintenance treatment with mood stabilizers. *Int. J. Neuropsychopharmacol., 6*: 269–275.

Bowden, C., Collins, M. A., McElroy, S. L., Calabrese, J. R., Swann, A. C., Weisler, R. H., & Wozniak, P. J. (2005a). Relationship of mania symptomatology to maintenance treatment response with divalproex, lithium or placebo. *Neuropsychopharmacology, 30*: 1932–1939.

Bowden, C., Grunze, H., Mullen, J., Brecher, M., Paulsson, B., jones, M., Vågerö, M., & Svensson, K. (2005b). A randomized double blind placebo controlled efficacy and safety study of quetiapine or lithium as monotherapy for mania in bipolar disorder. *J. Clin. Psychiatry, 66*: 111–121.

Bowden, C. L. (2000). The ability of lithium and other mood stabilizers to decrease suicide risk and prevent relapse. *Curr. Psychiatry Rep., 2*(6): 490–4.

Bowden, C. L. (2007). Spectrum of effectiveness of valproate in neuropsychiatry. *Expert Review of Neurotherapeutics 7*(1): 9–16.

Bowden, C. L., Brugger, A. M., Swann, A. C., Calabrese, J. R., Janicak, P. G., Dilsaver, S. C., Davis, J. M., Rush, A. J., & Small, J. G. (1994). Efficacy of divalproex vs lithium and placebo in the treatment of mania. *JAMA, 271*: 918–924.

Bowden, C. L., Calabrese, J. R., McElroy, S. L., Gyulai, L., Wassef, A., Petty, F., Pope H. G. Jr., Chou J. C., Keck P. E. Jr., Rhodes L. J., Swann A. C., Hirschfeld R. M., & Wozniak P. J. (2000). Randomized, placebo-controlled 12-month trial of divalproex and lithium in treatment of outpatients with bipolar I disorder. *Arch. Gen. Psychiatry, 57*: 481–489.

Bowden, C. L., Calabrese, J. R., Sachs, G., Yatham, L. N., Asghar, S. A., Hompland, M., Montgomery, P., Earl, N., Smoot, T. M., & DeVeaugh-Geiss, J. (2003). Placebocontrolled 18-month trial of lamotrigine and lithium maintenance treatment in recently manic or hypomanic patients with bipolar I disorder. Lamictal 606 Study Group. *Arch. Gen. Psychiatry. 60*: 392–400.

Bowden, C. L., Calabrese, J. R., et al. (2003). A placebo-controlled 18-month trial of lamotrigine and lithium maintenance treatment in recently manic or hypomanic patients with bipolar I disorder. *Arch. Gen. Psychiatry, 60*(4): 392–400.

Bowden, C. L., Swann, A. C., Calabrese, J. R., Rubenfaer, L. M., Wozniak, P. J., Collins, M. A., Abi-Saab, W., & Saltarelli, M. (2006). A randomized, placebo-controlled, multicenter study of divalproex sodium extended release in the treatment of acute mania. *J. Clin. Psychiatry, 67*(10): 1501–1510.

Brown, E. S., Nejtek, V. A., Perantie, D. C., & Bobadilla, L. (2002). Quetiapine in bipolar disorder and cocaine dependence. *Bipolar Disord. 4*(6): 406–411.

Brown, E. S., Nejtek, V. A., Perantine, D. C., Orsulak, P. J., & Bobadilla, L. (2003). Lamotrigine in patients with bipolar disorder and cocaine dependence. *J. Clin. Psychiatry, 64*: 197–201.

Burgess, S., Geddes, J., & Hawton, K., et al. (2001). Lithium for maintenance treatment of mood disorders (Cochrane Review), *Cochrane Database Systematic Reviews,* CD003013.

Calabrese, J. R., Bowden, C. L., Sachs, G. S., Ascher, J. A., Monaghan, E. & Rudd, G. D. (1999). A double-blind placebo-controlled study of lamotrigine monotherapy in outpatients with bipolar I depression. Lamictal 602 Study Group. *J. Clin. Psychiatry, 60*: 79–88.

Calabrese, J. R., Markovitz, P. J., Kimmel, S. E., & Wagner, S. C. (1992). Spectrum of efficacy of valproate in 78 rapid-cycling bipolar patients. *J. Clin. Psychopharmacol., 12*: 53–56.

Calabrese, J. R., Rapport, D. J., Youngstrom, E. A., Jackson, K., Bilali, S., & Findling, R. L. (2005a). New data on the use of lithium, divalproate, and lamotrigine in rapid cycling bipolar disorder. *Eur. Psychiatry, 20*: 92–95.

Calabrese, J. R., Shelton, M. D., Rapport, D. J., Youngstrom, E. A., Jackson, K., Bilali, S., Ganocy, S. J., & Findling, R. L. (2005b). A 20-month, double-blind, maintenance trial of lithium vs. divalproex in rapid-cycling bipolar disorder. *Am. J. Psychiatry 162*(11): 2152–2161.

Calabrese, J. R., Shelton, M. D., Rapport, D. J., Kimmel, S. E., & Elhaj, O., et al. (2002). Long-term treatment of bipolar disorder with lamotrigine. *J. Clin. Psychiatry, 63*(Suppl 10): 18–22.

Calabrese, J. R., Bowden, C. L., McElroy, S. L., Cookson, J., Andersen, J., Keck, P. E. Jr., Rhodes, L., Bolden-Watson, C., Zhou, J., & Ascher, J. A. (1999). Spectrum of activity of lamotrigine in treatment-refractory bipolar disorder. *Am. J. Psychiatry, 156*: 1019–1023.

Calabrese, J. R., Bowden, C. L., Sachs, G., Yatham, L. N., Behnke, K., Mehtonen, O. P., Montgomery, P., Ascher, J., Paska, W., Earl, N., & DeVeaugh-Geiss, J. (2003). Placebocontrolled 18-month trial of lamotrigine and lithium maintenance treatment in recently depressed patients with bipolar I disorder. Lamictal 605 Study Group. *J. Clin. Psychiatry, 64*: 1013–1024.

Calabrese, J. R., Bowden, C. L., et al. (2003). A placebo-controlled 18-month trial of lamotrigine and lithium maintenance treatment in recently depressed patients with bipolar I disorder. *J. Clin. Psychiatry, 64*(9): 1013–1024.

Calabrese, J. R., & Delucchi, G. A. (1990). Spectrum of efficacy of valproate in 55 patients with rapid-cycling bipolar disorder. *Am. J. Psychiatry, 147*(4): 431–434.

Calabrese, J. R., Goldberg, J. F., Ketter, T. A., Suppes, T., Frye, M., White, R., DeVeaugh-Geiss, A., & Thompson, T. R. (2006). Recurrence in bipolar I disorder: A post hoc analysis excluding relapses in two double-blind maintenance studies. *Biol. Psychiatry, 59*(11): 1061–1064.

Calabrese, J. R., Keck, P. E. Jr., Macfadden, W., Minkwitz, M., Ketter, T. A., Weisler, R. H., Cutler, A. J., McCoy, R., Wilson, E., & Mullen, J. (2005c). A randomized, double-blind, placebo-controlled trial of quetiapine in the treatment of bipolar I or II depression. *Am. J. Psychiatry, 162*(7): 1351–1360.

Calabrese, J. R., Kimmel, S. E., Woyshville, M. J., Rapport, D. J., Faust, C. J., Thompson, P. A., & Meltzer, H. Y. (1996). Clozapine for treatment-refractory mania. *Am. J. Psychiatry, 153*: 759–764.

Calabrese, J. R., Markovitz, P. J., Kimmel, S. E., & Wagner S. C. (1992). Spectrum of efficacy of valproate in 78 rapid-cycling bipolar patients. *J. Clin. Psychopharmacol., 12*(1 Suppl): 53S–56S.

Calabrese, J. R., Markovitz, P. J., et al. (1992). Spectrum of efficacy of valproate in 78 rapid-cycling bipolar patients. *J. Clin. Psychopharmacol., 12*: 53S–56S.

Calabrese, J. R., Meltzer, H. Y., & Markovitz, P. J., et al. (1991). Clozapine prophylaxis in rapid cycling bipolar disorder. *J. Clin. Psychopharmacol., 11*(6): 396–397.

Calabrese, J. R., Shelton, M. D., Rapport, D. J., Youngstrom, E. A., Jackson, K., Bilali, S., Ganocy, S. J., & Findling, R. L. (2005). A 20-month, double-blind, maintenance trial of lithium versus divalproex in rapid-cycling bipolar disorder. *Am. J. Psychiatry, 162*(11): 2152–2161.

Calabrese, J. R., Suppes, T., Bowden, C. L., Sachs, G. S., Swann, A. C., McElroy, S. L., Kusumakar, V., Ascher, J. A., Earl, N. L., Greene, P. L., & Monaghan, E. T. (2000). A double-blind, placebo-controlled, prophylaxis study of lamotrigine in rapid-cycling bipolar disorder. *J. Clin. Psychiatry, 61*: 841–850.

Calabrese, J. R., Vieta, E., El-Mallakh, R., Finding, R. L., Youngstrom, E. A., Elhaj, O., Gajani, P., & Pies, R. (2004). Mood state at study entry as predictor of risk of relapse and spectrum of efficacy in bipolar maintenance studies. *Biol. Psychiatry, 56*(12): 957–963.

Calabrese, J.R., Huffman, R.F., White, R.L., Edwards, S., Thompson, T.W., Ascher, J.A et al. Lamotrigine in the acute treatment of bipolar depression: results of five double-blind, placebo controlled clinical trails. Bipolar Disorders 2008; 10: 323–333.

Carlson, P. J., Merlock, M. C., & Suppes, T. (2004). Adjunctive stimulant use in patients with bipolar disorder: Treatment of residual depression and sedation. *Bipolar Disord., 6*: 416–420.

Carney, S. M., & Goodwin, D. C. (2005). Lithium-a continuing story in the treatment of bipolar disorder. *Acta Psychiatr. Scand., 111*(Suppl 426): 7–12.

Chengappa, R., K. N., Schwarzman, L. K., Hulihan, J. F., Xiang, J., & Roenthal, N. R. (2006). Adjunctive topiramate therapy in patients receiving a mood stabilizer for bipolar I disorder: a randomized, placebo-controlled trial. *J. Clin. Psychiatry, 67*(11): 1698–706.

Chou, J., & Fazzio, L. (2006). Maintenance treatment of bipolar disorder: applying research to clinical practice. *J. Psychiatric Pract., 12*(5): 283–299.

Cipriani, A., Pretty, H., Hawton, K., & Geddes, J. R. (2005). Lithium in the prevention of suicidal behavior and all-cause mortality in patients with mood disorders: a systematic review of randomized trials. *Am. J. Psychiatry, 162*: 1805–1819.

Cohn, J. B., Collins, G., Ashbrook, E., & Wernicke, J. F. (1989). A comparison of fluoxetine, imipramine and placebo in patients with bipolar depressive disorder. *Int. Clin. Psychopharmacol., 4*: 313–322.

Colom, F., Vieta, E., Martinez-Aran, A., Reinares, M., Goikolea, J. M., Benabarre, A., Torrent, C., Comes, M., Corbella, B., Parramon, G., & Corominas, J. (2003). A randomized trial on the efficacy of group psychoeducation in the prophylaxis of recurrences in bipolar patients whose disease is in remission. *Arch. Gen. Psychiatry, 60*: 402–407.

Colom, F., Vieta, E., Martínez-Arán, A., Reinares, M., Benabarre, A., & Gastó, C. (2000). Clinical factors associated with treatment noncompliance in euthymic bipolar patients. *J. Clin. Psychiatry, 61*: 549–555.

Conway, C. R., Chibnall, J. T., Nelson, L. A., McGuire, J. M., Abraham, P. F., Baram, V. Y., Grossberg, G. T., & Carroll, B. J. (2006). An open-label trial of adjunctive oxcarbazepine for bipolar disorder. *J. Clin. Psychopharmacol., 26*: 95–97.

Coppen, A., Peet, M., Bailey, J., Noguera, R., Burns, B. H., Swani, M. S., Maggs, R., & Gardner, R. (1973). Double-blind and open prospective studies on lithium prophylaxis in affective disorders. *Psychiatr. Neurol. Neurochir., 76*(6): 501–510.

Coryell, W., Winokur, G., Solomon, D., Shea, T., Leon, A., & Keller, M. (1997). Lithium and recurrence in a long-term follow up of bipolar affective disorder. *Psychol. Med., 27*: 281–289.

Cundall, R. L., Brooks, P. W., & Murray, L. G., et al. (1972). A controlled evaluation of lithium prophylaxis in affective disorders. *Psychol. Med. 2*(3): 308–311.

Dando, T. M., & Keating, G. M. (2006). Spotlight on quetiapine in acute mania and depression associated with bipolar disorder. *CNS Drugs, 20*(5): 429–431.

Davis, L. L., Bartolucci, A., & Petty, F. (2005). Divalproex in the treatment of bipolar depression:a placebo-controlled study. *J. Affect. Disord., 85*: 259–266.

Davis, L. L., Ryan, W., Adinoff, B., & Petty, F. (2000). Comprehensive review of the psychiatric uses of valproate. *J. Clin. Psychopharmacol., 20*(Suppl 1): 1S–17S.

Davis, L. L., Williams, R., & Cates, M. (2004). Divalproex sodium in the treatment of adults with bipolar disorder. *Expert. Rev. Neurother., 4*(3): 349–362.

Denicoff, K. D., Smith-Jackson, E. E., Disney, E. R., Ali, S. O., Leverich, G. S., & Post, R. M. (1997). Comparative prophylactic efficacy of lithium, carbamazepine and the combination in bipolar disorder. *J. Clin. Psychiatry, 58*: 470–478.

Denicoff, K. D., Smith-Jackson, E. E., Disney, E. R., Ali, S. O., Leverich, G. S., & Post, R. M. (1997). Comparative prophylactic efficacy of lithium, carbamazepine, and the combination in bipolar disorder. *J. Clin. Psychiatry, 58*(11): 470–478.

Dunner, D. L. (2004). Correlates of suicidal behavior and lithium treatment in bipolar disorder. *J. Clin. Psychiatry, 65*(Suppl 10): 5–10.

Endicott, J., Rajagopalan, K., Minkwitz, M., & Macfadden, W. (2007). A randomized, double-blind, placebo-controlled study of quetiapine in the treatment of bipolar I and II depression: improvements in quality of life. *Int. Clin. Psychopharmacol., 22*: 29–37.

Evins, E. (2003). Efficacy of newer anticonvulsant medications in bipolar spectrum mood disorders. *J. Clin. Psychiatry, 64*(Suppl 8): 9–14.

Fagiolini, A., Frank, E., Houck, P. R., Mallinger, A. G., Swartz, H. A., Buysse, D. J., Ombao, H., & Kupfer, D. J. (2002). Prevalence of obesity and weight change during treatment in patients with bipolar I disorder. *J. Clin. Psychiatry, 63*: 528–533.

Fagiolini, Frank, E., Scott, J. A., Turkin, S., & Kupfer, D. J. (2005). Metabolic syndrome in bipolar disorder: findings from the Bipolar Disorder Center for Pennsylvanians. *Bipolar Disord., 7*: 424–430.

Fawcett, J. (2003). Lithium combinations in acute and maintenance treatment of unipolar and bipolar depression. *J. Clin. Psychiatry, 64*(Suppl 5): 32–37.

Fehr, B. S., Ozcan, M. E., & Suppes, T. (2005). Low doses of clozapine may stabilize treatment-resistant bipolar patients. *Eur. Arch. Psychiatry Clin. Neurosci., 255*(1): 10–14.

Feighner, J., S. Targum, S. D., Bennett, M. E., Roberts, D L., Kensler, T. T., D'Amico, M. F., & Hardy, S. A., (1998). A double-blind, placebo controlled trial of nefazodone, in the treatment of patients hospitalized for major depression. *J. Clin. Psychiatry, 59*: 246–253.

Ferrier, I. N., Stanton, B. R., Kelly, T. P., & Scott, J. (1999). Neuropsychological function in euthymic patients with bipolar disorder. *Br. J. Psychiatry, 175:* 246–51.

Frankenburg, F., & Zanarini, M. (2002). Divalproex sodium treatment of women with borderline personality disorder and bipolar II disorder: a double-blind placebo-controlled pilot study. *J. Clin. Psychiatry, 63:* 442–446.

Frye, M. A., Ketter, T. A., Kimbrell, T. A., Dunn, R. T., Speer, A. M., Osuch, E. A., Luckenbaugh, D. A., Cora-Ocatelli, G., Leverich, G. S., & Post, R. M. (2000). A placebo-controlled study of lamotrigine and gapapentin monotherapy in refractory mood disorders. *J. Clin. Psychopharm., 20:* 607–614.

Frye, M. A., Yatham, L. N., Calabrese, J. R., Bowden, C. L., Ketter, T. A., Suppes, T., Adams, B. E., & Thompson, T. R. (2006). Incidence and time course of subsyndromal symptoms in patients with bipolar I disorder: an evaluation of 2 placebo-controlled maintenance trials. *J. Clin. Psychiatry, 67*(11): 1721–1728.

Geddes, J. R., Burgess, S., Hawton, K., Jamison, K., & Goodwin, G. M. (2004). Long-term lithium therapy for bipolar disorder: systematic review and meta-analysis of randomised controlled trials. *Am. J. Psychiatry, 161:* 217–222.

Gelenberg, A. J., Kane, J. M., Keller, M. B. Lavori, P., Rosenbaum, J. F., Cole, K., & Lavelle, J. (1989). Comparison of standard and low serum levels of lithium for maintenance treatment of bipolar disorder. *N. Engl. J. Med., 321:* 1489–1493.

Ghaemi, S., Hsu D. J., Rosenquist K. J., Pardo T. B., & Goodwin F. K. (2006). Extrapyramidal side effects with atypical neuroleptics in bipolar disorder. *Prog. Neuro-Psychopharmacol. Biol. Psychiatry, 30:* 209–213.

Ghaemi, S., Pardo, T. B., & Hsu, D. J. (2004). Strategies for preventing the recurrence of bipolar disorder. *J. Clin. Psychiatry, 65:* 16–23.

Ghaemi, S. N.,. Schrauwen, E., Klugman, J., Berv, D. A., Shirzadi, A. A., Pardo, T. B., & Goodwin, F. K. (2006). Long-term lamotrigine plus lithium for bipolar disorder: one year outcome. *J. Psychiatric Pract., 12*(5): 300–305.

Ghaemi, S. N., Hsu, D. J., Soldani, F., & Goodwin, F. K. (2003). Antidepressants in bipolar disorder: the case for caution. *Bipolar Disord., 5*(6): 421–433.

Ghaemi, S. N., Manwani, S. G., Katzow, J. J., Ko, J. Y., & Goodwin, F. K. (2001). Topiramate treatment of bipolar spectrum disorders: a retrospective chart review. *Ann. Clin. Psychiatry, 13*(4): 185–189.

Ghaemi, S. N., & Sachs, G. S. (1997). Long-term risperidone treatment in bipolar disorder: 6-month follow up. *Int. Clin. Psychopharmacol., 12:* 333–338.

Ghaemi, S. N., Zablotsky, B., Fillowski, M. M., Dunn, R. T., Pardo, T. B., Isemstein, E., & Baldassano, C. F. (2006). An open prospective study of zonisamide in acute bipolar depression. *J. Clin. Psychopharmacol., 26*(4): 385–388.

Goldberg, J., & Truman, C. (2003). Antidepressant-induced mania: an overview of current controversies. *Bipolar Disord., 5*(6): 407–420.

Goldberg, J. F., & Whiteside, J. E. (2002). The association between substance abuse and antidepressant-induced mania in bipolar disorder: A preliminary study. *J. Clin. Psychiatry, 63:* 791–795.

Gonzalez-Pinto, A., Mosquera, F., Alonso, M., López, P., Ramírez, F., Vieta, E., & Baldessarini, R. J. (2006). Suicidal risk in bipolar I disorder patients and adherence to long-term lithium treatment. *Bipolar Disord., 8*(5 Pt 2): 618–624.

Goodwin, D. C. (1994). Recurrence of mania after lithium withdrawal: implications for the use of lithiumin the treatment of bipolar affective disorder. *Br. J. Psychiatry, 164*: 149–152.

Goodwin, D. C. (2003). Rationale for using lithium in combination with other mood stabilizers in the management of bipolar disorder. *J. Clin. Psychiatry, 63*(Suppl 4): 18–24.

Goodwin, D. C., & Goldstein, M. J. (2003). Optimizing lithium treatment in bipolar disorder. *J. Psychiatric Pract., 9*(5): 333–343.

Goodwin F. K., Fireman, B., Simon, G. E., Hunkeler, E. M., Lee, J., & Revicki, D. (2003). Suicide risk in bipolar disorder during treatment with lithium and divalproex. *JAMA, 290*(11): 1467–1473.

Goodwin, G. M. (2003). Consensus Group of the British Association for Psychopharmacology. Evidence-based guidelines for treating bipolar disorder: recommendations from the British Association for Psychopharmacology. *J. Psychopharmacol., 17*: 149–173.

Goodwin, G. M. (2003). Evidence-based guidelines for treating bipolar disorder: recommendations from the British Association for Psychopharmacology. *J. Psychopharmacol., 17*: 149–173.

Goodwin, G. M., Bowden, C. L., Calabrese, J. R., Grunze, H., Kasper, S., White, R., Greene, P., & Leadbetter, R. (2004). Pooled analysis of 2 placebo-controlled 18-month trials of lamotrigine and lithium maintenance in bipolar I disorder. *J. Clin. Psychiatry, 65*: 432–441.

Gopal, S., Steffens, D. C., Kramer, M. L., & Olsen, M. K. (2005). Symptomatic remission in patients with bipolar mania: results from a double-blind, placebo-controlled trial of risperidone monotherapy. *J. Clin. Psychiatry, 66*(8): 1016–1020.

Grasela, T. H., Fiedler-Kelly, J., Cox, E., Womble, G. P., Risner, M. E., & Chen, C. (1999). Population pharmacokinetics of lamotrigine adjunctive therapy in adults with epilepsy. *J. Clin. Pharmacol., 39*(4): 373–384.

Groeper, K., & McCann, M. E. (2005). Topiramate and metabolic acidosis: a case series and review of the literature. *Paediatr. Anaesth., 15*: 167–170.

Grof, P. (2003). Selecting effective long-term treatment for bipolar patients: monotherapy and combinations. *J. Clin. Psychiatry, 64*(Suppl 5): 53–61.

Grunze, H., Kasper, S., Goodwin, G., Bowden, C., Möller, H. J., & WFSBP Task Force on Treatment Guidelines for Bipolar Disorders. (2004). The World Federation of Societies of Biological Psychiatry (WFSBP) Guidelines for the Biological Treatment of Bipolar Disorders. Part III: maintenance treatment. *World J. Biol. Psychiatry, 5*(3): 120–135.

Guberman, A. H., Besag, F. M., Brodie, M. J., Duchowny, M. S., Pellock, J. M., Richens, A., Stern, R. S., & Trevanthan, E. (1999). Lamotrigine associated rash: risk/benefit considerations in adults and children. *Epilepsia, 40*(7): 985–991.

Gyulai, L., Bowden, C. L., McElroy, S. L., Calabrese, J. R., Petty, F., Swann, A. C., Chou, J. C., Wassef, A., Risch, C. S., Hirschfeld, R. M., Nemeroff, C. B., Keck, P. E. Jr., Evans, D. L., & Wozniak, P. J. (2003). Maintenance efficacy of divalproex in the prevention of bipolar depression. *Neuropsychopharmacology, 28*(7): 1374–1382.

Hamilton, M. (1959). The assessment of anxiety states by rating. *Br. J. Med. Psychol., 32*(1): 50–55.

Harrigan, E. P., Miceli, J. J., Anziano, R., Watsky, E., Reeves, K. R., Cutler, N. R., Sramek, J., Shiovits, T., & Middle, M. (2004). A randomized evaluation of the effects of six antipsychotic agents on QTc, in the absence and presence of metabolic inhibition. *J. Clin. Psychopharmacol., 24*(1): 62–69.

Hellewell, J. (2006). A review of the evidence for the use of antipsychotics in the maintenance treatment of bipolar disorders. *J. Psychopharmacol., 20*(2): 39–45.

Henry, C., Sorbara, F., Lacoste, J., Gindre, C., & Leboyer, M. (2001). Antidepressant-induced mania in bipolar patients: identification of risk factors. *J. Clin. Psychiatry, 62*(4): 249–55.

Himmelhoch, J. M., Thase, M. E., Mallinger, A. G., & Houck, P. (1991). Tranylcypromine versus imipramine in anergic bipolar depression. *Am. J. Psychiatry, 148*(7): 910–916.

Hirschfeld, R. (2003). The efficacy of atypical antipsychotics in bipolar disorders. *J. Clin. Psychiatry, 64*(Suppl 8): 15–21.

Hirschfeld, R. (2005). Guideline watch: Practice guideline for the treatment of patients with bipolar disorder (2nd edition). Arlington, VA: American Psychiatric Association.

Hirschfeld, R. M., Eerdekens, M., Kalali, A. H., Canuso, C. M., Khan, A. A., Karcher, K., & Palumbo, J. M. (2006a). An open-label extension trial of risperidone monotherapy in the treatment of bipolar I disorder. *Int. Clin. Psychopharmacol., 21*(1): 11–20.

Hirschfeld, R. M., Weisler, R. H., Raines, S. R., & Macfadden, W. (2006b). Quetiapine in the treatment of anxiety in patients with Bipolar I or II Depressioin: a secondary analysis from a randomized, double-blind, placebo-controlled study. *J. Clin. Psychiatry, 67*(3): 335–362.

Hirschfeld, R. M., Baker, J. D., Wonzniak, P., Tracy, K., & Sommerville, K. W. (2003). The safety and early efficacy of oral-loaded divalproex versus standard-titration divalproex, lithium, olanzapine, and placebo in the treatment of acute mania associated with bipolar disorder. *J. Clin. Psychiatry, 64*(7): 841–846.

Hirschfeld, R. M. A., Keck, P. E. Jr., Kramer, M., Canuso, C., Eerdekens, M., & Grossman, F. (2004). Rapid antimanic effect of risperidone monotherapy: A 3-week multicenter, double-blind, placebo-controlled trial. *Am. J. Psychiatry, 161*(6): 1057–1065.

Honig, A., Hofman, A., Rozendall, N., & Dingemans, P. (1997). Psycho-education in bipolar disorder: effect of expressed emotion. *Psychiatr. Res., 72*(1): 17–22.

Houston, J. P., Ahl, J., Meyers, A. L., Kaiser, C. J., Tohen, M., & Baldessarini, R. J. (2006). Reduced suicidal ideation in bipolar I disorder mixed-episode patients in a placebo-controlled trial of olanzapine combined with lithium or divalproex. *J. Clin. Psychiatry, 67*(8): 1246–1252.

Howland, R. H. (1996). Induction of mania with serotonin reuptake inhibitors. *J. Clin. Psychopharmacol., 16*(6): 425–427.

Jacobsen, F. M. (1993). Low-dose valproate: a new treatment for cyclothymia, mild rapid cycling disorders, and premenstrual syndrome. *J. Clin. Psychiatry, 54*: 229–234.

Joffe, H., Cohen, L. S., Suppes, T., Hwang, C. H., Molay, F., Adams, J. M., Sachs, G. S., & Hall, J. E. (2006). Longitudinal follow-up of reproductive and metabolic features of valproate-associated polycystic ovarian syndrome features: A preliminary report. *Biol. Psychiatry, 60*(12): 1378–1381.

Judd, L. L., & Akiskal, H. S. (2003). Depressive episodes and symptoms dominate the longitudinal course of bipolar disorder. *Curr. Psychiatry Rep., 5*(6): 417–418.

Judd, L. L., Akiskal, H. S., Schettler, P. J., Coryell, W., Endicott, J., Maser, J. D., Solomon, D. A., Leon, A. C., & Keller, M. B. (2003). A prospective investigation of the natural history of the long-term weekly symptomatic status of bipolar II disorder. *Arch. Gen. Psychiatry, 60*(3): 261–269.

Judd, L. L., Akiskal, H. S., Schettler, P. J. Endicott, J., Solomon, D. A., Leon A. C., Rice, J. A., & Keller, M. B. (2002). The long-term natural history of the weekly symptomatic status of bipolar I disorder. *Arch. Gen. Psychiatry, 59*(6): 530–537.

Kanner, A. M., & Frey, M. (2000). Adding valproate to lamotrigine: a study of their pharmacokinetic interaction. *Neurology, 55*: 588–591.

Kaufman, K. R. (1998). Adjunctive tiagabine treatment of psychiatric disorders: Three cases. *Ann. Clin. Psychiatry, 10*: 181–184.

Keck, P. Jr., Bowden, C. L., Meinhold, J. M., Gyulai, L., Prihoda, T.J., Baker, J. D., & Wozniak, P. J. (2005). Relationship between serum valproate and lithium levels and efficacy and tolerability in bipolar maintenance therapy. *Int. J. Psychiatry Clin. Pract., 9*: 271–277.

Keck, P. E. Jr, Calabrese, J. R., McQuade, R. D., Carson, W. H., Carlson, B. X., Rollin, L. M., Marcus, R. N., Sanchez, R., & Aripiprazole study Group. (2006). A randomized, double-blind, placebo-controlled, 26 week trial of aripiprazole in recently manic patients with bipolar I disorder. *J. Clin. Psychiatry, 67*(4): 626–637.

Keck, P. Jr., & Mc Elroy, S. L. (2002). Carbamazepine and valproate in the maintenance treatment of bipolar disorder. *J. Clin. Psychiatry, 63*(Suppl 10): 13–17.

Keck, P. E. Jr., Mc Elroy, S. L., Strakowski, S. M., Bourne, M. L., & West, S. A. (1997). Compliance with maintenance treatment in bipolar disorder. *Psychopharmacol. Bull., 33*(1): 87–91.

Keck, P. E. Jr., Nabulsi, A. A., Taylor, J. L., Henke, C. J., Stanton, S. P., & Bennett, J. A. (1996). A pharmacoeconomic model of divalproex vs. lithium in te acute and prophylactic treatment of bipolar I disorder. *J. Clin. Psychiatry, 57*(5): 213–222.

Keck, P., Versiani, M., Potkin, S., West, S. A., Giller, E., Ice K., & Ziprasidone in Mania Study Group. (2003). Ziprasidone in the treatment of acute bipolar mania: a 3-week, placebo controlled, double-blind, randomized trial. *Am. J. Psychiatry, 160*: 741–748.

Keck, P. E., Mintz, L., McElroy, S. L., Freeman, M. P., Suppes, T., Frye, M. A., Altshuler, L. L., Kuppa, R., Nolen, W. A., Leverich, G. S., Denicoff, K. D., Grunze, H., Duan, N., & Post, R. M. (2002). A double-blind, placebo-controlled trial of eicosapentanoic acid in rapid cycling bipolar disorder. *Bipolar Disord., 4*: 26–27.

Keck, P. E., Marcus, R., Tourkodimitris, S., Ali, M., Liebeskind, A., Saha, A., & Ingenito, G. (2003). A placebo-controlled, double-blind study of the efficacy and safety of aripiprazole in patients with acute bipolar mania. *Am. J. Psychiatry, 160*(9): 1651–1658.

Keck, P. E., & McElroy, S. L. (2003). Bipolar disorder, obesity, and pharmacotherapy -associated weight gain. *J. Clin. Psychiatry, 64*: 1426–1435.

Keck, P. E. Jr., Mintz, J., Mcelroy, S. L., Freeman, M. P., Suppes, T., Frye, M. A., Altshuler, L. L., Kupka, R., Nolen, W. A., Leverich, G. S., Denicoff, K. D., Grunze, H., Duan, N., & Post, R. M. (2006). Double-blind, randomized, placebo-controlled trials of ethyl-eicosapentanoate in the treatment of bipolar depression and rapid cycling bipolar disorder. *Biol. Psychiatry, 60*(9): 1020–1022.

Keller, M. (2004). Improving the course of illness and promoting continuation of treatment of bipolar disorder. *J. Clin. Psychiatry, 65*(Suppl 15): 10–14.

Kemp, D. E., Gilmer, W. S., Fleck, J., Straus, J. L., Dago, P. L., & Karaffa, M. (2006). Aripiprazole augmentation in treatment-resistant bipolar depression: Early response and development of akathisia. *Prog. Neuro-Psychopharmacol. Biol. Psychiatry, 31*(2): 574–577.

Kessing, L., Sondergard, L., Kvist, K., & Andersen, P. K. (2005). Suicide risk in patients treated with lithium. *Arch. Gen. Psychiatry, 62*(8): 860–866.

Kessing, L. V., Hansen, M. G., Andersen, P. K., & Angst, J. (2004). The predictive effect of episodes on the risk of recurrence in depressive and bipolar disorders-a life-long perspective. *Acta. Psychiatr. Scand., 109*(5): 339–344.

Ketter, T., Houston, J. P., Adams, D. H., Risser, R. C., Meyers, A. L., Williamson D. J., & Tohen, M. (2006). Differential efficacy of olanzapine and lithium in preventing manic or mixed recurrence in patients with bipolar I disorder based on number of previous manic or mixed episodes. *J. Clin. Psychiatry, 67*(1): 95–101.

Ketter, T. A., Wang, P. W., Chandler, R. A., Culver, J. L., & Alarcon, A. M. (2006). Adjunctive aripiprazole in treatment-resistant bipolar depression. *Ann. Clin. Psychiatry, 18*(3): 169–172.

Khanna, S., Vieta, E., Lyons, B., Grossman, F., Eerdekens, M. & Kramer, M. (2005). Risperidone in the treatment of acute mania: double-blind, placebo-controlled study. *Br. J. Psychiatry, 187*: 229–234.

Kilbourne, A. M., Cornelius, J. R., Han, X., Pincus, H. A., Shad, M., Salloum, I., Conigliaro, J., & Haas, G. L. (2004). Burden of general medical conditions among individuals with bipolar disorder. *Bipolar Disord., 6*(5): 368–373.

Kleindienst, N., Engel, R. & Greil, W. (2005). Which clinical factors predict response to prophylactic lithium? A systematic review for bipolar disorders. *Bipolar Disord., 7*(5): 404–417.

Kleindienst, N., & Greil, W. (2000). Differential efficacy of lithium and carbamazepine in the prophylaxis of bipolar disorder: results of the MAP study. *Neuropsychobiology, 42*: 2–10.

Ko, C. H., & Kong, C. K. (2001). Topiramate-induced metabolic acidosis: report of two cases. *Dev. Med. Child Neurol., 43*(10): 701–704.

Kudla, D., Lambert, M., Domin, S., Kasper, S., & Naber, D. (2007). Effectiveness, tolerability, and safety of ziprasidone in patients with schizophrenia or schizoaffective disorder: Results of a multi-centre observational trial. *Eur. Psychiatry, 22*(3): 195–202.

Kukopulos, A., Reginaldi, D., Laddomada, P., Floris, G., Serra, G., & Tondo, L. (1980). Course of the manic-depressive cycle and changes caused by treatment. Pharmakopsychiatr. *Neuropsychopharmakol., 13*(4): 156–167.

Kupfer, D., Chengappa, K. N., Hirschfeld, R. M., Goldberg, J. F., Sachs, G. S., Grochocinski, V. J., Houck, P. R., & Kolar, A. B. (2001). Citalopram as adjunctive therapy in bipolar depression. *J. Clin. Psychiatry, 62*(12): 985–990.

Kushner, S. F., Khan, A., Lane, R., & Olson, W. H. (2006). Topiramate monotherapy in the management of acute mania: results of four double-blind placebo-controlled trials. *Bipolar Disord., 8*(1): 15–27.

Lambert, P. A., & Venaud G. (1992). Comparative study of valpromide versus lithium in treatment of affective disorders. *Nervure. 5*: 57–65.

Leverich, G. S., Altshuler, L. L., Frye, M. A., Suppes, T., McElroy, S. L., Keck, P. E. Jr., Kupka, R. W., Denicoff, K. D., Nolen, W. A., Grunze, H., Martinez, M. I., & Post, R. M. (2006). Risk of switch in mood polarity to hypomania or mania in patients with bipolar depression during acute and continuation trials of venlafaxine, sertraline, and bupropion as adjuncts to mood stabilizers. *Am. J. Psychiatry, 163*(2): 232–239.

Levy, W. O, Robichaux-Keene, N. R., & Nuez, C. (2004). No significant QTc interval changes with high-dose ziprasidone: a case series. *J. Psychiatric Pract., 10*(4): 227–232.

Li, J., McCombs, J. S., & Stimmel, G. L. (2002). Cost of treating bipolar disorder in the California Medicaid (Med-Cal) program. *J. Affect. Disord. 71*(1–3): 131–139.

Lingam, R., & Scott, J. (2002). Treatment non-adherence in affective disorders. *Acta Psychiatr. Scand., 105*: 164–172.

Maj, M., Pirozzi, R., Magliano, L., & Bartoli, L. (1998). Long-term outcome of lithium prophylaxis in bipolar disorder: a 5-year prospective study of 402 patients at a lithium clinic. *Am. J. Psychiatry, 155*(1): 30–35.

McAllister-Williams, R. H. (2006). Relapse prevention in bipolar disorder: a critical review of current guidelines. *J. Psychopharmacol., 20*(Suppl 2): 12–16.

McElroy, S., & Keck, P. Jr., (2000). Pharmacological agents for the treatment of acute bipolar mania. *Biol. Psychiatry, 48*: 539–557.

McElroy, S. L., Kotwal, R., Kaneria, R., & Keck, P. E. Jr. (2006). Antidepressants and suicidal behavior in bipolar disorder. *Bipolar Disord., 8*(5 Pt 2): 596–617.

McElroy, S. L., Kotwal, R., Malhotra, S., Nelson, E. B., Keck, P. E., & Nemeroff, C. B. (2004). Are mood disorders and obesity related? A review for the mental health professional. *J. Clin. Psychiatry, 65*(5): 634–651; quiz 730.

McElroy, S. L., Suppes, T., Keck P. E., Frye M. A., Denicoff K. D., Altshuler L. L., Brown E. S., Nolen W. A., Kupka R. W., Rochussen J., Leverich G. S., & Post R. M. (2000). Open-label adjunctive topiramate in the treatment of bipolar disorders. *Biol. Psychiatry, 47*(12): 1025–1033.

McElroy, S. L., Suppes, T., Keck, P. E. Jr., Black, D., Frye, M. A., Altshuler, L. L., Nolen, W. A., Kupka, R. W., Leverich, G. S., Walden, J., Grunze, H., & Post, R. M. (2005). Open-label adjunctive zonisamide in the treatment of bipolar disorders: a prospective trial. *J. Clin. Psychiatry, 66*(5): 617–624.

McElroy, S. L., Zarate, C. A., Cookson, J., Suppes, T., Huffman, R. F., Greene, P., & Ascher, J. (2004). A 52-week, open-label continuation study of lamotrigine in the treatment of bipolar depression. *J. Clin. Psychiatry, 65*(2): 204–210.

McIntyre, R. S., Brecher, M., Paulsson, B., Huizar, K., & Mullen, J. (2005). Quetiapine or haloperidol as monotherapy for bipolar mania: a 12-week, double blind, randomized, parallel group, placebo controlled trial. *Eur. Neuropsychopharmacol., 15*(5): 573–585.

McIntyre, R., Mancini, D. A., McCann, S., Srinivasan, J., Sagman, D., & Kennedy, S. H. (2002). Topiramate versus bupropion SR when added to mood stabilizer therapy for the depressive phase of bipolar disorder: a preliminary single-blind study. *Bipolar Disord., 4*(3): 207–213.

McIntyre, R., Riccardelli, R., Binder, C., & Kusumakar, V. (2005). Open label adjunctive topiramate in the treatment of unstable bipolar disorder. *Can. J. Psychiatry, 50*(7): 415–422.

Melia, P. I. (1970). Lithium prophylaxis. *Lancet, 2*(7680): 983.

Messenheimer, J., Lynette-Mullens, E. L., Giorgi, L., & Young, F. (1998). Safety review of adult clinical trial experience with lamotrigine. *Drug Saf., 1*(4)8: 281–296.

Miklowitz, D., Otto, M. W., Frank, E., Reilly-Harrington, N. A., Wisniewski, S. R., Kogan, J. N., Nierenberg, A. A., Calabrese, J. R., Marangell L. B., Gyulai, L., Araga, M., Gonzalez, J. M., Shirely, E. R., Thase M. E., & Sachs G. S. (2007). Psychosocial treatments for bipolar depression: a 1-year randomized trial from the systemic treatment enhancement program. *Arch. Gen. Psychiatry, 64*: 419–427.

Miklowitz, D., Simoneau, T. L., George, E. L., Richards, J. A., Kalbag, A., Sachs-Ericsson, N., & Suddath, R. (2000). Family-focused treatment of bipolar disorder: 1-year effects of a psychoeducational program in conjunction with pharmacotherapy. *Biol. Psychiatry, 48*(6): 582–592.

Miklowitz, D., & Taylor, D. O. (2006). Family-focused treatment of the suicidal bipolar patient. *Bipolar Disord., 8*: 640–651.

Miklowitz, D. J., Goldstein, M. J., Nuechterlein, K. H., Snyder, K. S., & Mintz, J. (1988). Family factors and the course of bipolar affective disorder. *Arch. Gen. Psychiatry, 45*(3): 225–231.

Milev, R., Abraham, G., & Zaheer, J. (2006). Add-on quetiapine for bipolar depression: a 12-month open-label trial. *Can. J. Psychiatry, 51*(8): 523–530.

Mishory, A., Winokur, M., & Bersudsky, Y. (2003). Prophylactic effect of phenytoin in bipolar disorder: a controlled study. *Bipolar Disord., 5*(6): 464–467.

Mishory, A., Yaroslavsky, Y., Bersudsky, Y., & Belmaker, R. H. (2000). Phenytoin as an antimanic anticonvulsant: a controlled study. *Am. J. Psychiatry, 157*(3): 463–465.

Moncrieff, J. (1997). Lithium: evidence reconsidered. *Br. J. Psychiatry, 171*: 113–9.

Morriss, R., & Mohammed, F. A. (2005). Metabolism, lifestyle and bipolar affective disorder. *J. Psychopharmacol., 19*: 94–101.

Muller-Oerlinghausen, B., Berghofer, A., & Ahrens, B. (2003). The antisuicidal and mortality-reducing effect of lithium prophylaxis: consequences for guidelines in clinical psychiatry. *Can. J. Psychiatry, 48*(7): 433–439.

Muller-Oerlinghausen, B., Felber, W., Berghofer, A., Lauterbach, E., & Ahrens, B. (2005). The impact of lithium long-term medication on suicidal behavior and mortality of bipolar patients. *Arch. Suicide Res., 9*(3): 307–319.

Muller-Oerlinghausen, B., Muser-Causemann, B., & Volk, J. (1992). Suicides and parasuicides in a high-risk patient group on and off lithium long-term medication. *J. Affect. Disord., 25*(4): 261–269.

Muzina, D. J., Elhaj, O., Gajwani, P., Gao, K., & Calabrese, J. R. (2005). Lamotrigine and antiepileptic drugs as mood stabilizers in bipolar disorder. *Acta Psychiatr. Scand., 111*(Suppl 426): 21–28.

Nasrallah, A., Ketter, T. A., & Kalali, A. H. (2006). Carbamazepine and valproate for the treatment of bipolar disorder: a review of the literature. *J. Affect. Disord., 9*(1–3): 69–78.

Nemeroff, C. B., Evans, D. L., Gyulai, L., Sachs, G. S., Bowden, C. L., Gergel, I. P., Oakes, R., & Pitts, C. D. (2001). Double-blind, placebo-controlled comparison of imipramine and paroxetine in the treatment of bipolar depression. *Am. J. Psychiatry, 158*(6): 906–912.

Newcomer, J. W. (2005). Second-generation (atypical) antipsychotics and metabolic effects: a comprehensive literature review. *CNS Drugs, 19*: 1–93.

Newcomer, J. W. (2007). Metabolic consideration in the use of antipsychotic medicationis: a review of recent evidence. *J. Clin. Psychiatry, 68*(Suppl. 1): 20–27.

Newcomer, J. W., & Haupt, D. W. (2006). The metabolic effects of antipsychotic medications. *Can. J. Psychiatry, 51*(8): 480–491.

O'Connell, R. A., Mayo, J. A., Flatow, L., Cuthbertson, B., & O'Brien, B. E. (1991). Outcome of bipolar disorder on long-term treatment with lithium. *Br. J. Psychiatry, 159*: 123–129.

Pae, C. U., Lee, K. U., Kim, J. J., Lee, C. U., Bahk, W. M., Lee, S. J., Lee, C., & Paik, I. H. (2004). Switching to quetiapine in patients with acute mania who were intolerant to risperidone. *Human Psychopharmacol: Clin. Exp., 19*(1): 47–51.

Pae, C. U., Kim, T. S., Kim, J. J., Lee, S. J., Lee, C. U., Lee, C., & Paik, I. H. (2005). Long-term treatment of adjunctive quetiapine for bipolar mania. *Prog. Neuropsychopharmacol. Biol. Psychiatry, 29*: 763–766.

Peet, M. (1994). Induction of mania with selective serotonin re-uptake inhibitors and tricyclic antidepressants. *Br. J. Psychiatry, 164*: 549–550.

Perlis, R., Ostacher, M. J., Patel, J. K., Marangell, L. B., Zhang, H., Wisniewski, S. R., Ketter, T. A., Miklowitz D. J., Otto, M. W., Gyulai, L., Reilly-Harrington, N. A., Nierenberg, A. A., Sachs, G. S., & Thase M. E. (2006a). Predictors of recurrence in bipolar disorder: primary outcomes from the systematic treatment enhancement program for bipolar disorder (STEP-BD). *Am. J. Psychiatry, 163*(2): 217–224.

Perlis, R., Welge, J. A., Vornik, L. A., Hirschfeld, R. M., & Keck, P. E. Jr. (2006b). Atypical antipsychotics in the treatment of maina: a meta-analysis of randomized, placebo controlled trials. *J. Clin. Psychiatry, 67*(4): 509–516.

Philippi, H., Boor, R., & Reitter, B. (2002). Topiramate and metabolic acidosis in infants and toddlers. *Epilepsia, 43*(7): 744–7.

Pini, S., Abelli, M., & Cassano, G. B. (2006). The role of quetiapine in the treatment of bipolar disorder. *Expert Opin. Pharmacother., 7*(7): 929–940.

Post, R., Altshuler Frye, M. A., Suppes, T., McElroy, S. L., Keck, P. E. Jr., Leverich, G. S., Kupka, R., Nolen, W. A., Luckenbaugh, D. A., Walden, J., & Grunze, H. (2005). Preliminary observations on the effectiveness of levetiracetam in the open adjunctive treatment of refractory bipolar disorder. *J. Clin. Psychiatry, 66*(3): 370–374.

Post, R. M., Altshuler, L. L., Frye, M. A., Suppes, T., McElroy, S., Keck, P. E. Jr., Leverich, G. S., Kupka, R., Nolen, W. A., & Grunze, H. (2006a). New findings from the Bipolar Collaborative Network: clinical implications for therapeutics. *Curr. Psychiatry Rep., 8*(6): 489–497.

Post, R. M., Altshuler, L.L., Leverich, G. S., Frye, M. A., Nolen, W. A., Kupka, R. W., Suppes, T., McElroy, S., Keck, P. E., Denicoff, K. D., Grunze, H., Walden, J., Kitchen, C. M., & Mintz, J. (2006b). Mood switch in bipolar depression: comparison of adjunctive venlafaxine, bupropion, and sertraline. *Br. J. Psychiatry, 189*: 124–131.

Post, R. M., Leverich, G. S., Altshuler, L. L., Frye, M. A., Suppes, T. M., Keck, P. E. Jr., McElroy, S. L., Kupka, R., Nolen, W. A., Grunze, H., & Walden, J. (2003). An overview of recent findings of the Stanley Foundation Bipolar Network (Part I). *Bipolar Disord., 5*(5): 310–319.

Post, R. M., Uhde, T. W., Roy-Byrne, P. P., & Joffe, R. T. (1986). Antidepressant effects of carbamazepine. *Am. J. Psychiatry, 143*(1): 29–34.

Potkin, S., Keck, P. E. Jr., Segal, S., Ice, K. & English, P. (2005). Ziprasidone in acute bipolar mania: a 21-day randomized, doubleblind, placebo-controlled replication trial. *J. Clin. Psychopharmacol.*, *25*(4): 301–310.

Priebe, S., Wildgrube, C., & Muller-Oerlinghausen, B. (1989). Lithium prophylaxix and expressed emotion. *Br. J. Psychiatry*, *154*: 396–399.

Prien, R. F., Klett, C. J., & Caffey, E. M. Jr. (1973). Lithium carbonate and imipramine in prevention of affective episodes. A comparison in recurrent affective illness. *Arch. Gen. Psychiatry*, *29*(3): 420–425.

Rendell, J., & Geddes, G. R. (2007). Risperidone in long-term treatment for bipolar disorder. *Cochrane Database Syst. Rev.*, *1*(CD004999): 1–6.

Rendell, J. M., Gijsman, H. J., Bauer, M. S., Goodwin, G. M., & Geddes, G. R. (2006). Risperidone alone or in combination for acute mania. *Cochrane Database Syst. Rev.*, *25*(1): CD004043.

Revicki, D., Paramore, L. C., Sommerville, K. W., Swann, A. C., & Zajecka, J. M., et al. (2003). Divalproex sodium versus olanzapine in the treatment of acute mania in bipolar disorder: health-related quality of life and medical cost outcomes. *J. Clin. Psychiatry*, *64*(3): 288–294.

Revicki, D. A., Hirschfeld, R. M., Ahearn, E. P., Weisler, R. H., Palmer, C., & Keck, P. E. Jr. (2005). Effectiveness and medical costs of divalproex versus lithium in the treatment of bipolar disorder: results of a naturalistic clinical trial. *J. Affect. Disord.*, *86*(2–3): 183–93.

Rosack, J. (2005). FDA orders new warning on atypical antipsychotics. *Psychiatric News*, *40*(9): 1.

Rucci, P., Frank, E., Kostelnik, B., Fagiolini, A., Mallinger, A. G., Swartz, H. A., Thase M. E., Siegil L., Wilson D., & Kupfer D. J. (2002). Suicide attempts in patients with bipolar I disorder during acute and maintenance phases of intensive treatment with pharmacotherapy and adjunctive psychotherapy. *Am. J. Psychiatry*, *159*(7): 1160–1164.

Sachs, G. S., Nierenberg, A.A., Calabrese, J., R., Marangell, L. B., Wisniewski, S. R., Gyulai, L., Friedman, E. S., Bowden, C. L., Fossey, M. D., Ostacher, M. J., Ketter, T. A., Patel, J., Hauser, P., Rapport, D., Martinez, J. M., Allen, M. H., Miklowitz, D. J., Otto, M. W., Dennehy, E. B., & Thase, M, E. (2007). Effectiveness of adjunctive antidepressant treatment for bipolar depression. *N. Engl. J. Med.*, *356*(17): 1711–1722.

Sachs, G. (2003). Unmet clinical needs in bipolar disorder. *J. Clin. Psychopharmacol.*, *23*(Suppl 1): S2–S8.

Sachs, G., Bowden, C., calabrese, J. R., Ketter, T., Thompson, T., White, R., & Bently, B. (2006). Effects of lamotrigine and lithium on body weight during maintenance treatment of bipolar I disorder. *Bipolar Disord.*, *8*(2): 175–181.

Sachs, G., Chengappa, K. N., Suppes, T., Mullen, J. A., Brecher, M., Devine, N. A., & Sweitzer, D. E. (2004). Quetiapine with lithium or divalproex for the treatment of bipolar mania: a randomized, double-blind, placebo-controlled study. *Bipolar Disord.*, *6*(3): 213–223.

Sachs, G., Sanchez, R., Marcus, R., Stock, E., McQuade, R., Carson W., Abou-Gharbia, N., Impellizzeri, C., Kaplita, S., Rollin, L., & Iwamoto, T. (2006). Aripiprazole in the treatment of acute manic or mixed episodes in patients with bipolar I disorder: a 3-week placebo-controlled study. *J. Psychopharmacol.*, *20*(4): 536–546.

Sachs, G. S., Lafer, B., Stoll, A. L., Banov, M., Thibault, A. B., Tohen, M., & Rosenbaum, J. F. (1994). A double-blind trial of bupropion versus desipramine for bipolar depression. *J. Clin. Psychiatry*, 55(9): 391–393.

Sachs, U. S., & Thase, M. E. (2000). Bipolar disorder therapeutics: maintenance treatment. *Biol. Psychiatry*, 48: 573–581.

Sajatovic, M., Davies, M., & Hrouda, D. R. (2004). Enhancement of treatment adherence among patients with bipolar disorder. *Psychiatr. Serv.*, 55(3): 264–269.

Saksa, J. R., Baker, C. B., & Woods, S. W. (2004). Mood-stabilizer-maintained, remitted bipolar patients: taper and discontinuation of adjunctive antipsychotic medication. *Gen. Hosp. Psychiatry*, 26(3): 233–236.

Sanger, T. M., Tohen, M., Vieta, E., Dunner, D. L., Bowden, C. L., Calabrese, J. R., Feldman, P. D., Jacobs, T. G., & Breier, A. (2003). Olanzapine in the acute treatment of bipolar I disorder with a history of rapid cycling. *J. Affect. Disord.*, 73(1–2): 155–161.

Schaffer, L. C., Schaffer, C. B., & Howe, J. (2002). An open case series on the utility of tiagabine as an augmentation in refractory bipolar outpatients. *J. Affect. Disord.*, 71(1–3): 259–263.

Schurhoff, F., Bellivier, F., Jouvent, R., Mouren-Simeoni, M. C., Bouvard, M., Allilaire, J. F., & Leboyer, M. (2000). Early and late onset bipolar disorders: two different forms of manicdepressive illness. *J. Affect. Disord.*, 58(3): 215–221.

Scott, J., & Pope, M. (2002). Self-reported adherence to treatment with mood stabilizers, plasma levels, and psychiatric hospitalization. *Am. J. Psychiatry*, 159: 1927–1929.

Severus, W. E., Kleindienst, N., & Greil, W. (2006). Re-evaluation of randomized controlled trials of lithium monotherapy. *Bipolar Disord.*, 8(5 Pt 1): 519–520; author reply 521.

Sharma, V., Persad, E., Mazmanian, D., & Karunaratne, K. (1993). Treatment of rapid cycling bipolar disorder with combination therapy of valproate and lithium. *Can. J. Psychiatry*, 38(2): 137–139.

Shelton, R. C., & Stahl, S. M. (2004). Risperidone and paroxetine given singly and in combination for bipolar depression. *J. Clin. Psychiatry*, 65: 1715–1719.

Sokolski, K. N., (2007). Adjunctive aripiprazole in bipolar I depression. *Ann. Pharmacother.*, 41(1): 35–40.

Solomon, D. A., Ryan, C. E., Keithner, G. I., Miller, I. W., Shea, M. T., Kazim, A., & Keller, M. B. (1997). A pilot study of lithium carbonate plus divalproex sodium for the continuation and maintenance treatment of patients with bipolar I disorder. *J. Clin. Psychiatry*, 58(3): 95–99.

Stoll, A. L., Severus, W. E., Freeman, M. P., Rueter, S., Zboyan, H. A., Diamond, E., Cress, K. K., & Marangell, L. B. (1999). Omega 3 fatty acids in bipolar disorder: A preliminary double-blind, placebo-controlled trial. *Arch. Gen. Psychiatry*, 56(5): 407–412.

Stowe, C. D., Bollinger, T., James, L. P., Haley, T. M., Griebel, M. L., & Farraf, H. C. 3rd. (2000). Acute mental status changes and hyperchloremic metabolic acidosis with long-term topiramate therapy. *Pharmacotherapy*, 20(1): 105–109.

Strober, M., Morrell, W., Lampert, C. & Burroughs, J. (1990). Relapse following discontinuation of lithium maintenance therapy in adolescents with bipolar I illness: a naturalistic study. *Am. J. Psychiatry*, 147(4): 457–461.

Sumiyoshi, T., Roy, A., Anil, A. E., Jayathilake, K., Erthugrul, A., & Meltzer, H. Y. (2004). A comparison of incidence of diabetes mellitus between atypical antipsychotic drugs: a survey for clozapine, risperidone, olanzapine, and quetiapine. *J. Clin. Psychopharmacol., 24*(3): 345–348.

Suppes, T., Baldessarini, R. J., Faedda, G. L., & Tohen, M. (1991). Risk of recurrence following discontinuation of lithium treatment in bipolar disorder. *Arch. Gen. Psychiatry, 48*(12): 1082–1088.

Suppes, T., Chisholm Dhavale, D., Frye, M. A., Altshuler, L. L., McElroy, S. L., Keck, P. E., Nolen, W. A., Kupka, R., Denicoff, K. D., Leverich, G. S., Rush, A. J., & Post, R. M. (2002). Tiagabine in treatment refractory bipolar disorder: a clinical case series. *Bipolar Disord., 4*(5): 283–289.

Suppes, T., Dennehy, E. B., Hirschfeld, R. M., Altshuler, L. L., Bowden, C. L., Calabrese, J. R., Crismon, M. L., Ketter, T. A., Sachs, G. S., & Swann, A. C. (2005). The Texas implementation of medication algorithms: update to the algorithms for treatment of bipolar I disorder. *J. Clin. Psychiatry, 66*(7): 870–886.

Suppes, T., Hirschfeld, R. M., Vieta, E., Raines, S., & Paulsson, B. (2007). Quetiapine for the treatemtn of bipolar II depression: analysis of data from two randomized, double-blind, placebo-controlled studies. *World J. Biol. Psychiarty, 11*: 1–14.

Suppes, T., McElroy, S. L., Gilbert, J., Dessain, E. C., & Cole, J. O. (1992). Clozapine in the treatment of dysphoric mania. *Biol. Psychiatry, 32*(3): 270–280.

Suppes, T., Mintz, J., McElroy, S. L., Altshuler, L. L., Kupka, R. W., Frye P. E. Jr., Nolen, W. A., Leverich, G. S., Grunze, H., Rush, A. J., & Pos,t R. M. (2005). Mixed hypomania in 908 patients with bipolar disorder evaluated prospectively in the Stanley Foundation Bipolar Treatment Network: a sex-specific phenomenon. *Arch. Gen. Psychiatry, 62*(10): 1089–1096.

Suppes, T., Ozcan, M. E., & Carmody, T. (2004). Response to clozapine of rapid cycling versus non-cycling patients with a history of mania. *Bipolar Disord., 6*(4): 329–332.

Suppes, T., Phillips, K. A., & Judd, C. R. (1994). Clozapine treatment of nonpsychotic rapid cycling bipolar disorder: a report of three cases. *Biol. Psychiatry, 36*(5): 338–340.

Suppes, T., Webb, A., Paul, B., Carmody, T., Kraemer, H., & Rush, A. J. (1999). Clinical outcome in a randomized 1-year trial of clozapine versus treatment as usual for patients with treatment-resistant illness and a history of mania. *Am. J. Psychiatry, 156*(8): 1164–1169.

Suppes, T., Kelly, D. I., Hynan, L. S., Snow, D. E., Sureddi, S., Foster, B., & Curley, E. (2007). Comparison of two anticonvulsants in a randomized, single-blind treatment of hypomanic symptoms in patients with bipolar disorder. *Aust. N Z J. Psychiatry, 41*(5): 397–402.

Suppes, T., Liu, S., Brecher, M., Paulsson, B., & Lazarus, A. (2008): Maintenance treatment in bipolar I disorder with quetiapine comcomitant with lithium/divalproex: A placebo controlled randomized multicentre trial. *Bipolar Disord., 10*(Suppl 1): 40.

Sussman, N. (2003). The implications of weight changes with antipsychotic treatment. *J. Clin. Psychopharmacol., 23*(Suppl 1): S21–S26.

Svarstad, B., Shireman, T. I., & Sweeney, J. K. (2001). Using drug claims data to assess the relationship of medication adherence with hospitalization and costs. *Psychiatric Serv., 52*(6): 805–811.

Swann, A. (2005). Long-term treatment in bipolar disorder. *J. Clin. Psychiatry,* 66(Suppl 1): 7–12.

Swann, A. C., Bowden, C. L., Calabrese, J. R., Dilsaver, S. C., & Morris, D. D. (2000). Mania: differential effects of previous depressive and manic episodes on response to treatment. *Acta Psychiatr. Scand.,* 101(6): 444–451.

Swann, A. C., Bowden, C. L., Clalbrese, J. R., Dilsaver, S. C., & Morris, D. D. (2002). Pattern of response to divalproex, lithium, or placebo in four naturalistic subtypes of mania. *Neuropsychopharmacology,* 26(4): 530–536.

Swann, A. C., Bowden, C. L., Morris, D., Calabrese, J. R., Petty, F., Small, J., Dilsaver S. C., & Davis J. M. (1997). Depression during mania. Treatment response to lithium or divalproex. *Arch. Gen. Psychiatry,* 54(1): 37–42.

Takeoka, M., Holmes, G. L., Thiele, E., Bourgeois, B. F., Helmers, S. L., Duffy, F. H., & Riviello, J. J. (2001). Topiramate and metabolic acidosis in pediatric epilepsy. *Epilepsia,* 42(3): 387–392.

Thase, M. E., Macfadden, W., Weisler, R. H., Chang, W., Paulsson, B., Khan, A., & Calabrese, J. R. (2006). Efficacy of quetiapine monotherapy in bipolar I and II depression: a double-blind, placebo-controlled study (the BOLDER II study). *J. Clin. Psychopharmacol,* 26(6): 600–609.

Thies-Flechtner, K., Muller-Oerlinghausen, B., Seibert, W., Walther, A., & Greil, W. (1996). Effect of prophylactic treatment on suicide risk in patients with major affective disorders. *Pharmacopsychiatry,* 29(3): 103–107.

Thompson, J. M., Gallagher, P., Hughes, J. H., Watson, S., Gray, J. M., Ferrier, I. N., & Young, A. H. (2005). Neurocognitive impairment in euthymic patients with bipolar affective disorder. *Br. J. Psychiatry,* 186: 32–40.

Tohen, M., Baker, R. W., Altshuler, L. L., Zarate, C. A., Suppes, T., Ketter, T. A., Milton, D. R., Risser, R., Gilmore, J. A., Breier, A., & Tollefson, G. A. (2002a). Olanzapine versus divalproex in the treatment of acute mania. *Am. J. Psychiatry,* 159(6): 1011–1017.

Tohen, M., Bowden, C. L., Calabrese, J. R., Lin, D., Forrester, T. D., Sachs, G. S., Koukopoulos, A., Yatham, L., & Grunze, H. (2006a). Influence of sub-syndromal symptoms after remission from manic or mixed episodes. *Br. J. Psychiatry,* 189: 515–519.

Tohen, M., Calabrese, J. R., Sachs, G. S., Banov, M. D., Detke, H. C., Risser, R., Baker, R. W., Chou, J. C., & Bowden, C. L. (2006b). Randomized, placebo-controlled trial of olanzapine as maintenance therapy in patients with bipolar I disorder responding to acute treatment with olanzapine. *Am. J. Psychiatry,* 163(2): 247–256.

Tohen, M., Chengappa, K. N., Suppes, T., Zarate, C. A. Jr., Calabrese, J. R., Bowden, C. L., Sachs, G. S., Kupfer, D. J., Baler, R. W., Risser, R. C., Ketter, E. L., Feldman, P. D., Tollefson, G. D., & Breier, A. (2002b). Efficacy of olanzapine in combination with valproate or lithium in the treatment of mania in patients partially nonresponsive to valproate or lithium monotherapy. *Arch. Gen. Psychiatry,* 59(1): 62–69.

Tohen, M., Chengappa, K. N., Suppes, T., Baker, R. W., Zarate, C. A., Bowden, C. L., Sachs, G. S., Kupfer, D. J., Ghaemi, S. N., Feldman, P. D., Risser, R. C., Evans, A. R., & Calabrese, J. R. (2004). Relapse prevention in bipolar I disorder: 18 month comparison of olanzapine plus mood stabiliser versus mood stabiliser alone. *Br. J. Psychiatry,* 184: 337–345.

Tohen, M., Greil, W., Calabrese, J. R., Sachs, G. S., yatham, L. N., Oerlinghausen, B. M., Koukopoulos, A., Cassano, G. B., Grunze, H., Licht, R. W., Dell'Osso, L., Evans, A. R., Risser, R., Baker, R. W., Crane, H., Dossenbauch, M. R., & Bowden, C. L., et al. (2005). Olanzapine versus lithium in the maintenance treatment of bipolar disorder: a 12-month, randomized, double-blind, controlled clinical trial. *Am. J. Psychiatry, 162*(7): 1281–1290.

Tohen, M., Jacobs, T. G., Grundy, S. L., McElroy, S. L., Banov, M. C., Janicak, P. G., Sanger, T., Risser, R., Zhang, F., Toma, V., Francis, J., Tollefson, G. D. & Breier, A. (2000). Efficacy of olanzapine in acute bipolar mania; a double-blind placebo controlled study. The olanzipine HGGW study group. *Arch. Gen. Pscyhiatry, 57*(9): 841–849.

Tohen, M., Ketter, T. A., Zarate, C. A., Suppes, T., Frye, M., Altshuler, L., Zajecka, J., Schuh, L. M., Risser, R. C., Brown, E., & Baker, R. W. (2003). Olanzapine versus divalproex sodium for the treatment of acute mania and maintenance of remission:a 47-week study. *Am. J. Psychiatry, 160*(7): 1263–1271.

Tohen, M., Greil, W., Calabrese, J. R., Sachs, G. S., Yatham, L. N., Oerlinghausen B. M., Koukopoulos, A., Cassano, G. B., Grunze, H., Licht, R. W., Dell'Osso, L., Evans, A. R., Risser, R., Baker, R. W., Crane, H., Dossenbauch, M. R., & Bowden, C. L. (2005). Olanzapine versus lithium in the maintenance treatment of bipolar disorder: a 12-month, randomized double-blind, controlled trail. *Am. J. Psychiatry, 162*(7): *1281-1290.*

Tohen, M., Sanger, T. M., McElroy, S. L., Tollefson, G. D., Chengappa, K. N., Daniel, D. G., Petty, F., Centorrino, F., Wang, R., Grundy, S. L., Greaney, M. G., Jacobs, T. G., David, S. R., & Toma, V. (1999). Olanzapine versus placebo in the treatment of acute mania.Olanzapine HGEH study group. *Am. J. Psychiatry, 156*(5): 702–709.

Tohen, M., Vieta, E., Calabrese, J. R., Ketter, T. A., Sachs, G., Bowden, C., Mitchell, P. B., Centorrino, F., Risser, R., Baker, R. W., Evans, A. R., Beymer, K., Dube, S., Tollefson, G. D., & Breier, A. (2003). Efficacy of olanzapine and olanzapine-fluoxetine combination in the treatment of bipolar I depression. *Arch. Gen. Psychiatry, 60*(11): 1079–1088.

Tohen, M., Zarate, C. A. Jr., Hennen, J., Khalsa, H. M., Strakowski, S. M., Gebre-Medhin, P., Salvatore, P., & Baldessarini, R. J. (2003b). The McLean-Harvard First-Episode Mania Study: prediction of recovery and first recurrence. *Am. J. Psychiatry, 160*(12): 2099–2107.

Tondo, L., Hennen, J., & Baldessarini, R. J. (2001). Lower suicide risk with long-term lithium treatment in major affective illness: a meta-analysis. *Acta Psychiatr. Scand., 104*(3): 163–172.

Tondo, L., Jamison, K. R., & Baldessarini, J. R. (1997). Effect of lithium maintenance on suicidal behavior in major mood disorders. *Ann. N Y Acad. Sci., 836*: 339–351.

Vaidya, N., Mahableshwarkar, A. R., & Shahid, R. (2003). Continuation and maintenance ECT in treatment-resistant bipolar disorder. *J. ECT, 19*(1): 10–16.

Vieta, E. (2005a). Improving treatment adherence in bipolar disorder through psychoeducation. *J. Clin. Psychiatry, 66*(Suppl 1): 24–29.

Vieta, E. (2005b). Mood stabilization in the treatment of bipolar disorder: focus on quetiapine. *Hum. Psychopharmacol., 20*(4): 225–236.

Vieta, E., Bourin, Sanchez, R., Marcus, R., Stock, E., McQuade, R., Carson, W., Abou-Gharbia, N., Swanink, R., & Iwamoto, T. (2005). Effectiveness of aripiprazole v. haloperidol in acute bipolar mania: double-blind, randomised, comparative 12-week trial. *Br. J. Psychiatry, 187*: 235–242.

Vieta, E., & Colom, F. (2004). Psychological interventions in bipolar disorder: From wishful thinking to an evidence-based approach. *Acta Psychiatr. Scand. Suppl.* 422: 34–38.

Vieta, E., Gasto, C., Colom, F., Reinares, M., Martinez-Aran, A., Benabarre, A., & Akiskal, H. S. (2001a). Role of risperidone in bipolar II: an open 6-month study. *J. Affect. Disord., 67*(1–3): 213–219.

Vieta, E., Manuel Goikolea, J., Martinez-Aran, A., Comes, M., Verger, K., Masramon, X., Sanchez-Moreno, J., & Colom, F. (2006). Double-blind, randomized, placebo-controlled, prophylaxis study of adjunctive gabapentin for bipolar disorder. *J. Clin. Psychiatry, 67*(3): 473–477.

Vieta, E., & Goikolea, J. M. (2005). Atypical antipsychotics: newer options for mania and maintenance therapy. *Bipolar Disord., 7*(Suppl 4): 21–33.

Vieta, E., Goikolea, J. M., Corbella, B., Benabarre, A., Reinares, M., Martinez, G., Fernadez, A., Colom, F., Martinez-Aran, A., & Torrent, C. (2001b). Risperidone safety and efficacy in the treatment of bipolar and schizoaffective disorders: results from a 6-month, multicenter, open study. *J. Clin. Psychiatry, 62*(10): 818–825.

Vieta, E., Herraiz, M., Fernadez, A., Gasto, C., Benabarre, A., Colom, F., Martinez-Aran, A., & Reinares, M. (2001c). Efficacy and safety of risperidone in the treatment of schizoaffective disorder: initial results from a large, multicenter surveillance study. Group for the Study of Risperidone in Affective Disorders (GSRAD). *J. Clin. Psychiatry, 62*(8): 623–630.

Vieta, E., Manuel Goikolea, J., Martinez-Aran, A., Comes, M., Masramon, X., Sanchez-Moreno, J., & Colom, F. (2006). A double-blind, randomized, placebo-controlled, prophylaxis study of adjunctive gabapentin for bipolar disorder. *J. Clin. Psychiatry, 67*(3): 473–477.

Vieta, E., Parramon, G., Padrell, E., Nieto, E., Martinez-Aran, A., Corbella, B., Colom, F., Reinares, M., Goikolea, J. M., & Torrent, C. (2002). Quetiapine in the treatment of rapid cycling bipolar disorder. *Bipolar Disord., 4*(5): 335–340.

Vieta, E., Reinares, M., Corbella, B., Benabarre, A., Gilaberte, I., Colom, F., Martinez-Aran, A., Gasto, C., & Tohen, (2001d). Olanzapine as long-term adjunctive therapy in treatment-resistant bipolar disorder. *J. Clin. Psychopharmacol., 21*(5): 469–473.

Vieta, E., Eggens, I., Persson, I., Paulsson, B., & Brecher, M. (2008). Efficacy and safety of quetiapine in combination with lithium/divalproex as maintenance treatment for bipolar I disorders. *Bipolar Disord., 10*(Suppl 1): 57.

Waddington, D., & McKenzie, I. P. (1994). Overdose rates in lithium-treated versus antidepressant-treated outpatients. *Acta Psychiatr. Scand., 90*(1): 50–52.

Watson, W. A., Litovitz, T. L., Klein-Schwartz, W., Rodgers, G. C. Jr., Youniss, J., Reid, N., Rouse, W. G., Rembert, R. S., & Borys, D. (2004). 2003 annual report of the American Association of Poison Control Centers Toxic Exposure Surveillance System. *Am. J. Emerg. Med., 22*(5): 335–404.

Weisler, R., Hirschfeld, R., Culter, A. J., Gazada, T., Ketter, T. A., Keck, P. E., Swann, A., & Kalali, A. (2006). Extended-release carbamazepine capsules as monotherapy in bipolar disorder: pooled results from two randomised, double-blind, placebo-controlled trials. *CNS Drugs, 20*(3): 219–231.

Weisler, R., Keck, P. E. Jr., Swann, A. C., Culter, A. J., Ketter, T. A., & Kalalia, A. H. (2005). Extended-release carbamazepine capsules as monotherapy for acute mania in bipolar disorder: a multicenter, randomized, double-blind, placebo-controlled trial. *J. Clin. Psychiatry, 66*(3): 323–330.

Wilner, A., Raymond, K., & Pollard, R. (1999). Topiramate and metabolic acidosis. *Epilepsia, 40*(6): 792–795.

Winsberg, M. E., DeGolia, S. G., Strong, C. M., & Ketter, T. A. (2001). Divalproex therapy in medication-naive and mood-stabilizer-naive bipolar II depression. *J. Affect. Disord., 67*(1–3): 207–212.

Wong, I., Mawer, G. E., & Sander, J. W. (1999). Factors influencing the incidence of lamotrigine-related skin rash. *Ann. Pharmacother., 33*(10): 1037–1042.

Worthington, J., J. 3rd., Kinrys, G., Wygant, L. E., & Pollack, M. H. (2005). Aripiprazole as an augmentor of selective serotonin reuptake inhibitors in depression and anxiety disorder patients. *Int. Clin. Psychopharmacol., 20*(1): 9–11.

Yatham, L. (2002). The role of novel antipsychotics in bipolar disorders. *J. Clin. Psychiatry, 63*(Suppl 3): 10–14.

Yatham, L. (2005). Atypical antipsychotics for bipolar disorder. *Psychiatr. Clin. North Am., 28*: 325–347.

Yatham, L. N. (2004). Newer anticonvulsants in the treatment of bipolar disorder. *J. Clin. Psychiatry, 65*(Suppl 10): 28–35.

Yatham, L. N., Binder, C., Riccardelli, R., Leblanc, J., Connolly, M., & Kusumakar, V. (2003). Risperidone in acute and continuation treatment of mania. *Int. Clin. Psychopharmacol., 18*(4): 227–235.

Yatham, L. N., Kennedy, S. H., O'donovan, C., Parikh, S., MacQueen, G., McIntyre, R., Sharma, V., Silverston, P., Alda, M., Baruch, P., Beaulieu, S., Daigneault, A., Milev, R., Young, L. T. Ravindran, A., Schaffer, A., Connolly, M., & Gorman, C. P. (2005). Canadian Network for Mood and Anxiety Treatments (CANMAT) guidelines for the management of patients with bipolar disorder: consensus and controversies. *Bipolar Disord., 7*(Suppl 3): 5–69.

Yatham, L. N., Kennedy, S. H. et al. (2005). Canadian Network for Mood and Anxiety Treatments (CANMAT) guidelines for the management of patients with bipolar disorder: consensus and controversies. *Bipolar Disord, 7*: 5–69.

Yatham, L. N. (2004). Newer anticonvulsants in the treatment of bipolar disorder. *J. Clin. Psychiatry, 65* (Suppl 10): 28–35.

Yatham, L. N. (2008). Current maintenance treatments for bipolar disorder. Presented at a Janssen-Ortho, Inc., satellite symposium, "Long term management of bipolar disorder". XVII CINP. Munich.

Yildiz, A., & Sachs, G. (2003). Do antidepressants induce rapid cycling? A gender-specific association. *J. Clin. Psychiatry, 64*: 814–818.

Young, R. C., Biggs, J. T., Ziegler, V. E., & Meyer, D. A. (1978). A rating scale for mania: reliability, validity and sensitivity. *Br. J. Psychiatry, 133*(5): 429–435.

Yumru, M., Savas, H. A., Kurt, E., Kaya, M. C., Selek, S., Savas, E., Oral, E. T., & Atagum, I. (2007). Atypical antipsychotics related metabolic syndrome in bipolar patients. *J. Affect. Disord., 98*(3): 247–252.

Zarate, C. A. Jr., Quiroz, J. A., Singh, J. B., Denicoff, K. D., De Jesus, G., Luckenbaugh, D. A., Charney, D. S., & Manji, H. K. (2005). An open-label trial of the glutamate-modulating agent riluzole in combination with lithium for the treatment of bipolar depression. *Biol. Psychiatry, 57*(4): 430–432.

Zarate, C. A., Jr., Rothschild, A., Fletcher, K. E., Mardrid, A., & Zapatel, J. (2000). Clinical predictors of acute response with quetiapine in psychotic mood disorders. *J. Clin. Psychiatry, 61*(3): 185–189.

Zarate, C. A. Jr., Rothschild, A., Fletcher, K. E., Mardrid, A., & Zapatel, J. (2000). Clinical predictors of acute response with quetiapine in psychotic mood disorders. *J. Clin. Psychiatry, 61*(3): 185–189.

Zarate, C. A. Jr., Tohen, M., banov, M. D., Weiss, M. K., & Cole, J. O. (1995). Is clozapine a mood stabilizer? *J. Clin. Psychiatry, 56*(3): 108–112.

Zornberg, G. L., & Pope, H. G. Jr. (1993). Treatment of depression in bipolar disorder: new directions for research. *J. Clin. Psychopharmacol., 13*(6): 397–408.

chapter six

Bipolar disorders in women: Special issues

Valerie H. Taylor
St. Joseph's Centre for Mountain Health Services

Meir Steiner
McMaster University
St. Joseph's Hospital

Claudio N. Soares
McMaster University

Contents

Introduction 154
Bipolar disorder across the female reproductive cycle............................ 155
    Menarche.. 155
    Menstrual cycle 156
Treatment strategies for menstrual related mood changes..................... 158
    Oral contraceptive pills... 158
    Mood stabilizers.. 159
Pregnancy 160
Treatment strategies during pregnancy 162
    Foundations for effective management...162
Pharmacotherapy during pregnancy and the postpartum 163
    Lithium... 163
        Clinical management 164
    Carbamazipine 164
        Clinical management... 165
    Valproate 165
        Clinical management... 166

Lamotrigine...167
    Clinical management..167
Antidepressants... 168
Menopause.. 168
Treatment strategies for menopausal related mood changes................. 169
Future directions 170
Summary... 170
References.. 171

Introduction

Gender plays a significant role in the development of major depression, a fact evidenced by lifetime prevalence rates as high as 21% in women compared with 12.7% in men (Kessler et al., 1994; Alonso et al., 2004). Although the diagnostic criteria for depression are the same for both sexes, women with depression more frequently experience guilt, anxiety, increased sleep, weight gain and comorbid eating disorders. In addition, women with bipolar disorder spend more symptomatic time in the depressive state compared to men with the same diagnosis (Perugi et al., 1990). The role of gender in bipolar disorder has not been studied to the same extent as has gender in other chronic mental illnesses (Leibenluft, 1996; Hendrick et al., 2000, 2003; Blehar et al., 1998; Weissman et al., 1988) but there are some specific features of bipolar disorder in women that set them apart from other patient populations. Women have a higher incidence of bipolar II disorder with lifetime prevalence rates ranging from 5% to 10% (Angst & Gamma, 2002; Tondo & Baldessarini, 1998); women also present with a higher incidence of rapid cycling episodes, mixed states and antidepressant-induced mania (Coryell, Endicott, & Keller, 1992; Swann, 2005; Burt & Rasgon, 2004; Taylor & Abrams, 1981; McElroy et al., 1995). Gender differences in patterns of substance abuse have also been described with both higher prevalence rates of alcoholism in women with bipolar disorder as compared to women without bipolar (Frye et al., 2003), and an increased amount of time spent in a depressed state among female alcoholics with bipolar disorder (Salloum et al., 2001). The presence of medical co-morbidities such as obesity, migraine and thyroid dysfunctions are also common in this population (Kuijpens et al., 2001) and clinicians should be aware of such vulnerabilities when contemplating treatment strategies. There is also evidence that in at least some women, hormonal changes associated with reproductive cyclicity may trigger mood episodes that further introduces multifactorial complexities in diagnosis and management.

Bipolar disorder across the female reproductive cycle

Menarche

Accumulated evidence has shown that approximately twice as many adult women are depressed as adult men (Weissman & Klerman, 1977; Nolen-Hoeksema, 1987; Weissman et al., 1984). In contrast, preadolescent boys are more likely to be depressed than preadolescent girls in both clinical samples (Kashani et al., 1982) and in the general population (Anderson et al., 1987; Rutter, 1986). Rates of depression seem to rise in girls during the transition into puberty (Ge et al., 1994; Petersen, Sarigiani & Kennedy, 1991) and it appears that sometime in adolescence a "switch" occurs and at least twice as many girls are depressed as boys. Data suggests that the onset of puberty, rather than chronological age, is linked to the increase in rates of depression in women (Angold, Costello, & Worthman, 1998) and that changes in the reproductive hormonal milieu play a role in the onset of affective disorders in women (Steiner, Born & Marton, 2000). Bipolar disorder is also an illness with a usual age of onset during the reproductive years and has an adolescent prevalence rate of approximately 1.0% (Lewinsohn, Klein & Seeley, 1995). Although there has been no identified gender difference in the prevalence of this illness, most studies on adolescents with major depression report rates of subsequent mania or hypomania that range from 19% to 49%, depending on illness severity and duration of follow up (Geller et al., 2001; Kovacs, 1996; Rao et al., 1995; Strober & Carlson, 1982). Given that in adult unipolar patients, women have been shown to be over represented in a cohort switching from unipolar depression to bipolar I or bipolar II, at rates of nearly 60% and 69%, respectively (Akiskal et al., 1995), the adolescent period may in fact be one of increased vulnerability for females with bipolar disorders. This theory is supported by recent work examining the impact of female reproductive hormones on the course of bipolar disorder. In this study, the onset of the illness occurred before menarche in 32% of women (Freeman et al., 2002). A study by Joffe et al. (2006b) also examined the association between menarche, menstrual dysfunction and bipolar disorder and concluded that women with bipolar disorder report early-onset menstrual dysfunction more often than healthy controls and women with unipolar depression. Further analysis of these data showed that women with bipolar disorder were 3.2 times more likely to report experiencing their first episode of illness prior to or within 5 years after menarche (Labad, Urretavizcaya & Crespo, 2006). This finding is consistent with the work of Lish and colleagues who observed that the peak age for symptom onset of bipolar disorder was adolescence. They also noted that while treatment was associated with less negative life events, 50% of study patients received no assistance for at least 5 years. This delay in receiving care was greatest when symptoms began in adolescence and was highest for females (Lish et al., 1994).

Menstrual cycle

There is accumulating evidence that some reproductive related hormonal changes in females may increase the risk of affective illness. This is most apparent in the association between menstrual cycle phase and mood, which may ultimately constitute the bases for the syndrome of premenstrual dysphoric disorder (PMDD) (American Psychiatric Association, 1994). Women with PMDD appear to be at higher risk for depression and other mood disorders (Yonkers, 1997) and alternatively, women with mood disorders may be more vulnerable to experience novel/emerging mood symptoms premenstrually (Endicott, 1993; Roy-Byrne et al., 1986; Rasgon et al., 2003). Reproductive hormones modulate various hormonal, neurotransmitter, and biologic clock systems, all of which have been implicated in the pathophysiology of affective disorders (Steiner, Dunn & Born, 2003). Gonadal steroids can modulate the central activity of serotonin, norepinephrine and gamma-amino butyric acid (Barnes & Mitchell, 2005) and it has been postulated that the fluctuations in estrogen and progesterone which occur during the female reproductive cycle play a role in the exacerbation of symptoms in a subset of women with bipolar disorder (Hendrick, Altshuler & Burt, 1996). This is supported by studies that have found an increase in suicide rates, increased severity of suicidal intent and increased rates of psychiatric hospitalization in woman with bipolar disorder during the premenstrual and menstrual phase of the cycle (Diamond et al., 1976; Rasgon et al., 2003; Blehar et al., 1998).

The relationship between the reproductive-endocrine system and bipolar illness in women is poorly defined and studies examining bipolar disorder and the menstrual cycle are far from definitive. Two retrospective studies reported that women with rapid-cycling bipolar disorder were morel likely to endorse premenstrual worsening (Diamond et al., 1976; Price & DiMarzio, 1986); and one case report describe a patient with bipolar II disorder who experienced monthly shifts in mood (Hendrick & Altshuler, 1998). While the over-representation in woman of rapid-cycling bipolar disorder has led to the hypothesis that alterations in female reproductive hormones may be in part responsible for this illness (Rasgon et al., 2003), prospective studies have not supported this association (Leibenluft et al., 1999; Wehr et al., 1988). Data on non-rapid cycling bipolar disorder is also mixed and while early reports suggest an association between mood and menstrual cycles (Luggin et al., 1984; Blehar et al., 1998; Endo et al., 1978) other studies have not found such association (Schmidt et al, 1990; Wehr et al., 1988).

The role of menstrual dysfunction in the clinical course and subsequent biological treatment of bipolar disorder is becoming an area of clinical focus and research interest. Menstrual dysfunction occurs in approximately 15–20% of the general population (Rowland et al., 2002; Singh, 1981; Bachmann & Kemmann, 1982) and the results of several small studies have documented rates in excess in this in women with affective illnesses (Rowland et al., 2002; McIntyre et al., 2003; O'Donovan et al., 2002; Rasgon et al., 2000; Bisaga et al., 2002).

While problems with menstrual dysfunction are not ubiquitous in women with bipolar disorder, it may be that this phenomenon represents a trait marker of hypothalamic-pituitary-gonadal (HPG) axis dysregulation in certain populations. This is supported by results of a study by Rasgon and colleagues that investigated the impact of the menstrual cycle on mood in women with bipolar disorder. In this study of 17 outpatients, significant mood changes were noted in relation to menstrual cycle phase, as well as a high rate of longer cycles (Rasgon et al., 2003). These finding replicate those of Leibenluft et al. (1999) who assessed prospectively mood changes in women with rapid-cycling bipolar disorder and found statistically significant relationships across all phases of the menstrual cycle with a variety of mood states.

Identification of menstrual irregularities is particularly relevant in women with bipolar disorder. If this phenomenon is present prior to initiation of treatment but is not identified it can in some instances erroneously contribute to patient noncompliance. For example, menstrual disturbances —including amenorrhea and oligomenorrhea—have been reported as a side effect of divalproex therapy, a drug used in the treatment of bipolar disorder (Rattya et al., 2001; Isojarvi et al., 1993; O'Donovan et al., 2002; Akdeniz et al., 2003). The primary research on divalproex has been done in a cross-sectional study of 238 women with epilepsy; and it documented a high prevalence of polycystic ovaries (43%) and menstrual disturbances in women receiving divalproex as compared with women treated with other anti convulsants (Isojarvi et al., 1993). These findings were replicated in a population-based study in which higher rates of menstrual disturbances and polycystic ovary syndrome (PCOS) were reported in women with bipolar disorder currently receiving divalproex (O'Donovan et al., 2002). A possible relationship between affective disorders and PCOS irrespective of treatment has also been suggested and is supported by work done by Matsunaga and Sarai (1993) who reported elevated serum luteinizing hormone levels and androgens in women with either a mood disorder or atypical psychosis who had never received divalproex treatment. Even without a link to PCOS, menstrual abnormalities in women with bipolar disorder may be a marker of metabolic abnormalities, including a predictor of increased risk for non-insulin dependent diabetes (Solomon et al., 2001) and warrant investigation.

While mood changes across the menstrual cycle may reflect medication effects, a study by Rasgon and colleagues that examined the relationship between PCOS and medication use in 22 outpatients with bipolar disorder suggests that other factors are also involved. The authors found that menstrual irregularities were common and present in all women taking lithium and 70% of women treated with divalproex (Rasgon et al., 2000) suggesting that women with bipolar disorder have higher rates of menstrual disturbance irrespective of treatment and in many cases preceding the diagnosis of bipolar disorder.

The frequency of menstrual abnormalities in women with bipolar disorder supports the concept of a trait-related liability for reproductive cycle associated symptoms that in some cases is mediated by the side effects of the medications used to treat the illness. A recent paper by Payne et al. (2007) found that rates of reproductive cycle-associated mood symptoms were reported with equal frequency in women with both unipolar depression and bipolar disorder, and in both these groups rates were more prevalent than in women who had never been mentally ill. Unlike woman with unipolar depression, however, in women with bipolar disorder the occurrence of one reproductive cycle-associated mood symptom did not predict the occurrence of others. One possible explanation is that diagnosis and treatment of bipolar disorder prevents some type of reproductive cycle-associated symptoms (Karadag et al., 2004). In support of this is the fact that women with bipolar disorder who receive treatment are more likely to be prescribed medication long term, while women with unipolar depression may take antidepressants only briefly or intermittently.

Treatment strategies for menstrual related mood changes

Oral contraceptive pills

Oral contraceptives (OC) and hormone therapies (HT) may modulate the menstrual cycle and influence mood symptoms (Oinonen & Mazmanian, 2002; Zweifel & O'Brien, 1997). In a study by Rasgon et al. (2003) examining the effects of the menstrual cycle on mood, women taking OCs did not have significant mood changes across the menstrual cycle while those not taking OC did, regardless of other therapeutic agents used. This finding is consistent with several studies that have reported the mood stabilizing effects of exogenous gonadal steroids in women with treatment resistant bipolar disorder (Hatotani et al., 1983; Price & DiMarzio, 1986; Chouinard, Steinberg & Steiner, 1987).

Similar effects were observed among women with PCOS where OC treatment was associated with decreased rates of depression (Pearlstein & Steiner, 2000).

The drug–drug interactions with concomitant medications needs to be considered when using OC in women with bipolar disorder. Both carbamazepine and topiramate induce cytochrome P450 activity and have been shown to decrease OC levels (Crawford, 2002) while the inhibitory action of OC may lead to higher serum concentrations of some atypical antipsychotics used in the bipolar treatment (Barnes & Mitchell, 2005). Conversely, a case report of seven women taking lamotrigine found a mean reduction in lamotrigine levels of 49% in women using OC (Sabers et al., 2001).

Mood stabilizers

While it constitutes a mainstay for the treatment of bipolar disorders, lithium has been shown to be ineffective as a treatment for the mood fluctuations associated with premenstrual syndrome (Singer, Cheng & Schou, 1974; Steiner, Haskett, Osmun & Carroll, 1980). Reports of menstrual cycle-related changes in lithium serum level have also been contradictory (Hendrick, Altshuler & Burt, 1996) but some research has indicated that breakthrough symptoms in the premenstrual phase in women with bipolar disorder might be related to subtheraputic lithium levels. This may indicate the existence of vulnerable subgroups of women in which improved drug response and more stable clinical course might be achieved if serum lithium levels were monitored for premenstrual decline (Kukopulos, Minnai & Muller-Oerlinghausen, 1985; Conrad & Hamilton, 1986).

The data on the efficacy of divalproex on premenstrual mood worsening is inconclusive (Jacobsen, 1993), but the impact of this agent on ovarian function is more definitive, and suggests an increased occurrence of reproductive-endocrine abnormalities, including hyperandrogenism, hyperinsulinemaia, and/or PCOS among women talking this medication. Most research has been conducted primarily in women taking divalproex for epileptic seizure control (Bilo et al., 1988; Herzog et al., 1986, 1991) and preliminary data in women with bipolar disorder have produced contradictory findings (Altshuler et al., 2004; McIntyre et al., 2003; O'Donovan et al., 2002; Rasgon et al., 2000). The general consensus, however, is that divalproex use is associated with reproductive-endocrine abnormalities in women with bipolar disorder (Joffe et al., 2006a). While guidelines are not yet available, the use of divalproex in reproductive-aged women should be preceded by a comprehensive assessment for obesity, menstrual abnormalities and hirsutism. In addition, patients being treated with divalproex should be further investigated if presenting with at least two of the following symptoms: hirsutism, menstrual disturbances, obesity, alopecia or infertility. The investigation should include a blood test for bioavailable testosterone and DHEA, with subsequent referral to a specialist (O'Donovan et al., 2002; Rasgon et al., 2000).

Proximity to puberty appears to increase vulnerability to perturbation of the reproductive-endocrine system; thus, adolescent girls with bipolar disorder may be at increased risk for developing PCOS when exposed to treatment with divalproex. Since there is increasing recognition that both divalproex (Papatheodorou et al., 1995; Garland & Behr, 1996; Geller & Luby, 1997) and lithium (Geller et al., 1998) are effective in the treatment of bipolar disorder in adolescents, regular monitoring in this population may be especially important.

The use of divalproex as the first choice for the treatment of bipolar in women during childbearing years carries an additional point for consideration; divalproex use has been associated with significant teratogenic risks, including neural tube defects, oral clefts lips, cardiovascular abnormalities, genitourinary defects and developmental delay (Alsdorf & Wyszynski, 2005). Given the significant number of unplanned pregnancies among young adults, the choice of using divalproex should be carefully reviewed by clinicians and their patients.

A case report on the efficacy of lamotrigine in a 30-year-old woman with treatment-resistant menstrually-entrained rapid cycling bipolar II disorder (Becker, Rasgon, Marsh, Glenn, & Ketter, 2004) brings attention to the potential use of lamotrigine in bipolar disorder associated with the menstrual cycle. Switching from divalproex to lamotrigine also resulted in a decrease in serum testosterone changes and a normalization of polycystic ovaries in a case report of three women with epilepsy, documenting that this medication has a more tolerable effect on reproductive variables than other mood stabilizers (Isojarvi & Tapanainen, 2000). In addition, lamotrigine appears to have a much safer profile in terms of teratogenic/ reproductive safety (Perucca, 2005).

Pregnancy

Historically, pregnancy had been thought to be "protective" against the risk of relapse of bipolar illness (Targum, Davenport & Webster, 1979; Kendell, Chalmers, & Platz, 1987; Grof et al., 2000; Sharma, Smith & Khan, 2004) but recent work has challenged this and the concept of bipolar illness improving during pregnancy is controversial (Pugh et al., 1963; Terp & Mortensen, 1998; Viguera et al., 2000; Viguera & Cohen, 1998; Freeman et al., 2002). A retrospective study by Grof et al. (2000) found that woman with lithium responsive bipolar disorder had fewer episodes during pregnancy compared to the 9-month periods before or after delivery, but the fact that all women in the study became pregnant before starting lithium treatment impacts the generalizability of this finding (Viguera et al., 2000). Research by Viguera et al. (2000) found that for women discontinuing lithium maintenance treatment, the recurrence rates in the first 40 weeks were similar in pregnant (52%) and non-pregnant women (58%); studies by Blehar et al. (1998) and Freeman et al. (2002) also found that 45–50% of women with bipolar disorder reported an exacerbation of their symptoms during pregnancy. While definitive conclusions regarding the impact of pregnancy on bipolar disorder cannot yet be made, what is evident is that pregnancy is not protective for all women with bipolar disorder (Viguera et al., 2000; Freeman et al., 2002).

Both the prepartum month and the immediate postpartum period are also times of increased vulnerability for mood symptoms and women with bipolar disorder are at higher risk during this time period (Brockington, Oates & Rose, 1990; Grof et al., 2000; Kendell, Chalmers & Platz, 1987; Terp & Mortensen, 1998; Viguera et al., 2000; Paffenbarger & McCabe, 1966). A nearly seven-fold higher risk of admission for a first episode of bipolar disorder and a nearly two-fold higher risk of recurrence have been described in puerperal women, compared with non-postpartum and pregnant women (Terp & Mortensen, 1998). Among women with bipolar disorder who elect to discontinue lithium therapy in the puerperium, the estimated risk of relapse is three-fold higher than that for nonpregnant, nonpuerperal women (Viguera et al., 2000). Symptom emergence during this time is quite often rapid and may commence a few weeks before (Grof et al., 2000) or within the first few weeks after parturition (Kendell, Chalmers & Platz, 1987; Viguera et al., 2000).

The postpartum time is also considered to be a period of high risk in women with bipolar disorder for the development of postpartum psychosis or postpartum depression (Freeman et al., 2002). Postpartum depression occurs after approximately 10–20% of all live births (Campbell & Cohn, 1991; Robinson & Stewart, 1986) and postpartum psychosis after 0.05–0.1% of all live births (Gitlin & Pasnau, 1989). These prevalence rates are significantly increased in women with bipolar disorder; Freeman et al. (2002) reported postpartum mood episodes in 67% of patients studied while Jefferson et al. found that 40–70% of untreated bipolar women may experience postpartum mania or depression (Jefferson, Greist & Ackerman, 1987). A postpartum manic episode is considered to be the most common cause of postpartum psychosis (Payne et al., 2007; Rapkin et al., 2003) and rates of postpartum psychosis increases from 10% to 20% in women with bipolar disorder (Kendell, Chalmers & Platz, 1987; Brockington et al., 1981). The risk of subsequent postpartum mood episodes also increases after the first initial presentation of a postpartum mood disorder, with an estimated subsequent risk ranging from 50% to 90% (Hunt & Silverstone, 1995; Reich & Winokur, 1970; Viguera et al., 2002). Interestingly, pregnancy and childbirth may also have adverse consequences in the spouse of women with a mood disorder, with paternal depression being highly correlated with maternal depression (Goodman, 2004; Matthey et al., 2001; Meighan et al., 1999).

Wellbeing during pregnancy can significantly impact the risk of psychiatric morbidity in the postpartum period. A relationship between mood during pregnancy and subsequent level of functioning in postpartum affective disorders has been repeatedly identified (Freeman et al., 2002), with mood changes in pregnancy representing a significant risk factor for serious postpartum problems (Halbreich, 2004). The risk of postpartum relapse is particularly high for those women who elect to discontinue prophylactic treatment; recurrence rates nearly tripled in women who discontinued lithium, as compared to non-pregnant women (Viguera et al., 2000). Women experiencing mood disturbances who are not treated or undertreated, particularly due to fear of fetal malformations, should be informed that partial and ineffective treatment (i.e. exposure to an untreated mood disturbances) also increases the risk of adverse maternal, as well as obstetrical and neonatal outcomes (Cohen et al., 1994; Federenko & Wadhwa, 2004; Nulman et al., 2002).

Treatment strategies during pregnancy

Foundations for effective management

The effective management of bipolar disorder during pregnancy requires a multi-disciplinary approach and should involve whenever possible the patient's treating clinician, family physician and obstetrician (Table 6.1). While biological management is easiest when the pregnancy is anticipated, this is rarely the case (Bergman et al., 1992). Either prior to, or post conception, a discussion with respect to the heritability of the illness, which is estimated to range from 1.5% to 10.2%, is important (Packer, 1992), as is education pertaining to the risks associated both with pharmacotherapy and drug discontinuation (Viguera & Cohen, 1998; Altshuler, Richards & Yonkers, 2003). The most important clinical factors that influence treatment planning during pregnancy are illness history and the reproductive risks of medications. Historical factors that should be identified include the patient's prior response to various medications, illness severity, and duration of euthymia while taking medication and while

Table 6.1 Management Strategies During Pregnancy

Planned pregnancy

Counseling regarding heritability of bipolar disorder.

Discuss risks of medication exposure during pregnancy versus risks of drug discontinuation: obtain details of illness severity and duration of euthymia while not receiving treatment. (Viguera et al., 1998; Altushuler et al., 2003; Barnes et al., 2005).

Develop management plans including treatment of recurrence during and after pregnancy (Ernst & Goldberg, 2002).

Medication use

Assess patient's risk of recurrence and avoid medication during pregnancy especially during first trimester, if possible (Iqbal et al., 2001).

Stable patients may be able to discontinue one or more medications before attempting to conceive and during first trimester (Freeman et al., 2002; Grof et al., 2000).

If medication is required, use monotherapy at minimally effective doses, if possible (Iqbal et al., 2001; Yonkers et al., 2004).

---

not taking medication, time to relapse after medication discontinuation, and time to recover with reintroduction of pharmacotherapy (Barnes & Mitchell, 2005).

Pharmacotherapy during pregnancy and the postpartum

Lithium

There are diverse opinions on lithium utilization in pregnancy. Some recommend discontinuing treatment prior to conception, restarting and then discontinuing again until the postnatal phase (Williams & Oke, 2000) while others suggested the maintenance of lithium treatment in women with severe illness but discontinuation in all other cases (Cohen et al., 1994). The incidence of major malformations in infants exposed to lithium during their fetal life ranges from 4% to 12%, while the rate in unexposed infants ranges from 2% to 4% (Cohen et al., 1994). The risk of Ebstein's anomaly (20 times more common with lithium) exists especially if the drug is taken during weeks 2–6 post conception (Cohen et al., 1994) however, the overall risk remains very low because of the rarity of the anomaly (0.1%–0.2%). Other types of lithium-related fetal and neonatal complications include: neonatal toxicity, premature delivery, floppy infant syndrome (Ananth, 1978; Schou, Amdisen, & Steenstrup, 1973), transient neurodevelopmental deficits, nephrogenic diabetes insipidus, thyroid dysfunctions and rarely, polyhydramnios (Mizrahi, Hobbs & Goldsmith, 1979; Nars & Girard, 1977).

Clinical management

As pregnancy advances, renal lithium excretion increases, and this may result in the need to increase lithium dosing (Williams & Oke, 2000). A number of factors including febrile illness, hyperemesis, sodium intake, reduced fluid intake and a change in blood volume during delivery can also impact lithium levels and require vigilant symptom and level monitoring (Williams & Oke, 2000) in order to avoid relapse or toxicity during delivery and the immediate postpartum period (Viguera et al., 2000; Cohen et al., 1994). It is also important that adequate hydration be maintained and the use of intravenous fluids be considered for patients in prolonged labor (Yonkers et al., 2004). Women taking lithium are vulnerable to changes in fluid volumes so it is important to monitor for signs of dehydration, and treat this condition accordingly. Any change in bipolar symptom control during pregnancy should result in a lithium level.

Lithium in breast-feeding: The American Academy of Pediatrics recommends that breast-feeding be undertaken with caution by women undergoing lithium treatment (Gartner, 1997). Lithium is secreted into breast milk (Skausig & Schou, 1977; Chaudron & Jefferson, 2000; Kaneko et al., 1999) and the diminished renal clearance in neonates can subsequently elevate serum levels. This is a concern given the propensity for rapid dehydration in neonates with febrile illnesses. It is also important that in a breast-fed infant exposed to lithium, lithium serum concentrations and CBC should be monitored (Yonkers et al., 2004).

Carbamazipine

The overall incidence of carbamazipine related fetal malformations ranges from 2.2% to 5.7% (Morrow et al., 2006) and include microcephaly, other craniofacial skeletal defects, growth retardation, cardiac defects and coagulopathies (Kaneko et al., 1999). In addition, an increased risk of spina bifida, ranging from 0.5% to 1.0% exists (Rosa, 1991; Jones et al., 1989). The use of oxcarbazepine, a structurally similar derivative of carbamazipine, theoretically may be less teratogenic than carbamazepine because it lacks epoxide metabolites, but to date no studies have been performed to rigorously examine this (Yonkers et al., 2004). Perinatnal exposure to oxcarbazepine has been associated with spontaneous abortion, amniotic bands, urogenital anomalies and mild facial dysplasia (Bulau et al., 1988; Artama et al., 2005).

Carbamazepine safety in breast-feeding: The American Academy of Pediatrics committee on medications in breast-feeding lists carbamazepine as being compatible with breast-feeding (American Academy of Pediatrics, 1994) while the American Academy of Neurology supports breast-feeding while undergoing carbamazepine treatment in selected cases (Holmes et al., 2001). The concentrations of this drug can range from 7% to 95% in breast milk and from 6% to 65% in infant serum (Chaudron & Jefferson, 2000) but there is only one case report describing minor adverse effects (poor suckling) in newborns exposed to carbamazepine via breast milk (Froescher et al., 1984). Two case reports on oxcarbamazipine have also not documented any adverse events but not enough data exists to confer a safety profile of this medication (Gentile, 2003, 2005; Bulau et al., 1988).

Clinical management

Carbamazipine should be used during pregnancy only if other options are lacking. Use in the first trimester has been shown to confer increased risk to the fetus of craniofacial abnormalities, fingernail hypoplasia; developmental retardation and a 0.5%–1% risk of neural tube defects. (Jones et al., 1989.) A recent metaanalysis involving 1255 cases of CBZ exposure confirmed an increased the rate of congenital anomalies; mainly neural tube defects, cardiovascular and urinary tract anomalies, and cleft palate. In total, a 2.89-fold increased risk of major congenital abnormalities was found in children of mothers treated with CBZ during pregnancy, as compared with children of healthy controls (Matalon et al., 2002). Expectant mothers incur a greater risk of serious side effects including Stevens-Johnson syndrome, hepatic failure and agranulocytosis if started on the medication while pregnant, since the risks of these side effects are highest in the first 8 weeks of treatment (Rzany et al., 1999).

Carbamazipine can also cause fetal vitamin K deficiency, increasing the risk of neonatal bleeding and mid-facial abnormalities and it is recommended that 20 mg/day of oral vitamin K be given to woman taking carbamazipine during the last month of pregnancy (Delgado-Escueta & Janz, 1992). Pediatricians should also administer 1 mg i.m. of vitamin K to neonates after in utero carbamazipine exposure. Oxcarbazepine should also only be used if all other options are lacking.

Valproate

Sodium valproate is considered a human teratogen and confers an approximately five-fold increased risk of major malformations and other serious pregnancy complications, especially if the compound is administered in the first trimester of pregnancy (Ernst & Goldberg, 2002; Wyszynski et al., 2005). Use of this compound during the first trimester is associated with an overall incidence of major malformations of 11%

(Kaneko et al., 1999), neural tube defect rates of about 5%–9% (Omtzigt et al., 1992; Kennedy & Koren, 1998; Jager-Roman et al., 1986) cognitive delays (Iqbal et al., 2001; Ardinger et al., 1988; Adab et al., 2004) skeletal malformations and cardiovascular abnormalities (Rodriguez-Pinilla et al., 2000; Koch et al., 1983). Coagulopathies, neonatal hypoglycemia, and hepatotoxicity have also been reported (Marcus et al., 2003; Kennedy & Koren, 1998).

The American Academy of Pediatrics committee on medications in breast-feeding lists valproate as being compatible with breast-feeding (American Academy of Pediatrics, 1994) and valproic acid concentrations range from less than 1% to 10% in breast milk and infant serum, and from undetectable levels to 40% in maternal serum (Chaudron et al., 2000; Kuller et al., 1996). Thrombocytopenic purpura and anemia were attributed to valproate exposure through placenta and breast milk (Stahl, Neiderud & Vinge, 1997).

Clinical management

In treatment of women with bipolar disorder, most experts recommend that valproate should be switched to another mood stabilizer before conception (American Academy of Neurology, 1998). However, since there is a significant number of unplanned pregnancies, the deleterious effects of exposure to this agent may occur prior to switching medications. In those who do continue on this medication, it is recommended that valproate should be dosed three to four times a day to avoid unpredictably high peak levels (Delgado-Escueta & Janz, 1992). As valproate levels are affected by the presence of other antiepileptic drugs that increase the activity of metabolic enzymes and in pregnancy, glucuronidation is induced, potentially leading to lower serum valproate levels, patients should be monitored closely to ensure therapeutic efficacy. It is important to note that valproate use during pregnancy may lead to additional adverse outcomes for the infant beyond the teratogenic risks already described. Exposure to valproate during pregnancy has been associated with impaired neurobehavior development, including lower verbal IQ and memory problems (Vinten et al., 2005).

Folate supplementation during pregnancy reduces the risk of neural tube defects and it is recommended that all women taking antiepileptic drugs consume a daily dose of 5 mg of folic acid before and during pregnancy or at least through the first trimester (Crawford et al., 1999). The American Academy of Neurology has recommended a more conservative dose of 3–4 mg/day of folic acid but has stated that the optimal dose has yet to be established (American Academy of Neurology, 1998). The patient's level of vitamin B_{12} should be measured before folate supplementation to assess for concurrent pernicious anemia, which can be masked with folate treatment. As vitamin K deficiency can occur, oral vitamin K be given to woman during the last month of pregnancy (Delgado-Escueta & Janz, 1992) and 1 mg i.m. of vitamin K to neonates after *in utero* carbamazipine exposure.

Lamotrigine

The International Lamotrigine Pregnancy Registry data suggests that major birth defects are observed in 2.9% of pregnant women exposed to lamotrigine monotherapy (Tennis & Eldridge, 2002; Cunnington, 2004; Cunnington & Tennis, 2005) while other studies have documented risk ranges between 2.1% and 7.7% (Morrow et al., 2006; Vajda et al., 2003; Calabrese et al., 2002). A substantially lower prevalence (to 0–2.4%) has been reported in the most recent updates of the Australian Registry of Antiepileptic Drugs (Vajda & Eadie, 2005; Vajda et al., 2004) and in a prospective study of women with epilepsy (Sabers et al., 2004). Only six studies have evaluated the neonatal consequences of lamotrigine exposure throughout breast-feeding (Rambeck et al., 1997; Tomson, Ohman & Vitols, 1997; Ohman, Vitols & Tomson, 2000; Liporace, Kao & D'Abreu, 2004; Gentile, 2005) and although a considerable amount of lamotrigine (2–5 mg/day) is excreted in breast milk, no untoward events were observed in the newborns. As some reports have indicated that lamotrigine concentration in breast-fed children can reach "therapeutic ranges" (Liporace, Kao & D'Abreu, 2004) it has been recommended that these babies should be monitored closely (Ohman, Vitols & Tomson., 2000).

Clinical management

Three recent studies have reported a decrease in lamotrigine levels of 60–65% of baseline between preconception and the second and third trimester of pregnancy in 35 epileptic women, 11 of which required a higher dose to maintain a therapeutic effect (Tran et al., 2002; de Haan et al., 2004; Petrenaite, Sabers & Hansen-Schwartz, 2005). Conversely, an increase in lamotrigine levels was observed in the last two trimesters, returning to preconception values in the postpartum period. Clinicians should also be aware of reports of hepatotoxicity in adults taking lamotrigine and concerns about the development of lamotrigine-related skin rash in a fetus or neonate whose antigen characteristics are different from those of the mother. An additional concern is that lamotrigine is metabolized exclusively by means of glucuronidation, a metabolic process that is very immature in the fetus and neonate. Two studies have found a significant increase in the clearance rate during pregnancy (Tran et al., 2002; Pennell et al., 2004). It is noteworthy that the rate of clearance returned to preconception levels rapidly after delivery, indicating the need for careful dose management in the early postpartum period.

Antidepressants

Antidepressant use during pregnancy is a source of controversy and decisions pertaining to the use or discontinuation of this treatment should be made by the physician and patient together. A number of reviews have provided evidence on the safety of exposure to selective serotonin reuptake inhibitors (SSRIs) (Einarson & Einarson, 2005; Hallberg & Sjoblom, 2005) during the first trimester. Recent reports on the use of paroxetine, however, have suggested an increased risk of cardiac defects in infants exposed to this medication early in pregnancy (1.5% compared with 1% in the general population) (GlaxoSmithKline). A recent study by Motherrisk however found rates of cardiac defects in both infants exposed to paroxetine and non-exposed infants to be similar (Einarson et al., 2007), findings that have been confirmed by other studies (Louik et al., 2007; Alwan et al., 2007). Adverse perinatal outcomes including low birth weight, prematuirty, and poor adaption have been reported in respect to fetal exposure to antidepressants (Zeskind & Stephens, 2004; Simon, Cunningham & Davis, 2002; Chambers et al., 1996) but these findings are contradicted by other studies that report no increase in adverse effects (Nulman et al., 2004; Suri et al., 2004; Pastuszak et al., 1993) The issue of neonatal withdrawal from anidepressants has also been an area of concern (Levinson-Castiel et al., 2006; Chambers et al., 2006) but this syndrome is mostly self-limiting and not life threatening (Levinson-Castiel et al., 2006; Koren et al., 2005). As it has been estimated that up to 20% of pregnant women suffer from some degree of depression (Flynn, Blow & Marcus, 2006), decisions regarding medication use needs to be balanced against the possible adverse effects of maternal illness on the fetus (Steer et al., 1992; Orr & Miller, 1995).

Menopause

Menopause is defined as the occurrence of 12 months of amenorrhea, while the menopause transition or perimenopause begins with variations in menstrual cycle length at the mean age of 47.5 years. While evidence supports the time between menarche and menopause as conferring the highest risk of depression in women (Kessler et al., 1993; Weissman et al., 1984) evidence supporting a heightened risk for depression during the menopause transition or postmenopausal years have been much more contradictory (Avis et al., 1994; Kaufert, Gilbert & Tate, 1992; Freeman et al., 2004; Schmidt, Haq & Rubinow, 2004; Harlow et al., 2003). Recent epidemiologic studies, however, consistently show an increased risk for developing depressive symptoms or clinical depression during this window of vulnerability (Freeman et al., 2006; Bromberger et al., 2007; Cohen et al., 2006; Cohen, Soares & Joffe, 2005).

Less work has focused on the effects of the menopause transition on bipolar disorder (Haynes & Parry, 1998); existing reports indicate that this reproductive milestone is associated with generally worsened mood symptoms (Marsh et al., 2007; Freeman et al., 2002; Blehar et al., 1998; Sajatovic et al., 2006). Blehar et al. examined the rates of perimenopausal symptoms in women with bipolar I disorder who participated in the NIMH Genetics Initiative Study and found that perimenopausal symptoms were present in 19% of the 186 women sample (Blehar et al., 1998). A study by Freeman and colleagues also reported on the impact of reproductive events on the course of bipolar disorder in 22 women who were either perimenopausal or menopausal (Freeman et al., 2002). In this study, 12 out of the 22 women reported a worsening of mood (increased depressive symptoms), ten women reported no change after the onset of menopause, three women with bipolar I disorder reported onset during or after perimenopause and there were no reports of improvement during this period. Other studies have also reported a worsening of mood symptoms, mostly depression, in postmenopausal women with bipolar disorder. A recent study by Payne et al. (2007) found that rates of perimenopausal symptoms were equivalent in women with either unipolar depression or bipolar disorder and were greater in women with mood disorders than in women who had never been mentally ill. Similar results were observed by Marsh and colleagues who, in a follow up of 47 women with bipolar disorder, found a higher frequency of depressive episodes during the menopausal transition in comparison to prior reproductive years (Marsh et al., 2007). It appears that the menopausal transition may be a time of increased frequency of depressive episodes in women with bipolar disorder.

Treatment strategies for menopausal related mood changes

Overall, the treatment of bipolar disorder in the perimenopause does not differ from treatment of this illness in the general population. While there have been studies demonstrating the antidepressant effects of estrogen therapy for depression (MDD) during perimenopause; its use, however, should be carefully considered along with other risks and benefits associated with hormone therapy use. Conversely, the use of hormonal interventions for the treatment of depressive disorders during postmenopausal years has not shown clinical efficacy, and even less convincing data are available for the treatment of bipolar disorder (Soares et al., 2005). It is important to consider, however, that estrogen use may offer additional benefits for postmenopausal women; neuroimaging studies suggest that estrogen may help preserving the hippocampal volume in postmenopausal women (Lord et al., 2006); its use has also been associated with protection of regional cerebral metabolism against metabolic decline (Rasgon et al., 2005).

A particular area of clinical relevance for this population pertains to the risk of osteoporosis (Soares & Taylor, 2007). When women reach menopause and their estrogen levels decrease, the rate of bone loss increases to 2–3% per year, placing them at increased risk of osteoporosis (Lata & Elliott, 2007). The National Osteoporosis Foundation has recommended guidelines for women with epilepsy who require anti-seizure medications, as these drugs can increase osteoporosis risk and as these same medications are used in the treatment of bipolar disorder, the same guidelines should apply. These guidelines include an adequate intake of dietary calcium (at least 1200 mg/day) and vitamin D (400–800 IU/day for individuals at risk of deficiency), as well as regular weight bearing and muscle strengthening exercises (McAuley et al., 2000). Other guidelines have suggested routine screening dual-energy x-ray absorptiometry (DEXA) to identify postmenopausal women with epilepsy and osteoporosis (Penovich, Eck & Economou, 2004) and these same management procedures should be followed in postmenopausal women with bipolar disorder.

Future directions

The treatment of bipolar disorder in women is complicated by a myriad of hormonal factors that are specific to this population, adding a degree of complexity to its biological management. The uniqueness of this patient population have led investigators to examine the role played by estrogen and how the hormonal milieu contributes to clinical presentation and management. An understanding of the role of the reproductive-related changes is especially important in the development of novel therapies specifically targeting this population. Estrogen, for example, has been shown to increase the expression of protein kinase C (PKC), an important extracellular messenger. The clinical relevance of this is unclear but it is worthwhile noting that both lithium and divalproex are PKC inhibitors (Manji & Lenox, 1999; Wang, Johnson & Friedman, 2001; Hahn et al., 2005), as is tamoxifen a selective estrogen receptor modulator. Tamoxifen is currently used in the treatment of estrogen receptor positive breast cancer and is being studied for its potential as an antimanic agent (Bebchuk et al., 2000).

Summary

The role played by hormonal changes in women who experience mood symptoms throughout their reproductive lifetime remains controversial.

What does seem clear is that while women with mood disturbances do not necessarily present with symptoms related to identifiable events within the developmental lifecycle, vulnerable subgroups may experience naturally occurring hormonal changes as triggers for mood symptoms. This hypothesis is supported by studies in which normal changes in hormone levels have been correlated with mood symptoms, particularly among those with a history of female-specific mood disturbances (e.g. severe PMS or postpartum depression) (Schmidt et al., 1998; Bloch et al., 2000; Daly et al., 2003). Thus mood changes across the female life cycle may reflect, in some women, a preexisting vulnerability to normal hormonal fluctuations. In addition, the impact of these hormone changes may still be modulated by medication effects, and the phenotypic heterogeneity of these disorders. To effectively treat this population physicians need to be aware of times of increased vulnerability, recognize female specific symptoms and evaluate the burden of risk associated with treatment, or lack of treatment, at different time points through out the reproductive lifecycle.

References

Adab, N., Kini, U., Vinten, J., Ayres, J., Baker, G., Clayton-Smith, J., Coyle, H., Fryer, A., Gorry, J., Gregg, J., Mawer, G., Nicolaides, P., Pickering, L., Tunnicliffe, L., & Chadwick, D. W. (2004). The longer term outcome of children born to mothers with epilepsy. *J. Neurol. Neurosurg. Psychiatry, 75*, 1575–1583.

Akdeniz, F., Taneli, F., Noyan, A., Yuncu, Z., & Vahip, S. (2003). Valproate-associated reproductive and metabolic abnormalities: are epileptic women at greater risk than bipolar women? *Prog. Neuropsychopharmacol. Biol. Psychiatry, 27*, 115–121.

Akiskal, H. S., Maser, J. D., Zeller, P. J., Endicott, J., Coryell, W., Keller, M., Warshaw, M., Clayton, P., & Goodwin, F. (1995). Switching from 'unipolar' to bipolar II. An 11-year prospective study of clinical and temperamental predictors in 559 patients. *Arch. Gen. Psychiatry, 52*, 114–123.

Alonso, J., Angermeyer, M. C., Bernert, S., Bruffaerts, R., Brugha, T. S., Bryson, H., de Girolamo, G., Graaf, R., Demyttenaere, K., Gasquet, I., Haro, J. M., Katz, S. J., Kessler, R. C., Kovess, V., Lépine, J. P., Ormel, J., Polidori, G., Russo, L. J., Vilagut, G., Almansa, J., Arbabzadeh-Bouchez, S., Autonell, J., Bernal, M., Buist-Bouwman, M. A., Codony, M., Domingo-Salvany, A., Ferrer, M., Joo, S. S., Martínez-Alonso, M., Matschinger, H., Mazzi, F., Morgan, Z., Morosini, P., Palacín, C., Romera, B., Taub, N., & Vollebergh, W. A. (2004). Prevalence of mental disorders in Europe: results from the European Study of the Epidemiology of Mental Disorders (ESEMeD) project. *Acta Psychiatr. Scand. Suppl.*, 21–27.

Alsdorf, R. & Wyszynski, D. F. (2005). Teratogenicity of sodium valproate. *Expert. Opin. Drug Saf., 4*, 345–353.

Altshuler, L., Rasgon, S., Elman, S., Bitran, J., Lablarca, R., & Saad, M. (2004). *Reproductive Endocrine Function in Women Treated for Bipolar Disorder: Reproductive Hormone Levels*. New York, NY: American Psychiatric Association.

Altshuler, L., Richards, M., & Yonders, K. (2003). Treating bipolar disorder during pregnancy. *Curr. Psychiatry, 2,* 14–26.

Alwan, S., Reefhuis, J., Rasmussen, S. A., Olney, R. S., & Friedman, J. M. (2007). Use of selective serotonin-reuptake inhibitors in pregnancy and the risk of birth defects. *N. Engl. J Med., 356,* 2684–2692.

American Academy of Neurology (1998). *Practice parameter: management issues for women with epilepsy (summary statement): Report of the Quality Stand Subcommittee of the American Academy of Neurology* (Rep. No. 51).

American Academy of Pediatrics (1994). Committee on drugs: the transfer of drugs and other chemicals into human milk. *Pediatrics, 93,* 137–50

American Psychiatric Association (1994). *Diagnostic and Statistical Manual of Mental Disorders DSM-IV.* (4th edn) Washington, DC: American Psychiatric Association.

Ananth, J. (1978). Side effects in the neonate from psychotropic agents excreted through breast-feeding. *Am. J. Psychiatry, 135,* 801–805.

Anderson, J. C., Williams, S., McGee, R., & Silva, P. A. (1987). DSM-III disorders in preadolescent children. Prevalence in a large sample from the general population. *Arch. Gen. Psychiatry, 44,* 69–76.

Angold, A., Costello, E. J., & Worthman, C. M. (1998). Puberty and depression: the roles of age, pubertal status and pubertal timing. *Psychol. Med, 28,* 51–61.

Angst, J. & Gamma, A. (2002). Prevalence of bipolar disorders: traditional and novel approaches. *Clin. Appr. Bipolar Disord., 1,* 10–14.

Ardinger, H. H., Atkin, J. F., Blackston, R. D., Elsas, L. J., Clarren, S. K., Livingstone, S., Flannery, D. B., Pellock, J. M., Harrod, M. J., Lammer, E. J., et al. (1988). Verification of the fetal valproate syndrome phenotype. *Am. J. Med. Genet., 29,* 171–185.

Artama, M., Auvinen, A., Raudaskoski, T., Isojarvi, I., & Isojarvi, J. (2005). Antiepileptic drug use of women with epilepsy and congenital malformations in offspring. *Neurology, 64,* 1874–1878.

Avis, N. E., Brambilla, D., McKinlay, S. M., & Vass, K. (1994). A longitudinal analysis of the association between menopause and depression. Results from the Massachusetts Women's Health Study. *Ann Epidemiol., 4,* 214–220.

Bachmann, G. A. & Kemmann, E. (1982). Prevalence of oligomenorrhea and amenorrhea in a college population. *Am. J. Obstet. Gynecol., 144,* 98–102.

Barnes, C. & Mitchell, P. (2005). Considerations in the management of bipolar disorder in women. *Aust. N. Z. J. Psychiatry, 39,* 662–673.

Bebchuk, J. M., Arfken, C. L., Dolan-Manji, S., Murphy, J., Hasanat, K., & Manji, H. K. (2000). A preliminary investigation of a protein kinase C inhibitor in the treatment of acute mania. *Arch. Gen. Psychiatry, 57,* 95–97.

Becker, O. V., Rasgon, N. L., Marsh, W. K., Glenn, T., & Ketter, T. A. (2004). Lamotrigine therapy in treatment-resistant menstrually-related rapid cycling bipolar disorder: a case report. *Bipolar Disord., 6,* 435–439.

Bergman, U., Rosa, F. W., Baum, C., Wiholm, B. E., & Faich, G. A. (1992). Effects of exposure to benzodiazepine during fetal life. *Lancet, 340,* 694–696.

Bilo, L., Meo, R., Nappi, C., Annunziato, L., Striano, S., Colao, A. M., Merola, B., & Buscaino, G. A. (1988). Reproductive endocrine disorders in women with primary generalized epilepsy. *Epilepsia, 29,* 612–619.

Bisaga, K., Petkova, E., Cheng, J., Davies, M., Feldman, J. F., & Whitaker, A. H. (2002). Menstrual functioning and psychopathology in a county-wide population of high school girls. *J. Am. Acad. Child Adolesc. Psychiatry, 41,* 1197–1204.

Blehar, M. C., DePaulo, J. R., Jr., Gershon, E. S., Reich, T., Simpson, S. G., & Nurnberger, J. I., Jr. (1998). Women with bipolar disorder: findings from the NIMH Genetics Initiative sample. *Psychopharmacol. Bull., 34,* 239–243.

Bloch, M., Schmidt, P. J., Danaceau, M., Murphy, J., Nieman, L., & Rubinow, D. R. (2000). Effects of gonadal steroids in women with a history of postpartum depression. *Am. J. Psychiatry, 157,* 924–930.

Brockington, I. F., Cernik, K. F., Schofield, E. M., Downing, A. R., Francis, A. F., & Keelan, C. (1981). Puerperal Psychosis. Phenomena and diagnosis. *Arch. Gen. Psychiatry, 38,* 829–833.

Brockington, I. F., Oates, M., & Rose, G. (1990). Prepartum psychosis. *J. Affect. Disord., 19,* 31–35.

Bromberger, J. T., Matthews, K. A., Schott, L. L., Brockwell, S., Avis, N. E., Kravitz, H. M., Everson-Rose, S. A., Gold, E. B., Sowers, M., & Randolph, J. F., Jr. (2007). Depressive symptoms during the menopausal transition: The Study of Women's Health Across the Nation (SWAN). *J. Affect. Disord., 103* (1–3), 267–272.

Bulau, P., Paar, W. D., & von Unruh, G. E. (1988). Pharmacokinetics of oxcarbazepine and 10-hydroxy-carbazepine in the newborn child of an oxcarbazepine-treated mother. *Eur. J. Clin. Pharmacol., 34,* 311–313.

Burt, V. K. & Rasgon, N. (2004). Special considerations in treating bipolar disorder in women. *Bipolar Disord., 6,* 2–13.

Calabrese, J. R., Shelton, M. D., Rapport, D. J., Kimmel, S. E., & Elhaj, O. (2002). Long-term treatment of bipolar disorder with lamotrigine. *J. Clin. Psychiatry, 63* (Suppl 10), 18–22.

Campbell, S. B. & Cohn, J. F. (1991). Prevalence and correlates of postpartum depression in first-time mothers. *J. Abnorm. Psychol., 100,* 594–599.

Chambers, C. D., Johnson, K. A., Dick, L. M., Felix, R. J., & Jones, K. L. (1996). Birth outcomes in pregnant women taking fluoxetine. *N. Engl. J. Med., 335,* 1010–1015.

Chambers, C. D., Hernandez-Diaz, S., Van Marter, L. J., Werler, M. M., Louik, C., Jones, K. L., & Mitchell, A. A. (2006). Selective serotonin-reuptake inhibitors and risk of persistent pulmonary hypertension of the newborn. *N. Engl. J. Med., 354,* 579–587.

Chaudron, L. H. & Jefferson, J. W. (2000). Mood stabilizers during breastfeeding: a review. *J. Clin. Psychiatry, 61,* 79–90.

Chouinard, G., Steinberg, S., & Steiner, W. (1987). Estrogen-progesterone combination: another mood stabilizer? *Am. J. Psychiatry, 144,* 826.

Cohen, L. S., Friedman, J. M., Jefferson, J. W., Johnson, E. M., & Weiner, M. L. (1994). A reevaluation of risk of in utero exposure to lithium. *JAMA, 271,* 146–150.

Cohen, L. S., Soares, C. N., & Joffe, H. (2005). Diagnosis and management of mood disorders during the menopausal transition. *Am. J. Med, 118* (Suppl 12B), 93–97.

Cohen, L. S., Soares, C. N., Vitonis, A. F., Otto, M. W., & Harlow, B. L. (2006). Risk for new onset of depression during the menopausal transition: the Harvard study of moods and cycles. *Arch. Gen. Psychiatry, 63,* 385–390.

Conrad, C. D. & Hamilton, J. A. (1986). Recurrent premenstrual decline in serum lithium concentration: clinical correlates and treatment implications. *J. Am. Acad. Child Psychiatry, 25,* 852–853.

Coryell, W., Endicott, J., & Keller, M. (1992). Rapidly cycling affective disorder. Demographics, diagnosis, family history, and course. *Arch. Gen. Psychiatry, 49,* 126–131.

Crawford, P. (2002). Interactions between antiepileptic drugs and hormonal contraception. *CNS Drugs, 16,* 263–272.

Crawford, P., Appleton, R., Betts, T., Duncan, J., Guthrie, E., & Morrow, J. (1999). Best practice guidelines for the management of women with epilepsy. The Women with Epilepsy Guidelines Development Group. *Seizure, 8,* 201–217.

Cunnington, M. C. (2004). The International Lamotrigine pregnancy registry update for the epilepsy foundation. *Epilepsia, 45,* 1468.

Cunnington, M. C., Tennis, P., & International Lamotrigine Pregnancy Registry Scientific Advisory Committee (2005). Lamotrigine and the risk for malformations in pregnancy. *Neurology, 64,* 955–960.

Daly, R. C., Danaceau, M. A., Rubinow, D. R., & Schmidt, P. J. (2003). Concordant restoration of ovarian function and mood in perimenopausal depression. *Am. J. Psychiatry, 160,* 1842–1846.

de Haan, G. J., Edelbroek, P., Segers, J., Engelsman, M., Lindhout, D., Dévilé-Notschaele, M., & Augustijn, P. (2004). Gestation-induced changes in lamotrigine pharmacokinetics: a monotherapy study. *Neurology, 63,* 571–573.

Delgado-Escueta, A. V. & Janz, D. (1992). Consensus guidelines: preconception counseling, management, and care of the pregnant woman with epilepsy. *Neurology, 42,* 149–160.

Diamond, S. B., Rubinstein, A. A., Dunner, D. L., & Fieve, R. R. (1976). Menstrual problems in women with primary affective illness. *Compr. Psychiatry, 17,* 541–548.

Einarson, A., Pistelli, A., DeSantis, M., Malm, H., Paulus, W. E., & Panchaud, A. (2007). Paroxetine use in pregnancy: Is there an association with congenital cardiac defects? In *Proceedings of the Teratology Society Meeting* (pp. 358). Pittsburg, PA.

Einarson, T. R. & Einarson, A. (2005). Newer antidepressants in pregnancy and rates of major malformations: a meta-analysis of prospective comparative studies. Pharmacoepidemiol. *Drug Saf., 14,* 823–827.

Endicott, J. (1993). The menstrual cycle and mood disorders. *J. Affect. Disord., 29,* 193–200.

Endo, M., Daiguji, M., Asano, Y., Yamashita, I., & Takahashi, S. (1978). Periodic psychosis recurring in association with menstrual cycle. *J. Clin. Psychiatry, 39,* 456–466.

Ernst, C. L. & Goldberg, J. F. (2002). The reproductive safety profile of mood stabilizers, atypical antipsychotics, and broad-spectrum psychotropics. *J. Clin. Psychiatry, 63* (Suppl 4), 42–55.

Federenko, I. S. & Wadhwa, P. D. (2004). Women's mental health during pregnancy influences fetal and infant developmental and health outcomes. *CNS. Spectr., 9,* 198–206.

Flynn, H. A., Blow, F. C., & Marcus, S. M. (2006). Rates and predictors of depression treatment among pregnant women in hospital-affiliated obstetrics practices. *Gen. Hosp. Psychiatry, 28,* 289–295.

Freeman, E. W., Sammel, M. D., Lin, H., & Nelson, D. B. (2006). Associations of hormones and menopausal status with depressed mood in women with no history of depression. *Arch. Gen. Psychiatry, 63,* 375–382.

Freeman, E. W., Sammel, M. D., Liu, L., Gracia, C. R., Nelson, D. B., & Hollander, L. (2004). Hormones and menopausal status as predictors of depression in women in transition to menopause. *Arch. Gen. Psychiatry, 61,* 62–70.

Freeman, M. P., Smith, K. W., Freeman, S. A., McElroy, S. L., Kmetz, G. E., Wright, R., & Keck, P. E. Jr. (2002). The impact of reproductive events on the course of bipolar disorder in women. *J. Clin. Psychiatry, 63*, 284–287.

Froescher, W., Eichelbaum, M., Niesen, M., Dietrich, K., & Rausch, P. (1984). Carbamazepine levels in breast milk. *Ther. Drug Monit., 6*, 266–271.

Frye, M. A., Altshuler, L. L., McElroy, S. L., Suppes, T., Keck, P. E., Denicoff, K., Nolen, W. A., Kupka, R., Leverich, G. S., Pollio, C., Grunze, H., Walden, J., & Post, R. M. (2003). Gender differences in prevalence, risk, and clinical correlates of alcoholism comorbidity in bipolar disorder. *Am. J. Psychiatry, 160*, 883–889.

Garland, E. J. & Behr, R. (1996). Hormonal effects of valproic acid? *J. Am. Acad. Child Adolesc. Psychiatry, 35*, 1424–1425.

Gartner L. (1997). Breastfeeding and the use of human milk. American Academy of Pediatrics Work Group on Breastfeeding. *Pediatrics, 100*, 1035–1039.

Ge, X., Conger, R. D., Lorenz, F. O., & Simons, R. L. (1994). Parents' stressful life events and adolescent depressed mood. *J. Health Soc. Behav., 35*, 28–44.

Geller, B., Cooper, T. B., Sun, K., Zimerman, B., Frazier, J., Williams, M., & Heath, J. (1998). Double-blind and placebo-controlled study of lithium for adolescent bipolar disorders with secondary substance dependency. *J. Am. Acad. Child Adolesc. Psychiatry, 37*, 171–178.

Geller, B. & Luby, J. (1997). Child and adolescent bipolar disorder: a review of the past 10 years. *J. Am. Acad. Child Adolesc. Psychiatry, 36*, 1168–1176.

Geller, B., Zimerman, B., Williams, M., Bolhofner, K., & Craney, J. L. (2001). Bipolar disorder at prospective follow-up of adults who had prepubertal major depressive disorder. *Am. J. Psychiatry, 158*, 125–127.

Gentile, S. (2003). Oxcarbazepine in pregnancy and lactation. *Clin. Drug Investig., 23*, 687.

Gentile, S. (2005). Lamotrigine in pregnancy and lactation. *Arch. Womens Ment. Health, 8*, 57–58.

Gitlin, M. J. & Pasnau, R. O. (1989). Psychiatric syndromes linked to reproductive function in women: a review of current knowledge. *Am. J. Psychiatry, 146*, 1413–1422.

GlaxoSmithKline. (2005). New safety information regarding paroxetine findings suggest increased risk over other antidepressants, of congenital malformations, following first trimester exposure to paroxetine 225. Available at http://www.gsk.ca/en/health_info/PAXIL_Pregnancy   DHCPL_EV4.pdf Accessed September 29, 2005.

Goodman, J. H. (2004). Paternal postpartum depression, its relationship to maternal postpartum depression, and implications for family health. *J. Adv. Nurs., 45*, 26–35.

Grof, P., Robbins, W., Alda, M., Berghoefer, A., Vojtechovsky, M., Nilsson, A., & Robertson, C. (2000). Protective effect of pregnancy in women with lithium-responsive bipolar disorder. *J. Affect. Disord, 61*, 31–39.

Hahn, C. G., Umapathy, Wang, H. Y., Koneru, R., Levinson, D. F., & Friedman, E. (2005). Lithium and valproic acid treatments reduce PKC activation and receptor-G protein coupling in platelets of bipolar manic patients. *J. Psychiatr. Res., 39*, 355–363.

Halbreich, U. (2004). Prevalence of mood symptoms and depressions during pregnancy: implications for clinical practice and research. *CNS Spectr., 9*, 177–184.

Hallberg, P. & Sjoblom, V. (2005). The use of selective serotonin reuptake inhibitors during pregnancy and breast-feeding: a review and clinical aspects. *J. Clin. Psychopharmacol., 25*, 59–73.

Harlow, B. L., Wise, L. A., Otto, M. W., Soares, C. N., & Cohen, L. S. (2003). Depression and its influence on reproductive endocrine and menstrual cycle markers associated with perimenopause: the Harvard Study of Moods and Cycles. *Arch. Gen. Psychiatry, 60*, 29–36.

Hatotani, N., Kitayama, I., Inoue, K., & Nomure, J. (1983). Psychoendocrine studies of recurrent psychoses. In N. Hatotani & J. Nomura (Eds.), *Neurobiology of Periodic Psychoses* (pp. 77–92). Tokyo: Igaku-Shoin.

Haynes, P. & Parry, B. L. (1998). Mood disorders and the reproductive cycle: affective disorders during the menopause and premenstrual dysphoric disorder. *Psychopharmacol. Bull., 34*, 313–318.

Hendrick, V. & Altshuler, L. L. (1998). Recurrent mood shifts of premenstrual dysphoric disorder can be mistaken for rapid-cycling bipolar II disorder. *J. Clin. Psychiatry, 59*, 479–480.

Hendrick, V., Altshuler, L. L., & Burt, V. K. (1996). Course of psychiatric disorders across the menstrual cycle. *Harv. Rev. Psychiatry, 4*, 200–207.

Hendrick, V., Altshuler, L. L., Gitlin, M. J., Delrahim, S., & Hammen, C. (2000). Gender and bipolar illness. *J. Clin. Psychiatry, 61*, 393–396.

Herzog, A. G. (1991). Reproductive endocrine considerations and hormonal therapy for women with epilepsy. *Epilepsia, 32* (Suppl 6), S27–S33.

Herzog, A. G., Seibel, M. M., Schomer, D. L., Vaitukaitis, J. L., & Geschwind, N. (1986). Reproductive endocrine disorders in women with partial seizures of temporal lobe origin. *Arch. Neurol., 43*, 341–346.

Hirschfeld, R. M., Calabrese, J. R., Weissman, M. M., Reed, M., Davies, M. A., Frye, M. A., Keck, P. E. Jr., Lewis, L., McElroy, S. L., McNulty, J. P., & Wagner, K. D. (2003). Screening for bipolar disorder in the community. *J. Clin. Psychiatry, 64*, 53–59.

Holmes, L. B., Harvey, E. A., Coull, B. A., Huntington, K. B., Khoshbin, S., Hayes, A. M., & Ryan, L. M. (2001). The teratogenicity of anticonvulsant drugs. *N. Engl. J. Med., 344*, 1132–1138.

Hunt, N. & Silverstone, T. (1995). Does puerperal illness distinguish a subgroup of bipolar patients? *J. Affect. Disord., 34*, 101–107.

Iqbal, M. M., Gundlapalli, S. P., Ryan, W. G., Ryals, T., & Passman, T. E. (2001). Effects of antimanic mood-stabilizing drugs on fetuses, neonates, and nursing infants. *South. Med. J., 94*, 304–322.

Isojarvi, J. I., Laatikainen, T. J., Pakarinen, A. J., Juntunen, K. T., & Myllyla, V. V. (1993). Polycystic ovaries and hyperandrogenism in women taking valproate for epilepsy. *N. Engl. J. Med., 329*, 1383–1388.

Isojarvi, J. I. & Tapanainen, J. S. (2000). Valproate, hyperandrogenism, and polycystic ovaries: a report of 3 cases. *Arch. Neurol., 57*, 1064–1068.

Jacobsen, F. M. (1993). Low-dose valproate: a new treatment for cyclothymia, mild rapid cycling disorders, and premenstrual syndrome. *J. Clin. Psychiatry, 54*, 229–234.

Jager-Roman, E., Deichl, A., Jakob, S., Hartmann, A. M., Koch, S., Rating, D., Steldinger, R., Nau, H., & Helge, H. (1986). Fetal growth, major malformations, and minor anomalies in infants born to women receiving valproic acid. *J. Pediatr., 108*, 997–1004.

Jefferson, J. W., Greist, J., & Ackerman, D. (1987). *Lithium Encyclopedia for Clinical Practice* (2nd edn.). Washington, DC: American Psychiatric Press.

Joffe, H., Cohen, L. S., Suppes, T., Hwang, C. H., Molay, F., Adams, J. M., Sachs, G. S., & Hall, J. E. (2006a). Longitudinal follow-up of reproductive and metabolic features of valproate-associated polycystic ovarian syndrome features: A preliminary report. *Biol. Psychiatry, 60,* 1378–1381.

Joffe, H., Kim, D. R., Foris, J. M., Baldassano, C. F., Gyulai, L., Hwang, C. H., McLaughlin, W. L., Sachs, G. S., Thase, M. E., Harlow, B. L., & Cohen, L. S. (2006b). Menstrual dysfunction prior to onset of psychiatric illness is reported more commonly by women with bipolar disorder than by women with unipolar depression and healthy controls. *J. Clin. Psychiatry, 67,* 297–304.

Jones, K. L., Lacro, R. V., Johnson, K. A., & Adams, J. (1989). Pattern of malformations in the children of women treated with carbamazepine during pregnancy. *N. Engl. J. Med., 320,* 1661–1666.

Kaneko, S., Battino, D., Andermann, E., Wada, K., Kan, R., Takeda, A., Nakane, Y., Ogawa, Y., Avanzini, G., Fumarola, C., Granata, T., Molteni, F., Pardi, G., Minotti, L., Canger, R., Dansky, L., Oguni, M., Lopes-Cendas, I., Sherwin, A., Andermann, F., Seni, M. H., Okada, M., & Teranishi, T. (1999). Congenital malformations due to antiepileptic drugs. *Epilepsy Res., 33,* 145–158.

Karadag, F., Akdeniz, F., Erten, E., Pirildar, S., Yucel, B., Polat, A., & Atmaca, M. (2004). Menstrually related symptom changes in women with treatment-responsive bipolar disorder. *Bipolar Disord., 6,* 253–259.

Kashani, J. H., Cantwell, D. P., Shekim, W. O., & Reid, J. C. (1982). Major depressive disorder in children admitted to an inpatient community mental health center. *Am. J. Psychiatry, 139,* 671–672.

Kaufert, P. A., Gilbert, P., & Tate, R. (1992). The Manitoba Project: a re-examination of the link between menopause and depression. *Maturitas, 14,* 143–155.

Kendell, R. E., Chalmers, J. C., & Platz, C. (1987). Epidemiology of puerperal psychoses. *Br. J. Psychiatry, 150,* 662–673.

Kennedy, D. & Koren, G. (1998). Valproic acid use in psychiatry: issues in treating women of reproductive age. *J. Psychiatry Neurosci., 23,* 223–228.

Kessler, R. C., McGonagle, K. A., Swartz, M., Blazer, D. G., & Nelson, C. B. (1993). Sex and depression in the National Comorbidity Survey. I: Lifetime prevalence, chronicity and recurrence. *J. Affect. Disord., 29,* 85–96.

Kessler, R. C., McGonagle, K. A., Zhao, S., Nelson, C. B., Hughes, M., Eshleman, S., Wittchen, H. U., Kendler, K. S. (1994). Lifetime and 12-month prevalence of DSM-III-R psychiatric disorders in the United States. Results from the National Comorbidity Survey. *Arch. Gen. Psychiatry, 51,* 8–19.

Koch, S., Jager-Roman, E., Rating, D., & Helge, H. (1983). Possible teratogenic effect of valproate during pregnancy. *J. Pediatr., 103,* 1007–1008.

Koren, G., Matsui, D., Einarson, A., Knoppert, D., & Steiner, M. (2005). Is maternal use of selective serotonin reuptake inhibitors in the third trimester of pregnancy harmful to neonates? *CMAJ, 172,* 1457–1459.

Kovacs, M. (1996). Presentation and course of major depressive disorder during childhood and later years of the life span. *J. Am. Acad. Child Adolesc. Psychiatry, 35,* 705–715.

Kuijpens, J. L., Vader, H. L., Drexhage, H. A., Wiersinga, W. M., van Son, M. J., & Pop, V. J. (2001). Thyroid peroxidase antibodies during gestation are a marker for subsequent depression postpartum. *Eur. J. Endocrinol., 145,* 579–584.

Kukopulos, A., Minnai, G., & Muller-Oerlinghausen, B. (1985). The influence of mania and depression on the pharmacokinetics of lithium: A longitundinal single-case study. *J. Affect. Disord., 8*, 159–166.

Kuller, J. A., Katz, V. L., McMahon, M. J., Wells, S. R., & Bashford, R. A. (1996). Pharmacologic treatment of psychiatric disease in pregnancy and lactation: fetal and neonatal effects. *Obstet. Gynecol., 87*, 789–794.

Labad, J., Urretavizcaya, M., & Crespo, J. M. (2006). Onset of unipolar depression or bipolar disorder prior or close to menarche. *J. Clin. Psychiatry, 67*, 2032.

Lata, P. F. & Elliott, M. E. (2007). Patient assessment in the diagnosis, prevention, and treatment of osteoporosis. *Nutr. Clin. Pract., 22*, 261–275.

Leibenluft, E. (1996). Women with bipolar illness: clinical and research issues. *Am. J. Psychiatry, 153*, 163–173.

Leibenluft, E., Ashman, S. B., Feldman-Naim, S., & Yonkers, K. A. (1999). Lack of relationship between menstrual cycle phase and mood in a sample of women with rapid cycling bipolar disorder. *Biol. Psychiatry, 46*, 577–580.

Lewinsohn, P. M., Klein, D. N., & Seeley, J. R. (1995). Bipolar disorders in a community sample of older adolescents: prevalence, phenomenology, comorbidity, and course. *J. Am. Acad. Child Adolesc. Psychiatry, 34*, 454–463.

Levinson-Castiel, R., Merlob, P., Linder, N., Sirota, L., & Klinger, G. (2006). Neonatal abstinence syndrome after in utero exposure to selective serotonin reuptake inhibitors in term infants. *Arch. Pediatr. Adolesc. Med., 160*, 173–176.

Liporace, J., Kao, A., & D'Abreu, A. (2004). Concerns regarding lamotrigine and breast-feeding. *Epilepsy Behav., 5*, 102–105.

Lish, J. D., me-Meenan, S., Whybrow, P. C., Price, R. A., & Hirschfeld, R. M. (1994). The National Depressive and Manic-depressive Association (DMDA) survey of bipolar members. *J. Affect. Disord., 31*, 281–294.

Lord, A., Kalimo, H., Eckman, C., Zhang, X. Q., Lannfelt, L., & Nilsson, L. N. (2006). The Arctic Alzheimer mutation facilitates early intraneuronal Abeta aggregation and senile plaque formation in transgenic mice. *Neurobiol. Aging, 27*, 67–77.

Louik, C., Lin, A. E., Werler, M. M., Hernandez-Diaz, S., & Mitchell, A. A. (2007). First-trimester use of selective serotonin-reuptake inhibitors and the risk of birth defects. *N. Engl. J. Med., 356*, 2675–2683.

Luggin, R., Bernsted, L., Petersson, B., & Jacobsen, A. T. (1984). Acute psychiatric admission related to the menstrual cycle. *Acta Psychiatr. Scand., 69*, 461–465.

Manji, H. K. & Lenox, R. H. (1999). Ziskind-Somerfeld Research Award. Protein kinase C signaling in the brain: molecular transduction of mood stabilization in the treatment of manic-depressive illness. *Biol. Psychiatry, 46*, 1328–1351.

Marcus, S. M., Flynn, H. A., Blow, F. C., & Barry, K. L. (2003). Depressive symptoms among pregnant women screened in obstetrics settings. *J. Womens Health (Larchmt.), 12*, 373–380.

Marsh, W. K., Templeton, A., Ketter, T. A., & Rasgon, N. L. (2007). Increased frequency of depressive episodes during the menopausal transition in women with bipolar disorder: Preliminary report. *J. Psychiatr. Res., 42* (3), 247–251.

Matalon, S., Schechtman, S., Goldzweig, G., & Ornoy, A. (2002). The teratogenic effect of carbamazepine: a meta-analysis of 1255 exposures. *Reproductive Toxicol., 16*, 9–17.

Matsunaga, H. & Sarai, M. (1993). Elevated serum LH and androgens in affective disorder related to the menstrual cycle: with reference to polycystic ovary syndrome. *Jpn. J. Psychiatry Neurol., 47*, 825–842.

Matthey, S., Barnett, B., Kavanagh, D. J., & Howie, P. (2001). Validation of the Edinburgh Postnatal Depression Scale for men, and comparison of item endorsement with their partners. *J. Affect. Disord., 64,* 175–184.

McAuley, J. W., Koshy, S. J., Moore, J. L., Peebles, C. T., & Reeves, A. L. (2000). Characterization and health risk assessment of postmenopausal women with epilepsy. *Epilepsy Behav., 1,* 353–355.

McElroy, S. L., Strakowski, S. M., Keck, P. E., Jr., Tugrul, K. L., West, S. A., & Lonczak, H. S. (1995). Differences and similarities in mixed and pure mania. *Compr. Psychiatry, 36,* 187–194.

McIntyre, R. S., Mancini, D. A., McCann, S., Srinivasan, J., & Kennedy, S. H. (2003). Valproate, bipolar disorder and polycystic ovarian syndrome. *Bipolar Disord., 5,* 28–35.

Meighan, M., Davis, M. W., Thomas, S. P., & Droppleman, P. G. (1999). Living with postpartum depression: the father's experience. *MCN Am. J. Matern. Child Nurs., 24,* 202–208.

Mizrahi, E. M., Hobbs, J. F., & Goldsmith, D. I. (1979). Nephrogenic diabetes insipidus in transplacental lithium intoxication. *J. Pediatr., 94,* 493–495.

Morrow, J., Russell, A., Guthrie, E., Parsons, L., Robertson, I., Waddell, R., Irwin, B., McGivern, R. C., Morrison, P. J., & Craig, J. (2006). Malformation risks of antiepileptic drugs in pregnancy: a prospective study from the UK Epilepsy and Pregnancy Register. *J. Neurol. Neurosurg. Psychiatry, 77,* 193–198.

Nars, P. W. & Girard, J. (1977). Lithium carbonate intake during pregnancy leading to large goiter in a premature infant. *Am. J. Dis. Child, 131,* 924–925.

Nolen-Hoeksema, S. (1987). Sex differences in unipolar depression: evidence and theory. *Psychol. Bull., 101,* 259–282.

Nulman, I., Rovet, J., Kennedy, D., Wasson, C., Gladstone, J., Fried, S., & Koren, G. (2004). Binge alcohol consumption by non-alcohol-dependent women during pregnancy affects child behavior, but not general intellectual functioning; a prospective controlled study. *Arch. Womens Ment. Health, 7,* 173–181.

Nulman, I., Rovet, J., Stewart, D. E., Wolpin, J., Pace-Asciak, P., Shuhaiber, S., & Koren, G. (2002). Child development following exposure to tricyclic antidepressants or fluoxetine throughout fetal life: a prospective, controlled study. *Am. J. Psychiatry, 159,* 1889–1895.

O'Donovan, C., Kusumakar, V., Graves, G. R., & Bird, D. C. (2002). Menstrual abnormalities and polycystic ovary syndrome in women taking valproate for bipolar mood disorder. *J. Clin. Psychiatry, 63,* 322–330.

Ohman, I., Vitols, S., & Tomson, T. (2000). Lamotrigine in pregnancy: pharmacokinetics during delivery, in the neonate, and during lactation. *Epilepsia, 41,* 709–713.

Oinonen, K. A. & Mazmanian, D. (2002). To what extent do oral contraceptives influence mood and affect? *J. Affect. Disord., 70,* 229–240.

Omtzigt, J. G., Los, F. J., Hagenaars, A. M., Stewart, P. A., Sachs, E. S., & Lindhout, D. (1992). Prenatal diagnosis of spina bifida aperta after first-trimester valproate exposure. *Prenat. Diagn., 12,* 893–897.

Orr, S. T. & Miller, C. A. (1995). Maternal depressive symptoms and the risk of poor pregnancy outcome. Review of the literature and preliminary findings. *Epidemiol. Rev., 17,* 165–171.

Packer, S. (1992). Family planning for women with bipolar disorder. *Hosp. Community Psychiatry, 43,* 479–482.

Paffenbarger, R. S., Jr. & McCabe, L. J., Jr. (1966). The effect of obstetric and peri-natal events on risk of mental illness in women of childbearing age. *Am. J. Public Health Nations Health, 56,* 400–407.

Papatheodorou, G., Kutcher, S. P., Katic, M., & Szalai, J. P. (1995). The efficacy and safety of divalproex sodium in the treatment of acute mania in adolescents and young adults: an open clinical trial. *J. Clin. Psychopharmacol., 15,* 110–116.

Pastuszak, A., Schick-Boschetto, B., Zuber, C., Feldkamp, M., Pinelli, M., Sihn, S., Donnenfeld, A., McCormack, M., Leen-Mitchell, M., Woodland, C., et al. (1993). Pregnancy outcome following first-trimester exposure to fluoxetine (Prozac). *JAMA, 269,* 2246–2248.

Payne, J. L., Roy, P. S., Murphy-Eberenz, K., Weismann, M. M., Swartz, K. L., McInnis, M. G., Nwulia, E., Mondimore, F. M., MacKinnon, D. F., Miller, E. B., Nurnberger, J. I., Levinson, D. F., DePaulo, J. R. Jr., & Potash, J. B. (2007). Reproductive cycle-associated mood symptoms in women with major depression and bipolar disorder. *J. Affect. Disord., 99,* 221–229.

Pearlstein, T. & Steiner, M. (2000). Non-antidepressant treatment of premenstrual syndrome. *J. Clin. Psychiatry, 61* (Suppl 12), 22–27.

Pennell, P. B., Newport, D. J., Stowe, Z. N., Helmers, S. L., Montgomery, J. Q., & Henry, T. R. (2004). The impact of pregnancy and childbirth on the metabo-lism of lamotrigine. *Neurology, 62,* 292–295.

Penovich, P. E., Eck, K. E., & Economou, V. V. (2004). Recommendations for the care of women with epilepsy. *Cleve. Clin. J. Med., 71* (Suppl 2), S49–S57.

Perucca, E. (2005). Birth defects after prenatal exposure to antiepileptic drugs. *Lancet Neurol., 4,* 781–786.

Perugi, G., Musetti, L., Simonini, E., Piagentini, F., Cassano, G. B., & Akiskal, H. S. (1990). Gender-mediated clinical features of depressive illness. The impor-tance of temperamental differences. *Br. J. Psychiatry, 157,* 835–841.

Petersen, A. C., Sarigiani, P., & Kennedy R. E. (1991). Adolescent depression: why more girls? *J. Youth Adoles., 20,* 247–271.

Petrenaite, V., Sabers, A., & Hansen-Schwartz, J. (2005). Individual changes in lam-otrigine plasma concentrations during pregnancy. *Epilepsy Res., 65,* 185–188.

Price, W. A. & DiMarzio, L. (1986). Premenstrual tension syndrome in rapid-cycling bipolar affective disorder. *J. Clin. Psychiatry, 47,* 415–417.

Pugh, T. F., Jerath, B. K., Schmidt, W. M., & Reed, R. B. (1963). Rates of mental dis-ease related to childbearing. *N. Engl. J. Med., 268,* 1224–1228.

Rambeck, B., Kurlemann, G., Stodieck, S. R., May, T. W., & Jurgens, U. (1997). Concentrations of lamotrigine in a mother on lamotrigine treatment and her newborn child. *Eur. J. Clin. Pharmacol., 51,* 481–484.

Rao, U., Ryan, N. D., Birmaher, B., Dahl, R. E., Williamson, D. E., Kaufman, J., Rao, R., & Nelson, B. (1995). Unipolar depression in adolescents: clinical outcome in adulthood. *J. Am. Acad. Child Adolesc. Psychiatry, 34,* 566–578.

Rapkin, A. J., Mikacich, J. A., & Moatakef-Imani, B. (2003). Reproductive mood disorders. *Prim Psychiatry, 10,* 31–40.

Rasgon, N., Bauer, M., Glenn, T., Elman, S., & Whybrow, P. C. (2003). Menstrual cycle related mood changes in women with bipolar disorder. *Bipolar Disord., 5,* 48–52.

Rasgon, N. L., Altshuler, L. L., Gudeman, D., Burt, V. K., Tanavoli, S., Hendrick, V., & Korenman, S. (2000). Medication status and polycystic ovary syndrome in women with bipolar disorder: a preliminary report. *J. Clin. Psychiatry, 61,* 173–178.

Rasgon, N. L., Silverman, D., Siddarth, P., Miller, K., Ercoli, L. M., Elman, S., Lavretsky, H., Huang, S. C., Phelps, M. E., & Small, G. W. (2005). Estrogen use and brain metabolic change in postmenopausal women. *Neurobiol. Aging, 26,* 229–235.

Rattya, J., Turkka, J., Pakarinen, A. J., Knip, M., Kotila, M. A., Lukkarinen, O., Myllylä, V. V., & Isojärvi, J. I. (2001). Reproductive effects of valproate, carbamazepine, and oxcarbazepine in men with epilepsy. *Neurology, 56,* 31–36.

Reich, T. & Winokur, G. (1970). Postpartum psychoses in patients with manic depressive disease. *J. Nerv. Ment. Dis., 151,* 60–68.

Robinson, G. E. & Stewart, D. E. (1986). Postpartum psychiatric disorders. *CMAJ, 134,* 31–37.

Rodriguez-Pinilla, E., Arroyo, I., Fondevilla, J., Garcia, M. J., & Martinez-Frias, M. L. (2000). Prenatal exposure to valproic acid during pregnancy and limb deficiencies: a case-control study. *Am. J. Med. Genet., 90,* 376–381.

Rosa, F. W. (1991). Spina bifida in infants of women treated with carbamazepine during pregnancy. *N. Engl. J. Med., 324,* 674–677.

Rowland, A. S., Baird, D. D., Long, S., Wegienka, G., Harlow, S. D., Alavanja, M., & Sandler, D. P. (2002). Influence of medical conditions and lifestyle factors on the menstrual cycle. *Epidemiology, 13,* 668–674.

Roy-Byrne, P. P., Rubinow, D. R., Hoban, M. C., Parry, B. L., Rosenthal, N. E., Nurnberger, J. I., & Byrnes, S. (1986). Premenstrual changes: a comparison of five populations. *Psychiatry Res., 17,* 77–85.

Rutter, M. (1986). Child psychiatry: looking 30 years ahead. *J. Child Psychol. Psychiatry, 27,* 803–840.

Rzany, B., Correia, O., Kelly, J. P., Naldi, L., Auquier, A., & Stern, R. (1999). Risk of Stevens-Johnson syndrome and toxic epidermal necrolysis during first weeks of antiepileptic therapy: a case-control study. Study Group of the International Case Control Study on Severe Cutaneous Adverse Reactions. *Lancet, 353,* 2190–2194.

Sabers, A., Buchholt, J. M., Uldall, P., & Hansen, E. L. (2001). Lamotrigine plasma levels reduced by oral contraceptives. *Epilepsy Res., 47,* 151–154.

Sabers, A., Dam, M., Rogvi-Hansen, B., Boas, J., Sidenius, P., Laue, F. M., Alving, J., Dahl, M., Ankerhus, J., & Mouritzen Dam, A. (2004). Epilepsy and pregnancy: lamotrigine as main drug used. *Acta Neurol. Scand., 109,* 9–13.

Sajatovic, M., Friedman, S. H., Schuermeyer, I. N., Safavi, R., Ignacio, R. V., Hays, R. W., West, J. A., & Blow, F. C. (2006). Menopause knowledge and subjective experience among peri- and postmenopausal women with bipolar disorder, schizophrenia and major depression. *J. Nerv. Ment. Dis., 194,* 173–178.

Salloum, I. M., Cornelius, J. R., Mezzich, J. E., Kirisci, L., Daley, D. C., Spotts, C. R., & Zuckoff, A. (2001). Characterizing female bipolar alcoholic patients presenting for initial evaluation. *Addict. Behav., 26,* 341–348.

Schmidt, P. J., Grover, G. N., Hoban, M. C., & Rubinow, D. R. (1990). State-dependent alterations in the perception of life events in menstrual-related mood disorders. *Am. J. Psychiatry, 147,* 230–234.

Schmidt, P. J., Haq, N., & Rubinow, D. R. (2004). A longitudinal evaluation of the relationship between reproductive status and mood in perimenopausal women. *Am. J. Psychiatry, 161,* 2238–2244.

Schmidt, P. J., Nieman, L. K., Danaceau, M. A., Adams, L. F., & Rubinow, D. R. (1998). Differential behavioral effects of gonadal steroids in women with and in those without premenstrual syndrome. *N. Engl. J. Med., 338,* 209–216.

Schou, M., Amdisen, A., & Steenstrup, O. R. (1973). Lithium and pregnancy. II. Hazards to women given lithium during pregnancy and delivery. *Br. Med. J.,* 2, 137–138.

Sharma, V., Smith, A., & Khan, M. (2004). The relationship between duration of labour, time of delivery, and puerperal psychosis. *J. Affect. Disord., 83,* 215–220.

Simon, G. E., Cunningham, M. L., & Davis, R. L. (2002). Outcomes of prenatal antidepressant exposure. *Am. J. Psychiatry, 159,* 2055–2061.

Singer, K., Cheng, R., & Schou, M. (1974). A controlled evaluation of lithium in the premenstrual tension syndrome. *Br. J. Psychiatry, 124,* 50–51.

Singh, K. B. (1981). Menstrual disorders in college students. *Am. J. Obstet. Gynecol., 140,* 299–302.

Skausig, O. B. & Schou, M. (1977). Breast feeding during lithium therapy. *Ugeskr. Laeger, 139,* 400–401.

Soares, C. N., Prouty, J., Born, L., & Steiner, M. (2005). Treatment of menopause-related mood disturbances. *CNS Spectr., 10,* 489–497.

Soares, C. N. & Taylor, V. (2007). Effects and management of the menopausal transition in women with depression and bipolar disorder. *J. Clin. Psychiatry, 68* (Suppl 9), 16–21.

Solomon, C. G., Hu, F. B., Dunaif, A., Rich-Edwards, J., Willett, W. C., Hunter, D. J., Colditz, G. A., Speizer, F. E., & Manson, J. E. (2001). Long or highly irregular menstrual cycles as a marker for risk of type 2 diabetes mellitus. *JAMA, 286,* 2421–2426.

Stahl, M. M., Neiderud, J., & Vinge, E. (1997). Thrombocytopenic purpura and anemia in a breast-fed infant whose mother was treated with valproic acid. *J. Pediatr., 130,* 1001–1003.

Steer, R. A., Scholl, T. O., Hediger, M. L., & Fischer, R. L. (1992). Self-reported depression and negative pregnancy outcomes. *J. Clin. Epidemiol., 45,* 1093–1099.

Steiner M., Born L., Marton P. (2000) Menarche and mood disorders in adolescence. In M. Steiner, K. A. Yonkers, E. Eriksson (Eds), Mood Disorders in Women (pp. 247–268). London, UK: Martin Dunitz Ltd.

Steiner, M., Dunn, E., & Born, L. (2003). Hormones and mood: from menarche to menopause and beyond. *J. Affect. Disord., 74,* 67–83.

Steiner, M., Haskett, R. F., Osmun, J. N., & Carroll, B. J. (1980). Treatment of premenstrual tension with lithium carbonate. A pilot study. *Acta Psychiatr. Scand., 61,* 96–102.

Strober, M. & Carlson, G. (1982). Bipolar illness in adolescents with major depression: clinical, genetic, and psychopharmacologic predictors in a three- to four-year prospective follow-up investigation. *Arch. Gen. Psychiatry, 39,* 549–555.

Suri, R., Altshuler, L., Hendrick, V., Rasgon, N., Lee, E., & Mintz, J. (2004). The impact of depression and fluoxetine treatment on obstetrical outcome. *Arch. Womens Ment. Health, 7,* 193–200.

Swann, A. C. (2005). Long–term treatment in bipolar disorder. *J. Clin. Psychiatry, 66* (Suppl 1), 7–12.

Targum, S. D., Davenport, Y. B., & Webster, M. J. (1979). Postpartum mania in bipolar manic-depressive patients withdrawn from lithium carbonate. *J. Nerv. Ment. Dis., 167,* 572–574.

Taylor, M. A. & Abrams, R. (1981). Gender differences in bipolar affective disorder. *J. Affect. Disord., 3,* 261–271.

Tennis, P. & Eldridge, R. R. (2002). Preliminary results on pregnancy outcomes in women using lamotrigine. *Epilepsia, 43,* 1161–1167.

Terp, I. M. & Mortensen, P. B. (1998). Post-partum psychoses. Clinical diagnoses and relative risk of admission after parturition. *Br. J. Psychiatry, 172,* 521–526.

Tomson, T., Ohman, I., & Vitols, S. (1997). Lamotrigine in pregnancy and lactation: a case report. *Epilepsia, 38,* 1039–1041.

Tondo, L. & Baldessarini, R. J. (1998). Rapid cycling in women and men with bipolar manic-depressive disorders. *Am. J. Psychiatry, 155,* 1434–1436.

Tran, T. A., Leppik, I. E., Blesi, K., Sathanandan, S. T., & Remmel, R. (2002). Lamotrigine clearance during pregnancy. *Neurology, 59,* 251–255.

Vajda, F., Lander, C., O'brien, T., Hitchcock, A., Graham, J., Solinas, C., Eadie, M., & Cook, M. (2004). Australian pregnancy registry of women taking antiepileptic drugs. *Epilepsia, 45,* 1466.

Vajda, F. J. & Eadie, M. J. (2005). Maternal valproate dosage and foetal malformations. *Acta Neurol. Scand., 112,* 137–143.

Vajda, F. J., O'Brien, T. J., Hitchcock, A., Graham, J., & Lander, C. (2003). The Australian registry of anti-epileptic drugs in pregnancy: experience after 30 months. *J. Clin. Neurosci., 10,* 543–549.

Viguera, A. C. & Cohen, L. S. (1998). The course and management of bipolar disorder during pregnancy. *Psychopharmacol. Bull., 34,* 339–346.

Viguera, A. C., Cohen, L. S., Baldessarini, R. J., & Nonacs, R. (2002). Managing bipolar disorder during pregnancy: weighing the risks and benefits. *Can. J. Psychiatry, 47,* 426–436.

Viguera, A. C., Nonacs, R., Cohen, L. S., Tondo, L., Murray, A., & Baldessarini, R. J. (2000). Risk of recurrence of bipolar disorder in pregnant and nonpregnant women after discontinuing lithium maintenance. *Am. J. Psychiatry, 157,* 179–184.

Vinten, J., Adab, N., Kini, U., Gorry, J., Gregg, J., & Baker, G. A. (2005). Neuropsychological effects of exposure to anticonvulsant medication in utero. *Neurology, 64,* 949–954.

Wang, H. Y., Johnson, G. P., & Friedman, E. (2001). Lithium treatment inhibits protein kinase C translocation in rat brain cortex. *Psychopharmacology (Berl), 158,* 80–86.

Wehr, T. A., Sack, D. A., Rosenthal, N. E., & Cowdry, R. W. (1988). Rapid cycling affective disorder: contributing factors and treatment responses in 51 patients. *Am. J. Psychiatry, 145,* 179–184.

Weissman, M. M. & Klerman, G. L. (1977). Sex differences and the epidemiology of depression. *Arch. Gen. Psychiatry, 34,* 98–111.

Weissman, M. M., Leaf, P. J., Holzer, C. E., III, Myers, J. K., & Tischler, G. L. (1984). The epidemiology of depression. An update on sex differences in rates. *J. Affect. Disord., 7,* 179–188.

Weissman, M. M., Leaf, P. J., Tischler, G. L., Blazer, D. G., Karno, M., Bruce, M. L., & Florio, L. P. (1988). Affective disorders in five United States communities. *Psychol. Med., 18,* 141–153.

Williams, K. & Oke, S. (2000). Lithium and pregnancy. *Psychiatr. Bull., 24,* 229–231.

Wyszynski, D. F., Nambisan, M., Surve, T., Alsdorf, R. M., Smith, C. R., & Holmes, L. B. (2005). Increased rate of major malformations in offspring exposed to valproate during pregnancy. *Neurology, 64,* 961–965.

Yonkers, K. A. (1997). The association between premenstrual dysphoric disorder and other mood disorders. *J. Clin. Psychiatry, 58* (Suppl 15), 19–25.

Yonkers, K. A., Wisner, K. L., Stowe, Z., Leibenluft, E., Cohen, L., Miller, L., Manber, R., Viguera, A., Suppes, T., & Altshuler, L. (2004). Management of bipolar disorder during pregnancy and the postpartum period. *Am. J. Psychiatry, 161,* 608–620.

Zeskind, P. S. & Stephens, L. E. (2004). Maternal selective serotonin reuptake inhibitor use during pregnancy and newborn neurobehavior. *Pediatrics, 113,* 368–375.

Zweifel, J. E. & O'Brien, W. H. (1997). A meta-analysis of the effect of hormone replacement therapy upon depressed mood. *Psychoneuroendocrinology, 22,* 189–212.

chapter seven

Bipolar disorder in children and adolescents

Joris Berwaerts
Johnson & Johnson Pharmaceutical Research and Development

Stanley Kutcher
Dalhousie University

Vivek Kusumakar
Dalhousie University
Johnson & Johnson Pharmaceutical Research and Development

Contents

Background 185
Epidemiology 186
Clinical presentation 186
Comorbidity with other DSM-IV disorders 189
Treatment 190
    Mood stabilizers 191
    Atypical antipsychotics 194
    Antidepressants 198
    Nonpharmacological interventions 198
References 199

Background

Bipolar disorder has been typically described as beginning in late adolescence or early adulthood. However, family reports, clinical experience and research findings suggest prepubertal and early adolescent onset of depressive and/or manic symptoms in a significant proportion of subjects with bipolar disorder. There are few reliable statistics on the incidence of pediatric bipolar disorder, but recent studies suggest a rapid increase in the diagnosis of childhood bipolar disorder in clinics (Moreno et al., 2007). Whether a diagnosis of childhood bipolar disorder can be validly and reliably made or not remains a highly controversial area with significant debate in the academic and lay press. Central to this controversy lies whether or not the episodic or chronic presentation of irritability, mood lability, aggression and reduced sleep in children, who are often diagnosed with bipolar disorder, truly represents a childhood-onset of bipolar disorder as described in adults.

Epidemiology

The lifetime prevalence estimates for bipolar disorder are approximately between 0.4% and 2.1%. In the National Comorbidity Survey Replication Study, the prevalence estimates varied significantly with age across different types of bipolar disorder. The lifetime prevalence was 1.0% for bipolar type I, 1.1% for bipolar type II and 2.4% for subthreshold bipolar disorder (Merikangas et al., 2007). Data from the Epidemiologic Catchment Area (ECA) survey indicated a 1-year prevalence rate of 1.4 % among young adults between 18 and 44 years. Epidemiological studies of bipolar disorder in children are limited. Community studies estimate 1% prevalence in youths. However, bipolar disorder affects an estimated 1–2% of adolescents worldwide with significant disparity in diagnostic rates across countries (Soutullo et al., 2005).

Clinical presentation

Classic bipolar illness, as described by Kraepelin and currently reflected in the DSM-IV-TR criteria, is characterized by discrete episodes of mania and depression. One of the earliest definitions in the diagnosis of prepubertal bipolar disorder was agreed upon by experts at the National Institute of Mental Health Roundtable in 2001. Two different phenotypes in children were defined: "narrow" and "broad". Children with the narrow-phenotype have the classic symptoms of episodes of mania and depression, although many of these children experience rapid cycling of their mood states and fail to meet the 4- to 7-day criteria for hypomania, thereby qualifying for a diagnosis of bipolar disorder not otherwise specified (NOS). Children with the broad phenotype present with irritability, mood lability, temper outbursts, hyperactivity, and poor concentration in a non-episodic illness pattern (National Institute of Mental Health [NIMH], 2001). The debate centers on whether bipolar disorder in children is the same as that seen in adults with implication for the treatment, prognosis and long-term outcome of the condition.

The narrow-phenotype is attributed to those who meet the full DSM-IV criteria for mania/hypomania including the duration criteria of 7 days and 4 days, respectively, and also have the hallmark symptom of elevated and expansive mood or grandiosity and decreased need for sleep. The broader phenotype consists of non-episodic chronic illness without the hallmark symptoms of elated mood or grandiosity associated with the narrow-phenotype but with irritability and hyperarousal. An intermediate phenotype has also been defined, which includes symptoms of short duration (1–3 days) and the presence of episodic irritable mania or hypomania meeting the duration criteria without elation (Leibenluft et al., 2003). The intermediate and the broad phenotypes correspond to the bipolar disorder NOS category in the DSM-IV.

Results from studies in bipolar disorder have not been consistent, in part due to different diagnostic definitions and methodology in these studies. In a series of studies by Biederman and colleagues, children with juvenile mania most often present with irritability rather than euphoria (Biederman, 2006). Irritability has also been shown to predict adulthood depressive disorder (Brotman et al., 2006). In a 4-year longitudinal study of bipolar disorder in children, Geller et al. (2004) required the presence of elation and grandiosity, a cycle of manic symptoms possibly as short as 4 hours, with at least one cycle daily for 2 weeks defined as meeting DSM-IV criteria for mania (intermediate type). They found that the diagnosis of mania in pre-adolescents was reliable and stable over 4 years, with subjects' long-term course and outcome resembling that of severe and poor-outcome adult bipolar disorder. The time to relapse after recovery was 40 weeks. Subjects had high rates of comorbidity with ADHD, although it was possible to specifically diagnose bipolar disorder by the identification of the unique symptom of euphoria/elation. Low ratings of maternal warmth predicted a shorter time to relapse, whereas psychosis was associated with greater chronicity. Whether these children will continue to develop a typical or atypical form of bipolar disorder or other disorder is an ongoing area of research. Other symptoms that are consistently seen in pediatric bipolar disorder are increase in energy and grandiosity. Episodic irritability, with periods of calm extending to weeks, is more suggestive of underlying bipolar disorder than chronic or continual irritability and aggression. Symptoms that are not frequently seen in pediatric bipolar disorder include flight of ideas, and hypersexuality (Youngstrom et al., 2008). However, symptoms of hypersexuality, in the absence of sexual abuse, is more likely to occur in the context of bipolar disorder. Symptoms that are non-specific and are not very helpful to diagnose bipolar disorder in children include difficulty in concentration, high motor activity, aggression, lack of insight and bizarre appearances.

A frequently asked question to child psychiatrists is whether childhood-onset bipolar disorder is a distinct disorder from adult-onset bipolar disorder as described in adults?

The criteria defined by (Robins & Guze, 1970) to define distinct disorders include: common phenomenology, longitudinal stability of the disorder, familial aggregation, biological underpinning and treatment response.

Phenomenology: As discussed above, the symptoms in childhood-onset bipolar disorder that have high (>75%) overlap with the adult-onset version include elation or euphoria, grandiosity, increase in energy, distractibility, irritable mood, and pressured speech. Symptoms that overlap to a lesser degree (50–75%) include racing thoughts, decreased need for sleep and poor judgment. Symptoms that overlap in less than 50% of subjects include flight of ideas and hypersexuality (Youngstrom et al., 2008).

Familial Aggregation: Recent studies suggest a tenfold increase in risk for developing bipolar disorder in relatives of adults with bipolar disorder compared with control subjects (Merikangas & Low, 2004; Hillegers et al., 2005). Studies using pediatric subjects diagnosed with bipolar disorder as probands have found significantly higher rates of bipolar disorder, but also of other mood disorders among relatives (Althoff et al., 2005). Recently, a study comparing the axis I diagnoses in parents of children with narrow-phenotype bipolar disorder and parents of youth with severe mood dysregulation found that, parents of youth with narrow-phenotype bipolar disorder were significantly more likely to be diagnosed with bipolar disorder suggesting narrow-phenotype bipolar disorder may be distinct from severe mood dysregulation in terms of familial aggregation. Additionally, the familiality of narrow-phenotype bipolar disorder in children and adult DSM-IV bipolar disorder is high (Brotman et al., 2007).

Biological Abnormalities: Brain imaging is a useful tool in understanding the neurobiology of bipolar disorder. Morphometric studies in children with bipolar show deficits in the parietal and temporal regions in areas involved in attentional control, facial recognition, and verbal and declarative memory (Frazier et al., 2005; Chang et al., 2006a; DelBello et al., 2006). These findings are similar to those seen in adult bipolar disorder. A recent imaging study compared healthy children, and children with "atypical psychosis" who had an initial presentation marked by mood dysregulation and transient psychosis. Subjects who developed bipolar disorder showed subtle, regionally specific, bilaterally asymmetrical cortical changes. Cortical grey matter increased over the left temporal cortex and decreased bilaterally in the anterior (and subgenual) cingulate cortex. The neurodevelopmental trajectory was similar to the group of children who did not develop bipolar disorder suggesting that this pattern of cortical development may reflect affective dysregulation (lability) in general (Gogtay et al., 2007).

A study comparing the behavioral and psychophysiological corre-lates of irritability among children with broad- and narrow-phenotype bipolar disorder suggests that, while irritability is an important feature of severe mood dysregulation and narrow-phenotype bipolar disorder, the pathophysiology of irritability may differ among the groups and is influ-enced by oppositional defiant disorder (ODD) severity (Rich et al., 2006). The two groups also showed differences in cognitive flexibility with the narrow-phenotype being much slower to adapt (Dickstein et al., 2007).

Preliminary magnetic resonance spectroscopy studies show abnor-malities consistent with glutamine metabolism in anterior cingulate cor-tex glia in unmedicated children with bipolar disorder similar to that in adults but not in medicated children with bipolar disorder (Moore et al., 2007).

These findings suggest that child and adult forms of bipolar disorder likely have common symptoms that are longitudinally consistent, have similar underlying neurobiology, have high familial aggregation and that the form is likely to represent childhood-onset of adult bipolar disorder. Ongoing studies of genetics and neurobiology will undoubtedly add fur-ther clarity to this issue.

Comorbidity with other DSM-IV disorders

Psychiatric comorbidity seems to be a rule rather than an exception in bipolar disorder. This may, of course, not be true co-morbidity, but simply an artifact of diagnosis because of common symptoms and phenomenology between different conditions.

Current studies suggest that peri-pubertal onset of bipolar disor-der is often characterized by continuous, rapid-cycling, irritable, and mixed mood symptom states. Although there is a symptom overlap with disruptive behavior disorders, particularly attention deficit hyper-activity disorder (ADHD) or ODD, these disruptive behavior disorders are characterized by onset before the age of 7 years, while the mood symptoms of bipolar disorder are poorly diagnosable before the age of 10. In contrast, later adolescent- or adult-onset bipolar disorder tends to begin with silent depressive symptoms and an abrupt onset of clas-sic manic or hypomanic symptoms, with an episodic pattern with rela-tively stable, calm, euthymic periods between episodes. There is also less co-occurring ADHD or ODD among those with later onset illness. On the other hand children and adolescents with ADHD appear to be only modestly at increased risk for bipolar disorders (Reich et al., 2005; Singh et al., 2006). There is some additional data that children and ado-lescents with bipolar disorder and ADHD tend to be less responsive to drugs used in the treatment of acute mania (Consoli et al., 2007).

Borderline personality symptoms in adolescence, particularly in the presence of a history of traumatic early attachment and abuse, can be characterized by biphasic mood dysregulation and turbulent behaviors. Akiskal (1996) has postulated that this is a form of "soft" bipolar disorder or bipolar disorder type II. There is no consensus in the field about this.

Treatment

Treatment for bipolar disorder should only be instituted after establishing the diagnosis by longitudinal observation, including the maintenance of a mood, activity and sleep diary, over weeks or months if required.

When there is a question whether the young person has ADHD or bipolar disorder even after detailed assessments and longitudinal observation, it is more pragmatic to institute a trial of medications for ADHD. This is because medications for ADHD are usually of a short half-life and efficacy and tolerability can be assessed within days, if not hours, unlike mood stabilizing medications, which take longer to show efficacy. However, care should be taken not to use supra-therapeutic doses of psychostimulants as this may trigger hypo/mania-like symptoms.

In a young person who presents with borderline symptoms, a trial of mood stabilizers may be worthwhile in addition to robust cognitive and behavioral therapy only if biphasic mood dysregulation is present in an episodic manner, with intervening periods of calm and reasonable interpersonal functioning.

So far, only a limited number of placebo-controlled trials of mood stabilizers and atypical antipsychotics have been conducted in children and adolescents with bipolar disorder. Up to this point, data documenting the efficacy and safety of these agents in the pediatric population was based mainly on retrospective chart reviews and small prospective studies. More recently, data have become available from double-blind placebo-controlled trials with aripiprazole, olanzapine and risperidone demonstrating the efficacy of atypical antipsychotics in pediatric mania. While most agents have only been evaluated for the treatment of acute mania, studies are currently being conducted to document their efficacy and safety as maintenance therapy and for the treatment of bipolar depression in children and adolescents.

Aripiprazole and risperidone are approved for the treatment of pediatric mania by the US FDA. Lithium is approved for the treatment of adolescent bipolar disorder in the US, largely on the basis of its efficacy in adult bipolar disorder. The benefit-risk of lithium has not been adequately demonstrated in placebo-controlled trials in the pediatric population. None of the agents is currently authorized by the US FDA for the treatment of bipolar disorder in all its phases, particularly for depression or prevention of recurrent mood episodes. The consensus from the data currently available to document the efficacy and safety of various agents supports the use of mood stabilizers and atypical antipsychotics, as monotherapy or adjunctive therapy, for the treatment of acute mania in the pediatric population (McClellan et al., 2007).

Mood stabilizers

Lithium is the only mood stabilizer currently authorized by the US FDA for the treatment of acute mania in adolescents and children ≥12 years of age. It was originally authorized for this indication on the basis of data from clinical trials in adult subjects. The benefit-risk of lithium has not been adequately demonstrated in placebo-controlled trials in the pediatric population. In 1998, Geller et al. published the data from the first placebo-controlled trial of lithium over a period of 6 weeks as monotherapy for the treatment of adolescents with bipolar disorder with comorbid substance abuse (Geller et al., 1998). With response defined as a Children's Clinical Global Assessment Scale score ≥65 at endpoint, lithium was found statistically superior to placebo for the rate of response (46.2% and 8.3% of subjects, respectively): six of 13 subjects assigned to treatment with lithium had a significant reduction in positive urine drug screens after 6 weeks compared to one out of 12 subjects receiving placebo. Kowatch et al. (2000) presented the data from an open-label, randomized controlled trial of the mood stabilizers, lithium, divalproex sodium, and carbamazepine, over a period of 6 weeks in the treatment of 42 children and adolescents aged 8–18 years presenting with an acute manic or mixed episode. With response defined as a reduction from baseline in Young Mania Rating Scale (YMRS) score of ≥50% at endpoint, the response rates were 53%, 38%, and 38% for divalproex sodium, lithium, and carbamazepine, respectively ($p=0.60$). The authors concluded that the three mood stabilizers evaluated had large effect sizes for the treatment of manic symptoms in children and adolescents with bipolar I or bipolar II disorder with response rates similar to those reported in clinical trials of adult subjects with acute mania.

In 2003, Kafantaris et al. reported the data from a large open-label trial of lithium for the treatment of adolescents presenting with an acute manic or mixed episode that served as lead-in for a subsequent randomized, placebo-controlled withdrawal trial (Kafantaris et al., 2003). In the open-label trial, 100 adolescents received treatment with lithium for 4 weeks, with 46 subjects receiving concomitant antipsychotic medication for associated psychosis or severe aggression. With response defined as a reduction from baseline in YMRS score of ≥50% at endpoint, the response rate was reported as 55%. This led the authors to conclude that treatment with lithium for 4 weeks was effective for the acute stabilization of manic symptoms in adolescents. In the randomized, placebo-controlled withdrawal trial, 19 subjects who had previously responded to open-label lithium were assigned to continuation of lithium monotherapy for 2 weeks, while 21 subjects received placebo after a 3-day taper period (Kafantaris et al., 2004). There was no statistically significant difference in the rate of exacerbation of symptoms between the two treatment groups (52.6% and 61.9%, respectively). This study did not demonstrate the maintenance of efficacy of lithium and its ability to prevent relapse in adolescent mania.

In 2003, Findling et al. also reported the data from a long-term, open-label trial of lithium in combination with divalproex sodium for the treatment of children and adolescents aged 5–17 years inclusive with a recent manic or hypomanic episode that served as lead-in for a subsequent randomized withdrawal trial (Findling et al., 2003). In the open-label trial, 90 children and adolescents received the combination for up to 20 weeks. With response defined as a reduction in YMRS score from baseline at endpoint of ≥50%, the response rate in this study was 71%. In addition, 47% of subjects met a priori criteria for remission. This led the authors to conclude that symptoms of mania and depression can be treated safely and effectively with the combination of lithium and divalproex sodium in children and adolescents with bipolar disorder. In the randomized withdrawal trial, 30 subjects who had previously responded to open-label combination therapy were assigned to lithium monotherapy, and 30 subjects received monotherapy with divalproex sodium for up to 76 weeks in a double-blind, double-dummy fashion (Findling et al., 2005). There was no statistically significant difference in the time to recurrence of emerging mood symptoms between the two treatment groups (mean (SE): 114 (57.4) days and 112 (56) days, respectively). This led the authors to conclude that divalproex sodium was not superior to lithium as maintenance treatment in children and adolescents who had been stabilized first with combination therapy. In a subsequent open-label trial, 34 of the 38 (89%) subjects who had experienced a recurrence of mood symptoms during monotherapy with either lithium or divalproex sodium in the double-blind trial were stabilized successfully with the combination of lithium and divalproex sodium (Findling et al., 2006). Four subjects required adjunctive therapy with antipsychotic medications for the treatment of residual mood symptoms or aggression.

A recently published open-label trial evaluated the safety and effectiveness of lithium as monotherapy over a 6-week period in the treatment of 27 adolescents with bipolar I disorder presenting with an acute depressive episode (with or without psychotic features) (Patel et al., 2006). With response defined as a reduction from baseline in Children's Depression Rating Scale-Revised (CDRS-R) score of ≥50% at endpoint, the response rate was reported as 48%. The authors concluded that lithium may be effective for the treatment of an acute depressive episode in adolescents with bipolar disorder (pending confirmation in controlled clinical trials).

Adverse events that are commonly reported with lithium used alone or in combination with other medications in children and adolescents with bipolar disorder include nausea, abdominal discomfort, diarrhea, polyuria, polydipsia, tremor, acne, hypothyroidism, cognitive dysfunction and weight gain. Campbell et al. (1991) noted that these adverse events are more commonly reported by younger (5–9 years of age) than older children. Long-term treatment with lithium may also result in nephrogenic diabetes mellitus and cardiac conduction defects, including atrioventricular block and sinoatrial block. During long-term treatment with lithium, thyroid, renal, and cardiac functions should be re-evaluated periodically. Lithium has not been demonstrated as having a positive benefit-risk profile from data from controlled studies. Lithium should be used with particular care in young people, ensuring that serum levels do not exceed 1 mmol/l and noting that lower serum levels may be adequate (0.5–0.8 mmol/l) for maintenance treatment. The lethality of lithium in overdose, a not uncommon problem in adolescence, should not be underestimated.

To date, there are only a small number of published controlled clinical trials of divalproex sodium as monotherapy or as part of combination therapy in the treatment of children and adolescents with bipolar disorder. In published prospective, open-label trials of divalproex sodium as monotherapy in the treatment of children (≥5 years of age) and adolescents with or without comorbid ADHD presenting with an acute manic or mixed episode, response rates ranged between 61 and 80% (Campbell et al., 1991; Wagner et al., 2002; Pavuluri et al., 2005; Scheffer et al., 2005). In addition to the controlled clinical trials involving lithium specified above (Kowatch et al., 2000; Findling et al., 2005), and the clinical trials that evaluated the efficacy and safety of quetiapine as monotherapy and adjunctive therapy in the treatment of acute manic or mixed episodes in adolescents with bipolar I disorder as described later (DelBello et al., 2002, 2006), data are available from one double-blind, placebo-controlled trial to evaluate the efficacy and safety of an extended-release formulation of divalproex sodium as monotherapy for a duration of 4 weeks in the treatment of 144 adolescents with bipolar I disorder who presented with an acute manic or mixed episode (Segal, 2008). In this trial, the extended-release formulation of divalproex sodium failed to separate from placebo for the primary efficacy variable, i.e. change from baseline to the final evaluation in YMRS score, and other efficacy measures. In as yet unpublished data of a double-blind placebo-controlled trial of lithium and valproate in adolescent mania, valproate, but not lithium, demonstrated efficacy (Kowatch et al., personal communication).

Adverse events reported with the use of divalproex sodium in the treatment of pediatric subjects with bipolar disorder include sedation, tremor, nausea, weight gain, low platelets, blood dyscrasias, hepatotoxicity, pancreatitis, and neural tube effects as a result of intrauterine exposure. Divalproex sodium has also been associated with the development of androgenization and polycystic ovary disease in young females (Azorin & Findling, 2007). The benefit-risk of valproate has not been adequately established in published literature through controlled trials both in acute mania and for maintenance treatment. Further, there is no evidence of its efficacy in treating or preventing relapse of bipolar depression.

Data documenting the safety and efficacy of carbamazepine in the treatment of children and adolescents with an acute manic or mixed episode is limited to individual case reports and the controlled clinical trial of lithium specified above (Kowatch et al., 2000). Similarly, data illustrating the safety and efficacy of lamotrigine in children and adolescents with bipolar disorder is limited to case reports and a single uncontrolled, open-label trial in 20 adolescents presenting with an acute depressive episode with lamotrigine used as monotherapy over a period of 8 weeks (Chang et al., 2006b). With response defined as a reduction from baseline in CDRS-R score of $\geq 50\%$ at endpoint, the response rate was reported as 63%. The most commonly reported adverse events were headache, fatigue, and nausea, with none of the subjects reporting a serious rash. However, the risk of Steven-Johnson's Syndrome or a serious exfoliative skin rash with lamotrigine and carbamazepine should not be underestimated. A double-blind, placebo-controlled trial to evaluate the efficacy and safety of topiramate as monotherapy in the treatment of 230 (planned) children and adolescents aged 6–17 years presenting with an acute manic or mixed episode for a duration of 4 weeks was discontinued early when adult mania trials failed to demonstrate the efficacy of topiramate (DelBello et al., 2005). In this trial that was discontinued after only 56 subjects were enrolled, topiramate was well tolerated with the most commonly reported adverse events being somnolence, insomnia, nausea, diarrhea, and decreased appetite.

Atypical antipsychotics

There is a growing body of evidence to suggest that atypical antipsychotics are safe and efficacious as monotherapy or adjunctive therapy to mood stabilizers in the treatment of children and adolescents with bipolar I disorder presenting with an acute manic or mixed episode. The data currently available to document the efficacy and safety of atypical antipsychotics in this population is arguably of higher methodological quality than that of mood stabilizers, as the data often originate from double-blind, active- or placebo-controlled trials. Consequently, two atypical antipsychotics, risperidone and aripiprazole, are currently authorized by the US FDA for use as monotherapy in the short-term treatment of acute manic and mixed episodes in children and adolescents aged 10–17 years inclusive.

Two prospective, open-label trials documented the safety and efficacy of risperidone used as monotherapy over a period of 8 weeks in 30 children and adolescents aged 6–17 years and 16 preschool-age children aged 4–6 years, respectively, presenting with an acute manic or mixed episode (Biederman et al., 2005a, 2005b). With response defined as a reduction in YMRS score from baseline at endpoint of ≥50%, the response rates in these studies were 50% and 53%, respectively. A recently completed double-blind, placebo-controlled trial evaluated the efficacy and safety of risperidone in two dose ranges (0.5–2.5 mg/day and 3–6 mg/day, respectively) as monotherapy in the treatment of 169 children and adolescents aged 10–17 years presenting with an acute manic or mixed episode for a duration of 3 weeks (Pandina et al., 2007). Response rates (i.e. ≥50% reduction from baseline in YMRS score) were significantly higher for both dose ranges of risperidone (59% and 63%) relative to placebo (26%) ($p=0.002$ and $p<0.001$, respectively). The most commonly reported adverse events in the risperidone dose groups were headache, somnolence, and fatigue. The incidence of potentially prolactin-related adverse events was low for both dose groups of risperidone, and there were no glucose- or lipid metabolism-related adverse events in either group. Mean changes from baseline to endpoint in bodyweight were 0.65 kg, 1.9 kg, and 1.4 kg for the placebo, and risperidone low- and high- dose range groups, respectively. A long-term, open-label trial evaluated the safety and efficacy of risperidone used as adjunctive therapy to lithium or divalproex sodium (assigned sequentially) over a period of 6 months in 37 children and adolescents aged 4–17 years presenting with an acute manic or mixed episode (Pavuluri et al., 2004). In this study, response rates (i.e. ≥50% reduction from baseline in YMRS score) were 80.0% and 82.4% in subjects assigned to the combinations of risperidone+lithium and risperidone+divalproex sodium, respectively. Another long-term, open-label trial evaluated the safety and efficacy of risperidone used as adjunctive therapy over a period of 1 year in 38 children and adolescents aged 5–18 years who presented with an acute manic or mixed episode and failed to respond to monotherapy with lithium for 8 weeks (Pavuluri et al., 2006). In this study, the response rate after augmentation with risperidone in the 21 subjects who initially failed to respond to lithium monotherapy was 85.7%. Data were recently presented to document the successful use of a long-acting injectable formulation of risperidone as maintenance treatment in two subjects with bipolar disorder aged 12 and 14 years, respectively, who had previously failed treatment with oral risperidone due to non-adherence (Fu-I et al., 2008).

Two open-label trials evaluated the safety and efficacy of olanzapine as monotherapy over a period of 8 weeks in 23 children and adolescents aged 5–14 years and 15 preschool-age children aged 4–6 years, respectively, presenting with an acute manic or mixed episode (Frazier et al., 2001; Biederman et al., 2005a). Response rates (i.e. ≥50% reduction from baseline in YMRS score) in these studies were 74% and 33%, respectively. A double-blind, placebo-controlled trial also evaluated the efficacy and safety of olanzapine as monotherapy in the treatment of 161 adolescents aged 13–17 years presenting with an acute manic or mixed episode over a period of 3 weeks (Tohen et al., 2007). The response rate (i.e. ≥50% reduction from baseline in YMRS score) was significantly higher in subjects assigned to treatment with olanzapine relative to placebo (44.8% and 18.5%, $p=0.002$). The mean change from baseline in bodyweight at the 3-week time point was significantly greater for subjects receiving olanzapine relative to those receiving placebo (3.7 kg vs. 0.3 kg), with a statistically significant difference in the incidence of weight gain ≥7% from baseline (41.9% vs. 1.9%). The mean changes from baseline to endpoint in prolactin, fasting blood glucose, fasting total cholesterol, uric acid, and liver transaminase levels were also significantly greater in subjects assigned to treatment with olanzapine.

A double-blind, randomized, controlled trial evaluated the efficacy and safety of quetiapine relative to divalproex sodium as monotherapy in the treatment of 50 adolescents presenting with an acute manic or mixed episode over a period of 4 weeks (DelBello et al., 2006). With response defined as a Clinical Global Impression-Bipolar Disorder-Improvement score ≤2 at endpoint, the response rate was significantly higher in the quetiapine group than in the divalproex sodium group (72% and 40%, $p=0.02$). There were no significant differences between the treatment groups in the rates of adverse events. The most commonly reported adverse events in both groups were sedation, dizziness, and gastrointestinal upset. Another double-blind, placebo-controlled trial evaluated the efficacy and safety of quetiapine used as adjunctive therapy to divalproex sodium over a period of 6 weeks in 30 adolescents presenting with an acute manic or mixed episode (Delbello et al., 2002). With response defined as a reduction in YMRS score from baseline at endpoint of ≥50%, the response rate was significantly higher in the quetiapine group than in the placebo group (87% and 53%, $p=0.05$). Sedation, rated as mild or moderate, was significantly more common in the quetiapine group.

A prospective, open-label trial documented the safety and efficacy of ziprasidone used as monotherapy over a period of 8 weeks in 21 children and adolescents aged 6–17 years presenting with an acute manic or mixed episode (Biederman et al., 2007a). The response rate (i.e. ≥50% reduction from baseline in YMRS score) in this study was 33%. Only 67%

of subjects completed the study. The most commonly reported adverse events were sedation, headache, and gastrointestinal upset. There were no significant changes from baseline at endpoint in metabolic parameters or QTc interval. An open-label, blinded-rater, randomized, controlled trial to evaluate the efficacy and safety of two titration regimens of ziprasidone as monotherapy in the treatment of 60 children and adolescents aged 10–17 years presenting with an acute manic or mixed episode over a period of 6 weeks is currently ongoing (Saxena, 2008).

Two recently published open-label trials documented the safety and efficacy of aripiprazole used as monotherapy over a period of 6 weeks and 8 weeks, respectively, in 10 children and adolescents aged 8–17 years with comorbid ADHD and 19 children and adolescents aged 6–17 years, respectively, presenting with an acute manic or mixed episode (Biederman et al., 2007b; Tramontina et al., 2007). Response rates in these studies (i.e. ≥30% and ≥50% reduction from baseline in YMRS score) were 70% and 79%, respectively. A double-blind, placebo-controlled trial evaluated the efficacy and safety of aripiprazole at two fixed doses (10 mg/day and 30 mg/day, respectively) used as monotherapy in the treatment of 296 children and adolescents aged 10–17 years presenting with an acute manic or mixed episode over a period of 4 weeks (Bristol-Myers Squibb Company, 2008). Both doses of aripiprazole were superior to placebo for the mean changes from baseline at endpoint in YMRS score ($p<0.0001$) (with no data on response rates currently available). The most commonly reported adverse events in the aripiprazole dose groups were somnolence, extrapyramidal disorder, fatigue, nausea, akathisia, blurred vision, salivary hypersecretion, and dizziness. The proportions of subjects with weight gain ≥7% from baseline were 3.3%, 3.2%, and 9.4% in the placebo, and aripiprazole 10-mg and 30-mg dose groups, respectively. There were no clinically important differences in the mean changes from baseline at endpoint in prolactin, and fasting cholesterol and triglyceride levels.

To date, there have been no randomized controlled trials to directly compare the efficacy and safety of different atypical antipsychotics for the treatment of acute manic or mixed episodes in children and adolescents with bipolar disorder. An analysis of the data from prospective, open-label trials of atypical antipsychotics used as monotherapy over a period of 8 weeks suggested that the treatment effect on the basis of Clinical Global Impression scores is greatest for risperidone, followed by ziprasidone, quetiapine and olanzapine (Biederman et al., 2006). A pooled analysis of short-term trials of mood stabilizers and atypical antipsychotics indicated that most of these agents are associated with an increase in bodyweight (Correll, 2007). The unanswered question is: may these agents increase the risk of development of metabolic syndrome and future cardiovascular morbidity and mortality if treatment with the agents is continued over a prolonged period of time? Combination of an atypical antipsychotic and mood stabilizer seems to be associated with a greater risk of age-inappropriate weight gain than treatment with one or even two mood stabilizers. Data are insufficient to gauge the risk of weight gain due to monotherapy with atypical antipsychotics relative to treatment with one or two mood stabilizers. Among atypical antipsychotics, monotherapy with olanzapine is associated with a greater increase in bodyweight than any of the other atypical antipsychotics (Biederman et al., 2006).

Antidepressants

Recent deliberations by the US FDA with regard to the possible relationship of antidepressant use and suicidality in children and adolescents have incited debate as to the safety of these agents in the treatment of pediatric depression, especially major depressive disorder in children (Vasa et al., 2006). There are currently no randomized controlled trials of antidepressants in children and adolescents with bipolar disorder. Current practice recommends that treatment with antidepressants be initiated for the treatment of depressive symptoms in children and adolescents with bipolar disorder only in conjunction with a mood stabilizer because of their potential to cause patients to "switch" into mania (McClellan et al., 2007).

Nonpharmacological interventions

Electroconvulsive therapy (ECT) is an effective treatment of mania and depression in adults with bipolar disorder but is only considered for patients who do not respond to standard medicinal treatment. Data documenting the safety and efficacy of ECT in children and adolescents is very limited. Current practice restricts the use of ECT to adolescents with well-characterized bipolar I disorder who have severe symptomatology, have exhausted other treatment options with no response, or for whom pharmacotherapy is contraindicated (McClellan et al., 2007).

Psychosocial interventions are a critical component in the overall management of children and adolescents with bipolar disorder (McClellan et al., 2007). These interventions help ameliorate the negative impact of the bipolar disorder on family and peer relationships and augment symptom remission in children and adolescents with comorbid oppositional defiant or conduct disorders. The following four types of psychotherapeutic intervention have been evaluated and found beneficial in the management of bipolar disorder in children and adolescents: psychoeducation, family-focused therapy, cognitive behavioral therapy, and interpersonal social rhythm therapy.

References

Akiskal, H.S. 1996. The prevalent clinical spectrum of bipolar disorders: beyond DSM-IV. *J. Clin. Psychopharmacol,* 16(2 Suppl 1): 4S–14S.
Althoff, R. R., S. V. Faraone, et al. (2005). Family, twin, adoption, and molecular genetic studies of juvenile bipolar disorder. *Bipolar Disord., 7* (6): 598–609.
Azorin, J. M. and R. L. Findling (2007). Valproate use in children and adolescents with bipolar disorder. *CNS Drugs, 21* (12): 1019–33.
Biederman, J. (2006). The evolving face of pediatric mania. *Biol. Psychiatry, 60* (9): 901–2.
Biederman, J., E. Mick, et al. (2005a). Open-label, 8-week trial of olanzapine and risperidone for the treatment of bipolar disorder in preschool-age children. *Biol. Psychiatry, 58* (7): 589–94.
Biederman, J., E. Mick, et al. (2005b). An open-label trial of risperidone in children and adolescents with bipolar disorder. *J. Child Adolesc. Psychopharmacol., 15* (2): 311–7.
Biederman, J., E. Mick, et al. (2006). Comparative efficacy of atypical antipsychotics in youth with bipolar disorder. 159th Annual Meeting of the American Psychiatric Association in Toronto, Canada from May 20 through 25, 2006.
Biederman, J., E. Mick, et al. (2007a). A prospective open-label treatment trial of ziprasidone monotherapy in children and adolescents with bipolar disorder. *Bipolar Disord., 9* (8): 888–94.
Biederman, J., E. Mick, et al. (2007b). An open-label trial of aripiprazole monotherapy in children and adolescents with bipolar disorder. *CNS Spectr., 12* (9): 683–9.
Bristol-Myers Squibb Company. (2008). United States Prescribing Information of Abilify (Aripiprazole). From http://packageinserts.bms.com/pi/pi_abilify.pdf.
Brotman, M. A., L. Kassem, et al. (2007). Parental diagnoses in youth with narrow phenotype bipolar disorder or severe mood dysregulation. *Am. J. Psychiatry, 164* (8): 1238–41.
Brotman, M. A., M. Schmajuk, et al. (2006). Prevalence, clinical correlates, and longitudinal course of severe mood dysregulation in children. *Biol. Psychiatry, 60* (9): 991–7.
Campbell, M., R. R. Silva, et al. (1991). Predictors of side effects associated with lithium administration in children. *Psychopharmacol. Bull., 27* (3): 373–80.
Chang, K., N. Adleman, et al. (2006a). Will neuroimaging ever be used to diagnose pediatric bipolar disorder? *Dev. Psychopathol., 18* (4): 1133–46.
Chang, K., K. Saxena, et al. (2006b). An open–label study of lamotrigine adjunct or monotherapy for the treatment of adolescents with bipolar depression. *J. Am. Acad. Child Adolesc. Psychiatry, 45* (3): 298–304.
Consoli, A., A. Bouzamondo, et al. (2007). Comorbidity with ADHD decreases response to pharmacotherapy in children and adolescents with acute mania: evidence from a metaanalysis. *Can. J. Psychiatry, 52* (5): 323–8.
Correll, C. U. (2007). Weight gain and metabolic effects of mood stabilizers and antipsychotics in pediatric bipolar disorder: a systematic review and pooled analysis of short-term trials. *J Am. Acad. Child Adolesc. Psychiatry, 46*(6): 687–700.
DelBello, M. P., C. M. Adler, et al. (2006). The neurophysiology of childhood and adolescent bipolar disorder. *CNS Spectr., 11* (4): 298–311.

Delbello, M. P., R. L. Findling, et al. (2005). A pilot controlled trial of topiramate for mania in children and adolescents with bipolar disorder. *J. Am. Acad. Child Adolesc. Psychiatry, 44* (6): 539–47.

DelBello, M. P., R. A. Kowatch, et al. (2006). A double-blind randomized pilot study comparing quetiapine and divalproex for adolescent mania. *J. Am. Acad. Child Adolesc. Psychiatry, 45* (3): 305–13.

Delbello, M. P., M. L. Schwiers, et al. (2002). A double-blind, randomized, placebo-controlled study of quetiapine as adjunctive treatment for adolescent mania. *J. Am. Acad. Child Adolesc. Psychiatry, 41* (10): 1216–23.

Dickstein, D. P., E. E. Nelson, et al. (2007). Cognitive flexibility in phenotypes of pediatric bipolar disorder. *J. Am. Acad. Child Adolesc. Psychiatry, 46* (3): 341–55.

Findling, R. L., N. K. McNamara, et al. (2003). Combination lithium and divalproex sodium in pediatric bipolarity. *J. Am. Acad. Child Adolesc. Psychiatry, 42* (8): 895–901.

Findling, R. L., N. K. McNamara, et al. (2005). Double-blind 18-month trial of lithium versus divalproex maintenance treatment in pediatric bipolar disorder. *J. Am. Acad. Child Adolesc. Psychiatry, 44* (5): 409–17.

Findling, R. L., N. K. McNamara, et al. (2006). Combination lithium and divalproex sodium in pediatric bipolar symptom re-stabilization. *J. Am. Acad. Child Adolesc. Psychiatry, 45* (2): 142–8.

Frazier, J. A., J. Biederman, et al. (2001). A prospective open-label treatment trial of olanzapine monotherapy in children and adolescents with bipolar disorder. *J. Child Adolesc. Psychopharmacol., 11* (3): 239–50.

Frazier, J. A., J. L. Breeze, et al. (2005). Cortical gray matter differences identified by structural magnetic resonance imaging in pediatric bipolar disorder. *Bipolar Disord., 7* (6): 555–69.

Fu-I, L., A. Stravogiannis, et al. (2008). Risperidone long-acting injection helping treatment adherence and symptom control of pediatric bipolar patients. 3rd Biennial Conference of the International Society for Bipolar Disorders. New Delhi and Agra, India.

Geller, B., T. B. Cooper, et al. (1998). Double-blind and placebo-controlled study of lithium for adolescent bipolar disorders with secondary substance dependency. *J. Am. Acad. Child Adolesc. Psychiatry, 37* (2): 171–8.

Geller, B., R. Tillman, et al. (2004). Four-year prospective outcome and natural history of mania in children with a prepubertal and early adolescent bipolar disorder phenotype. *Arch. Gen. Psychiatry, 61* (5): 459–67.

Gogtay, N., A. Ordonez, et al. (2007). Dynamic mapping of cortical development before and after the onset of pediatric bipolar illness. *J. Child Psychol. Psychiatry, 48* (9): 852–62.

Hillegers, M. H., C. G. Reichart, et al. (2005). Five-year prospective outcome of psychopathology in the adolescent offspring of bipolar parents. *Bipolar Disord., 7* (4): 344–50.

Kafantaris, V., D. J. Coletti, et al. (2003). Lithium treatment of acute mania in adolescents: a large open trial. *J. Am. Acad. Child Adolesc. Psychiatry, 42* (9): 1038–45.

Kafantaris, V., D. J. Coletti, et al. (2004). Lithium treatment of acute mania in adolescents: a placebo-controlled discontinuation study. *J. Am. Acad. Child Adolesc. Psychiatry, 43* (8): 984–93.

Kowatch, R. A., T. Suppes, et al. (2000). Effect size of lithium, divalproex sodium, and carbamazepine in children and adolescents with bipolar disorder. *J. Am. Acad. Child Adolesc. Psychiatry, 39* (6): 713–20.

Leibenluft, E., D. S. Charney, et al. (2003). Defining clinical phenotypes of juvenile mania. *Am. J. Psychiatry, 160* (3): 430–7.

McClellan, J., R. Kowatch, et al. (2007). Practice parameter for the assessment and treatment of children and adolescents with bipolar disorder. *J. Am. Acad. Child Adolesc. Psychiatry, 46* (1): 107–25.

Merikangas, K. R., H. S. Akiskal, et al. (2007). Lifetime and 12-month prevalence of bipolar spectrum disorder in the National Comorbidity Survey replication. *Arch. Gen. Psychiatry, 64* (5): 543–52.

Merikangas, K. R. & N. C. Low. (2004). The epidemiology of mood disorders. *Curr. Psychiatry Rep., 6* (6): 411–21.

Moore, C. M., J. Biederman, et al. (2007). Mania, glutamate/glutamine and risperidone in pediatric bipolar disorder: a proton magnetic resonance spectroscopy study of the anterior cingulate cortex. *J. Affect. Disord., 99* (1–3): 19–25.

Moreno, C., G. Laje, et al. (2007). National trends in the outpatient diagnosis and treatment of bipolar disorder in youth. *Arch. Gen. Psychiatry, 64* (9): 1032–9.

NIMH (2001). National Institute of Mental Health research roundtable on prepubertal bipolar disorder. *J. Am. Acad. Child Adolesc. Psychiatry, 40* (8): 871–8.

Pandina, G., M. DelBello, et al. (2007). Risperidone for the treatment of acute mania in bipolar youth. 154th Annual Meeting of the American academy of Child and Adolescent Psychiatry. Boston, MA.

Patel, N. C., M. P. DelBello, et al. (2006). Open-label lithium for the treatment of adolescents with bipolar depression. *J. Am. Acad. Child Adolesc. Psychiatry, 45* (3): 289–97.

Pavuluri, M. N., D. B. Henry, et al. (2004). Open-label prospective trial of risperidone in combination with lithium or divalproex sodium in pediatric mania. *J. Affect. Disord., 82* (Suppl 1): S103–11.

Pavuluri, M. N., D. B. Henry, et al. (2005). Divalproex sodium for pediatric mixed mania: a 6-month prospective trial. *Bipolar Disord., 7* (3): 266–73.

Pavuluri, M. N., D. B. Henry, et al. (2006). A one-year open-label trial of risperidone augmentation in lithium nonresponder youth with preschool-onset bipolar disorder. *J. Child Adolesc. Psychopharmacol., 16* (3): 336–50.

Reich, W., R. J. Neuman, et al. (2005). Comorbidity between ADHD and symptoms of bipolar disorder in a community sample of children and adolescents. *Twin Res. Hum. Genet., 8* (5): 459–66.

Rich, B. A., D. T. Vinton, et al. (2006). Limbic hyperactivation during processing of neutral facial expressions in children with bipolar disorder. *Proc. Natl. Acad. Sci. USA, 103* (23): 8900–5.

Robins, E., & Guze, S.B. 1970. Establishment of diagnostic validity in psychiatric illness: its application to schizophrenia. *Am. J. Psychiatry, 126*(7): 983–7.

Saxena, K. (2008). Ziprasidone in pediatric bipolar disorder: a 6-week, open-label comparison of rapid vs. slow dose titration. Clinicaltrials.gov.

Scheffer, R. E., R. A. Kowatch, et al. (2005). Randomized, placebo-controlled trial of mixed amphetamine salts for symptoms of comorbid ADHD in pediatric bipolar disorder after mood stabilization with divalproex sodium. *Am. J. Psychiatry, 162* (1): 58–64.

Segal, S. (2008). A double-blind, placebo-controlled trial to evaluate the safety and efficacy of Depakote ER for the treatment of mania associated with bipolar disorder in children and adolescents [online]. Available from URL: http://pdf.clinicalstudyresults.org/documents/company-study_1561_0.pdf. Accessed November 26, 2008.

Singh, M. K., M. P. DelBello, et al. (2006). Co-occurrence of bipolar and attention-deficit hyperactivity disorders in children. *Bipolar Disord.*, *8* (6): 710–20.

Soutullo, C. A., K. D. Chang, et al. (2005). Bipolar disorder in children and adolescents: international perspective on epidemiology and phenomenology. *Bipolar Disord.*, *7* (6): 497–506.

Tohen, M., L. Kryzhanovskaya, et al. (2007). Olanzapine versus placebo in the treatment of adolescents with bipolar mania. *Am. J. Psychiatry, 164* (10): 1547–56.

Tramontina, S., C. P. Zeni, et al. (2007). Aripiprazole in juvenile bipolar disorder comorbid with attention-deficit/hyperactivity disorder: an open clinical trial. *CNS Spectr. 12* (10): 758–62.

Vasa, R. A., A. R. Carlino, et al. (2006). Pharmacotherapy of depressed children and adolescents: current issues and potential directions. *Biol. Psychiatry, 59* (11): 1021–8.

Wagner, K. D., E. B. Weller, et al. (2002). An open-label trial of divalproex in children and adolescents with bipolar disorder. *J. Am. Acad. Child Adolesc. Psychiatry, 41* (10): 1224–30.

Youngstrom, E. A., B. Birmaher, et al. (2008). Pediatric bipolar disorder: validity, phenomenology, and recommendations for diagnosis. *Bipolar Disord., 10* (1 Pt 2): 194–214.

chapter eight

Bipolar disorder in the elderly

Jaskaran Singh
University of Vermont
Johnson & Johnson Pharmaceutical Research and Development

Vivek Kusumakar
Dalhousie University
Johnson & Johnson Pharmaceutical Research and Development

Martha Sajatovic
Case Western Reserve University

Contents

Background 204
Epidemiology 204
Sociodemographic correlates.. 205
Psychiatric and medical comorbidity.. 205
Course of illness: Influence of age on the presentation of illness 206
Vascular risk factors in late onset bipolar disorder 207
Symptoms and diagnosis of late life bipolar disorder............. 208
Pathogenesis 209
    Neuroimaging studies.. 209
    Neuropsychological studies 209
Treatment.. 210
Lithium 211
    Divalproex.. 212
    Lamotrigine.. 212
    Carbamazepine 213
    Antipsychotic agents.. 213
    Psychotherapy 215
Service utilization.. 215
Duration of treatment... 216

Conclusion 216
References...217

Background

Bipolar disorder typically begins in late adolescence or early adulthood; however, *de novo* presentation of symptoms that meet DSM-IV criteria for bipolar disorders is both challenging to diagnose and to treat. Onset of symptoms in late life is often considered secondary to vascular disorders, traumatic brain injury or occasionally an adverse drug reaction. Although rare, concluding that onset of bipolar disorder at an older age is secondary to vascular disorder etc. is risky and likely erroneous. On the other hand, longitudinal studies of the phenomenology of bipolar disorder suggest some differences in phenomenology, course, comorbidities, and outcome and importantly the need for health care services.

Epidemiology

Community studies of prevalence of bipolar disorder among community-based/population-based samples consistently indicate that the prevalence of bipolar disorder declines in late life. Data from the Epidemiologic Catchment Area (ECA) survey indicated a 1-year prevalence rate of 0.1% among adults over age 65. This is much lower than the prevalence among young adults (18–44 years; 1.4%) and middle-aged adults (45–64 years; 0.4%) (Weisman et al., 1988). According to the ECA data, depression and schizophrenia are about 14 and three times more common than bipolar disorder in the elderly, respectively. In the National Comorbidity Survey Replication study, the prevalence estimates varied significantly with age for most disorders; however, it is remarkably reduced with age for bipolar I and II disorders. In this study, the overall lifetime prevalence of DSM-IV bipolar I, bipolar II, and subthreshold bipolar disorders combined was 3.9%. This is highest in the 18–29 age group (5.9%) and lowest in the above-60 age group (1.0%) (Kessler et al., 2005).

In summary, it appears from existing data that bipolar disorder becomes less common with age in community samples. Reasons for this decline in prevalence may include factors related to the disorder (e.g. excess mortality, recovery) and/or the interaction with aging and case-finding methods (e.g. institutionalization, cohort differences in symptom reporting). However, bipolar disorder appears to account for roughly the same proportion of admissions to psychiatric facilities among older adults as younger adults (approximately 8–10%), and possibly the same proportion of outpatient and psychiatric emergency diagnoses.

Sociodemographic correlates

A majority of studies, but not all (Kessing, 2006) have found that older people with bipolar disorder were more likely to be women, by a ratio of about 2 to 1 (reviewed in Depp & Jeste, 2004). In the National Comorbidity Survey replication study, the sociodemographic correlates of bipolar disorder were modest. No significant differences were found for sex, race/ethnicity or family income.

In the National Comorbidity Survey replication study, the median age of onset (i.e. the 50th percentile on the age of onset percentile) for bipolar disorder was 25 years. New onset of bipolar disorder at age 57 was 5% and at age 65 was 1% (Kessler et al., 2005). This dramatic decrease in prevalence with age was similar to drug abuse, drug dependence and post traumatic stress disorder. The decrease in prevalence rates was much less marked for other disorders.

A number of studies have reported that older adults report a later onset of affective symptoms and mania than mixed-age groups. Although their onset is considerably later, older adults report experiencing some form of affective disturbance for a mean of 10–20 years (Sajatovic et al., 2005; Merikangas et al., 2007).

Studies of family history of bipolar disorder comparing early versus late onset bipolar disorder have been inconclusive. Family history of affective disorder was more common in older adults, which is contrary to expectation and deserves further investigation (Tohen, Shulman & Satlin, 1994; Hays et al., 1998). It is unclear if there is any difference in the genetic epidemiology of early onset vs. late onset bipolar disorder.

Psychiatric and medical comorbidity

Psychiatric comorbidity seems to be a rule rather than an exception in bipolar disorder. The only significant comorbidity that is reduced in older subjects with bipolar disorder compared with younger subjects from the NCS-replication study was substance abuse or dependence (Merikangas et al., 2007).

There are few data to determine whether older people have different rates of other psychiatric comorbidities. In an epidemiological community survey of 84 elderly subjects (>65 years) compared with 1327 younger adults with bipolar disorder and 8121 elderly subjects with bipolar disorder, comorbid axis 1 disorders were found to be common among elderly individuals with bipolar disorder (Goldstein, Herrmann & Shulman, 2006). Elderly subjects with bipolar disorder had lifetime prevalence of 38.1% for alcohol use disorders, 15.5% for dysthymia, 20.5% for generalized anxiety disorder and 19% for panic disorder. In this study, elderly subjects with bipolar disorder were much more likely to have alcohol use disorders, dysthymia, generalized anxiety disorder and panic disorder compared to elderly subjects without bipolar disorder. However, elderly subjects with bipolar disorder had lower rate of alcohol use disorders, and comparable rates of dysthymia, generalized anxiety disorder or panic disorder compared to younger subjects with bipolar disorder.

Similarly, an analysis of a Veterans Health Administrative database found high rates of comorbidity in population of 16,330 elderly subjects (>60 years) with bipolar disorder. Substance abuse was seen is 8.9%, PTSD in 5.4% and dementia in 4.5% of elder veterans (Sajatovic, Blow & Iqnacio, 2006). Comorbid anxiety may have serious consequences, since in older adult populations with depression, the presence of comorbid anxiety is associated with more severe depressive symptoms, more chronic medical illness, greater functional impairment, and lower quality of life. While this has not been shown in prospective studies for elderly subjects with bipolar disorder, the data from the veterans database documenting increased hospitalization and outpatient services suggest that it may be critically important to diagnose and treat comorbid anxiety disorder (Sajatovic & Kales, 2006). Regarding substance use, these data suggest that even though the rates of alcohol and substance use disorders are lower in the elderly with bipolar disorder, they are still significantly higher than an age-matched population and suggest that screening for alcohol and substance use disorders should be part of screening of elderly subjects with bipolar disorder.

Emerging clinical evidence also indicates that a number of chronic systemic medical disorders are highly prevalent among bipolar probands. For example, migraine headaches cardiovascular disorders, and diabetes are frequently cited comorbid conditions (Fenn et al., 2005; Osby et al., 2001). However in clinical practice the temporal onset of disorders is often unclear. It is also often unclear whether a comorbid condition is caused by adverse drug reactions. At this time, no published systematic studies are available specifically for elderly bipolar subjects. It is also unclear as to how these conditions affect the health related quality of life in this population.

In contrast, a consistently higher rate of neurologic illness was present in late-onset mania/bipolar disorder. Other differences, such as presence of psychotic features, social support, mixed episodes, and treatment response are reported in too few studies to allow firm conclusions.

Course of illness: Influence of age on the presentation of illness

A number of small studies have reported difference in clinical presentation between subjects presenting with bipolar disorder with early onset versus late onset (summarized in Depp & Jeste, 2004). Studies have found that patients with late-onset bipolar disorder more often presented with mania, have a higher prevalence of mixed episodes, and are more likely to have psychotic features. However, in larger systematic reviews of studies these differences have been less obvious. Kessing's review of subjects in the Danish registry suggests that older patients with bipolar disorder present less often with psychotic manic episodes and more often with depressive episodes (Kessing, 2006). These differences in presentation were more obvious in studies done in inpatients and not obvious in outpatients. This finding has not been replicated by other studies suggesting that there are only small differences between early and late onset bipolar disorder; however, late onset bipolar disorder are more likely to have comorbidities, cognitive disorders and higher mental health services needs (Almeida, 2004; Depp et al., 2005; Sajatovic et al., 2005).

A great majority of studies did not report ethnicity of their samples, and therefore the ethnic distribution in bipolar disorder in older age is uncertain. The prevalence of psychotic features in older people versus younger vary between the studies (Depp et al., 2005; Schulze et al., 2002; Kessing, 2006). Overall, older people appeared to have psychotic features at the same frequency as younger people. Contrary to clinical observations, mixed features were no more common in older people in one study. In the few studies that have made direct comparisons between younger and older people, there was some evidence for mania to be less intense in severity and there is a possible trend for more time spent asymptomatic in older age (Young et al., 2007b) (although older adults may have longer hospital stays, possibly due to multiple comorbid disorders).

Vascular risk factors in late onset bipolar disorder

There is a significant body of literature suggesting that head injuries, stroke, intra cranial space occupying lesions that effect the fronto-cortico-limbic circuit may present with a mania-like syndrome and that these patients are often diagnosed with late onset bipolar disorder (Jampala & Abrams, 1983; Berthier et al., 1996; Cassidy & Carroll, 2002; Chemerinski & Levine, 2006).

The challenge for the clinician is when should vascular factors be considered in the differential diagnosis when an elderly patient presents with a new-onset mania-like syndrome? Are the symptoms of mania different from those of early-onset bipolar disorder? What kind of work-up should be done for an accurate diagnosis and subsequently is the treatment and health service need different from that of early-onset bipolar disorder?

There is no clear distinction in the literature as to what constitutes early onset vs. late onset. The majority of studies in patients 65 years or older have used 50–60 years as a cutoff for defining late onset. While there are no large community-based epidemiological studies evaluating the prevalence of cerebrovascular risk factors in subjects with early vs. late-onset bipolar disorder, studies from small clinical samples suggest between 6 and 50% of subjects with late onset mania have one or more cerebrovascular risk factors (Cassidy & Carroll, 2002; Klumpers et al., 2004; Sajatovic et al., 2005; Chemerinski & Levine, 2006). The inpatient studies are likely to overestimate the prevalence since they are often referred or have a more severe presentation and multiple co-occurring disorders. However, since the course of illness, management of symptoms of mania and health care services needs are different, a clinician may find it useful to assess vascular risk factors that may contribute to the presentation of bipolar disorder with onset in later life.

The Framingham stroke risk score has been shown to be a useful way for assessing this risk (Subramaniam, Dennis & Byrne, 2006) and may be a scale that can be used in clinical practice.

Symptoms and diagnosis of late life bipolar disorder

While the diagnostic criteria for bipolar disorder presenting in late life are similar to those of bipolar disorder with adult onset, co-occurring illnesses and adverse effects of medications can complicate the diagnosis in those presenting with onset in late life.

The evaluation of subjects presenting with depression, agitation, and mania-like symptoms requires a detailed assessment of symptoms and use of drugs that may be associated with mania (for example antidepressants, alcohol, anticholinergics, antiparkinsonian medications, corticosteroids, amphetamines, benzodiazepines, opiates etc.), laboratory assessment (chemistry, thyroid functions, vitamin B12, folate, drug screen etc.). Family history of bipolar disorder may predict a higher likelihood of bipolar disorder in this case.

Clinical scales such as the Mood Disorders Questionnaire (MDQ) (Hirschfeld et al., 2000) may be useful in obtaining a past history of manic episodes from the patient and family members. The Hachinski Ischemic Scale with a score greater than 4 may be indicative of a vascular etiology (Moroney et al., 1997). The Mini Mental State Examination (MMSE, Folstein, Folstein & McHugh, 1975) is a cognitive performance examination that is widely utilized in clinical practice and has research applications (Gildengers, 2004). However literature on rating scale application in elderly with bipolar disorder is extremely limited (Young et al., 2007a).

Patients with agitated bipolar I depression, compared to those with non-agitated depression, tend to have the first psychiatric contact at a later age and be hospitalized more frequently (Maj et al., 2003). It is often difficult to differentiate between agitated major depression and mixed bipolar disorder. Subjects with at least two symptoms of mania/hypomania are more likely to have bipolar disorder, especially racing thoughts, pressured speech and increased motor activity while elation and grandiosity are not as common in mixed bipolar disorder in the elderly (Maj et al., 2006).

Pathogenesis

Neuroimaging studies

Several studies have reported structural changes in the brain in late-onset bipolar disorder. Initial studies reported an increase in ventricle brain ratio; however, this has not been seen consistently, nor is it specific to this disorder. Bipolar patients who are older have been reported to have greater cerebral sulcus widening (Young, 2005a) and white matter hyperintensities (de Asis et al., 2006). While these are not specific to bipolar disorder, they are commonly seen in vascular disorders, which may contribute to the onset of bipolar disorder in later life.

Diffusion-weighted imaging (DWI) can quantitatively assess the microstructural integrity of white matter using the average apparent diffusion coefficient (ADC(av)), a measure of the extent to which water molecules move freely within tissue. It has shown increased sensitivity in detecting brain white matter disease compared to traditional T2-weighted MRI. In a pilot study of eight subjects with bipolar disorder compared with subjects with other neurological disorders, subjects with bipolar disorder had microstructural changes consistent with decreased white matter integrity (Regenold et al., 2006). The imaging findings are supported by post-mortem tissue examination in subjects with depression and bipolar disorder suggesting white matter lesions(Regenold et al., 2007). Taken together, these findings suggest that onset bipolar disorder in later life is often associated with white matter lesions, possibly vascular in origin.

Neuropsychological studies

Studies using neuropsychological test have not been conclusive in differentiating late-onset bipolar disorder (Subramaniam et al., 2007). Simple bed side tests such as the Mini Mental Score Examination (MMSE) did not differentiate between a group of inpatients with unipolar depression and bipolar disorder subjects (Harvey et al., 1997). However, subjects with a primary vascular disorder were excluded. Young et al. (2006) reported that elderly subjects with bipolar disorder had lower MMSE scores, but these scores do not correlate with increase in the severity of manic symptoms. Burt and colleagues (2000) assessed inpatients with unipolar and bipolar depression referred for ECT, comparing bipolar and unipolar elderly to a group of younger patients with affective disorders. There was no difference in global measures between older unipolar and bipolar patients. Older patients, however, did poorer than younger bipolar patients in memory performance especially delayed recall.

While there is a dearth of studies with neuropsychological tests in bipolar disorder with late-life onset, they are an important part of a clinician's armamentarium in the differential diagnosis and in determining service needs especially where vascular risk factors are suspected.

Treatment

There is limited data on the treatment of late-life bipolar disorder. Current treatment guidelines for bipolar disorder do not include recommendations for late-life bipolar disorder. There has been one pilot study using a standardized treatment algorithm for the treatment of bipolar disorder in the elderly leading the authors to conclude that this approach is feasible and a larger study is needed. However, only 10% of participants achieved recovery from symptoms. However, the higher comorbidity, number of treatments, and drug interactions make it very difficult to standardize treatment in this population. There are a number of recent comprehensive reviews for the treatment of bipolar disorder in the elderly (Aziz, Lorberg & Tampi, 2006; Fenn et al., 2006; Sajatovic, 2002) and treatment of comorbidity (Singh & Zarate, 2006). Some of the salient features are discussed here.

The treatment for bipolar disorder include mood stabilizers such as lithium, anticonvulsants such as valproic acid, lamotrigine, and carbamazepine, antipsychotic agents, antidepressants, psychotherapy and electroconvulsive therapy. It should be noted, however, that there is an increased rate of overall mortality and also cerebrovascular adverse events in elderly patients with dementia treated with antipsychotics.

Goals of treatment as in younger adults include resolution of symptoms in the acute episode, prevention of recurrence in the long term, and restoration of health related quality of life.

Elderly patients often have slower metabolism and clearance rates, and are consequently more sensitive to the adverse effects of medications; the basic principle of "start low and go slow" is useful to keep in mind. Although the majority of studies of efficacy of pharmacotherapy have been completed in younger adults, the same medications often are effective in treating elderly patients with BP. The dosing considerations for the elderly are discussed:

Lithium

Although there are no controlled trials of efficacy of lithium for older bipolar patients, lithium is still considered a first-line treatment in bipolar disorder, particularly for those with classical mania and minimal neurological impairment (Schaffer & Gravey, 1984). Older patients who are frail or have numerous medical problems such as cardiovascular or renal problems are not good candidates for lithium therapy as they are at greater risk for lithium toxicity. There is also increasing research interest in whether lithium may delay or attenuate Alzheimer's disease.

Lithium is eliminated renally. Therefore, reduced renal clearance (frequently seen in the elderly), reduced volume of distribution or drug interactions may affect the pharmacokinetics of lithium. Lithium has a narrow therapeutic index and the elderly are more sensitive to its effects. Maintenance levels in the elderly (0.4–0.7 mEq/L) should be lower than those recommended in adults (0.6–1.2 mEq/L). The half-life of lithium has been reported to increase from 24 to 36 hours in the elderly. The dosage level should be determined individually taking into consideration individual's frailty, concomitant drugs, renal function, age and medical condition. Lithium clearance in patients with chronic renal disease decreases by a mean of 25%. The recommendation for the dose of lithium in reduced renal function can be based upon glomerular filtration rate (GFR):

- GFR 10–50 ml/min, 50–75% of the usual dose given at the normal dosage interval.
- GFR less than 10 ml/min, 25–50% of the usual dose given at the normal dosage interval.

Drug Interactions: Caution should be used when lithium is used concomitantly with diuretics, angiotensin-converting enzyme inhibitors, calcium channel blockers, NSAIDS and Cox-2 inhibitors as they may increase serum lithium levels with risk of lithium toxicity. Patients receiving such combined therapy should have serum lithium levels monitored closely and the lithium dosage adjusted if necessary.

The concomitant administration of lithium with selective serotonin reuptake inhibitors should be undertaken with caution as this combination has been reported to result in symptoms such as diarrhea, confusion, tremor, dizziness, and agitation.

Divalproex

Divalproex sodium (comprised of sodium valproate and valproic acid) is approved by the FDA for the treatment of mania. Divalproex has also been evaluated for its efficacy in relapse prevention (Tohen et al., 2004; Bowden et al., 2006). No controlled trials have evaluated its efficacy in elderly subjects. Retrospective case reviews have suggested its efficacy in elderly subjects with bipolar disorder (Noaghiul, Narayan & Nelson, 1998; Chen et al., 1999; Mordecai, Sheikh & Glick, 1999). Case reports have also described amelioration of mania-like symptoms after traumatic brain injury (Yassa & Cvejic, 1994; Monji et al., 1999; Tariot, 2003). A number of studies have also assessed the effect of divalproex on agitation and aggression in subjects with dementia (Tariot et al., 2005; Porsteinsson, 2006; Herrmann et al., 2007). Overall, they have found limited benefit, increased sensitivity to somnolence and decreased overall tolerability.

In regards to pharmacokinetics, protein binding of valproate is reduced in the elderly, in patients with chronic hepatic diseases, in patients with renal impairment, and in the presence of other drugs (e.g. aspirin). The capacity of elderly patients (age range: 68–89 years) to eliminate valproate has been shown to be reduced compared to younger adults. Intrinsic clearance is reduced by 39%; the free fraction is increased by 44%. Since the free fraction is pharmacologically active, this would suggest use of lower doses in the elderly.

Divalproex coadministration has been shown to increase the elimination half-life of lamotrigine from 26 to 70 hours (a 165% increase). The dose of lamotrigine should be reduced when co-administered with valproate. Serious skin reactions (such as Stevens-Johnson syndrome and toxic epidermal necrolysis) have been reported with concomitant lamotrigine and valproate administration.

Due to a decrease in unbound clearance of valproate and possibly a greater sensitivity to somnolence in the elderly, the starting dose should be reduced in elderly bipolar patients (125–500 mg/day). Dosage should be increased more slowly (no more than 500 mg/day) and with regular monitoring for fluid and nutritional intake, dehydration, somnolence, and other adverse events. Dose reductions or discontinuation of valproate should be considered in patients with decreased food or fluid intake and in patients with excessive somnolence. The blood level including the unbound fraction should be monitored in this population. The ultimate therapeutic dose should be achieved on the basis of both tolerability and clinical response.

Lamotrigine

Lamotrigine is indicated for the maintenance treatment of bipolar I disorder to delay the time to occurrence of mood episodes (depression, mania, hypomania, mixed episodes) in patients treated for acute mood episodes with standard therapy. The effectiveness of lamotrigine in the acute treatment of mood episodes has not been fully established. The sub-analyses from the mixed age studies show similar efficacy and tolerability of lamotrigine as in younger patients.

Lamotrigine is metabolized hepatically and has few drug interactions with the notable exception for divalproex, as discussed earlier. The mean half-life and clearance in the elderly is similar to younger subjects. Specific manufacturer's guidelines for starting lamotrigine in combination with divalproex should be followed in order to reduce the risk of Stevens-Johnson syndrome and toxic epidermal necrolysis.

Carbamazepine

The FDA has recently approved carbamazepine extended release (CBZ-ERC) for bipolar I disorder, acute manic and mixed episodes in adults. Of the 443 randomized patients in the pooled population, 240 completed the studies. Forty-two percent of CBZ-ERC-treated patients did not complete the studies, compared with 50% of placebo-treated patients. Overall it is not considered to be as effective as other agents such as lithium, divalproex. In addition to symptoms of mania, it may also have effects on symptoms of depression.

Carbamazepine is known to induce hepatic isozymes, therefore it is useful to measure levels of carbamazepine 3–4 weeks after it has been initiated and also assess the dose of other concomitant drugs that may be affected by the isozyme induction.

No age-related changes in pharmacokinetics with carbamazepine are reported.

In general, dose selection for an elderly patient should be cautious, usually starting at the low end of the dosing range, reflecting the greater frequency of decreased hepatic, renal, or cardiac function, and of concomitant disease or other drug therapy. The dosing should be titrated for efficacy and tolerability, generally between 6 and 12 mcg/ml. Electrolytes, complete blood count should be monitored every 3–6 months to monitor for potential hyponatremia, white blood cell count and neutropenia.

Antipsychotic agents

Among second-generation antipsychotics, risperidone, olanzapine, ziprasidone, quetiapine, and aripiprazole are indicated for the short-term treatment of acute manic or mixed episodes associated with bipolar I disorder. Studies with paliperidone are ongoing.

Risperidone and olanzapine also have an indication for the treatment of acute manic or mixed episodes associated with bipolar I disorder in combination with lithium or divalproex.

In addition, olanzapine is indicated for the maintenance treatment of bipolar disorder while olanzapine/fluoxetine combination is indicated for the treatment of bipolar I depression. Quetiapine has, in addition to mania, an indication for the treatment of bipolar I depression.

Published information about these agents in elderly subjects is lacking and information is extrapolated from studies of mixed age populations. It should be noted that there is an increased rate of overall mortality and also cerebrovascular adverse events in elderly patients with dementia treated with antipsychotics.

The second-generation antipsychotics have improved upon the first generation in reducing the risk for extrapyramidal syndrome and tardive dyskinesia and subsequently use of anticholinergic agents, which may lead to cognitive impairment in this vulnerable patient population. However, a number of the second-generation antipsychotics are associated with weight gain, hyperglycemia and dyslipidemia. Recently the FDA has placed a black box warning on all of the second-generation antipsychotics referring to the use in elderly patients with dementia with increased risk of mortality at the rate of 1.6–1.7 compared to those treated with placebo as well as an increase in risk of cerebrovascular events. This warning is not mentioned for elderly bipolar patients, however extra care needs to be used in subjects with onset of bipolar disorder in later life where a vascular etiopathogenesis is suspected.

Since choosing an antipsychotic agent is complex and few empirical data are available to guide treatment, a survey was conducted of experts in the field to recommend use of antipsychotics in elderly subjects (Alexopoulos et al., 2004). The expert consensus panel on the use of antipsychotics in the elderly recommends the following regarding the treatment of mania in the elderly:

- For mild-moderate geriatric nonpsychotic mania, the first-line recommendation is a mood stabilizer alone and discontinuation of the antidepressant if the patient is taking one.
- For severe nonpsychotic mania in the elderly, the experts recommend a mood stabilizer plus an antipsychotic (57%; first line) or a mood stabilizer alone (48%; first line) and would discontinue any antidepressant the patient is receiving.
- For psychotic mania in the elderly, treatment of choice is a mood stabilizer plus an antipsychotic (98%; first line) and continuing it for 3-month before attempting to taper and discontinue. Risperidone (1.25–3.0 mg/day) and olanzapine (5–15 mg/day)

were first-line options in combination with a mood stabilizer for mania with psychosis, with quetiapine (50–250 mg/day) high second line.

It must be noted that additional data on risks and benefits of use of antipsychotic agents in older adults have continued to accumulate and must be factored into clinical decision-making as to best biologic treatments for older adults with either manic or depressive bipolar symptoms.

For patients with diabetes, dyslipidemia, or obesity, the experts recommended avoiding clozapine, olanzapine, and conventional antipsychotics (especially low- and mid-potency). Quetiapine is recommended as first line for a patient with Parkinson's disease. Clozapine, ziprasidone, and conventional antipsychotics (especially low- and mid-potency) should be avoided in patients with QTc prolongation or congestive heart failure. For patients with cognitive impairment, constipation, diabetes, diabetic neuropathy, dyslipidemia, xerophthalmia, and xerostomia, the experts preferred risperidone, with quetiapine high second line.

Dosing recommendations for use of any antipsychotic must be individualized based upon the patient's circumstances, especially in view of multiple drug interactions, reduced renal clearance and multiple co-occurring conditions.

Psychotherapy

In the last two decades there has been a dramatic increase in high quality, well controlled research of focused psychotherapy and psychoeducation in patients with bipolar disorder (Sachs et al., 2001; Ball et al., 2006; Frank, Gonzalez & Fagiolini, 2006; Frank, 2007; Miklowitz et al., 2007). There is accumulating evidence that family-focused therapy, interpersonal and social rhythm therapy, and cognitive behavior therapy have significant benefit as augmenting agents to pharmacotherapy for maintenance therapy in bipolar disorder. There is little research, however, in elderly subjects with bipolar disorder, and it is unknown if the response in the elderly would be any different. However given the low risk and significant benefits in adults, these therapies are likely to have a positive impact on elderly subjects with bipolar disorder.

Service utilization

Bipolar disorder is associated with substantial disability in older adults. Remission of bipolar disorder was associated with significant but incomplete improvement in functioning, whereas psychotic and depressive symptoms and cognitive impairment seemed to contribute to lower health related quality of life (Malhi et al., 2007). Even euthymic elderly patients with bipolar disorder show decrements in information processing speed and executive functioning and often perform more poorly on activities of daily living (Gildengers et al., 2007).

Relapse and rehospitalization are common among elderly manic patients with early-onset and late-onset bipolar disorder (Lehmann & Rabins, 2006). The strongest predictors of psychiatric hospitalization was the presence of an alcohol use disorder (Brooks et al., 2006) or dementia (Sajatovic, Blow & Iqnacio, 2006).

Duration of treatment

There is a paucity of data for long-term studies in the elderly. Current literature based upon expert consensus suggests that only mood stabilizers such as lithium, lamotrigine, valproate be used indefinitely, while additional treatments such as antidepressants, benzodiazepines and antipsychotics be used for the short-term treatment of an episode and subsequently gradually tapered off and discontinued over a period of 6–12 weeks (Young et al., 2004; Young, 2005b).

Conclusion

Bipolar disorder becomes less common with age in community epidemiology studies. Reasons for this decline in prevalence may include factors related to the disorder (e.g. excess mortality, recovery) and/or the interaction with aging and case-finding methods (e.g. institutionalization). However, bipolar disorder appears to account for roughly the same proportion of admissions to psychiatric facilities among older adults as younger adults. Comorbidity is the rule rather than the exception in elderly subjects with bipolar disorder, with alcohol use disorders being the most prominent. This is also related to high rates of hospitalization and increases in health care services needs and costs.

Current research suggests that the presentation of early-onset bipolar disorder in the elderly is not that different from bipolar disorder in the young. However late-onset bipolar disorder has a higher likelihood of a vascular etiology. In late-onset (>50 years age) bipolar disorder a comprehensive medical, neurological, neuropsychological examination may be useful in helping diagnosing the exact etiology and guide treatment.

Finally, there is little data from controlled trials in bipolar disorder in the elderly, specifically bipolar disorder with onset in later life. There is even less evidence for the treatment of mania secondary to vascular disorders or traumatic brain injury. Since this is a vulnerable population with multiple co-occurring disorders and multiple medication use, considerable caution should be used when adding new medications. Lower doses and slow titration rates may help improve tolerance, and the therapy should be individualized.

Research in this population undoubtedly will help improve the care of elderly subjects with bipolar disorder and will help inform treatment of bipolar disorder across the life-cycle.

References

Alexopoulos, G.S., Streim, J., Carpenter, D., & Docherty, J.P. (2004). Using antipsychotic agents in older patients. *J. Clin. Psychiatry, 65* (Suppl 2): 5–99; discussion 100–2; quiz 103–4.

Almeida, O.P. (2004). Bipolar disorder with late onset: an organic variety of mood disorder?. *Rev. Bras. Psiquiatr., 26* (Suppl 3): 27–30.

Aziz, R., Lorberg, B., & Tampi, R.R. (2006). Treatments for late-life bipolar disorder. *Am. J. Geriatr. Pharmacother., 4* (4): 347–64.

Ball, J.R., Mitchell, P.B., Corry, J.C., Skillecom, A., Smith, M., & Malhi, G.S. (2006). A randomized controlled trial of cognitive therapy for bipolar disorder: focus on long-term change. *J. Clin. Psychiatry, 67* (2): 277–86.

Berthier, M.L., Kulisevsky, J., Gironell, A., & Fernandez Beritez, J.A. (1996). Poststroke bipolar affective disorder: clinical subtypes, concurrent movement disorders, and anatomical correlates. *J. Neuropsychiatry Clin. Neurosci., 8* (2): 160–7.

Bowden, C.L., Swann, A.C., Calabrese, J.R., Rubenfaer, L.M., Wozniak, P.J., Collins, M.A., Abi-Saab, W., & Saltarelli, M. (2006). A randomized, placebo-controlled, multicenter study of divalproex sodium extended release in the treatment of acute mania. *J. Clin. Psychiatry, 67* (10): 1501–10.

Brooks, J.O., 3rd, Hoblyn, J. C., Kraemer, H.C., & Yesavage, J.A. (2006). Factors associated with psychiatric hospitalization of individuals diagnosed with dementia and comorbid bipolar disorder. *J. Geriatr. Psychiatry Neurol., 19* (2): 72–7.

Burt, T.P.J., Peyser, S., Clark, J., & Sackheim, H. (2000). Learning and memory in bipolar and unipolar major depression: effects of aging. *Neuropsychiatr. Neuropsychol. Behav. Neurol., 13*: 246–53.

Cassidy, F., & Carroll, B.J. (2002). Vascular risk factors in late onset mania. *Psychol. Med., 32* (2): 359–62.

Chemerinski, E., & Levine, S.R. (2006). Neuropsychiatric disorders following vascular brain injury. *Mt. Sinai J. Med. 73* (7): 1006–14.

Chen, S.T., Altshuler, L.L., Melnyk, K.A., Erhart, S.M., Miller, E., & Mitz, J. (1999). Efficacy of lithium vs. valproate in the treatment of mania in the elderly: a retrospective study. *J. Clin. Psychiatry, 60* (3): 181–6.

de Asis, J.M., Greenwald, B.S., Alexopoulos, G.S., Kiosses, D.N., Ashtari, M., Heo, M., & Young, R.C. (2006). Frontal signal hyperitensities in mania in old age. *Am. J. Geriatr. Psychiatry, 14* (7): 598–604.

Depp, C.A., & Jeste, D.V. (2004). Bipolar disorder in older adults: a critical review. *Bipolar Disord., 6* (5): 343–67.

Depp, C.A., Lindamer, L.A., Folsom, D.P., Gilmer, T., Hough, R.L., Garcia, P., & Jeste, D.V. (2005). Differences in clinical features and mental health service use in bipolar disorder across the lifespan. *Am. J. Geriatr. Psychiatry*, 13 (4): 290–8.

Fenn, H.H., Bauer, M.S., Altshuler, L., Evans, D.R., Williford, W.O., & Kilbourne, A.M., et al. (2005). Medical comorbidity and health-related quality of life in bipolar disorder across the adult age span. *J. Affect. Disord.*, 86: 47–60.

Fenn, H.H., Sommer, B.R., Ketter, T.A., & Alldredge, B. (2006). Safety and tolerability of mood-stabilising anticonvulsants in the elderly. *Expert Opin. Drug Saf.*, 5 (3): 401–16.

Folstein, M.F., Folstein, S.E., McHugh, P.R. (1975). Mini-Mental State: a practical method for grading the cognitive state of patients for the clinician. *J. Psychiatr. Res.*, 112: 189–98.

Frank, E. (2007). Interpersonal and social rhythm therapy: a means of improving depression and preventing relapse in bipolar disorder. *J. Clin. Psychol.*, 63 (5): 463–73.

Frank, E., Gonzalez, J.M., & Fagiolini, A. (2006). The importance of routine for preventing recurrence in bipolar disorder. *Am. J. Psychiatry*, 163 (6): 981–5.

Gildengers, A.G., Butters, M.A., & Seligman, K., et al. (2004). Cognitive impairment in late life bipolar disorders. *Am J Psychiatry* 161: 736–738.

Gildengers, A.G., Butters, M.A., Chisholm, D., Rogers, J.C., Holm, M.B., Ghalla, R.K., Seligman, K., Dew, M.A., Reynolds, C.F. 3rd, Kupfer, D.J., & Mulsant, B.H. (2007). Cognitive functioning and instrumental activities of daily living in late-life bipolar disorder. *Am. J. Geriatr. Psychiatry*, 15 (2): 174–9.

Goldstein, B.I., Herrmann, N., & Shulman, K.I. (2006). Comorbidity in bipolar disorder among the elderly: results from an epidemiological community sample. *Am. J. Psychiatry*, 163 (2): 319–21.

Harvey, P.P.P., Parrella, M., White, L., & Davidson, M. (1997). Symptom severity and cognitive impairment in chronically hospitalised geriatric patients with affective disorders. *Br. J. Psychiatry*, 170: 369–74.

Hays, J.C., Krishnan, K.R., George, L.K., & Blazer, D.G. (1998). Age of first onset of bipolar disorder: demographic, family history, and psychosocial correlates. *Depress Anxiety*, 7 (2): 76–82.

Herrmann, N., Lanctot, K.L., Rothenburg, L.S., & Eryavec, G. (2007). A placebo-controlled trial of valproate for agitation and aggression in Alzheimer's disease. *Dement. Geriatr. Cogn. Disord.*, 23 (2): 116–9.

Hirschfeld, R.M., Williams, J. B., Spitzer, R.L., Calabrese, J.R., Flynn, L., Keck, P.E., Jr., Lewis, L., McElroy, S.L., Post, R.M., Rapport, D.J., Russell, J.M., Sachs, G.S., & Zajecka, J. (2000). Development and validation of a screening instrument for bipolar spectrum disorder: the Mood Disorder Questionnaire. *Am. J. Psychiatry*, 157 (11): 1873–5.

Jampala, V.C., & Abrams, R. (1983). Mania secondary to left and right hemisphere damage. *Am. J. Psychiatry*, 140 (9): 1197–9.

Kessing, L.V. (2006). Diagnostic subtypes of bipolar disorder in older versus younger adults. *Bipolar Disord.*, 8 (1): 56–64.

Kessler, R.C., Berglund, P., Demler, O., Jin, R., Merikangas, K.R., & Walters, E.E. (2005). Lifetime prevalence and age-of-onset distributions of DSM-IV disorders in the National Comorbidity Survey Replication. *Arch. Gen. Psychiatry*, 62 (6): 593–602.

Klumpers, U.M., Boom, K., Janssen, F.M., Tulen, J.H., & Loonen, A.J. (2004). Cardiovascular risk factors in outpatients with bipolar disorder. *Pharmacopsychiatry*, 37 (5): 211–6.

Lehmann, S.W., & Rabins, P.V. (2006). Factors related to hospitalization in elderly manic patients with early and late-onset bipolar disorder. *Int. J. Geriatr. Psychiatry, 21* (11): 1060–4.

Maj, M., Pirozzi, R., Magliano, L., & Bartoli, L. (2003). Agitated depression in bipolar I disorder: prevalence, phenomenology, and outcome. *Am. J. Psychiatry, 160* (12): 2134–40.

Maj, M., Pirozzi, R., Magliano, L., Fiorillo, A., & Bartoli, L. (2006). Agitated unipolar major depression: prevalence, phenomenology, and outcome. *J. Clin. Psychiatry, 67* (5): 712–9.

Malhi, G.S., Ivanovski, B., Hadzi-Pavlovic, D., Mitchell, P.B., Vieta, E., & Sachdev, P. (2007). Neuropsychological deficits and functional impairment in bipolar depression, hypomania and euthymia. *Bipolar Disord., 9* (1–2): 114–25.

Merikangas, K.R., Akiskal, H.S., Angst, J., Greenberg, P.E., Hirschfeld, R.M., Petukhova, M., & Kessler, R.C.. (2007). Lifetime and 12-month prevalence of bipolar spectrum disorder in the national comorbidity survey replication. *Arch. Gen. Psychiatry, 64* (5): 543–52.

Miklowitz, D J., Otto, M.W., Frank, E., Reilly-Harrington, N.A., Wisniewski, S.R., Kogan, J.N., Nierenberg, A.A., Calabrese, J.R., Marangell, L.B., Gyulai, L., Araga, M., Gonzales, J.M., Shirley, E.R., Thase, M.E., & Sachs, G.S. (2007). Psychosocial treatments for bipolar depression: a 1-year randomized trial from the Systematic Treatment Enhancement Program. *Arch. Gen. Psychiatry, 64* (4): 419–26.

Monji, A., Yoshida, I., Koga, H., Toshiro, K., & Tashiro, N. (1999). Brain injury-induced rapid-cycling affective disorder successfully treated with valproate. *Psychosomatics, 40* (5): 448–9.

Mordecai, D.J., Sheikh, J.I., & Glick, I.D. (1999). Divalproex for the treatment of geriatric bipolar disorder. *Int. J. Geriatr. Psychiatry, 14* (6): 494–6.

Moroney, J.T., Bagiella, E., Desmond, D.W., Hachinski, V.C., Molsa, P.K., Gustafson, L., Brun, A., Fischer, P., Erkinjuntti, T., Rosen, W., Paik, M.C., & Tatemichi, T.K. (1997). Meta-analysis of the Hachinski Ischemic Score in pathologically verified dementias. *Neurology, 49* (4): 1096–105.

Noaghiul, S., Narayan, M., & Nelson, J.C. (1998). Divalproex treatment of mania in elderly patients. *Am. J. Geriatr. Psychiatry, 6* (3): 257–62.

Osby, U., Brandt, L., Correia, N., Ekbom, A., & Sparen, P., (2001). Excess mortality in bipolar and unipolar disorder in Sweden. *Arch. Gen. Psychiatry, 58*: 844–50.

Porsteinsson, A.P. (2006). Divalproex sodium for the treatment of behavioural problems associated with dementia in the elderly. *Drugs Aging, 23* (11): 877–86.

Regenold, W.T., D'Agostino, C.A., Ramesh, N., Hasnain, M., Roys, S., & Gullapalli, R.P. (2006). Diffusion-weighted magnetic resonance imaging of white matter in bipolar disorder: a pilot study. *Bipolar Disord., 8* (2): 188–95.

Regenold, W.T., Phatak, P., Marano, C.M., Gearhart, L., Viens, C.H., & Hisley, K.C. (2007). Myelin staining of deep white matter in the dorsolateral prefrontal cortex in schizophrenia, bipolar disorder, and unipolar major depression. *Psychiatry Res, 151* (3): 1791–88.

Sachs, G.S., Yan, L.J., Swann, A.C., & Allen, M.H. (2001). Integration of suicide prevention into outpatient management of bipolar disorder. *J. Clin. Psychiatry, 62* (Suppl 25): 3–11.

Sajatovic, M., (2002). Treatment of bipolar disorder in older adults. *Int. J. Geriatr. Psychiatry, 17*: 865–73.

Sajatovic, M., Bingham, C.R., Campbell, E.A., & Fletcher, D.F. (2005). Bipolar disorder in older adult inpatients. *J. Nerv. Ment. Dis., 193* (6): 417–9.

Sajatovic, M., Blow, F.C., & Iqnacio, R.V. (2006). Psychiatric comorbidity in older adults with bipolar disorder. *Int. J. Geriatr. Psychiatry, 21* (6): 582–7.

Sajatovic, M., Blow, F.C., Iqnacio, R.V., & Kales, H.C. (2005). New-onset bipolar disorder in later life. *Am. J. Geriatr. Psychiatry, 13* (4): 282–9.

Sajatovic, M., & Kales, H.C. (2006). Diagnosis and management of bipolar disorder with comorbid anxiety in the elderly. *J. Clin. Psychiatry, 67* (Suppl 1): 21–7.

Schaffer, C.B., & Gravey, M.J. (1984). Use of lithium in acutely manic elderly patients. *Clin. Gerontol., 3*: 58–60.

Schulze, T.G., Muller, D.J., Krauss, H., Gross, M., Fragerau-Lefevre, H., & Illes, F., et al. (2002). Further evidence for age of onset being an indicator for severity in bipolar disorder. *J. Affect. Disord., 68*: 343–45.

Singh, J.B., & Zarate, C.A., Jr. (2006). Pharmacological treatment of psychiatric comorbidity in bipolar disorder: a review of controlled trials. *Bipolar Disord., 8* (6): 696–709.

Subramaniam, H., Dennis, M.S., & Byrne, E.J. (2007). The role of vascular risk factors in late onset bipolar disorder. *Int J Geriatr Psychiatry, 22* (8): 733–7.

Tariot, P.N. (2003). Valproate use in neuropsychiatric disorders in the elderly. *Psychopharmacol. Bull., 37* (Suppl 2): 116–28.

Tariot, P.N., Raman, R., Jakimovich, L., Schneider, L., Porsteinsson, A., Thomas, R., Mintzer, J., Brenner, R., Schafer, K., & Thal, L. (2005). Divalproex sodium in nursing home residents with possible or probable Alzheimer Disease complicated by agitation: a randomized, controlled trial. *Am. J. Geriatr. Psychiatry, 13* (11): 942–9.

Tohen, M., Chengappa, K.N., Suppes, T., Baker, R.W., Zarate, C.A., Bowden, C.L., Sachs, G.S., Kupfer, D.J., Ghaemi, S.N., Feldman, P.D., Risser, R.C., Evans, A.R., & Calabrese, J.R. (2004). Relapse prevention in bipolar I disorder: 18-month comparison of olanzapine plus mood stabiliser v. mood stabiliser alone. *Br. J. Psychiatry, 184*: 337–45.

Tohen, M., Shulman, K.I., & Satlin, A. (1994). First-episode mania in late life. *Am. J. Psychiatry, 151* (1): 130–2.

Weissman, M.M., Leaf, P.J., Tischler, G.L., Blazer, D.G., Karno, M., Bruce, M.L., & Florio, L.P. (1998). Affective disorders in five United States communities. *Psychol Med., 18* (1): 141–53.

Yassa, R., & Cvejic, J. (1994). Valproate in the treatment of posttraumatic bipolar disorder in a psychogeriatric patient. *J. Geriatr. Psychiatry Neurol., 7* (1): 55–7.

Young, RC. (2005a). Bipolar disorder in older persons: perspectives and new findings. *Am. J. Geriatr. Psychiatry, 13* (4): 265–7.

Young, R.C. (2005b). Evidence-based pharmacological treatment of geriatric bipolar disorder. *Psychiatr. Clin. North Am., 28* (4): 837–69.

Young, R.C., Gyulai, L., Mulsant, B.C., Flint, A., Beyer, J.L., Shulman, K.I., & Reynolds, C.F. 3 rd. (2004). Pharmacotherapy of bipolar disorder in old age: review and recommendations. *Am. J. Geriatr. Psychiatry, 12* (4): 342–57.

Young, R.C., Kiosses, D., Heo, M., Schulbberg, H.C., Murphy, C., Klimstra, S., Deasis, J.M., & Alexopoulos, G.S. (2007a). Age and ratings of manic psychopathology. *Bipolar Disord., 9* (3): 301–4.

Young R.C., Peasley-Miklus, C., & Shulberg, H.C. (2007b). Mood rating scales and the psychopathology of old age. In: *Bipolar Disorder in Later Life* (pp 17–26). Sajatovic M. and Blow F.C. (Eds). Johns Hopkins University Press, Baltimore, MD.

Young, R.C., Murphy, C.F., Heo, M., Schulberg, H.C., & Alexopoulos, G.S. (2006). Cognitive impairment in bipolar disorder in old age: literature review and findings in manic patients. *J. Affect. Disord., 92* (1): 125–31.

chapter nine

Comorbidity in bipolar disorder: Assessment and treatment

Joseph F. Goldberg
Mount Sinai School of Medicine

Contents

Introduction 221
DSM-IV and the hierarchical ordering of symptoms: either/or or
    both/and? 223
Alcohol and substance use disorders 224
Self-medication hypothesis 231
Impact on long-term course and clinical features 232
Treatment 233
Anxiety disorders 236
Panic disorder 237
Obsessive-compulsive disorder (OCD) 237
Generalized anxiety disorder (GAD) 238
Social phobia 239
Posttraumatic stress disorder (PTSD) 239
Eating disorders 240
Attention-deficit/hyperactivity disorder (ADHD) 240
Personality disorders 241
Treatment 243
Medical comorbidities 244
Clinical recommendations for diagnostic assessment
    and treatment 245
Conclusions 246
References 247

Introduction

It has often been said that comorbidity represents the rule more than the exception in bipolar disorder. Observational studies indicate that about two-thirds of individuals with bipolar disorder have at least one additional Axis I diagnosis, while nearly half have two or more (McElroy et al., 2001). From a diagnostic standpoint, the frequent comorbidity of other psychiatric problems in tandem with bipolar illness may partly contribute to the oft-noted lengthy delays from initial symptom onset to actual diagnosis, or the frequent "misdiagnosis" of other conditions (Lish et al., 1994; Hirschfeld et al., 2003). Clear diagnostic impressions may be difficult to formulate even by the most experienced clinicians when presentations of bipolar disorder are complicated by prominent comorbid conditions. Furthermore, unclear chronologies among multiple disorders can easily confuse distinctions between "primary" and "secondary" diagnoses when affective, anxiety, substance-related, or personality disorder features become confluent.

Comorbid psychopathology is a leading contributor to poor treatment response (Black et al., 1988) and long-term chronicity (Judd et al., 2002), yet studies of effective treatments for comorbidly ill patients with bipolar disorder remain few and far between. An obvious irony exists in that the great majority of individuals with bipolar disorder have comorbid disorders, yet almost all clinical therapeutic trials for bipolar disorder routinely exclude such patients from participation because they are deemed "nonprototypical".

Accurate recognition and treatment for complex, comorbid forms of bipolar disorder represents a substantial unmet clinical challenge. Outcome studies reveal that in routine practice, only about 60% of individuals with comorbid forms of bipolar disorder receive at least minimally adequate doses of mood stabilizing medications (Simon et al., 2004), suggesting potential undertreatment of their affective symptoms. The presentations, management, and treatment outcomes for comorbidly ill patients with bipolar disorder may well differ from those patients without comorbidities, accounting in part for disparities between the optimal efficacy of treatment for "pristine" cases (i.e. *does* a treatment work?) relative to treatment effectiveness in "real world" patients (i.e., *how well* does an efficacious treatment work under ordinary circumstances?).

This chapter will consider the phenomenology of comorbid psychiatric and medical problems commonly seen in individuals with bipolar disorder. Consideration will first be paid to findings from epidemiologic studies on prevalence rates for distinct comorbid conditions, as well as the implications of comorbidities with respect to clinical course and outcome. Finally, data will be reviewed from existing clinical pharmacotherapy and psychotherapy trials for distinct groups of comorbidly ill individuals with bipolar disorder, with recommendations for appropriate management.

DSM-IV and the hierarchical ordering of symptoms: either/or or both/and?

DSM-IV diagnoses are made by satisfying formal operational criteria sets. Yet, nosologic controversies arise when criteria overlap among multiple disorders.

Sometimes, complex symptom constellations can be explained parsimoniously by a single underlying condition rather than several disparate problems (such as weakness, vision problems, pain and urinary incontinence attributable to multiple sclerosis; or arthritis, dermatitis and kidney disease due to systemic lupus erythematosus). In certain situations, deducing a single unifying explanation for clinical phenomena becomes a necessity (as when determining *the* cause of chest pain). At other times, it becomes reasonable to consider the presence of two or more disorders with different pathophysiologies arises when a single diagnosis fails to account for a complex clinical presentation (Hilliard et al., 2004).

It can be especially difficult in psychiatry to subsume varied clinical phenomena under a single rubric since etiologies remain largely speculative, symptoms are often non-pathognomonic, and broad dimensions of psychopathology (such as impulsivity or anxiety) can span across multiple illness constructs. While DSM-IV permits multiple coexistent diagnoses, it also encourages clinicians to make a differential diagnosis before venturing to identify comorbidities through its proviso that symptoms must not be better accounted for by another disorder. In bipolar disorder, this caveat poses special challenges because of the broad, multidimensional nature of symptoms. For example, when is alcohol or substance abuse a manifestation of reckless indiscretions during mania or an independent condition separable from an affective episode? When do cognitive problems related to sustained attention and distractibility reflect a core symptom of mania versus a free-standing, independent diagnosis of attention-deficit disorder? When does mood instability and impulsive aggression reflect the psychopathology of bipolar disorder, borderline personality, or both? Where one draws the line in differentiating multiple "comorbid" conditions from one disorder with complex, varied forms thus remains the subject of debate.

As described further below, corroboration for suspected comorbid diagnoses may come from features beyond than the rigorous assessment of cross-sectional symptoms—such as the longitudinal course of illness, response to treatment, and familial co-segregation of related conditions.

Alcohol and substance use disorders

Several lines of evidence suggest that alcohol and substance use or dependence often are the most frequently encountered comorbidities in people with bipolar disorder. As summarized in Table 9.1, the prominence of comorbid substance use disorders is illustrated by several large-scale population surveys conducted during the past two decades: first, in the Epidemiologic Catchment Area Survey ($n=20,291$), 71% of individuals with bipolar disorder met a lifetime diagnosis of alcohol abuse or dependence (Regier et al., 1990). In the National Comorbidity Survey ($n=9282$), lifetime prevalence rates of any substance use disorder were higher among individuals with bipolar I (61%) or bipolar II (48%) disorder than in any other Axis I diagnosis (Kessler et al., 1997). Similarly, the more recent National Epidemiologic Survey on Alcohol and Related Conditions (NESARC; $n=43,093$) cited a 14-fold increase for any drug dependence among individuals with a history of mania, with a 58% lifetime prevalence rate of alcohol abuse or dependence in people with bipolar disorder (Grant et al., 2004).

Alcohol and drug use in general have risen in the United States since World War II (Grant, 1997; Warner et al., 1995), although little is known about changes in prevalence rates across decades specifically among individuals with bipolar disorder. In a case registry from the Bipolar Disorders Research Program at the Weill-Cornell Medical Center (Goldberg et al., 1999b), a breakdown of substances of abuse among bipolar disorder patients with substance use disorders revealed alcoholism in 28%, cocaine in 12%, cannabis in 10%, opiates in 4%, and other substances in 7%; two or more substances of abuse were found in 16% of the study group. Feinman and Dunner (1996) found amphetamines to be the most frequently abused psychoactive substance (26% of dual-diagnosis bipolar disorder patients from a private practice setting), followed by alcoholism (20%) and cocaine (9%) or cannabis (9%).

From the standpoint of gender, comorbid alcohol and substance abuse appears equally likely among men and women with bipolar disorder. As compared to the general population, however, findings from the Stanley Bipolar Network reveal a risk for lifetime alcoholism that is about 6 times higher in bipolar women than nonbipolar women, whereas alcoholism in bipolar men appears only about twice as likely as in nonbipolar men (Frye et al., 2003). Alcoholic bipolar women also demonstrate higher rates of comorbid posttraumatic stress disorder (PTSD) as compared to non-alcoholic bipolar women (Levander et al., 2007). Correspondingly, in findings from the NESARC cohort, associations between hypomania and any drug use were stronger among women than men (Conway et al., 2006); in addition, among NESARC subjects with both bipolar disorder

Table 9.1 Published Prevalence Rates of Comorbid Axis I Disorders with Bipolar Disorder

Comorbidity	Investigations	N	Prevalence
Alcohol or substance abuse and dependence	• McLean First Episode Psychosis (Strakowski et al., 1993)	60	17% drug abuse/dependence, 27% alcohol abuse/dependence
	• Cornell Bipolar Program (Goldberg et al., 1999)	204	28% alcohol abuse/dependence, 34% drug abuse/dependence
	• University of Cincinnati Mania Project (McElroy et al., 1995)	71	39% alcohol abuse/dependence, 32% drug abuse/dependence
	• McLean-Harvard First Episode Mania Study (Baethge et al., 2005)	112	33% with any substance use disorder.
	• NIMH CDS (Winokur et al., 1995)	231	37% with alcoholism at study entry; 5% at 5-year follow-up
	• SBRN (Frye et al., 2003)	267	Alcoholism in 38%
	• SBRN (McElroy et al., 2001)	288	Substance use disorder in 42%
	• University of Cincinnati First-Episode Mania Study (Strakowski et al., 2005)	144	42% with co-occuring alcohol abuse or dependence
	• STEP-BD (Weiss et al., 2005)	1000	45% current or lifetime substance use disorder
	• Western Psychiatric Institute & Clinic (Chengappa et al., 2000)	89	58% with alcohol or substance abuse or dependence
	• NESARC (Grant et al., 2004)	43,093	58% of bipolar patients from among 43,093 community respondents
	• NCS (Kessler et al., 1997)	9282	61% of bipolar I, 48% of bipolar II disorder patients, from among 9282 community respondents
	• ECA (Regier et al., 1990)	20,291	71% of bipolar patients, from among 20,291 community respondents

(continued)

Table 9.1 Published Prevalence Rates of Comorbid Axis I Disorders with Bipolar Disorder (*Continued*)

Comorbidity	Investigations	N	Prevalence
Panic disorder	• McLean Hospital First Episode (Strakowski et al., 1992)	41	5%
	• McLean First Episode Psychosis (Strakowski et al., 1993)	60	7%
	• ECA (Chen & Dilsaver, 1995a)	168	21%
	• SBRN (McElroy et al., 2001)	288	20%
	• Otago Bipolar Genetic Study (Edmonds et al., 1998)	64	27%
	• University of Verona (Pini et al., 1997)	24	37%
	• MGH (Simon et al., 2003)	122	38%
Social phobia	• University of Verona (Pini et al., 1997)	24	0%
	• McLean First Episode Psychosis (Strakowski et al., 1993)	60	7%
	• University of Pisa (Pini et al., 2006)	189	13%
	• SBRN (McElroy et al., 2001)	288	16%
	• St. Joseph's Hospital, Ontario, Canada (Boylan et al., 2004)	138	17%
	• MGH (Simon et al., 2003)	122	31%

Disorder	Study	n	%
Obsessive-compulsive disorder	• Tirat Carmel Israel First Episode Mania (Pashminian et al., 2006)	56	2%
	• Otago Bipolar Genetic Study (Edmonds et al., 1998)	64	2%
	• University of Toronto (Krüger et al., 2000)	143	7%
	• McLean First Episode Psychosis (Strakowski et al., 1993)	60	8%
	• University of Cincinnati Mania Project (McElroy et al., 1995)	71	10%
	• McLean First Episode (Strakowski et al., 1992)	41	17%
	• MGH (Simon et al., 2003)	122	13%
	• ECA (Chen & Dilsaver, 1995b)	167	21%
	• SBRN (McElroy et al., 2001)	288	35%
	• University of Bochum, Germany (Krüger et al., 1995)	145	39%
Generalized anxiety disorder	• SBRN (McElroy et al., 2001)	288	3%
	• MGH (Simon et al., 2003)	122	27%
	• St. Joseph's Hospital, Ontario, Canada (Boylan et al., 2004)	138	31%
	• University of Verona (Pini et al., 1997)	24	32%
	• NCS (Kessler et al., 1997)	59	43%

(continued)

Table 9.1 Published Prevalence Rates of Comorbid Axis I Disorders with Bipolar Disorder (*Continued*)

Comorbidity	Investigations	N	Prevalence
Eating disorders	• SBRN (McElroy et al., 2001)	288	6%
	• University of Pisa (Cassano et al., 1998)	47	6%
	• McLean First Episode (Strakowski et al., 1992)	41	7%
	• McLean First Episode Psychosis (Strakowski et al., 1993)	60	7%
	• Otago Bipolar Genetic Study (Edmonds et al., 1998)	64	7%
	• University of Cincinnati Mania Project (McElroy et al., 1995)	71	9%
	• University of Bochum, Germany (Krüger et al., 1996)	61	13%
	• McMaster University (MacQueen et al., 2003)	139	15%
	• University of Pisa (Ramacciotti et al., 2005)	51	27%
Personality disorders	• University of Colorado (George et al., 2003)	52	29%
	• NESARC (Grant et al., 2005)	100	30% with cluster B
	• Cornell Bipolar Program (Garno et al., 2005)	52	38%
	• UCLA (Kaye et al., 2002)	56	48%
	• University of Cincinnati First-Episode Mania Study (Dunayevich et al., 2000)		

PTSD	• McLean First Episode Psychosis (Strakowski et al., 1993)	60	2%
	• SBRN (McElroy et al., 2001)	288	7%
	• University of Cincinnati Mania Project (McElroy et al., 1995)	71	17%
	• MGH (Simon et al., 2003)	122	19%
	• University of Cincinnati First-Episode Mania Study (Strakowski et al., 1998)	77	21%
	• Cornell Bipolar Program (Goldberg & Garno, 2005)	100	24%
ADHD	• STEP-BD (Nierenberg et al., 2005)	1000	10%
	• Cukurova University, Turkey (Tamam et al., 2006)	44	16%
	• NIMH CDS (Winokur et al., 1993)	189	21%
	• University of Cincinnati (Patel et al., 2006)	27 adolescents	22%
	• University of Cincinnati (Soutullo et al., 2002)	80 adolescents	49%
	• University of Cincinnati (West et al., 1995)	14 adolescents	57%
	• University of Texas Southwestern Med. Ctr. (Kowatch et al., 2000)	42 adolescents	71%; 85% among prepubertal

Abbreviations: ECA=Epidemiologic Catchment Area Survey; MGH=Massachusetts General Hospital Bipolar Disorders Research Program; NCS=National Comorbidity Study; NESARC=National Epidemiologic Study of Alcohol Related Conditions; NIMH CDS=National Institute of Mental Health Collaborative Depression Study; SBRN=Stanley Foundation Bipolar Research Network; STEP-BD=Systematic Treatment Enhancement Program for Bipolar Disorder Bipolar Research Network.

and alcoholism, men were more likely to seek treatment for alcoholism, whereas women were more likely to seek treatment for mood symptoms, suggesting a gender-specific potential for under-treatment of the corresponding comorbidity (Goldstein & Levitt, 2006a).

Reasons for elevated rates of alcohol abuse or dependence in people with bipolar disorder are manifold. While there is some evidence suggesting an increased prevalence of alcoholism among first-degree relatives of bipolar probands (Winokur et al., 1996; Biederman et al., 2000), findings in this area have been inconsistent. Winokur and colleagues (1995) observed that family histories of alcoholism were no higher for bipolar probands with versus without comorbid alcoholism, supporting the view that alcoholism may often represent a secondary phenomenon (rather than an independent disorder) in patients with bipolar illness. Further supporting that perspective is the finding that alcoholism was more likely to remit when accompanied by bipolar disorder as compared to alcoholism without bipolar disorder (Winokur et al., 1995). In genetically dense families with bipolar disorder, comorbid alcohol and substance use disorders show strong familial patterns (Schulze et al., 2006). Alcoholism and attempted suicide together have also been reported to cluster within subsets of bipolar families (Potash et al., 2000; Schulze et al., 2006).

One of the most robust finding to date about alcoholism and bipolar illness has been an observed earlier age at onset for bipolar disorder when accompanied by alcoholism (Winokur et al., 1995; Feinman & Dunner, 1996; Strakowski et al., 1996). Moreover, when alcoholism *precedes* the onset of bipolar disorder (and bipolar disorder has a later age at onset), the overall prognosis appears better (Strakowski et al., 1996)—despite a greater propensity toward mixed states (Strakowski et al., 2005). By contrast, bipolar disorder preceding the onset of alcoholism has been associated with a slower recovery, more prolonged affective symptoms, and poorer outcome (Goldstein & Levitt, 2006c; Strakowski et al., 1996).

Further, more recent corroboration for these observations comes from the NIMH STEP-BD database. In univariate analyses, comorbid substance use disorders were associated with fewer days of euthymia, more days of mania and depression, and more extensive histories of suicide attempts (Fossey et al., 2006; Weiss et al., 2005). However, in a multifactorial regression model, none of these features remained significant after controlling for the confounding effects of age at onset. Similarly, in findings from the NESARC cohort, subjects with adolescent-onset bipolar disorder were more likely to develop later substance abuse as an illness complication, in contrast to less frequent substance misuse seen in adult-onset bipolar disorder (Goldstein & Levitt, 2006b).

Self-medication hypothesis

There are likely no simple rationales to explain the high prevalence of co-occurring alcohol or substance misuse with bipolar disorder. Nevertheless, some patients and clinicians embrace the assumption that substance misuse represents an effort to "self-medicate" an underlying mood disorder—with the implication that more effective management of the mood disorder would in itself remedy substance misuse as a secondary phenomenon. As appealing as this idea may seem, there has been little empirical study either to support or refute this clinical assumption. Some authors have taken the more frequent chronology of bipolar disorder *preceding* alcoholism as suggestive of a self-medication process (Preisig et al., 2001), although little attention has been paid to the likely mediating influence of factors such as impulsivity, relief of boredom, sensation-seeking, refusal to acknowledge personal accountability for one's actions, and denial of alcoholism as its own illness (Bizzarri et al., 2007).

In perhaps the most systematic assessment of the relationship between substance misuse and mood symptoms in bipolar disorder, data from the University of Cincinnati First-Episode Mania Study reveal that the proportion of time spent with alcohol symptoms or syndromes was significantly associated with depressive but not manic or mixed state symptoms (Strakowski et al., 2000). By contrast, time spent with cannabis abuse was significantly associated with mania but not depression or mixed states (Strakowski et al., 2007). Interestingly, a similar pattern linking alcohol abuse with bipolar depression and cannabis abuse with bipolar mania has been described elsewhere in first-episode mania (Baethge et al., 2005). The fraction of time with alcohol and cannabis abuse in the University of Cincinnati cohort also was significantly interrelated. In the University of Cincinnati Bipolar Disorders program, a stronger correlation was observed for alcohol abuse temporally *following* an affective relapse (T–β=0.88) than *preceding* an affective relapse (T–β=0.39) (Strakowski et al., 2000).

Longitudinal studies concurrently tracking mood and alcohol-related symptoms in patients with bipolar disorder reveal no clear temporal correlations between alcohol use and mood symptoms, although when alcoholism precedes the onset of bipolar disorder, moderate positive correlations have been found between age at bipolar disorder onset and affective symptoms (Fleck et al., 2006)—again pointing to age at onset of bipolar disorder as an important mediator of clinical course. In related outcome studies after a first lifetime hospitalized manic episode, affective relapse at one year follow-up occurred independent of alcohol relapse in 54% of bipolar patients who had alcoholism at index admission, and occurred independent of substance abuse relapse in 39% of those who had active substance abuse at their index hospitalization (Strakowski et al., 1998b).

Another perspective on the "self-medication" hypothesis comes from psychosocial intervention studies conducted by Weiss and colleagues (2004, 2007). Using patient self-assessments of reasons for substance use, two-thirds of dual-diagnosis bipolar disorder patients connected their drug use with their subjective improvement of at least one affective symptom—most often, depression or racing thoughts. A structured group psychotherapy, in turn, was most effective against drug relapse for that subgroup who perceived their drug use as an effort to relieve affective symptoms (Weiss et al., 2004).

Uncertainties about whether alcohol or substance misuse reflects a "primary" versus "secondary" condition are often compounded by the effects of illness chronicity, treatment nonresponse, and functional disability in multi-episode patients. Studies focusing on first lifetime episodes of mania partly help minimize potential artifacts of chronicity by examining substance use patterns unconfounded by the effects of multiple affective recurrences. Notably, in the Harvard-McLean First Episode Mania Study, the prevalence of lifetime alcohol or substance abuse or dependence was 33% (Baethge et al., 2005)—still higher than the roughly 13% lifetime prevalence of alcohol dependence in the general population (Grant, 1997) but nevertheless only about half of that seen among multi-episode patients with bipolar disorder.

Impact on long-term course and clinical features

Comorbid alcohol and substance use disorders have been associated with numerous and diverse negative outcome states in patients with bipolar disorder. These include:

- Slower and less extensive recovery (both in *first episode mania patients* (Strakowski et al., 1998a; and *multi-episode patients* (Tohen, Waternaux & Tsuang, 1990; Weiss et al., 2005))
- Higher relapse rates (Winokur et al., 1995; Delbello et al., 2007)
- More frequent Emergency Department visits (Goldstein, Velyvis & Parikh, 2006) and hospitalizations (Cassidy, Ahearn & Carroll, 2001)
- Increased risk for suicidal ideas and behaviors (Goldberg et al., 1999a, 1999b)
- More impulsivity and violent behavior (Salloum et al., 2002)
- Greater occupational impairment (Tohen, Waternaux & Tsuang, 1990)
- More extensive treatment nonadherence (Goldberg et al., 1999b; Keck et al., 1998; Strakowski et al., 1998a)
- More frequent mixed states than pure manias in bipolar disorder patients with comorbid alcoholism (Goldberg et al., 1999a)

- Greater anxiety comorbidity (Baethge et al., 2005; Mitchell, Brown & Rush, 2007)
- Diminished quality of life (Singh et al., 2005)
- More extensive service utilization (Goldstein et al., 2006)

While each of the foregoing correlates of alcohol or drug abuse adversely affects the course of bipolar disorder, complex inter-relationships among certain of these factors merit closer attention. For example, alcoholism and mixed states each likely contribute independently to protracted recovery and suicidal behavior in patients with bipolar disorder, although Goldberg and colleagues (1999a) showed that above and beyond the presence of mixed or dysphoric mania, alcoholism poses an approximate four-fold independent increased risk for suicidal behavior in bipolar disorder.

A further adverse consequence of alcohol dependence involves its impact on neurocognitive function. While the neurotoxic effects of alcohol in general have long been associated with the progressive development of global cognitive deficits, individuals with bipolar disorder represent a particularly vulnerable population in light of the prevalence of cognitive impairment central to the diagnosis of bipolar disorder itself, even during periods of euthymia (Martinez-Aran et al., 2004). Van Gorp and colleagues (1998) found that regardless of the presence or absence of comorbid alcoholism, patients with bipolar disorder displayed poorer verbal memory than normal control subjects, although bipolar patients with alcoholism had more extensive deficits in executive function.

Treatment

As previously noted, most randomized controlled intervention trials in bipolar disorder exclude prospective subjects with comorbid alcohol or drug use disorders. Early observational studies suggested that the presence of alcohol or substance misuse may be associated with a poor antimanic response to lithium but possibly better response to certain anticonvulsants (divalproex or carbamazepine) (Goldberg et al., 1999b). Small open trials also have reported beneficial outcomes with adjunctive lamotrigine for bipolar disorder patients with alcohol dependence (Rubio, Lopez-Munoz & Alamo, 2006) or cocaine dependence (Brown et al., 2006), leading to improvement from baseline in manic, depressive and alcohol craving symptoms. Elsewhere, open-label adjunctive quetiapine has preliminarily been reported to reduce affective symptoms as well as craving, but not drug use, among bipolar disorder patients with cocaine dependence (Brown et al., 2002). Quetiapine also has been shown to help diminish anxiety, insomnia and other symptoms related to withdrawal during opiate detoxification (Pinkofsky et al., 2005).

Depression is common among individuals with substance use disorders, and naturalistic outcome data from the STEP-BD found that antidepressant use is especially common among dual-diagnosis bipolar disorder patients—despite reports elsewhere that substance abuse comorbidity may pose a risk factor for antidepressant-induced mania or hypomania (Goldberg & Whiteside, 2002; Manwani et al., 2006). Only 0.4% of STEP-BD patients with comorbid alcohol or drug abuse/dependence were noted to have received a pharmacotherapy specific to substance abuse, such as disulfiram, naltrexone, methadone or buprenorphine (Simon et al., 2004).

There exists only a small controlled trial literature on the treatment of patients with bipolar disorder and substance use disorders. One early randomized study of adolescent patients with bipolar disorder and substance abuse found better overall functioning and less substance use (by toxicology screens) in subjects taking lithium than placebo (Geller et al., 1998). That study is notable not only for its overall positive finding, but moreover, because of its suggestion that lithium may be effective for adolescent dual-diagnosis patients with bipolar disorder, despite reports of lithium's less robust effect in adult dual-diagnosis populations (Goldberg et al., 1999b).

As noted in Table 9.2, Salloum and colleagues (2005) conducted a randomized 26-week comparison of divalproex plus treatment as usual ($n = 27$) versus placebo plus treatment as usual ($n = 25$) in adult bipolar outpatients with current alcoholism. Treatment groups did not differ significantly in depressive or manic symptoms over time, however, subjects taking divalproex had a significantly lower proportion of heavy drinking days, fewer drinks per heavy drinking day, and fewer drinks per drinking day. Divalproex also was associated with a significantly longer time until sustained heavy drinking (defined as at least three consecutive days of five or more drinks per day in men or four or more drinks per day in women). While neuropharmacologic mechanisms remain speculative about the specific effect of divalproex on symptoms of alcoholism, the findings suggest a role for divalproex potentially to reduce drinking behavior regardless of its effect on mood symptoms in bipolar disorder. Of particular concern among individuals with alcoholism, those with hepatic enzyme levels greater than three times the upper limit of normal may be poor candidates for divalproex. Other studies have suggested that among alcoholic bipolar patients, medication adherence appears to be significantly higher with divalproex than lithium (Weiss et al., 1998).

Finally, mention is warranted of the anti-alcoholism effects reported with topiramate. While this novel anticonvulsant has demonstrated little difference from placebo in the treatment of bipolar mania (Kushner et al., 2006), it was associated with a substantial reduction in drinking behavior and craving during a 12-week placebo-controlled trial in 150

Table 9.2 Randomized Intervention Trials for Bipolar Disorder with Axis I Comorbidities

Condition	Authors	Design	Outcome
Adolescent comorbid substance abuse	Geller et al., 1998	6-week comparison of lithium ($n=13$) or placebo ($n=12$) in outpatients	Fewer positive drug screens, lower global assessment of functioning scores with lithium than placebo
Adult comorbid alcohol dependence	Salloum et al., 2005	26-week comparison of divalproex+treatment as usual ($n=27$) versus placebo+treatment as usual ($n=25$)	Longer time to heavy drinking with divalproex than placebo
Adult comorbid substance dependence	Weiss et al., 2007	20 weeks of Integrated Group Therapy (IGT) ($n=31$) versus group drug counseling ($n=31$)	Fewer days of substance use at 3-month follow-up for IGT
Adult comorbid anxiety symptoms in bipolar depression	Tohen et al., 2003	8-week comparison of olanzapine-fluoxetine combination (OFC) ($n=86$) versus placebo ($n=377$) or olanzapine ($n=370$)	Greater reduction in Hamilton Anxiety scale scores with OFC than placebo
	Calabrese et al., 2005	8-week comparison of quetiapine 300 mg ($n=172$) or 600 mg ($n=170$) or placebo ($n=169$)	Greater reduction in Hamilton Anxiety scale scores with quetiapine (either dose) than placebo
	Davis, Bartolucci & Petty, 2005	8-week comparison of divalproex ($n=13$) or placebo ($n=12$)	Greater reduction in Hamilton Anxiety scale scores with divalproex than placebo
Comorbid ADHD	Scheffer et al., 2005	4-week randomized crossover comparison of mixed amphetamine salts versus placebo ($n=30$) after 8 weeks of open divalproex	Greater clinical global impressions improvement scores with mixed amphetamine salts than placebo

non-bipolar subjects with alcohol dependence, at a dose of up to 300 mg/day (Johnson et al., 2003). In addition, although cognitive impairment is a known potential adverse effect of topiramate, its incidence in this study was only 18%. The efficacy of topiramate for symptoms of alcoholism specifically accompanying bipolar disorder has not been studied, although it may nevertheless warrant consideration for its possible anti-alcoholism effect when used as part of a broader thymoleptic regimen for such dual-diagnosis patients.

Anxiety disorders

Anxiety disorders vie with substance use disorders as the most prevalent comorbid condition seen among individuals with bipolar disorder (see Table 9.1), occurring in slightly over half of individuals with bipolar disorder in the NESARC study (Grant et al., 2005). In the STEP-BD, 32% of study participants had at least one comorbid anxiety disorder, which was associated with fewer days well, a diminished likelihood for recovery from depression, earlier relapse, and greater functional impairment (Otto et al., 2006). Clinically, it is often difficult for clinicians to discriminate between comorbid anxiety and more fundamental signs of psychomotor agitation or activation due to mania.

Historically, anxiety disorders have long been linked with mood disorders, drawing particular attention because of their negative prognostic implications. Panic disorder, for example, confer an approximate 18-fold increased risk for suicidal ideation or attempts, independent of depressive features, among patients with other psychiatric disorders (Weissman et al., 1989). More specifically among individuals with bipolar disorder, coexistent anxiety disorders have been suggested to mediate the emergence of suicidal ideation or behaviors due to increased ruminations, as well as lower emotional processing among men (Simon et al., 2007). Anxiety also has been associated with loss of insight about psychiatric symptoms and a diminished capacity to recognize treatment response (Pini et al., 2003), as well as fewer days well, lower probability of recovery from depression, faster relapse, poorer quality of life, and poorer functional outcome as compared to bipolar disorder patients without comorbid anxiety disorders (Otto et al., 2006).

Though pharmacotherapy is often considered fundamental to the treatment of severe anxiety symptoms, it is important to keep in mind that cognitive therapy and other structured forms of psychotherapy represent effective but often under-utilized adjunctive treatments specific to anxiety (as well as depressive) symptoms in patients with bipolar disorder. Moreover, to date there have been no published placebo-controlled trials specifically designed to treat comorbid anxiety disorders in patients with bipolar illness. As shown in Table 9.2, several placebo-controlled clinical trials have reported favorable changes in Hamilton Anxiety Scale ratings as secondary analyses within the context of treating acute bipolar depression.

Panic disorder

Rates of panic disorder co-occurring with bipolar disorder range from 5% to 38% (see Table 9.1) and are more than twice as high in bipolar disorder as in unipolar depression (Simon et al., 2003). Comorbid panic disorder may be especially common among elderly women with bipolar disorder (Goldstein, Herrmann & Shulman, 2006). In contrast to social phobia, it appears to persist during hypomanic episodes (Perugi et al., 2001).

Interestingly, data from the NIMH Genetics Initiative suggest a familial association of panic disorder within bipolar pedigree families; thus, MacKinnon and colleagues (2002) found an approximate 1.5-fold increased likelihood for panic disorder in mood-disordered first-degree relatives of bipolar probands, suggesting that panic disorder may be a familial trait that may co-segregate with bipolar disorder.

The anticonvulsant gabapentin has demonstrated efficacy relative to placebo for panic disorder patients in general (Pande et al., 2000b), even though its utility specific for mania or depression has not been demonstrated in bipolar disorder (Frye et al., 2000; Pande et al., 2000a). In fact, there has been some suggestion that global improvement with gabapentin among patients with bipolar disorder may largely be attributable to its incidental beneficial effects for comorbid anxiety symptoms, notably panic disorder or generalized anxiety disorder (Perugi et al., 2002).

Obsessive-compulsive disorder (OCD)

OCD has been reported in 2–39% of individuals with bipolar disorder (see Table 9.1), and appears more than twice as likely to occur in bipolar than unipolar disorder (Simon et al., 2003). There is literature to suggest that OCD precedes bipolar disorder in about half of cases (Zutshi, Kamath & Reddy, 2007) yet still may be relatively rare (about 2%) in first-episode mania patients (Pashinian et al., 2006). OCD has been reported to co-occur with generalized anxiety disorder or social phobia more often than in non-bipolar OCD (Zutshi, Kamath & Reddy, 2007). In the ECA study, bipolar disorder patients with OCD were about twice as likely as those without OCD also to have panic disorder (37% vs 17%, respectively) (Chen & Dilsaver, 1995b). OCD also has been suggested to arise in conjunction with bipolar II disorder, chronic depression, and suicidality in patients with bipolar disorder (Krüger, Braunig & Cooke, 2000).

OCD symptoms may worsen during depression more clearly than during mania (Zutshi, Kamath & Reddy, 2007) and may be more frequent in patients with mixed than pure manias (McElroy et al., 1995). The course of comorbid OCD following a first hospitalization for mania appears to correspond closely to the course of affective symptoms in bipolar disorder (Strakowski et al., 1998b). OCD-bipolar patients, as compared to non-OCD bipolar patients, may show a more episodic and depression-prone course of illness (Perugi et al., 2002), more lifetime suicide attempts (Krüger, Braunig & Cooke, 2000), and more extensive comorbid substance abuse and/or panic disorder (Perugi et al., 2002).

Of obvious concern from a therapeutic standpoint is the question of whether traditional pharmacotherapies for uncomplicated OCD—namely, selective serotonin reuptake inhibitors (SSRIs), often at higher doses than used for unipolar depression—are safe (with respect to the potential for induction of mania or cycle acceleration) and as effective as in OCD without bipolar disorder. The absence of any controlled or even large open trials of SSRIs for OCD in patients with bipolar disorder makes it difficult to address either issue empirically, although naturalistic follow-up data point to an elevated risk for switches to mania with tricyclic (i.e. clomipramine) or SSRI antidepressants (Perugi et al., 2002). Moreover, since SSRIs have not shown greater efficacy than placebo for the treatment of bipolar depression (Nemeroff et al., 2001; Sachs et al., 2007), it may be premature to assume that results from non-bipolar disorder populations are generalizable to bipolar disorder populations. Some authorities advocate first pursuing anxiolytic mood stabilizing agents (such as quetiapine or other atypical antipsychotics (Gao et al., 2006) and anxiolytic anticonvulsants such as divalproex or gabapentin (Freeman, Freeman & McElroy, 2002)) when feasible before assuming the need for adjunctive serotonergic antidepressants.

Generalized anxiety disorder (GAD)

GAD has been reported to occur in 3–43% of individuals with bipolar disorder (see Table 9.1) and may be three times more common in adults with bipolar disorder than unipolar depression (Simon et al., 2003). It has been associated with comorbid alcohol abuse but more rarely with cocaine dependence (Mitchell, Brown & Rush, 2007). Oftentimes, the autonomic hyperarousal associated with GAD (including features such as irritability, tension and apprehension) may be difficult to distinguish from features of hypomania.

To the extent that anxiolytic psychotropic agents (such as certain anticonvulsants or atypical antipsychotics) are effective for GAD symptoms without destabilizing mood, they may offer an advantage over more traditional antidepressants as first-line interventions for dual-diagnosis bipolar disorder patients. Augmentation with standard antidepressants having known efficacy for GAD (such as some SSRIs) may be advisable in the absence of manic or hypomanic symptoms. Adjunctive use of the mixed serotonergic-noradrenergic antidepressant venlafaxine, approved by the US Food and Drug Administration for the treatment of GAD, likely merits particularly close monitoring in light of reports about its dramatically elevated risk for inducing mania or hypomania in depressed bipolar patients (Post et al., 2006).

Social phobia

Social phobia has been identified in 0–31% of individuals with bipolar disorder (see Table 9.1). Its presence has been linked with elevated rates of substance use disorders, early age at onset of bipolar disorder, and heightened interpersonal sensitivity, obsessiveness, phobic anxiety and paranoid thinking (Pini et al., 2006). Retrospective studies suggest that social phobia more often precedes rather than follows the onset of hypomania in bipolar II disorder, and may remit alongside the resolution of affective symptoms (Perugi et al., 2001).

Anxiolytic anticonvulsants such as gabapentin (Pande et al., 1999) or pregabalin (Pande et al., 2004) with demonstrated efficacy in social phobia may warrant consideration within a broader pharmacotherapy regimen when social phobia co-occurs with bipolar disorder.

Posttraumatic stress disorder (PTSD)

Lifetime prevalence rates of PTSD vary from about 7% to 8% in the Stanley Bipolar Network (McElroy et al., 2001) and the National Comorbidity Survey (Kessler et al., 1995) to 21% in the Cincinnati First Episode Mania Study (Strakowski et al., 1998) and 24% in the Cornell Bipolar Disorders Research Program (Goldberg & Garno, 2005). Following a first lifetime hospitalization for mania, subsequent symptoms of comorbid PTSD appear divergent from the course of affective symptoms, in contrast to a greater conformity of course between affective symptoms and OCD in bipolar disorder (Strakowski et al., 1998b).

Comorbid PTSD has been identified in 2–24% of adults with bipolar disorder (see Table 9.1), with an elevated risk among those who report histories of severe childhood abuse (Brown et al., 2005; Goldberg & Garno, 2005). Its prevalence appears twice as likely among bipolar women as bipolar men (Baldassano et al., 2005). PTSD has been linked with adult cocaine (but not alcohol) dependence (Mitchell, Brown & Rush, 2007), more severe global illness severity, and more frequent hospitalizations as compared to patients with only PTSD or only bipolar disorder (Thatcher et al., 2007). As with other comorbid anxiety disorders, the use of serotonergic antidepressants to target PTSD symptoms is largely unexplored in patients with bipolar disorder and demands caution. Preliminary randomized trials support the utility of several anticonvulsants, including lamotrigine and topiramate, for at least some dimensions of PTSD symptoms, such as re-experiencing or avoidance/numbing (Hertzberg et al., 1999; Tucker et al., 2007).

Eating disorders

There has been growing interest in points of clinical overlap between bipolar disorder and eating disorders, particular binge-eating disorder, based in part on conceptual parallels between dysregulation of eating and mood, impulsivity and compulsivity, and increased goal-directed activity and exercise (McElroy et al., 2005). Family-genetic studies also reveal a disproportionate elevation of bipolar disorder among relatives of anorexia nervosa probands (Gershon et al., 1984). Reported prevalence rates of eating disorders among individuals with bipolar disorder range from 6–27% (see Table 9.1). Cross-sectional studies suggest that bipolar disorder more often precedes the onset of binge-eating disorders, rather than the reverse, and that eating disorder may represent the use of food in efforts to modulate emotional dysregulation (Ramacciotti et al., 2005). Bulimia is substantially rarer in men than women with bipolar disorder (Baldassano et al., 2005).

High-dose SSRIs, commonly used to treat bulimia nervosa in patients without bipolar disorder, have not been studied either for their safety or efficacy in those with bipolar disorder. In addition, though few treatments have systematically been studied for binge-eating disorder, preliminary controlled data suggest some potential benefit with the anticonvulsant topiramate (McElroy et al., 2007).

Attention-deficit/hyperactivity disorder (ADHD)

Published rates of comorbid ADHD with bipolar disorder range from about 10–20% in retrospectively assessed adults to up to 85% in prepubertal and adolescent samples (see Table 9.1). The co-occurrence of bipolar disorder with ADHD remains particularly controversial since the cognitive dimensions of bipolar disorder by definition often involve distractibility, and impaired attention may be a trait phenomenon that is independent of mood state for a substantial proportion of individuals with bipolar disorder (Bora, Vahip & Akdeniz, 2006; Martinez-Aran et al., 2004;

Najt et al., 2005). The differentiation between ADHD and bipolar disorder has been suggested to rest on (a) cardinal symptoms of mania that are significantly rarer in ADHD (i.e. elation, grandiosity, racing thoughts/flight of ideas, decreased need for sleep, hypersexuality; by contrast, irritability, hyperactivity, rapid speech and distractibility are comparatively nonspecific between bipolar disorder and ADHD; Geller et al., 1998, 2002); (b) the rarity of psychosis or suicidality in ADHD as compared to bipolar disorder (Geller et al., 1998); (c) the episodic (bipolar) versus persistent (ADHD) nature of symptoms; and (d) the more probable onset of ADHD symptoms before age 7 with a later age at onset for bipolar disorder (Masi et al., 2006).

In the STEP-BD, comorbid ADHD was more common among men (15%) than women (6%), bipolar I than II patients, and a younger age at onset (Nierenberg et al., 2005). In addition, STEP-BD patients with comorbid AHDH also had higher prevalence rates of social phobia, PTSD, and alcohol or drug abuse/dependence. Among adolescent first-episode mania patients, comorbid ADHD has been associated with higher rates of syndromic relapse (Delbello et al., 2007).

Effective pharmacotherapy strategies for true dual-diagnosis patients with ADHD and bipolar disorder generally involve combined treatment with psychostimulants after beginning mood stabilizing agents. Notably, open label treatment with divalproex in a study of 40 children and adolescents with comorbid bipolar disorder and ADHD produced an antimanic response in 80%, but with minimal change in ADHD symptoms; responders for whom mixed amphetamine salts were then added to divalproex had significantly greater improvement in ADHD symptoms, without worsening of manic symptoms, as compared to those who then took divalproex plus placebo (Scheffer et al., 2005).

Small open trial data also exist involving the addition of atomoxetine to mood stabilizers for children with comorbid bipolar disorder and ADHD; despite the potential hazard for a noradrenergic agent to induce mania or hypomania, it appeared to be safe and well-tolerated, although larger and more systematic studies are needed in ADHD subjects at risk for mood destabilization by antidepressants (Hah & Chang, 2005).

Personality disorders

It has been estimated that comorbid personality disorders, based on assessments of longitudinal history, are identifiable in about 30–50% of patients with documented bipolar I or II disorder (see Table 9.1), particularly cluster B (e.g. borderline, narcissistic) disorders when contrasted with unipolar depressed patients, according to European studies (Mantere et al., 2006; Schiavone et al., 2004).

There has long been debate about the validity of diagnosing personality disorders as separable entities from other aspects of psychopathology in people with chronic mood disorders such as bipolar illness. One source of controversy involves the parsing of non-pathognomonic features such as mood instability, chaotic relationships, or dramatic interpersonal styles as more accurately reflecting an independent personality disorder versus stigmata of a poorly regulated mood disorder. Overlapping mood-versus personality-based symptoms are especially difficult to disentangle when one appreciates that (a) in most patients with bipolar disorder, mood symptoms first arise before age 18 (Perlis et al., 2004), (b) subsyndromal symptoms often persist between full affective syndromes in bipolar disorder (Altshuler et al., 2006), and (c) longstanding affective symptoms taint attitudes and expectations about oneself relative to one's capabilities, and impact important relationships and developmental milestones during formative years. Some authors have suggested on largely theoretical grounds that "dramatic" or cluster B personality disorders may be variants, rather than comorbidities, of bipolar disorder (MacKinnon & Pies, 2006), although there has been little empirical study to address their points of formal overlap and contrast.

Deltito and colleagues (2001) retrospectively examined various correlates of bipolar disorder, including family history, temperament, and response to antidepressants, in a small group ($n = 16$) of mostly female adults ages 20–72, for whom approximately one-third had a history of spontaneous manic or hypomanic episodes. Elsewhere, in a prospective 4-year follow-up of 196 patients with borderline personality disorder and 433 with other personality disorders, Gunderson and colleagues (2006) found a 19.4% prevalence rate of DSM-IV bipolar disorder among individuals with borderline personality disorder—higher than seen in other personality disorders, but with no clear influence on course of illness relative to patients with borderline personality disorder alone. Another report, based on patients seen in an outpatient private practice setting in Italy, found borderline personality traits in almost half of individuals with bipolar II disorder, significantly higher than seen in unipolar depressed patients (Benazzi, 2006). In this latter study, factor analysis identified a dimension of affective instability (comprised of unstable mood, unstable relationships, unstable self-image, chronic emptiness, and anger) common in patients with bipolar disorder plus borderline traits, but a separate dimension of impulsivity (comprised of impulsivity, suicidal behavior, avoidance of abandonment, paranoid ideation) linked with borderline traits but unrelated to a bipolar II diagnosis.

A related line of investigation suggests that trait hostility is more common in bipolar disorder when borderline personality disorder coexists (Garno, Gunawardane & Goldberg, 2008), although trait impulsivity and aggression both appear to be more common in borderline personality disorder than in bipolar disorder alone (Henry et al., 2001). Comorbid cluster B personality disorders have been associated with an increased risk for suicide attempts (Garno et al., 2005), perhaps mediated by trait aggression.

Comorbid personality disorders among individuals with bipolar disorder have been associated with more extensive residual affective symptoms as well as impaired functional outcome (George et al., 2003; Loftus & Jaeger, 2006), and appear to contribute as an independent factor to risk for suicidal behavior (Garno et al., 2005). Axis II comorbidity also has been linked with comorbid alcohol and substance use disorders, more elaborate pharmacotherapy, and occupational disability (Kay et al., 2002), as well as slower time until recovery (Swartz et al., 2005). Antisocial personality disorder among individuals with bipolar illness also has been associated with cocaine (but not alcohol) dependence (Mitchell, Brown & Rush, 2007).

Psychotherapy is widely considered essential to the successful treatment of serious personality disorders, although there has been little systematic study of its effects specifically in individuals with comorbid bipolar disorder. Most existing structured psychotherapies for bipolar disorder (such as cognitive-behavioral therapy or interpersonal/social rhythm therapy) target depressive or related affective symptoms, although often the interpersonal correlates of bipolar disorder (such as stress responsivity or reactions to negative expressed emotion) represent core elements of the psychotherapy process. In recent years, psychotherapies such as dialectical behavior therapy (DBT) have been developed to target emotional dysregulation, impulsivity, maladaptive behaviors and coping strategies, chronic suicidality, and interpersonal conflicts common in cluster B personality disorders. There is likely value in adapting such psychotherapy approaches for bipolar disorder patients when prominent features suggestive of comorbid maladaptive personality traits are evident.

Treatment

Pharmacotherapy has generally been regarded as providing only moderate benefit for symptoms related to severe personality disorders co-occurring with bipolar disorder (Swartz et al., 2005), and little data exists to examine the relative benefits of pharmacotherapy with versus without adjunctive psychotherapy (or psychotherapy with versus without adjunctive pharmacotherapy) specifically targeting maladaptive personality traits. One retrospective analysis of lamotrigine for bipolar disorder identified a subgroup with comorbid borderline personality disorder and found that about 40% had a significant reduction in active DSM-IV criteria for borderline personality disorder (Preston et al., 2004). Other anticonvulsants, such as divalproex, have been shown to exert benefits on dimensions of psychopathology such as impulsivity and aggression in patients with borderline personality disorder (Hollander et al., 2003), and as such may represent a useful strategy for symptoms that may overlap personality and affective disorders.

Medical comorbidities

A number of specific medical comorbidites have been identified as being disproportionately elevated among individuals with bipolar disorder, including migraine (up to 20–25%; McIntyre et al., 2006; Mahmood, Romans & Silverstone, 1999), asthma (up to 15%; McIntyre et al., 2006), heart disease (nearly 10%; McIntyre et al., 2006) and diabetes (7–9% (Cassidy, Ahearn & Carroll, 1999; McIntyre et al., 2006), about three times higher than seen in the general population). Excess medical comorbidity has been associated with increased service utilization, social and occupational disability, and an overall more severe course of illness in bipolar disorder (McIntyre et al., 2006). Subclinical hypothyroidism has been described in bipolar mixed or rapid cycling patients, and bipolar women appear more likely than bipolar men overall to have thyroid disease (Baldassano et al., 2005).

One of the more remarkable observations about the longitudinal course of bipolar disorder has been the finding that the diagnosis of bipolar disorder itself is associated with increased likelihood of mortality not only from suicide and accidents, but also from excess cardiopulmonary and other circulatory disorders (Angst et al., 2002; Ösby et al., 2001; Weeke, Juel & Vaeth, 1987) and other serious medical conditions (Ösby et al., 2001). Follow-up studies suggest an approximate two-fold increased risk for cerebrovascular accidents (Lin, Tsai & Lee, 2007). Some authors have speculated about the possibility of adverse effects related to systemic inflammation (as evidenced by leukocytosis) and nonhepatic tissue damage (reflected by elevated hepatic enzyme levels) in bipolar disorder patients studied post-mortem (Tsai et al., 2005). Overall, natural causes of death carry an approximate two-fold increased standardized mortality ratio among individuals with bipolar disorder as compared to the general population (Ösby et al., 2001).

Some authors have suggested that excess mortality from natural causes among individuals with bipolar disorder may be an epiphenomenon due to factors such as increased smoking, obesity, or sedentary lifestyle, although depression itself is considered a direct risk factor for coronary heart disease, potentially via a serotonergic effect on platelet aggregation (Ösby et al., 2001). It is also possible that individuals with bipolar disorder may be more likely than non-bipolar medically ill patients to seek or receive rigorous primary medical care and to have poorer adherence to nonpsychotropic drugs prescribed for chronic medical conditions.

Medical comorbidities also have been associated with more severe and extensive depressive features in bipolar disorder, as well as a slower time until recovery from depression (Thompson et al., 2006).

Clinical recommendations for diagnostic assessment and treatment

The following points for consideration may be useful in the evaluation and management of individuals with bipolar disorder and possible comorbid psychiatric or substance use disorders:

1. In any mood disorder patient with poor response to traditional pharmacotherapy, consider the presence of factors that may complicate the presumed primary diagnosis—including psychosis, alcohol or substance use disorders, medical comorbidities, other Axis I disorders, and comorbid Axis II disorders.
2. When considering a diagnosis of bipolar disorder in patients with prominent or active substance use disorders, assure that a prior period of abstinence can be identified in which symptoms of mania or hypomania previously existed. Bipolar disorder may be wrongly diagnosed as present in half or more of individuals who present with mood instability and substance use disorders (Goldberg et al., 2009; Stewart & El-Mallakh, 2007).
3. Attempt to clarify the extent to which current symptoms are likely attributable to an affective illness versus a comorbid condition (e.g. paranoia and rapid speech during acute cocaine intoxication; autonomic hyperarousal due to an anxiety disorder; distractibility due to ADHD). Identify corroborating signs that form symptom constellations rather than isolated symptoms. (For example, distractible thinking in the presence of psychosis or sleeplessness would be more parsimoniously explained within the context of mania rather than by an additional diagnosis.)
4. Consider the role of longitudinal course of illness when attempting to discriminate symptoms attributable to bipolar disorder versus comorbid psychopathology (e.g. symptoms of a possible comorbid personality disorder should arise in early adolescence, appear as chronic traits rather than intermittent states, and should be evident independent of mood symptoms or psychomotor disturbances).
5. Consider the extent to which cognitive or motor symptoms may reflect iatrogenic phenomena versus comorbid conditions (e.g. "anxiety" attributable to a comorbid anxiety disorder versus substance withdrawal versus akathisia among individuals taking antipsychotic

medication; or, compulsive overeating attributable to psychotropic medications versus a freestanding eating disorder). Generating *differential* diagnoses for possible comorbid features stimulates broadened thought about possible explanations.

6. In the case of symptoms that potentially overlap multiple conditions, a hierarchical approach involves initially treating the potentially more serious condition and determining whether or not suspected comorbid phenomena remain as residual features. A classic example involves treating mania or hypomania and observing the degree of change in attentional complaints or motor agitation before assuming the presence of comorbid ADHD. Randomized data support the efficacy and safety of psychostimulants sequenced after mood stabilization with divalproex for dual-diagnosis bipolar disorder with ADHD (Scheffer et al., 2005).

7. Before using medications that can aggravate a comorbid condition (e.g. high-dose SSRIs for OCD in patients with bipolar disorder), optimize mood stabilizing agents first, carefully monitor changes in affective symptoms, and taper or withdraw co-therapies if they prove to destabilize mood. When possible, favor co-therapies that exert more neutral effects on mood (e.g. anxiolytic anticonvulsants rather than serotonergic antidepressants for comorbid anxiety).

8. In bipolar disorder patients with substance abuse, exercise caution if choosing to prescribe controlled substances for additional comorbidities (e.g. psychostimulants for ADHD; benzodiazepines for anxiety disorders) and monitor their safety, abuse potential, and demonstrable efficacy.

9. Discontinue ineffective co-therapies to minimize the unnecessary accrual of multiple agents with additive adverse effects and potential pharmacokinetic interactions.

10. Avoid pitfalls of oversimplification (e.g. automatically ascribing substance abuse to "self-medication" of bipolar disorder rather than identifying it as a freestanding comorbid illness requiring its own treatment).

11. Incorporate structured psychotherapies when appropriate as potential alternatives or adjuncts to additional pharmacotherapies (e.g. CBT for comorbid panic disorder).

Conclusions

Likely the most important aspect of comorbidity in bipolar disorder is recognizing its presence. It is possible, though as yet not empirically demonstrated, that the emergence of comorbid psychopathology could be minimized by anticipating risks for illness complexity (such as early age at onset for bipolar disorder) and minimizing delays to initiating effective mood stabilizing agents. Careful and rigorous diagnostic assessments require an awareness of common comorbid conditions in bipolar disorder and a thoughtful effort to discriminate comorbid conditions (such as anxiety or alcoholism) from fundamental affective symptoms (such as agitation or behavioral indiscretions during hypomania).

Treatment regimens for complex forms of bipolar illness hinge on the integrative use of complementary pharmacotherapies that do not exacerbate or worsen affective symptoms, and often require extrapolation from studies in non-bipolar populations. Knowledge about specific role for individual or group-based adjunctive psychotherapies—particularly for comorbid anxiety or substance use disorders—is instrumental to optimal comprehensive care. Parsimonious pharmacotherapy involves identifying putative mood stabilizing agents that may exert additional psychotropic benefits for comorbid conditions—such as divalproex for comorbid alcoholism, migraine or cluster B personality disorders; or anxiolytic anticonvulsants (such as gabapentin) or atypical antipsychotics (such as quetiapine) targeting prominent anxiety features; and devising complementary medication combinations that collectively address global presentations of psychopathology.

References

Altshuler LL, Post RM, Black DO, Keck PE Jr., Nolen WA, Frye MA, Suppes T, Grunze H, Kupka RW, Leverich GS, McElroy SL, Walden J, & Mintz J. (2006). Subsyndromal depressive symptoms are associated with functional impairment in patients with bipolar disorder: results of a large, multi-site study. *J. Clin. Psychiatry*, 67: 1551–1560.

Angst F, Stassen HH, Clayton PJ, & Angst J. (2002). Mortality of patients with mood disorders: follow-up over 34–38 years. *J. Affect. Disord.*, 68: 167–181.

Baethge C, Baldessarini RJ, Khalsa HM, Hennen J, Salvatore P, & Tohen M. (2005). Substance abuse in first-episode bipolar I disorder: indications for early intervention. *Am. J. Psychiatry*, 162: 1008–1010.

Baldassano CF, Marangell LB, Gyulai L, Ghaemi SN, Joffe H, Kim DR, Sagduyu K, Truman CJ, Wisniewski SR, Sachs GS, & Cohen LS. (2005). Gender differences in bipolar disorder: retrospective data from the first 500 STEP-BD participants. *Bipolar Disord.*, 7: 465–470.

Benazzi F. (2006). Borderline personality-bipolar spectrum relationship. *Prog. Neuropsychopharmacol. Biol. Psychiatry*, 30: 68–74.

Biederman J, Faraone SV, Wozniak J, & Monuteaux MC. (2000). Parsing the association between bipolar, conduct and substance use disorders: a familial risk analysis. *Biol. Psychiatry*, 48: 1037–1044.

Bizzarri JV, Sbrana A, Rucci P, Ravani L, Massei GJ, Gonnelli C, Spagnolli S, Doria MR, Raimondi F, Endicott J, Dell'Osso L, & Cassano GB. (2007). The spectrum of substance abuse in bipolar disorder: reasons for use, sensation seeking and substance sensitivity. *Bipolar Disord.*, 9: 213–220.

Black DW, Winokur G, Bell S, Nasrallah H, & Hulbert J. (1988). Complicated mania: comorbidity and immediate outcome in the treatment of mania. *Arch. Gen. Psychiatry*, 45: 232–236.

Bora E, Vahip S, & Akdeniz F. (2006). Sustained attention deficits in manic and euthymic patients with bipolar disorder. *Prog. Neuropsychopharmacol. Biol. Psychiatry*, 30: 1097–1102.

Boylan KR, Bieling PJ, Marriott M, Begin H, Young LT, & MacQueen GM. (2004). Impact of comorbid anxiety disorders on outcome in a cohort of patients with bipolar disorder. *J. Clin. Psychiatry*, 65: 1106–1113.

Brown ES, Nejtek VA, Perantie DC, & Bobadilla L. (2002). Quetiapine in bipolar disorder and cocaine dependence. *Bipolar Disord.*, 4: 406–411.

Brown ES, Perantie DC, Dhanani N, Beard L, Orsulak P, & Rush AJ. (2006). Lamotrigine for bipolar disorder and comorbid cocaine dependence: a replication and extension study. *J. Affect. Disord.*, 93: 219–222.

Brown GR, McBride L, Bauer MS, Williford WO, & Cooperative Studies Program 430 Study Team. (2005). Impact of childhood abuse on the course of bipolar disorder: a replication study in US veterans. *J. Affect. Disord.*, 89: 57–67.

Calabrese JR, Keck PE Jr., Macfadden W, Minkwitz M, Ketter TA, Weisler RH, Cutler AJ, McCoy R, Wilson E, & Mullen J. (2005). A randomized, double-blind, placebo-controlled trial of quetiapine in the treatment of bipolar I or II depression. *Am. J. Psychiatry*, 162: 1351–1360.

Cassano GB, Pini S, Saettoni M, Rucci P, & Dell'Osso L. (1998). Occurrence and clinical correlates of psychiatric comorbidity in patients with psychotic disorders. *J. Clin. Psychiatry*, 59: 60–68.

Cassidy F, Ahearn E, & Carroll BJ. (1999). Elevated frequency of diabetes mellitus in hospitalized manic-depressive patients. *Am. J. Psychiatry*, 156: 1417–1420.

Cassidy F, Ahearn EP, & Carroll BJ. (2001). Substance abuse in bipolar disorder. *Bipolar Disord.*, 3: 181–188.

Chen YW, & Dilsaver SC. (1995a). Comorbidity of panic disorder in bipolar illness: evidence from the Epidemiologic Catchment Area Survey. *Am. J. Psychiatry*, 152: 280–282

Chen YW, & Dilsaver SC. (1995b). Comorbidity for obsessive-compulsive disorder in bipolar and unipolar disorders. *Psychiatry Res.*, 59: 57–64.

Chengappa KNR, Levine J, Gershon S, & Kupfer DJ. (2000). Lifetime prevalence of substance or alcohol abuse and dependence among subjects with bipolar I and II disorders in a voluntary registry. *Bipolar Disord.*, 2: 191–195.

Conway KP, Compton W, Stinson FS, & Grant BF. (2006). Lifetime comorbidity of DSM-IV mood and anxiety disorders and specific drug use disorders: results from the National Epidemiologic Survey on Alcohol and Related Conditions. *J. Clin. Psychiatry*, 67: 247–257.

Davis LL, Bartolucci A, & Petty F. (2005). Divalproex in the treatment of bipolar depression: a placebo-controlled study. *J. Affect. Disord.*, 85: 259–266.

Delbello MP, Hanseman D, Adler CM, Fleck DE, & Strakowski SM. (2007). Twelve-month outcome of adolescents with bipolar disorder following first hospitalization for a manic or mixed episode. *Am. J. Psychiatry*, 164: 582–590.

Deltito J, Martin L, Riefkohl J, Austria B, Kissilenko A, Corless C, & Morse P. (2001). Do patients with borderline personality disorder belong to the bipolar spectrum? *J. Affect. Disord.*, 67: 221–228.

Dunayevich E, Sax KW, Keck PE, McElroy SL, Sorter MT, McConville BJ, & Strakowski SM. (2000). Twelve-month outcome in bipolar patients with and without personality disorders. *J. Clin. Psychiatry*, 61: 134–139.

Edmonds LK, Mosley BJ, Admiraal AJ, Olds RJ, Romans SE, Silverstone T, & Walsh AE. (1998). Familial bipolar disorder: preliminary results from the Otago Familial Bipolar Genetic Study. *Aust. N Z J. Psychiatry*, 32: 823–829.

Feinman JA, & Dunner DL. (1996) The effect of alcohol and substance abuse on the course of bipolar affective disorder. *J. Affect. Disord.*, 37: 43–49.

Fleck DE, Arndt S, Delbello MP, & Strakowski SM. (2006). Concurrent tracking of alcohol use and bipolar disorder symptoms. *Bipolar Disord.*, 8: 338–344.

Fossey MD, Otto MW, Yates WR, Wisniewski SR, Gyulai L, Allen MH, Miklowitz DJ, Coon KA, Ostacher MJ, Neel JL, Thase ME, Sachs GS, & Weiss RD; Step-BD Investigators. (2006). Validity of the distinction between primary and secondary substance use disorder in patients with bipolar disorder: data from the first 1000 STEP-BD participants. *Am. J. Addict.*, 15: 138–143.

Freeman MP, Freeman SA, & McElroy SL. (2002). The comorbidity of bipolar and anxiety disorders: prevalence, psychobiology, and treatment issues. *J. Affect. Disord.*, 68: 1–23.

Frye MA, Altshuler LL, McElroy SL, Suppes T, Keck PE, Denicoff K, Nolen WA, Kupka R, Leverich GS, Pollio C, Grunze H, Walden J, & Post RM. (2003). Gender differences in prevalence, risk, and clinical correlates of alcoholism comorbidity in bipolar disorder. *Am. J. Psychiatry*, 160: 883–889.

Frye MA, Ketter TA, Kimbrell TA, Dunn RT, Speer AM, Osuch EA, Luckenbaugh DA, Cora-Ocatelli G, Leverich GS, & Post RM. (2000). A placebo-controlled study of lamotrigine and gabapentin monotherapy in refractory mood disorders. *J. Clin. Psychopharmacol.*, 20: 607–614.

Gao K, Muzina D, Gajwani P, & Calabrese JR. (2006). Efficacy of typical and atypical antipsychotics for primary and comorbid anxiety symptoms or disorders: a review. *J. Clin. Psychiatry*, 67: 1327–1340.

Garno JL, Goldberg JF, Ramirez PM, & Ritzler BA. (2005). Bipolar disorder with comorbid cluster B personality disorder features: impact on suicidality. *J. Clin. Psychiatry*, 66: 339–345.

Garno JL, Gunawardane N, & Goldberg JF. (2008). Predictors of trait aggression in bipolar disorder. *Bipolar Disord.*, 10: 285–292.

Geller B, Zimerman B, Williams M, Delbello MP, Bolhofner K, Craney JL, Frazier J, Beringer L, & Nickelsburg MJ. (2002). DSM-IV mania symptoms in a prepubertal and early adolescent bipolar disorder phenotype compared to attention-deficit hyperactive and normal controls. *J. Child Adolesc. Psychopharmacol.*, 12: 11–25.

Geller B, Williams M, Zimerman B, Frazier J, Beringer L, & Warner KL. (1998). Prepubertal and early adolescent bipolarity differentiate from ADHD by manic symptoms, grandiose delusions, ultra-rapid or ultradian cycling. *J. Affect. Disord.*, 51: 81–91.

George EL, Miklowitz DJ, Richards JA, Simoneau TL, & Taylor DO. (2003). The comorbidity of bipolar disorder and axis II personality disorders: prevalence and clinical correlates. *Bipolar Disord.*, 5: 115–122.

Gershon ES, Schreiber JL, Hamovit JR, Dibble ED, Kaye W, Nurnberger JI Jr., Andersen AE, & Ebert M. (1984). Clinical findings in patients with anorexia nervosa and affective illness in their relatives. *Am. J. Psychiatry*, 141: 1419–1422.

Goldberg JF, & Garno JL. (2005). Development of posttraumatic stress disorder in adult bipolar patients with histories of severe childhood abuse. *J. Psychiatr. Res.*, 39: 595–601.

Goldberg JF, Garno JL, Callahan AM, Kearns DL, Kerner B, Ackerman SH. (2009). Overdiagnosis of bipolar disorder among substance use disorder inpatients with mood instability. *J. Clin. Psychiatry*, Jan. 7, epublication ahead of print.

Goldberg JF, Garno JL, Kocsis JH, Leon AC, Portera L, & Whiteside JE. (1999a). Correlates of suicidal ideation in dysphoric mania. *J. Affect. Disord.*, 56: 75–81.

Goldberg JF, Garno JL, Leon AC, Kocsis JH, & Portera L. (1999b). A history of substance abuse complicates remission from acute mania in bipolar disorder. *J. Clin. Psychiatry*, 60: 733–740.

Goldberg JF, & Whiteside JE. (2002). The association between substance abuse and antidepressant-induced mania in bipolar disorder: a preliminary report. *J. Clin. Psychiatry*, 63: 791–795.

Goldstein BI, Herrmann N, & Shulman KI. (2006). Comorbidity in bipolar disorder among the elderly: results from an epidemiological community sample. *Am. J. Psychiatry*, 163: 319–321.

Goldstein BI, & Levitt AJ. (2006a). A gender-focused perspective on health service utilization in comorbid bipolar I disorder and alcohol use disorders: results from the National Epidemiologic Survey on Alcohol and Related Conditions. *J. Clin. Psychiatry*, 67: 925–932.

Goldstein BI, & Levitt AJ. (2006b). Further evidence for a developmental subtype of bipolar disorder defined by age at onset: results from the National Epidemiologic Survey on Alcohol and Related Conditions. *Am. J. Psychiatry*, 163: 1633–1636.

Goldstein BI, & Levitt AJ. (2006c). Factors associated with temporal priority in comorbid bipolar I disorder and alcohol use disorders: results from the National Epidemiologic Survey on Alcohol and Related Conditions. *J. Clin. Psychiatry*, 67: 643–649.

Goldstein BI, Velyvis VP, & Parikh SV. (2006). The association between moderate alcohol use and illness severity in bipolar disorder: a preliminary report. *J. Clin. Psychiatry*, 67: 102–106.

Grant BF. (1997). Prevalence and correlates of alcohol use and DSM-IV alcohol dependence in the United States: results of the National Longitudinal Alcohol Epidemiologic Survey. *J. Stud. Alcohol*, 58: 464–473.

Grant BF, Stinson FS, Dawson DA, Chou SP, Dufour MC, Compton W, Pickering RP, & Kaplan K. (2004). Prevalence and co-occurrence of substance use disorders and independent mood and anxiety disorders: results from the National Epidemiologic Survey on Alcohol and Related Conditions. *Arch. Gen. Psychiatry*, 61: 807–816.

Grant BF, Stinson FS, Hasin DS, Dawson DA, Chou SP, Ruan WJ, & Huang B. (2005). Prevalence, correlates, and comorbidity of bipolar I disorder and Axis I and II disorders: results from the National Epidemiological Survey on Alcohol and Related Conditions. *J. Clin. Psychiatry*, 60: 1205–1215.

Gunderson JG, Weinberg I, Daversa MT, Kueppenbender KD, Zanarini MC, Shea MT, Skodol AE, Sanislow CA, Yen S, Morey LC, Grilo CM, McGlashan TH, Stout RL, & Dyck I. (2006). Descriptive and longitudinal observations on the relationship of borderline personality disorder and bipolar disorder. *Am. J. Psychiatry*, 163: 1173–1178.

Hah M, & Chang K. (2005). Atomoxetine for the treatment of attention-deficit/ hyperactivity disorder in children and adolescents with bipolar disorders. *J. Child Adolesc. Psychopharmacol.*, 15: 996–1004.

Henry C, Mitropoulou V, New AS, Koenigsberg HW, Silverman J, & Siever LJ. (2001). Affective instability and impulsivity in borderline personality and bipolar II disorders: similarities and differences. *J. Psychiatr. Res.*, 35: 307–312.

Hertzberg MA, Butterfield MI, Feldman ME, Beckham JC, Sutherland SM, Connor KM, & Davidson JR. (1999). A preliminary study of lamotrigine for the treatment of posttraumatic stress disorder. *Biol. Psychiatry*, 45: 1226–1229.

Hilliard AA, Weinberger SE, Tierney LM Jr., Midthun DE, & Saint S. (2004). Occam's Razor versus Saint's Triad. *N. Engl. J. Med.*, 350: 599–603.

Hirschfeld RM, Lewis L, & Vornik LA. (2003). Perceptions and impact of bipolar disorder: How far have we really come? Results of the national depressive and manic-depressive association 2000 survey of individuals with bipolar disorder. *J. Clin. Psychiatry*, 64: 161–174.

Hollander E, Tracy KA, Swann AC, Coccaro EF, McElroy SL Wozniak P, Sommerville KW, & Nemeroff CB. (2003). Divalproex in the treatment of impulsive aggression: efficacy in Cluster B personality disorders. *Neuropsychopharmacology*, 28: 1186–1197.

Johnson BA, Ait-Daoud N, Bowden CL, DiClemente CC, Roache JD, Lawson K, Javors MA, & Ma JZ. (2003). Oral topiramate for treatment of alcohol dependence: a randomised controlled trial. *Lancet*, 361: 1677–1685.

Judd LL, Akiskal HS, Schettler PJ, Endicott J, Maser J, Solomon DA, Leon AC, Rice JA, & Keller MB. (2002). The long-term natural history of the weekly symptomatic status of bipolar I disorder. *Arch. Gen. Psychiatry*, 59: 530–537.

Kay JH, Altshuler LL, Ventura J, & Mintz J. (2002). Impact of axis II comorbidity on the course of bipolar illness in men: a retrospective chart review. *Bipolar Disord.*, 4: 237–242.

Keck PE Jr., McElroy SL, Strakowski SM, West SA, Sax KW, Hawkins JM, Bourne ML, & Haggard P. (1998). Twelve-month outcome of patients with bipolar disorder following hospitalization for a manic or mixed episode. *Am. J. Psychiatry*, 155: 646–652.

Kessler RC, Crum RM, Warner LA, Nelson CB, Schulenberg J, & Anthony JC. (1997). Lifetime co-occurrence of DSM-III-R alcohol abuse and dependence with other psychiatric disorders in the National Comorbidity Survey. *Arch. Gen. Psychiatry*, 54: 313–321.

Kessler RC, Rubinow DR, Holmes C, Abelson JM, & Zhao S. (1997). The epidemiology of DSM-III-R bipolar I disorder in a general population survey. *Psychol. Med.*, 27: 1079–1089.

Kowatch RA, Suppes T, Carmody TJ, Bucci JP, Hume JH, Kromelis M, Emslie GJ, Weinberg WA, & Rush AJ. (2000). Effect size of lithium, divalproex sodium, and carbamazepine in children and adolescents with bipolar disorder. *J. Am. Acad. Child Adolesc. Psychiatry*, 39: 713–720.

Krüger S, Braunig P, & Cooke RG. (2000). Comorbidity of obsessive-compulsive disorder in recovered inpatients with bipolar disorder. *Bipolar Disord.,* 2: 71–74.

Krüger S, Cooke RG, Hasey GM, Jorna T, & Persad E. (1995). Comorbidity of obsessive-compulsive disorder in bipolar disorder. *J. Affect. Disord.,* 34: 117–120.

Krüger S, Shugar G, & Cooke RG. (1996). Comorbidity of binge eating disorder and the partial binge eating syndrome with bipolar disorder. Int. *J. Eat. Disord.,* 19: 45–52.

Kushner SF, Khan A, Lane R, & Olson WH. (2006). Topiramate monotherapy in the management of acute mania: results of four double-blind placebo-controlled trials. *Bipolar Disord.,* 8: 15–27.

Levander E, Frye MA, McElroy S, Suppes T, Grunze H, Nolen WA, Kupka R, Keck PE Jr., Leverich GS, Altshuler LL, Hwang S, Mintz J, & Post RM. (2007). Alcoholism and anxiety in bipolar I women with and without alcoholism. *J. Affect. Disord.,* 101: 211–217.

Lin HC, Tsai SY, & Lee HC. (2007). Increased risk of developing stroke among patients with bipolar disorder after an acute mood episode: a six-year follow-up study. *J. Affect. Disord.,* 100: 49–54.

Lish JD, Dime-Meenan S, Whybrow PC, Price RA, & Hirschfeld RM. (1994). The National Depressive and Manic-Depressive Association (DMDA). survey of bipolar members. *J. Affect. Disord.,* 31: 281–294.

Loftus ST, & Jaeger J. (2006). Psychosocial outcome in bipolar I patients with a personality disorder. *J. Nerv. Ment. Dis.,* 194: 967–970.

Mackinnon DF, & Pies R. (2006). Affective instability as rapid cycling: theoretical and clinical implications for borderline personality and bipolar spectrum disorders. *Bipolar Disord.,* 8: 1–14.

MacKinnon DF, Zandi PP, Cooper J, Potash JB, Simpson SG, Gershon E, Nurnberger J, Reich T, & DePaulo JR. (2002). Comorbid bipolar disorder and panic disorder in families with a high prevalence of bipolar disorder. *Am. J. Psychiatry,* 159: 30–35.

Mahmood T, Romans S, & Silverstone T. (1999). Prevalence of migraine in bipolar disorder. *J. Affect. Disord.,* 52: 239–241.

Mantere O, Melartin TK, Suominen K, Rytsala HJ, Valtonen HM, Arvilommi P, Leppämäki S, & Isometsä ET. (2006). Differences in Axis I and II comorbidity between bipolar I and II disorders and major depressive disorder. *J. Clin. Psychiatry,* 67: 584–593.

MacQueen GM, Marriott M, Begin H, Robb J, Joffe RT, & Young LT. (2003). Subsyndromal symptoms assessed in longitudinal, prospective follow-up of a cohort of patients with bipolar disorder. *Bipolar Disord.,* 5: 349–355.

Manwani SG, Pardo TB, Albanese MJ, Zablotsky B, Goodwin FK, & Ghaemi SN. (2006). Substance use disorder and other predictors of antidepressant-induced mania: a retrospective chart review. *J. Clin. Psychiatry,* 67: 1341–1345.

Martinez-Aran A, Vieta E, Reinares M, Colom F, Torrent C, Sanchez-Moreno J, Benabarre A, Goikolea JM, Comes M, & Salamero M. (2004). Cognitive function across manic or hypomanic, depressed, and euthymic states in bipolar disorder. *Am. J. Psychiatry,* 161: 262–270.

Masi G, Perugi G, Toni C, Millepiedi S, Mucci M, Bertini N, & Pfanner C. (2006). Attention-deficit hyperactivity disorder – bipolar comorbidity children and adolescents. *Bipolar Disord.,* 8: 373–381.

McElroy SL, Altshuler LL, Suppes T, Keck PE Jr., Frye MA, Denicoff KD, Nolen WA, Kupka RW, Leverich GS, Rochussen JR, Rush AJ, & Post RM. (2001). Axis I psychiatric comorbidity and its relationship to historical illness variables in 288 patients with bipolar disorder. *Am. J. Psychiatry,* 158: 420–426.

McElroy SL, Hudson JI, Capece JA, Beyers K, Fisher AC, Rosenthal NR, Topiramate Binge Eating Disorder Research Group. (2007). Topiramate for the treatment of binge eating disorder associated with obesity: a placebo-controlled study. *Biol. Psychiatry,* 61: 1039–1048.

McElroy SL, Kotwal R, Keck PE Jr., & Akiskal HS. (2005). Comorbidity of bipolar disorder and eating disorders: distinct or related disorders with shared dysregulation? *J. Affect. Disord.,* 86: 107–127.

McElroy SL, Strakowski SM, Keck PE Jr., Tugrul KL, West SA, & Lonczak HS. (1995). Differences and similarities in mixed and pure mania. *Compr. Psychiatry,* 36: 187–194.

McIntyre RS, Konarski JZ, Soczynska JK, Wilkins K, Panjwani G, Bouffard B, Bottas A, & Kennedy SH. (2006). Medical comorbidity in bipolar disorder: implications for functional outcomes and health service utilization. *Psychiatr. Serv.,* 57: 1140–1144.

Mitchell JD, Brown ES, & Rush AJ. (2007). Comorbid disorders in patients with bipolar disorder and concomitant substance dependence. *J. Affect. Disord.,* 102: 281–287.

Najt P, Glahn D, Bearden CE, Hatch JP, Monkul ES, Kaur S, Villarreal V, Bowden C, & Soares JC. (2005). Attention deficits in bipolar disorder: a comparison based on the Continuous Performance Task. *Neurosci. Lett.,* 379: 122–126.

Nemeroff CB, Evans DL, Gyulai L, Sachs GS, Bowden Cl, & Gergel IP. (2001). Double-blind placebo-controlled comparison of imipramine and paroxetine in the treatment of bipolar depression. *Am. J. Psychiatry,* 158: 906–912.

Nierenberg AA, Miyahara S, Spencer T, Wisniewski SR, Otto MW, Simon N, Pollack MH, Ostacher MJ, Yan L, Siegel R, & Sachs GS; STEP-BD Investigators. (2005). Clinical and diagnostic implications of lifetime attention deficit/hyperactivity disorder comorbidity in adults with bipolar disorder: data from the first 1000 STEP-BD participants. *Biol. Psychiatry,* 57: 1467–1573.

Ösby U, Brandt L, Correia N, Ekbom A, & Sparen P. (2001). Excess mortality in bipolar and unipolar disorder in Sweden. *Arch. Gen. Psychiatry,* 58: 844–850.

Otto MW, Simon NM, Wisniewski SR, Miklowitz DJ, Kogan JN, Reilly-Harrington NA, Frank E, Nierenberg AA, Marangell LB, Sagduyu K, Weiss RD, Miyahara S, Thas ME, Sachs GS, & Pollack MH; STEP-BD Investigators. (2006). Prospective 12-month course of bipolar disorder in out-patients with and without comorbid anxiety disorders. *Br. J. Psychiatry,* 189: 20–25.

Pande AC, Davidson JR, Jefferson JW, Janney CA, Katzelnick DJ, Weisler RH, Greist JH, & Sutherland SM. (1999). Treatment of social phobia with gabapentin: a placebo-controlled study. *J. Clin. Psychopharmacol.,* 19: 341–348.

Pande AC, Crockatt JG, Janney CA, Werth JL, & Tsaroucha G. (2000). Gabapentin in bipolar disorder: a placebo-controlled trial of adjunctive therapy. *Bipolar Disord.,* 2 (3 Part 2): 249–255.

Pande AC, Feltner DE, Jefferson JW, Davidson JR, Pollack M, Stein MB, Lydiard RB, Futterer R, Robinson P, Slomkowski M, DuBoff E, Phelps M, Janney CA, & Werth JL. (2004). Efficacy of the novel anxiolytic pregabalin in social anxiety disorder: a placebo-controlled, multi-center study. *J. Clin. Psychopharmacol.,* 24: 141–149.

Pande AC, Pollack MH, Crockatt J, Greiner M, Chouinard G, Lydiard RB, Taylor CB, Dager SR, & Shiovitz T. (2000). Placebo-controlled study of gabapentin treatment of panic disorder. *J. Clin. Psychopharmacol.*, 20: 467–471.

Pashinian A, Faragian S, Levi A, Yeghiyan M, Gasparyan K, Weizman R, Weizman A, Fuchs C, & Poyurovsky M. (2006). Obsessive-compulsive disorder in bipolar patients with first manic episode. *J. Affect. Disord.*, 94: 151–156.

Patel NC, DelBello MP, Bryan HS, Adler CCM, Kowatch RA, Stanford K, & Strakowski SM. (2006). Open-label lithium for the treatment of adolescents with bipolar depression. *J. Am. Acad. Child Adolesc. Psychiatry*, 34: 289–297.

Perlis RH, Miyahara S, Marangell LB, Wisniewski SR, Ostacher M, DelBello MP, Bowden CL, Sachs GS, & Nierenberg AA; STEP-BD Investigators. (2004). Long-term implications of early onset in bipolar disorder: data from the first 1000 participants in the Systematic Treatment Enhancement Program for Bipolar Disorder (STEP-BD). *Biol. Psychiatry*, 55: 875–881.

Perugi G, Toni C, Frare F, Ruffolo G, Moretti L, Torti C, & Akiskal HS. (2002). Effectiveness of adjunctive gabapentin in resistant bipolar disorder: is it due to anxious-alcohol abuse comorbidity? *J. Clin. Psychopharmacol.*, 22: 584–591.

Perugi G, Akiskal HS, Toni C, Simionini E, & Gemignani A. (2001). The temporal relationship between anxiety disorders and (hypo)mania: a retrospective examination of 63 panic, social phobic and obsessive-compulsive patients with comorbid bipolar disorder. *J. Affect. Disord.*, 67: 199–206.

Perugi G, Toni C, Frare F, Travierso MC, Hantouche E, & Akiskal HS. (2002). Obsessive-compulsive bipolar comorbidity: a systematic exploration of clinical features and treatment outcome. *J. Clin. Psychiatry*, 63: 1129–1134.

Pini S, Cassano GB, Simonini E, Savino M, Russo M, & Montgomery SA. (1997). Prevalence of anxiety disorders comorbidity in bipolar depression. *J. Affect. Disord.*, 42: 145–153.

Pini S, Dell'Osso L, Amador XF, Mastrocinque C, Saettoni M, & Cassano GB. (2003). Awareness of illness in patients with bipolar I disorder with and without comorbid anxiety disorders. *Aus. N Z J. Psychiatry*, 37: 355–361.

Pini S, Maser JD, Dell'Osso L, Abelli M, Muti M, Gesi C, & Cassano GB. (2006). Social anxiety disorder comorbidity in patients with bipolar disorder: a clinical replication. *J. Anxiety Disord.*, 20: 1148–1157.

Pinkofsky HB, Hahn AM, Campbell FA, Rueda J, Daley DC, & Douaihy AB. (2005). Reduction of opioid withdrawal symptoms with quetiapine. *J. Clin. Psychiatry*, 66: 1285–1288.

Post RM, Altshuler LL, Leverich GS, Frye MA, Nolen WA, Kupka RW, Suppes T, McElroy S, Keck PE, Denicoff KD, Grunze H, Walden J, Kitchen CM, & Mintz J. (2006). Mood switch in bipolar depression: comparison of adjunctive venlafaxine, bupropion and sertraline. *Br. J. Psychiatry*, 189: 124–131.

Potash JB, Kane HS, Chiu YF, Simpson SG, MacKinnon DF, McInnis MG, McMahon FJ, & DePaulo JR Jr. (2000). Attempted suicide and alcoholism in bipolar disorder: clinical and familial relationships. *Am. J. Psychiatry*, 157: 2058–2050.

Preisig M, Fenton BT, Stevens DE, & Merikangas K. (2001). Familial relationship between mood disorders and alcoholism. *Compr. Psychiatry*, 42: 87–95.

Preston GA, Marchant BK, Reimherr FW, Strong RE, & Hedges DW. (2004). Borderline personality disorder in patients with bipolar disorder and response to lamotrigine. *J. Affect. Disord.*, 79: 297–303.

Ramacciotti CE, Paoli RA, Marcacci G, Piccinni A, Burgalassi A, Dell'Osso L, & Garfinkel PE. (2005). Relationship between bipolar illness and binge-eating disorders. *Psychiatr. Res.*, 135: 165–170.

Regier DA, Farmer ME, Rae DS, Locke BZ, Keith SJ, Judd LL, & Goodwin FK. (1990). Comorbidity of mental disorders with alcohol or other drug abuse. Results from the Epidemiologic Catchment Area (ECA) study. *JAMA*, 264: 2511–2518.

Rubio G, Lopez-Munoz F, & Alamo C. (2006). Effects of lamotrigine in patients with bipolar disorder and alcohol dependence. *Bipolar Disord.*, 8: 289–293.

Sachs GS, Nierenberg AA, Calabrese JR, Marangell LB, Wisniewski SR, Gyulai L, Friedman ES, Bowden CL, Fossey MD, Ostacher MJ, Ketter TA, Patel J, Hauser P, Rapport D, Martinez JM, Allen MH, Miklowitz DJ, Otto MW, Dennehy EB, & Thase ME. (2007). Effectiveness of adjunctive antidepressant treatment for bipolar depression. *N. Engl. J. Med.*, 356: 1711–1722.

Salloum IM, Cornelius JR, Daley DC, Kirisci L, Himmelhoch JM, & Thase ME. (2005). Efficacy of valproate maintenance in patients with bipolar disorder and alcoholism. *Arch. Gen. Psychiatry*, 62: 37–45.

Salloum IM, Cornelius JR, Mezzich JE, & Kirisci L. (2002). Impact of concurrent alcohol misuse on symptom presentation of acute mania at initial evaluation. *Bipolar Disord.*, 4: 418–421.

Scheffer RE, Kowatch RA, Carmody T, & Rush AJ. (2005). Randomized, placebo-controlled trial of mixed amphetamine salts for symptoms of comorbid ADHD in pediatric bipolar disorder after mood stabilization with divalproex sodium. *Am. J. Psychiatry*, 162: 58–64.

Schiavone P, Dorz S, Conforti D, Scarso C, & Borgherini G. (2004). Comorbidity of DSM-IV personality disorders in unipolar and bipolar affective disorders: a comparativce study. *Psychol. Rep.*, 95: 121–128.

Schulze TG, Hedeker D, Zandi P, Rietschel M, & McMahon FJ. (2006). What is familial about familial bipolar disorder? Resemblance among relatives across a broad spectrum of phenotypic characteristics. *Arch. Gen. Psychiatry*, 63: 1368–1376.

Simon NM, Otto MW, Weiss RD, Bauer MS, Miyahara SR, Thase ME, Kogan J, Frank E, Nierenberg AA, Calabrese JR, Sachs GS, & Pollack MH; STEP-BD Investigators. (2004). Pharmacotherapy for bipolar disorder and comorbid conditions: baseline data from STEP-BD. *J. Clin. Psychopharmacol.*, 24: 512–520.

Simon NM, Pollack MH, Ostacher MJ, Zalta AK, Chow CW, Fischmann D, Demopulos CM, Nierenberg AA, & Otto MW. (2007). Understanding the link between anxiety symptoms and suicidal ideation and behaviors in outpatients with bipolar disorder. *J. Affect. Disord.*, 97: 91–99.

Simon NM, Smoller JW, Fava M, Sachs G, Racette SR, Perlis R, Sonawalla S, & Rosenbaum JF. (2003). Comparing anxiety disorders and anxiety-related traits in bipolar disorder and unipolar depression. *J. Psychiatr. Res.*, 37: 187–192.

Singh J, Mattoo SK, Sharan P, & Basu D. (2005). Quality of life and its correlates in patients with dual diagnosis of bipolar affective disorder and substance dependence. *Bipolar Disord.*, 7: 187–191.

Soutullo CA, DelBello MP, Ochsner JE, McElroy SL, Taylor SA, Strakowski SM, & Keck PE Jr. (2002). Severity of bipolarity in hospitalized manic adolescents with a history of stimulant or antidepressant treatment. *J. Affect. Disord.*, 70: 323–327.

Stewart C, & El-Mallakh RS. (2007). Is bipolar disorder overdiagnosed among patients with substance abuse? *Bipolar Disord.*, 9: 646–648.

Strakowski SM, Delbello MP, Fleck DE, Adler CM, Anthenelli RM, Keck PE Jr., Arnold LM, & Amicone J. (2005). Effects of co-occurring alcohol abuse on the course of bipolar disorder after a first hospitalization for mania. *Arch. Gen. Psychiatry*, 62: 851–858.

Strakowski SM, Delbello MP, Fleck DE, Adler CM, Anthenelli RM, Keck PE Jr., Arnold LM, & Amicone J. (2007). Effects of co-occurring cannabis use disorders on the course of bipolar disorder after a first hospitalization for mania. *Arch. Gen. Psychiatry*, 64: 57–64.

Strakowski SM, DelBello MP, Fleck DE, & Arndt S. (2000). The impact of substance abuse on the course of bipolar disorder. *Biol. Psychiatry*, 48: 477–485.

Strakowski SM, Tohen M, Stoll AL, Faedda GL, & Goodwin DC. (1992). Comorbidity in mania at first hospitalization. *Am. J. Psychiatry*, 149: 554–556.

Strakowski SM, Tohen M, Stoll AL, Faedda GL, Mayer PV, Kolbrener ML, & Goodwin DC. (1993). Comorbidity in psychosis at first hospitalization. *Am. J. Psychiatry*, 150: 752–757.

Strakowski SM, Keck PE Jr., McElroy SL, Lonczak HS, & West SA. (1995). Chronology of comorbid and principal syndromes in first-episode psychosis. *Compr. Psychiatry*, 36: 106–112.

Strakowski SM, Keck PE Jr., McElroy SL, West SA, Sax KW, Hawkins JM, Kmetz GF, Upadhyaya VH, Tugrul KC, & Bourne ML. (1998a). Twelve-month outcome after a first hospitalization for affective psychosis. *Arch. Gen. Psychiatry*, 55: 49–55.

Strakowski SM, McElroy SL, Keck PE Jr., & West SA. (1996). The effects of antecedent substance abuse on the development of first-episode psychotic mania. *J. Psychiatr. Res.*, 30: 59–68.

Strakowski SM, Sax KW, McElroy SL, Keck PE Jr., Hawkins JM, & West SA. (1998b). Course of psychiatric and substance abuse syndromes co-occurring with bipolar disorder after a first psychiatric hospitalization. *J. Clin. Psychiatry*, 59: 465–471.

Swartz HA, Pilkonis PA, Frank E, Proietti JM, & Scott J. (2005). Acute treatment outcomes in patients with bipolar I disorder and co-morbid borderline personality disorder receiving medication and psychotherapy. *Bipolar Disord.*, 7: 192–197.

Tamam L, Tuglu C, Karatas G, & Ozcan S. (2006). Adult attention deficit hyperactivity disorder in patients with bipolar I disorder in remission: a preliminary study. *Psych. Clin. Neurosci.*, 60: 480–485.

Thatcher JW, Marchand WR, Thatcher GW, Jacobs A, & Jensen C. (2007). Clinical characteristics and health service use of veterans with comorbid bipolar disorder and PTSD. *Psych. Serv.*, 58: 703–707.

Thompson WK, Kupfer DJ, Fagiolini A, Scott JA, & Frank E. (2006). Prevalence and clinical correlates of medical comorbidities in patients with bipolar I disorder: analysis of acute-phase data from a randomized controlled trial. *J. Clin. Psychiatry*, 67: 783–788.

Tohen M, Waternaux CM, & Tsuang MT. (1990). Outcome in mania: a 4-year prospective follow-up of 75 patients utilizing survival analysis. *Arch. Gen. Psychiatry*, 47: 1106–1111.

Tohen M, Vieta E, Calabrese J, Ketter TA, Sachs GS, Bowden C, Mitchell PB, Centorrino F, Risser R, Baker RW, Evans AR, Beymer K, Dube S, Tollefson GD, & Breier A. (2003). Efficacy of olanzapine and olanzapine-fluoxetine combination in the treatment of bipolar I depression. *Arch. Gen. Psychiatry*, 60: 1079–1088.

Tsai SY, Lee CH, Kuo CJ, & Chen CC. (2005). A retrospective analysis of risk and protective factors for natural death in bipolar disorder. *J. Clin. Psychiatry*, 66: 1586–1591.

Tucker P, Trautman RP, Wyatt DB, Thompson J, Wu SC, Capece JA, & Rosenthal NR. (2007). Efficacy and safety of topiramate monotherapy in civilian post-traumatic stress disorder: a randomized, double-blind, placebo-controlled study. *J. Clin. Psychiatry*, 68: 201–206.

Van Gorp WG, Altshuler L, Theberge DC, Wilkins J, & Dixon W. (1998). Cognitive impairment in euthymic bipolar patients with and without prior alcohol dependence. A preliminary study. *Arch. Gen. Psychiatry*, 55: 41–46.

Warner LA, Kessler RC, Hughes M, Anthony JC, & Nelson CB. (1995). Prevalence and correlates of drug use and dependence in the United States. Results from the National Comorbidity Survey. *Arch. Gen. Psychiatry*, 52: 219–229.

Weeke A, Juel K, & Vaeth M. (1987). Cardiovascular death and manic-depressive psychosis. *J. Affect. Disord.*, 13: 287–292.

Weiss RD, Kolodziej M, Griffin ML, Najavits LM, Jacobson LM, & Greenfield SF. (2004). Substance use and perceived symptom improvement among patients with bipolar disorder and substance dependence. *J. Affect. Disord.*, 79: 279–283.

Weiss RD, Ostacher MJ, Otto MW, Calabrese JR, Fossey M, Wisniewski SR, Bowden CL, Nierenberg AA, Pollack MH, Salloum IM, Simon NM, Thase ME, & Sachs GS; for STEP-BD Investigators. (2005). Does recovery from substance use disorder matter in patients with bipolar disorder? *J. Clin. Psychiatry*, 66: 730–735.

Weiss RD, Griffin ML, Kolodjziej ME, Greenfield SF, Najavits LM, Daley DC, Doreau HR, & Hennen JA. (2007). A randomized trial of integrated group therapy versus group drug counseling for patients with bipolar disorder and substance dependence. *Am. J. Psychiatry*, 164: 100–107.

Weiss RD, Greenfield SF, Najavits LM, Soto JA, Wyner D, Tohen M, & Griffin ML. (1998). Medication compliance among patients with bipolar disorder and substance use disorder. *J. Clin. Psychiatry*, 59: 172–174.

Weissman MM, Klerman GL, Markowitz JS, & Ouellette R. (1989). Suicidal ideation and suicide attempts in panic disorder and attacks. *N. Engl. J. Med.*, 321: 1209–1214.

West SA, McElroy SL, Strakowski SM, Keck PE Jr., & McConville BJ. (1995). Attention deficit hyperactivity disorder in adolescent mania. *Am. J. Psychiatry*, 152: 271–273.

Winokur G, Coryell W, Akiskal HS, Maser JD, Keller MB, Endicott J, & Mueller T. (1995). Alcoholism in manic-depressive (bipolar) illness: familial illness, course of illness, and the primary-secondary distinction. *Am. J. Psychiatry*, 152: 365–372.

Winokur G, Coryell W, Endicott J, & Akiskal H. (1993). Further distinctions between manic-depressive illness (bipolar disorder) and primary depressive disorder. *Am. J. Psychiatry*, 150: 1176–1181.

Winokur G, Coryell W, Endicott J, Keller M, Akiskal H, & Solomon D. (1996). Familial alcoholism in manic-depressive (bipolar) illness. *Am. J. Med. Genet.*, 67: 197–201.

Zutshi A, Kamath P, & Reddy YC. (2007). Bipolar and nonbipolar obsessive-compulsive disorder: a clinical exploration. *Compr. Psychiatry*, 48: 245–251.

chapter ten

Lithium in the treatment of bipolar disorder

Joseph Levine
Ben Gurion University of the Negev

K.N. Roy Chengappa
University of Pittsburgh School of Medicine

Contents

Historical notes.. 260
Lithium in acute mania 262
Pre-DSM era open studies 263
Double-blind studies 263
    Lithium versus placebo... 263
        1952–1967 (DSM-I)... 263
        1968–1979 (DSM-II).. 264
        1980–1993 (DSM-III and DSM-III-R) 265
        1994–1999 (DSM-IV) 265
    Lithium versus antipsychotic drugs 265
        1968–1979 (DSM-II).. 265
        1980–1986 (DSM-III) 267
        1987–1993 (DSM-III-R) 267
        1994–1999 (DSM-IV) 267
        2000–2006 (DSM-IV-TR)... 268
    Lithium versus anticonvulsants 268
        1987–1993 (DSM-III-R) 268
        1994–1999 (DSM-IV)... 269
        2000–2006 (DSM-IV-TR)... 269
Lithium in bipolar depression... 270
Lithium in mixed and dysphoric manic episodes.......................... 272
Lithium maintenance therapy of bipolar disorder........................ 272
    1952–1967 (DSM-I)... 272
        Open trials.. 272

1968–1979 (DSM-II).. 273
   Prospective trials.. 273
   Discontinuation trials..274
1980–1986 (DSM-III) 274
   Prospective trials 274
   Discontinuation studies 275
1987–1993 (DSM-III-R) 275
   Prospective trials.. 275
1994–1999 (DSM-IV) 276
   Meta-analysis.. 276
   Prospective trials.. 276
2000–2006 DSM-IV-TR.. 276
   Meta-analysis.. 276
Prospective trials.. 277
   Lithium versus atypical antipsychotics.............................. 277
   Lithium versus lamotrigine.. 277
Lithium in rapid cycling bipolar disorder.................................... 279
Predictors of lithium response in bipolar disorder 279
   Acute mania or mixed episode 279
     Paranoid and depressive symptomatology 279
   Rapid cycling.. 279
   Acute bipolar depression.. 280
   Prophylaxis 280
   Lithium efficacy in different age groups 281
Lithium in the prevention of suicidality....................................... 282
New clinical issues with lithium treatment.................................. 283
   Point-of-care (POC) test for lithium levels 283
Clinical decision-making and lithium treatment......................... 284
   General recommendations as to indication for lithium use 286
References.. 286

Historical notes

As with many other psychotropic drugs, lithium was discovered by serendipity. In a short essay entitled, *The History of Lithium*, Cade (1970) describes the background against which he made the discovery of lithium's specific effects in bipolar illness, his working hypothesis, as well as the unexpected way in which these effects were found.

> *Lithium has an erratic history in medicine...The alkali itself was discovered by Arfvedson in 1817.... Lithium salts were introduced to medicine by A.B. Garrod in 1859*

> *for the treatment of gout… Culbreth in 1927 stated that*
> *lithium bromide is the most hypnotic of all bromides. My*
> *discovery of the specific antimanic effect of lithium ion*
> *was unexpected but to be retrospectively percipient for*
> *a moment, inevitable by-product of experimental work I*
> *was doing to test a hypothesis regarding the etiology of*
> *manic depressive illness. Could mania be a state analo-*
> *gous to thyrotoxicosis and myxoedema, mania being a*
> *state of intoxication by a normal product of the body cir-*
> *culating in excess, whilst melancholia is the correspond-*
> *ing deprivative condition? …for this purpose guinea pigs*
> *were used and fresh urine (of manic patients) was injected*
> *intraperitonealy… it soon became evident that some spec-*
> *imens of urine from manic patients were far more toxic*
> *than any of control specimens from normal persons…*

In an attempt to uncover such a toxic metabolite, Cade examined first the role of creatinine and urea, although he hypothesized that a different, third metabolite may be the toxic one. Cade planned to inject his laboratory animals with an aqueous solution of uric acid. However as uric acid is not soluble in water, Cade used the most soluble urate–an aqueous solution of a lithium salt. While examining the effect of the lithium salt itself on the animals, to his surprise he noticed that "… *although fully conscious (the animals), they became extremely lethargic and unresponsive to stimuli… it may seem a long way from lethargy in guinea pigs to the control of manic patients but…*" and here Cade describes in length his experiments with lithium in manic patients. Interestingly Cade never found the hypothesized toxic metabolite he was looking for, but he opened the way for what is still considered the "gold standard" treatment of bipolar illness. Cade (1949) in a small series of cases reported remarkable therapeutic effects for the manic patients, while schizophrenic and chronic depressive patients failed to demonstrate any changes. Thus, Cade was the first to notice a specific effect for lithium in bipolar disorder.

Cade later studied the effect of other related alkali metals such as rubidium and cesium along with cerium, lanthanum, neodymium and strontium and praseodymium. Cade even examined the effect of strontium in three manic, seven acute schizophrenic, two psychotic depressed, and 10 chronic schizophrenic patients. Four of the acute schizophrenic patients showed rapid improvement within a few days, and this was true for two out of the three manic patients. None of the chronic schizophrenic patients or the psychotic depressive patients improved. Cade concludes his historical lecture (Cade, 1970) stating, "*That lithium, a simple inorganic ion, can reverse a major psychotic reaction (manic episode) must have, quite apart from its substantial therapeutic value, profound theoretical significance in unraveling the mystery of the so-called functional psychoses. It must be regarded as a major research tool. Strontium may also prove to have a similar value for research in this field even if it has only minor therapeutic value."* Cade, using the terminology of his time (i.e. psychotic reaction), was right about the major role of lithium in a host of studies trying to unravel the mechanisms underlying bipolar illness. Strontium, however, raised no interest, and no further research was done with this agent.

Lithium in acute mania

The study of lithium in acute mania included several phases, some of them overlapping. The drug was first studied openly in small-scale studies, many of them lacking clear diagnostic criteria and well defined rating scales. After initial positive results were reported, placebo controlled double-blind studies followed. As these studies demonstrated evidence for the efficacy of lithium in bipolar mania, a series of controlled studies compared it with traditional antipychotics, and also reported antimanic effects. After a lag of about two decades (the 1970s and the 1980s) the marketing of the new antiepileptic and antipsychotic agents, spurred new double-blind studies comparing lithium to these drugs. In the large majority of studies, lithium was shown to be highly effective in acute mania, although more recent naturalistic studies reported lower improvement rates, and some authors even suggested that the benefit of response is compromised by side effects appearing in the early phases of treatment.

One of the main problems in comparing and assessing the results of various studies is that different diagnostic criteria and rating scales were used. We will present here the results of the first two open studies conducted prior to the publication of the Diagnostic Statistical Manual (DSM) I (American Psychiatric Association, 1952) to be followed by double-blind studies during DSM-I era, 1952–1967 (American Psychiatric Association, 1952); DSM-II era, 1968–1979 (American Psychiatric Association, 1968); DSM-III era, 1980–1986 (American Psychiatric Association, 1980); DSM-III-R era, 1987–1993 (American Psychiatric Association, 1987); DSM-IV era; 1994–1999 (American Psychiatric Association, 1994a) and the DSM-IV-TR era; 2000 (American Psychiatric Association, 2000). While not all the double-blind studies used this diagnostic system, and some studies published during a certain period were conducted in a previous one, we felt that such an organization may serve as an appropriate framework enabling follow-up and assessment of response rates over these time periods.

Pre-DSM era open studies

Two pioneering open studies were conducted during the pre-DSM era. The first one by Cade (1949) included 10 manic patients, all of whom improved following lithium treatment. No clear diagnostic and assessment criteria were presented. Cade's description of the first case of mania ever to be treated with lithium illustrates the magnitude of the breakthrough associated with this new treatment:

> *this was a little wizened man of 51 who had been in a state of chronic manic excitement for 5 years. He was amiably restless, dirty, destructive, mischievous and interfering. He enjoyed preeminent nuisance value in a backward for all those years and bid fair to remain there for the rest of his life. He commenced treatment with lithium citrate 1200 mg tid on 29 March 1948. On the fourth day the optimistic therapist thought he saw some change... by the fifth day it was clear he was in fact more settled, tidier, less disinhibited and less distractible. From that day on there was a steady improvement... He remained well and left hospital (after housing was arranged) on 9 July, 1948... taking maintenance dose of lithium carbonate 300 mg bid.*

The second open study was that of Noack and Trautner (1951). These authors studied openly 30 manic patients. Twenty-five patients responded well (83%) to lithium treatment. Both of these pioneering studies reported very high response rates to lithium. When comparing their results to results of more recent studies, one should bear in mind the expectation associated with these investigations, the open design utilized, and the fact that patients were lithium naïve.

Double-blind studies

Lithium versus placebo

1952–1967 (DSM-I)

Schou et al. (1954) studied 38 manic (30 typical and eight atypical) patients in Denmark in a partially open and partially placebo-controlled double-blind design. The dose of lithium used resulted in serum lithium levels of 0.5–2.0 meq/L. Clinical response was determined by a three point global severity scale. Fourteen patients showed a positive response (37%), 18 a possible response (47%), and six had no response (16%). Schou (1959) also conducted a large open study in which 91 of 119 (76%) manic patients improved. On the role of Schou in introducing lithium treatment for mania, Cade (1970) wrote: *"The person who has done most to achieve this recognition by validating and extending my original observation has been Mogens Schou in Denmark."*

Maggs (1963) studied 28 acute manic patients. However, the diagnostic criteria used for patient selection was not specified. Lithium or placebo was each given for 2 weeks in a cross-over design. Two weeks of no drug elapsed between crossing from one drug to another. The Wittenborn Scale for Manic State and Schizophrenic Excitement was used to assess the results. Ten patients dropped out of the study; eight due to uncooperativeness and two due to lithium toxicity. Lithium was found to be superior to placebo. The strengths of this study were the use of a rating scale and its blindness. Its weakness was the high drop-out rate and the cross-over design, which might have biased its results and the short duration of the treatment period.

1968–1979 (DSM-II)

Bunney et al. (1968) studied two patients in a longitudinal double-blind fashion demonstrating the sensitivity of manic symptoms to short periods of withdrawal from lithium treatment. The rating scale used was a 24-item mania scale measuring the core as well as other symptoms associated with mania. Diagnosis was made by the Mayer Gross definition of mania (Gershon and Shopsin, 1973). This longitudinal follow-up demonstrated the reappearance or increase of manic symptoms within 24 hours of lithium discontinuation.

Goodwin, Murphy and Bunney (1969) studied 30 manic-depressive patients in a double-blind placebo-controlled fashion. This group included 12 manic patients. Doses of lithium used were 900–1800 mg daily. Patients' serum lithium level was above 0.8 and below 1.2 meq/L. Nurses rating scales were employed. Eight of the 12 manic patients had a complete response (67%), one had partial response, and three worsened. The symptomatology of the three patients who worsened seemed to correspond more closely with schizoaffective disorder than with bipolar mania.

Stokes et al. (1971), studied 38 manic patients in a double-blind, placebo-controlled cross-over design. Patients were selected for the study after diagnostic consensus was obtained by three psychiatrists. Lithium was given at 0.5 meq/kg/day in four divided doses. Mean serum lithium was 0.93 meq/L. Data was analyzed for 98 manic periods (56 on lithium and 42 on placebo), each of 7–10 days. Seventy-five % of the 56 lithium-treated episodes responded to lithium treatment, while only 40.5% of the 42 placebo-treated episodes responded to placebo. However, this study has significant flaws. The period chosen for each period of treatment may be too short to examine lithium anti-manic effect. There was no washout period between the placebo and lithium periods that may attenuate a carry-over or withdrawal effect, and the rating scale used was not well defined. Nevertheless, this study added to the growing body of studies on lithium efficacy in acute mania.

1980–1993 (DSM-III and DSM-III-R)

The above studies established the role of lithium as the gold standard treatment for acute mania. No placebo-controlled studies of lithium effect in acute mania were performed during these years.

1994–1999 (DSM-IV)

Bowden et al. (1994) conducted a double-blind placebo-controlled, randomly assigned prospective parallel group study comparing lithium, valproic acid, and placebo in acute mania. No neuroleptics were used, and rescue medication was lorazepam allowed in the first week of the study. One hundred and seventy-nine patients were treated for 3 weeks with either lithium, divalproex, or placebo in a 1:2:2 ratio. Dosage of lithium was increased if tolerated, resulting in up to 1.5 mmol/L. The primary outcome measure was the Mania Rating Scale derived from the Schedule for Affective Disorders and Schizophrenia (SADS). Intent to treat analysis included 35 patients on lithium, 68 patients on divalproex, and 73 patients on placebo. Thirty-three % of the lithium treated patients, 30% of the divalproex treated patients, and 51% of the placebo treated patients terminated prematurely due to lack of efficacy. More than 50% improvement was noticed in 49%, 48% and 25% of patients on lithium, divalproex, and placebo, respectively.

Lithium versus antipsychotic drugs

1968–1979 (DSM-II)

Johnson et al. (1968; 1971) compared the effect of lithium versus chlorpromazine in 21 manic-depressive patients and 13 excited schizoaffective patients. Lithium blood levels were maintained above 1.0 meq/L and medications were given for 14–21 days. Rating scales included the Brief Psychiatric Rating Scale (BPRS), and Clinical Global Impression Scale. Specific features of the manic symptomatology including excitability were more responsive to lithium, while motor activity was more responsive to chlorpromazine, suggesting that lithium treatment may be more specific to mania.

Spring et al. (1970) studied in a double-blind design 14 acute manic patients randomly assigned to treatment with lithium or chlorpromazine. Lithium treatment in the first week was 1800 mg daily, and could subsequently be raised up to 3000 mg daily. Chlorpromazine dose could be adjusted up to 1600 mg daily. Six of seven patients who started on lithium responded, while only three of the five patients starting with chlorpromazine had a therapeutic response. Interestingly, the two chlorpromazine failures were switched to lithium and also responded. While the results are impressive for such a small study, regrettably these authors did not report how they defined response. Although not statistically significant, lithium was found to be more effective than chlorpromazine for the treatment of typical manic symptoms such as motor hyperactivity, flight of ideas, euphoria, expansiveness and pressured speech.

Platman (1970) studied 23 manic patients in double-blind fashion. Patients were randomized to either lithium or chlorpromazine treatment, each after 2 weeks of lead in placebo treatment. Plasma lithium levels were maintained at 0.8 meq/L. The mean daily dose of lithium was 1800 mg, and for chlorpramazine it was 870 mg. Thirteen patients were treated with lithium and ten with chlorpromazine. Ten patients dropped out of the study. Clinical change was evaluated blindly with the Psychiatric Evaluation Form. After 3 weeks of treatment, lithium seemed to be superior to chlorpromazine, but statistical significance was not reached.

The Veterans Administration and the National Institute of Mental Health initiated a collaborative project on lithium involving 18 US centers (Prien, Caffey and Klett, 1972). One of its objectives was to compare the efficacy of lithium and chlorpromazine in the treatment of bipolar manic and schizoaffective patients. After a lead-in period of 3–5 days, patients were randomly assigned to lithium or chlorpromazine for 3 weeks. The BPRS and Multidimensional Psychiatric Scale were used to evaluate the results. Data from 225 patients was analyzed. No major differences between the two drugs were found among study completers, however, a large proportion of the patients treated with lithium terminated prematurely because of lack of cooperativeness, lack of improvement (at least some of it may be attributed to delay in lithium therapeutic effect), or toxicity, while this was true for only 8% of the chlorpromazine-treated patients. Patients defined as highly active were improved by both drugs.

Shopsin et al. (1975) compared lithium, haloperidol and chlorpromazine in severely ill hospitalized manic patients, in a double-blind study design, with random treatment assignment. All drugs showed similar efficacy on most clinical measures. The authors suggest however, that the scales used were not sensitive enough to measure the manic psychopathlogy, as the majority of lithium treated patients met discharge criteria at the end of the trial, but this was not true for patients receiving anti-psychotic drugs. The authors suggested that lithium and haloperidol significantly improved the manic symptoms without sedation, while chlorpromazine, on the other hand, seemed to produce considerable sedation, contributing less to improving the underlying manic symptoms. They also suggested that while haloperidol had rapid impact on behavioral-motor activity, lithium tended to act more evenly on the entire manic clinical picture.

Takahashi et al. (1975) conducted a multi-center trial comparing lithium and chlorpromazine in a double-blind controlled design in a series of 80 Japanese patients with endogenous manic psychosis. The dosages employed were at a ratio of 4:1 (lithium:chlorpromazine). Lithium was found to be superior to chlorpromazine in physicians' overall ratings. The onset of therapeutic effects of lithium in 65% of the patients occurred within 10 days. Lithium, but not chlorpromazine, was found to improve mood and pressured speech.

1980–1986 (DSM-III)
Garfinkel, Stancer and Persad (1980) studied lithium plus placebo versus haloperidol plus placebo versus the combination of lithium and haloperidol in a double-blind study with random treatment assignment. Each treatment was administered for 3 weeks, in 21 severely ill manic patients. The subjects on placebo and haloperidol and the subjects on lithium and haloperidol significantly improved after 7 days of treatment in comparison to the lithium and placebo treated group. The authors concluded that haloperidol is superior to lithium in the treatment of acutely severe hospitalized manic patients, and mentioned that the combination of haloperidol and lithium was not superior to haloperidol and placebo.

1987–1993 (DSM-III-R)
No studies comparing lithium and neuroleptics were reported during these years. Such studies had to wait until the development and marketing efforts of the atypical antipsychotics.

1994–1999 (DSM-IV)
Segal, Berk and Brook (1998) studied 45 inpatients diagnosed by DSM-IV as bipolar manic patients in a randomized, controlled, double-blind study of either 6 mg daily of risperidone, 10 mg daily of haloperidol or 800–1200 mg daily of lithium. Similar improvement was reported for all the three groups after 4 weeks of treatment as determined by Global Assessment of Functioning (GAF), Clinical Global Impression (CGI), and BPRS (mean BPRS improvement scores: lithium=9, haloperidol=5, risperidone=6.5) scales.

Berk, Ichim and Brook (1999) compared lithium to olanzapine in mania in a double-blind randomized controlled trial. Thirty patients meeting DSM-IV criteria for mania were randomly assigned to receive either lithium or olanzapine for 4 weeks. No significant differences were found between these treatments. Olanzapine was however, significantly superior to lithium on the CGI-severity scale at week 4. The authors suggest that olanzapine appears to be at least as effective as lithium in the treatment of mania.

2000–2006 (DSM-IV-TR)

Bowden et al. (2005) evaluated the efficacy of lithium versus quetiapine versus placebo in the treatment of hospitalized patients with mania in a multi-center, double-blind, parallel-group, and 12-week study. Patients with diagnosis of bipolar I disorder in their manic episode were randomly assigned to receive quetiapine (titrated up to 800 mg/day based on tolerance), placebo, or lithium. Results showed that more patients in the quetiapine (72/107) and lithium (67/98) treatment arms completed the study compared with the placebo group (35/97). Improvement in YMRS score was significantly greater for quetiapine than placebo at day 7 and the difference between groups continued to increase over time to day 21 and to endpoint at day 84. Lithium-treated patients improved significantly compared with placebo patients similar to quetiapine treated patients. The authors concluded that quetiapine and lithium demonstrated superior efficacy to placebo in patients with bipolar mania.

Comparison of these various studies is not an easy task, as different time points and rating scales were used. However, since some of the above studies suggested lithium to be superior to antipsychotic agents, and others suggested the superiority of antipsychotic agents, while still others found no difference, it seems logical to sum up the reviewed studies by stating that; overall, there are no overwhelming differences between these drugs in the treatment of bipolar mania. It appears, however, that typical neuroleptics tend to influence primarily the behavioral motor signs (haloperidol) or produce sedation (chlorpromazine), while lithium tends to affect the core manic symptoms in a more even way. This may have lead to the observation of Segal, Berk and Brook (1998) that haloperidol may have an advantage over lithium in the first week of treatment for hospitalized severely ill manic patients, and the clinical impression is that these neuroleptic agents may help in decreasing combativeness and agitation, and other signs of motoric over activity. As to atypical antipsychotic agents it seems that they are at least as effective in treating acute mania as lithium and clinical trial data suggest that the combination of lithium with an atypical antipsychotic agent (i.e. quetiapine or olanzapine or risperidone) may be superior to lithium administered alone in the treatment of acute mania (see Sachs et al., 2002, 2004; Tohen et al., 2002).

Lithium versus anticonvulsants

1987–1993 (DSM-III-R)

Lerer et al. (1987) conducted a double-blind study comparing lithium and carbamazepine in acute mania. Fourteen patients were assigned randomly to each group. BPRS, CGI, and Beigel–Murphy Manic State Rating Scales were employed. A more consistent level of improvement across patients was found for lithium compared to a minority of good responders in the carbamazepine group.

Small et al. (1991) studied 52 hospitalized manic patients who were randomized to either carbamazepine or lithium treatment after 2 weeks of drug withdrawal. The subjects were followed for 8 weeks. No difference was found between the two groups. The researchers had the impression that patients treated with carbamazepine were more manageable than those treated with lithium, while lithium-treated patients remained longer in a follow-up phase. The authors concluded that monotherapy with either drug may not be sufficient for hospitalized manic patients.

Freeman et al. (1992) studied 27 DSM-III-R manic patients in a 3-week randomized, double-blind parallel study comparing the efficacy of valproate and lithium. BPRS, GAF and SADS-C were used as rating scales. Nine of the 14 (64%) patients treated with valproate and 12 out of the 14 (86%) patients treated with lithium responded favorably, suggesting that both drugs are effective in the treatment of acute mania.

1994–1999 (DSM-IV)

Emilien et al. (1996) conducted a meta-analysis comparing the efficacy of lithium, valproic acid and carbamazepine in the treatment of mania. The analysis included only randomized double-blind controlled clinical trials in which the therapeutic plasma level of lithium was 0.4–1.5 mmol/L. Effect sizes were measured by the odds ratio using the Mantel-Haenszel method. No significant difference was observed among the three drugs.

Bowden et al. (1994) conducted a double-blind placebo-controlled, randomly assigned study comparing lithium, valproic acid, and placebo in acute mania on 179 patients. The dosage of lithium was increased, if tolerated, to 1.5 mmol/L (a detailed description of this study appears in the section of lithium versus placebo). Bowden analyzed the effect size for the efficacy of each treatment arm in a later publication (Bowden et al., 1997). Effect size for the improvement score in the Manic Syndrome Score was 0.79 for lithium and 1.01 for divalproex, compared with only 0.37 for placebo. Effect size for the improvement score at the Behavior and Ideation Score (BIS) was 0.62 for lithium, and 0.67 for divalproex, compared with only 0.25 for placebo. These results suggest that both drugs are effective in the treatment of mania compared to placebo.

2000–2006 (DSM-IV-TR)

Hirschfeld et al. (2003) evaluated the early efficacy of oral-loaded divalproex in acute mania versus standard-titration divalproex, lithium, olanzapine, or placebo by the use of a pooled analysis of 348 subjects from three randomized, double-blind, parallel-group, active- or placebo-controlled studies. Subjects were inpatients diagnosed with bipolar I disorder-acute manic phase (DSM-III-R or -IV and SADS-Change Version). Patients were administered oral-loaded divalproex (20 or 30 mg/kg/day on days 1 and 2 followed by 20 mg/kg/day, and increased at physician's discretion), standard-titration divalproex initiated at 250 mg t.i.d. and titrated to 40–150 mg/mL, lithium (300 mg t.i.d. initial dose) titrated to 0.4–1.5 meq/L, olanzapine (10 mg q.d. initial dose) up to 20 mg/day, or placebo. The results suggested the oral loading of divalproex leads to a more rapid antimanic effect when compared with standard-titration divalproex, lithium, or placebo and is better tolerated than olanzapine and as well tolerated as lithium or standard-titration divalproex.

In summary, lithium was demonstrated to be effective in the treatment of mania. Some clinicians treat manic patients with lithium alone, while others may start with combined lithium and antipsychotic treatment, or may add lithium after the first few days of neuroleptic treatment. To some extent this depends on the acuity of the presenting manic episode and the symptom clusters that are behavioral issues (for instance, agitation, combativeness, extreme motor activity) or the need to target other symptoms such as lack of need for sleep, suicidality and anxiety among others. Alternatively, clinicians may use divalproex or carbamazepine, or in certain cases, combine each one of them with lithium, i.e. lithium and divalproex or lithium and carbamazepine.

Lithium in bipolar depression

Although the hallmark of bipolar illness may be its manic episode, this disorder is also characterized by depressive episodes. Six placebo-controlled trials examined lithium efficacy in bipolar depression (Goodwin and Jamison, 1990). Goodwin, Murphy and Bunney (1969) studied the role of lithium in 13 bipolar depressed patients, and reported that in ten cases there was indication of some response. Stokes et al. (1971) reported that lithium administration for bipolar depressive episodes of up to 10 days resulted in a significant trend towards response compared with placebo. Eighteen of their 38 patients demonstrated depressive episodes. Eleven patients with 17 depressive episodes were treated with lithium, while 15 patients with 21 depressive episodes were treated with placebo. Fifty-nine % of the lithium treated episodes improved as compared to 48% of the placebo treated episodes. Goodwin et al. (1972) studied 40 bipolar depressed patients reporting that 80% of these patients responded. Noyes, Dempsey and Blum (1974) reported that six of six bipolar depressed patients responded to lithium. Baron et al. (1975) studied nine bipolar depressed patients of whom seven responded, and Mendels (1975) reported that nine of 13 bipolar depressed patients responded to lithium treatment. Overall, response rates of bipolar depression to lithium treatment seemed to exceed

70%. All these studies suggested that lithium has antidepressant effects in bipolar depression. Interestingly, some of these studies also reported lithium's effects on unipolar depression which were lower than in bipolar depression, and in general fell under 50% of response rate. Other studies in depressed individuals compared lithium to the classical tricyclic antidepressants. Fieve, Platman and Plutchick (1968), Mendels (1975), Watanabe, Ishino and Otsuki (1975) and Worrall et al. (1979) compared the efficacy of lithium to either imipramine (three studies) or desipramine in samples containing bipolar depressed and unipolar depressed patients. Although the majority of these studies suggested that lithium is at least as effective as the tricyclic antidepressants (see also review by Srisurapanont, Yatham and Zis (1995)), the study of Fieve, Platman and Plutchick (1968)—the only one comparing both lithium and tricyclic drug to placebo—reported only a mild antidepressant effect for lithium.

In a review of the treatment studies of acute bipolar depression conducted prior to 1995, Srisurapanont, Yatham and Zis (1995) reported that in seven of eight placebo-controlled cross-over studies, lithium was superior to placebo with a mean response rate of 76%; relapses occurred in 38–70% of patients (mean: 52%) when placebo was substituted for lithium. The authors noted that in one study, response rates were better for imipramine compared with lithium (response rate of 58% vs. 32%). In two augmentation studies where lithium was added to anti-depressant resistant patients, or to carbamazepine resistant patients, response rates increased by 36% and 46%, respectively. The authors concluded that the benefits of lithium monotherapy or lithium augmentation are impressive for bipolar depression, and that no hypomanic or manic switching was noted.

In a more recent study, Nemeroff et al. (2001) compared the efficacy and safety of paroxetine versus imipramine versus placebo in the treatment of bipolar depression in adult outpatients who had been on lithium in a double-blind, placebo-controlled study. A total of 117 depressed bipolar patients were randomly assigned to each of the treatment for 10 weeks. Some patients may have received either carbamazepine or valproate in combination with lithium for control of manic symptoms prior to the onset of index depressive episode. No statistically significant difference was noticed among the three groups in overall efficacy. However, both paroxetine and imipramine were superior to placebo in patients who had low serum lithium levels (≤ 0.8 meq/L) but not in those that had higher serum lithium levels. Compared with imipramine, paroxetine resulted in a lower incidence of adverse events, most notably emergence of manic symptoms. The authors concluded that antidepressants may not be useful adjunctive therapy for bipolar depressed patients with high serum lithium levels. However, the authors suggest that antidepressant therapy may be beneficial for patients who cannot tolerate high serum lithium levels or who have symptoms that are refractory to the antidepressant effects of lithium.

Lithium in mixed and dysphoric manic episodes

Only a few studies examined the role of lithium in mixed and dysphoric mania. Clothier, Swann and Freeman (1992) reported that both lithium and valproate were found to be equally effective in the control of depressed mood or anxiety associated with a manic episode. Swann et al. (1997) reported that in a parallel group, placebo controlled, double-blind, multi-center study of lithium and divalproex for mania (Bowden et al., 1994), depressive symptoms were associated with poor antimanic response to lithium and better response to divalproex. Mixed patients were also suggested to have a poor response to lithium treatment varying between 29% and 42% (Himmelhoch et al., 1976; de Montigny et al., 1981; Secunda et al., 1985; Swann et al., 1986; Prien, 1988; Dilsaver et al., 1993b; Soares & Gershon, 1998).

Interestingly, although the existence of depressive symptoms during mania seems to lower responsivity to lithium, lithium has a role in the treatment of resistant depression and its addition to ongoing antidepressant treatment was suggested to reverse refractoriness to treatment (Prien, Caffey, & Klett, 1972; Heninger, Charney, & Sternberg, 1983). In this regard, lithium has been added to anti-depressant resistant bipolar depressed patients or to carbamazepine resistant bipolar depressed patients as noted earlier and shown benefits (Srisurapanont, Yatham, & Zis, 1995).

In summary, lithium seems to have a modest therapeutic effect in the treatment of bipolar depression. It is also generally less effective in dysphoric and mixed manic states. In such instances, other anticonvulsant mood stabilizers may be more effective, and atypical antipsychotic agents have also shown efficacy in mixed mania.

Lithium maintenance therapy of bipolar disorder

The issue of long-term prevention or prophylaxis of illness episodes is of utmost importance for this cycling disorder. A variety of studies to be detailed here corroborate the effectiveness of lithium as an important prophylactic agent for this disorder. These studies will be grouped as open versus double-blind, or prospective versus discontinuation studies.

1952–1967 (DSM-I)

Open trials

Three open studies suggested that lithium may be effective in the prophylaxis of bipolar disorder (Hartigan, 1963; Baastrup, 1964; Baastrup & Schou, 1967).

1968–1979 (DSM-II)

During the 1970s a series of double-blind studies were conducted to examine the possible efficacy of lithium in the prophylaxis of bipolar disorder. Goodwin (1994) summarized these studies calculating the recurrence rates over a 1 year period for placebo to be 81%, but only 34% for lithium. These included both prospective and discontinuation studies.

Prospective trials

Coppen et al. (1971) conducted a parallel group, randomized, prospective trial that included 17 patients on lithium and 21 on placebo, who were followed for 4–6 months. The recurrence rates were 18% in the lithium group and 95% in the placebo one.

Prien, Caffey and Klett (1973a) conducted a parallel group, randomized, prospective trial with patients admitted to hospital for the treatment of a manic episode. One hundred and one patients were on lithium, and 104 patients were on placebo. The duration of the study was 24 months. The recurrence rates were 43% in the lithium group and 80% on placebo. The recurrence rates of manic and depressive episodes were 32% and 16% on lithium, and 68% and 26% on placebo.

Prien, Caffey and Klett (1973b) conducted a parallel group, randomized, prospective trial in patients admitted for hospitalization due to the occurrence of depressive episodes. Eighteen patients were on lithium, 13 patients on placebo. The duration of the study was 5–24 months with a recurrence rate on lithium of 28% and on placebo 77%. Percent recurrence of manic and depressive episodes for lithium was 11% and 22%, for placebo 38% and 62%, respectively.

Stallone et al. (1973) conducted a parallel group, randomized, prospective trial. Twenty-five patients were on lithium, and 27 patients were on placebo, for a study duration of up to 28 months. The recurrence rates on lithium were 44%, and on placebo 93%. The recurrence rates for manic and depressive episodes were 20% and 28% in the lithium group, and 56% and 48% in the placebo group, respectively.

Dunner and Fieve (1976) conducted a parallel group, randomized, prospective trial in bipolar II patients. Sixteen patients were on lithium and 24 patients on placebo. The study duration was up to 36 months. Recurrence rates for manic and depressive episodes on lithium were 6% and 56%, and on placebo 25% and 50%, respectively.

Fieve, Kumbarachi and Dunner (1976) conducted a parallel group, randomized, prospective trial in bipolar patients. Seventeen patients were on lithium and 18 patients on placebo. They were followed for up to 53 months. The recurrence rates for manic and depressive episodes on lithium were 59% and 29%, while on placebo they were 94% and 44%, respectively. Fieve, Kumbarachi and Dunner (1976) also studied bipolar II patients. Seven patients were on lithium and 11 patients on placebo, and those were followed for up to 53 months. The recurrence rates for manic and depressive episodes on lithium were 0% and 57%, and on placebo were 9% and 64%, respectively.

Discontinuation trials

Baastrup et al. (1970) studied 22 patients on placebo, and 28 patients on lithium. The duration of the study was up to 5 months. The recurrence rates of illness episodes were 0% on lithium and 55% on placebo. The recurrence rates of manic episodes for lithium and placebo were 0% and 27%, respectively. The recurrence rates for depressive episodes for lithium and placebo were 0% and 23%, respectively.

Melia (1970) studied seven patients on lithium and eight patients on placebo for a period of 24 months. Percent recurrence on lithium was 57%, and on placebo 78%. Cundall, Brooks and Murray (1972) studied 12 patients on lithium and 12 patients on placebo, who were followed for 6 months. The recurrence rates on lithium were 33%, and on placebo 83%. The recurrence rates of manic and depressive episodes in the lithium group were 8% and 25%, and in the placebo group 75% and 42%, respectively.

Hullin, McDonald, and Allsopp (1972) studied 18 patients on lithium and 18 patients on placebo, who were followed for 6 months. The recurrence rates were 6% on lithium, and 33% on placebo.

1980–1986 (DSM-III)

Prospective trials

Coppen et al. (1983) studied 72 patients in a prospective double-blind fashion. Patients continued with their ongoing lithium treatment or received a 25–50% reduction in their lithium dosage resulting in plasma levels of 0.45–0.79 mmol/L. The patients on the reduced dose had fewer side effects, including hand tremors, and decreased thyroid stimulating hormone (TSH) blood levels. They also had significantly decreased affective morbidity. The authors suggested that there may be an advantage in keeping maintenance blood lithium levels at about 0.6 mml/L.

Prien et al. (1984) studied 117 bipolar patients receiving either lithium, imipramine, or both in a long-term double-blind study. Lithium carbonate and the combination were found superior to imipramine in preventing the manic recurrence, and equally effective to imipramine in preventing depressive episodes.

Discontinuation studies

Christodoulou and Lykouras (1982) abruptly discontinued prophylactic treatment in a placebo-controlled, double-blind design in 18 manic-depressive patients for a total period of 18 days. Side effects were significantly reduced, no withdrawal symptoms were noted, and three patients relapsed within 4 days.

1987–1993 (DSM-III-R)

Prospective trials

Luszanat, Murphy and Nunn (1988) studied the long-term effects of lithium versus carbamazepine in 44 bipolar patients, both initiated during an acute manic phase. There was a high drop-out rate. Both drugs were found to have prophylactic properties, although lithium appeared to be more effective in the treatment of acute mania.

Gelenberg et al. (1989) compared standard and low serum lithium levels in the maintenance treatment of 94 bipolar disorder patients, in a prospective randomized double-blind trial. Standard plasma levels were defined as 0.8–1.0 mml/L, while low levels were defined as 0.4–0.6 mml/L. Six of 47 (13%) patients assigned to standard versus 18 of 47 (38%) assigned to low levels relapsed. The authors recommend that standard range of lithium plasma levels rather than low range should be used in maintenance lithium therapy.

Abou-Saleh and Coppen (1990) conducted a prospective double-blind lithium dose reduction study in patients receiving lithium prophylactic therapy over 1 year. Lithium dose was reduced by up to 50%. No association between lithium dose/level and affective morbidity was found among patients on standard or low lithium levels. Dose reduction was associated with decreased plasma TSH levels, and decreased side effects, including tremor and weight gain. Interestingly, elderly patients had significantly increased affective morbidity in the low versus standard dose group. Coxhead, Silverstone and Cookson (1992) studied 31 bipolar patients in a double-blind design over 1 year. All patients had previously been stable on lithium. Sixteen patients remained on lithium, and 15 were switched to carbamazepine. Relapse occurred in eight of the patients on lithium and six of those on carbamazepine. Most of the carbamazepine patients relapsed within 1 month of the switch. The authors suggested relapse in this study was likely to be due to lithium withdrawal.

Keller et al. (1992) studied bipolar patients demonstrating a sub-syndromal clinical picture in a double-blind fashion. Low (0.4–0.6 mmol/L) versus standard (0.8–1.0 mmol/L) lithium levels were compared and the results showed a 2.6 fold higher risk for recurrence in the low dose regimen.

1994–1999 (DSM-IV)

Meta-analysis

Dardennes et al. (1995) conducted a meta-analysis to compare the efficacy of lithium and carbamazepine prophylaxis. This meta-analysis included four randomized, double-blind controlled studies demonstrating significant heterogeneity. The analysis could not confirm the equipotency of carbamazepine and lithium in maintenance therapy. The authors concluded that the prophylactic efficacy of carbamazepine remained questionable.

Prospective trials

Jensen et al. (1995) compared prophylactic treatment with lithium given every second day (median dose 800 mg/day, plasma level 0.6–0.7 mmol/L) compared with daily dosing (median dose 1200 mg/day, plasma level 0.6–0.7 mmol/L) in a double-blind fashion. Fifty bipolar patients were included. The authors found that the risk of relapse increased three times in the "every second day" lithium treatment group compared with daily treatment. Interestingly, Jensen et al. (1996) reported that alternate day dosing schedule with lithium did not result in significant reduction in side-effects.

Maj et al. (1998) studied prospectively 402 bipolar patients analyzing the long-term outcome of lithium prophylaxis. These authors reported that at the end of 5 years 28% were no longer taking lithium, 23% were taking lithium and had no recurrence, and 38% were taking lithium and had at least one recurrence.

Greil and Kleindienst (1999a) reported in a randomized clinical trial comparing the efficacy of lithium versus carbamazepine—each given for 2.5 years—in 114 patients with bipolar I disorder, that lithium is superior to carbamazepine on several outcome criteria. These authors also used the same study design in 57 patients with bipolar II or bipolar NOS disorders reporting no significant difference between lithium and carbamazepine prophylaxis (Greil and Kleindienst, 1999b).

Kulhara et al. (1999) conducted a retrospective chart review in 118 bipolar patients (who were enlisted between 1989 and 1990) and prospectively followed up until 1995. Mean follow up was approximately 11 years (range 2–27). Patients had mean of 0.43 relapses per year while on lithium, which was significantly less than pre-lithium episode frequency. About half of the subjects were good responders to lithium. It is of note that the patients also utilized other psychotropic medications and this may have affected the results.

2000–2006 DSM-IV-TR

Meta-analysis

A Cochrane Review by Burgess et al. (2001) surveyed nine maintenance or prophylaxis randomized controlled trials comparing lithium with placebo. Subjects were males and females of all ages diagnosed as suffering from mood disorders. Discontinuation studies were not included. There were 825 patients who were randomly assigned to lithium or placebo. This systematic review suggests that lithium is an efficacious maintenance treatment for bipolar disorder. In unipolar disorder the evidence of lithium efficacy was less robust.

Prospective trials

Lithium versus atypical antipsychotics

Tohen et al. (2004) explored whether olanzapine plus either lithium or valproate reduces the rate of relapse, compared with lithium or valproate alone. Patients achieving syndromic remission after 6 weeks of treatment with olanzapine plus either lithium (0.6–1.2 mmol/L) or valproate (50–125 mg/ml) received lithium or valproate plus either olanzapine 5–20 mg/day (combination therapy) or placebo (monotherapy), and were followed in a double-masked trial for 18 months. Time to relapse into mania or depression although not significantly different for syndromic relapse (median for combination therapy 94 days for monotherapy 40.5 days), was significantly different for symptomatic relapse (median for combination therapy 163 days, for monotherapy 42 days; $P = 0.02$).

Tohen et al. (2005) studied olanzapine versus lithium as a maintenance treatment in bipolar disorder in a 12-month, randomized, double-blind, and controlled clinical trial. Patients diagnosed with bipolar disorder (manic or mixed), a history of two or more manic or mixed episodes within 6 years, and a Young Mania Rating Scale total score ≥20 entered the study. All patients received initially an open-label co-treatment with olanzapine and lithium for 6–12 weeks. Those meeting symptomatic remission criteria were randomly assigned to 52 weeks of double-blind monotherapy with olanzapine, 5–20 mg/day ($N = 217$), or lithium (blood level: 0.6–1.2 meq/L) ($N = 214$). Symptomatic relapse/recurrence occurred in 30% of olanzapine-treated and 39% of lithium-treated patients. Secondary results suggested that compared with lithium, olanzapine had significantly lower risks of manic or mixed episode relapse/recurrence. Depression relapse/recurrence occurred in 16% of olanzapine-treated and 11% of lithium-treated patients. These results suggest that olanzapine was significantly more effective than lithium in preventing manic or mixed episode relapse/recurrence in patients acutely stabilized with olanzapine and lithium co-treatment. Both agents were found to be comparable in preventing depression relapse/recurrence.

Lithium versus lamotrigine

Calabrese et al. (2003) conducted a placebo-controlled 18-month trial of lamotrigine and lithium maintenance treatment in recently depressed patients with bipolar I disorder. Initially during an 8- to 16-week open-label phase, lamotrigine was added to current therapy for currently or recently depressed bipolar I outpatients whereas other psychotropic drugs were gradually withdrawn. Four hundred and sixty three patients who were stabilized on the open-label phase were then randomly assigned to lamotrigine, lithium (0.8–1.1 meq/L), or placebo for up to 18 months. Results showed that lamotrigine and lithium were superior to placebo for the prevention of mood episodes in bipolar I patients, with lamotrigine mainly effective against recurrence of depression and lithium mainly effective against recurrence of mania.

Bowden et al. (2003) conducted a placebo-controlled 18-month trial of lamotrigine and lithium maintenance treatment in recently manic or hypomanic patients with bipolar I disorder. Initially during an 8- to 16-week open-label phase, lamotrigine was added to current therapy for currently or recently depressed bipolar I outpatients whereas other psychotropic drugs were gradually withdrawn. One hundred and seventy five patients who were stabilized on the open-label phase were then randomly assigned to lamotrigine, lithium (0.8–1.1 meq/L), or placebo for up to 18 months. Results showed that both lamotrigine and lithium were superior to placebo in the prevention of relapse or recurrence of mood episodes. The authors also state that "the results also indicate that lamotrigine is an effective maintenance treatment for bipolar disorder, particularly for prophylaxis of depression". In the Bowden et al. study (2003), the index episode while entering the study was hypomanic/manic, and in the Calabrese et al. (2003) study, the index episode for entry was major depression, and it can be said, that while both agents prevented future mood episodes, lamotrigine was more effective in preventing depressive episodes, whereas lithium was more effective against manic recurrences.

In summary, data emerging from the above studies suggested that lithium is an effective treatment in the prevention of future bipolar episodes, especially hypomanic or manic recurrences, and less effective against depressive recurrences. Some studies suggested that lithium plasma levels of 0.8–1.0 meq/L, if tolerated, are more effective than lower levels, but may be associated with more side effects. Some authors suggested that there are cases in which the response to lithium prophylaxis decreases with time, while in other instances it may not continue to be effective upon reinstitution of treatment after discontinuation, though one study suggested this not to be the case (Coryell et al., 1998). Some authors even called into question the role of lithium in maintenance therapy of the bipolar illness (Akhondzadeh et al., 1999). Grof (1999) suggested that a group of patients with classical bipolar illness have a good long-term prophylactic response to lithium treatment. Based on recent lamotrigine maintenance studies, it was suggested that when one compares lithium with lamotrigine, lamotrigine is more effective against recurrences of depression whereas lithium is a more effective maintenance agent against manic recurrences. While early data suggest that atypical antipsychotic agents are slightly more effective than lithium in preventing manic recurrences, more substantial data is needed to evaluate the role of the atypical antipsychotic agents versus lithium in the prevention of manic/mixed/depressive episodes of bipolar illness.

Lithium in rapid cycling bipolar disorder

Rapid cycling bipolar disorder is defined as more than four illness episodes in a year by DSM-IV (American Psychiatric Association, 1994a). These patients generally have lower response to lithium compared to non-rapid cycling bipolar disorder patients (Dunner & Fieve, 1974; Kukopulos et al., 1980). Bipolar disorder with a rapid cycling course seems to respond to other mood stabilizers including divalproex (Bowden et al., 1994) or carbamazepine or lamotrigine. Head to head comparisons with lithium or with each other for the anticonvulsants are not available to the extent to form an informed opinion in rapid cycling bipolar illness. Further, the role of atypical antipsychotics in treating or modifying rapid cycling bipolar illness remains to be determined.

Predictors of lithium response in bipolar disorder

Acute mania or mixed episode

Paranoid and depressive symptomatology

Murphy and Beigel (1974) suggested that paranoid destructive manic patients respond less well to lithium, however Swann et al. (1986) who studied paranoid-irritable manic patients did not concur. Cohen, Khan and Coz (1989) suggested that depressive symptomatology and earlier age of onset might be related to decreased response. However, since these authors had small numbers of subjects, their findings should be interpreted with caution. Swann et al. (1986) suggested that more severe forms of mania, high anxiety and depression might be associated with decreased response to lithium. In addition, patients exhibiting mixed or dysphoric mania seem to respond less to lithium (McElroy et al., 1992; Dilsaver et al., 1993a, 1993b).

Rapid cycling

Approximately 20% of bipolar patients demonstrate rapid cycling. This group of patients responded less well to lithium prophylactic treatment

(Post et al., 1990). However, Maj (1992) reported that a certain subgroup of these patients may respond more favorably to lithium treatment compared to other subgroups.

Acute bipolar depression

Bipolar depression compared with unipolar depression seemed to respond well to lithium treatment (Goodwin and Jamison, 1990). Jefferson (1996) suggested that some clinicians reported that bipolar patients with reverse vegetative symptoms such as anergia, increased sleep, and appetite may be more responsive to lithium treatment compared to bipolar patients with anxiety, insomnia, and anorexia.

Prophylaxis

Grof et al. (1983, 1993, 1999) suggested that course of illness with periods of euthymia, mania-depression-euthymia course, absence of rapid cycling, positive family history for bipolar disorder, absence of personality disorder, and diagnosis of primary bipolar disorder (i.e. not secondary to organic cause) predicts a good prophylactic response to lithium.

Faedda et al. (1991), in agreement with Grof et al. (1983, 1993, 1999), suggested that the mania-depression-euthymia course is related to good response to lithium prophylaxis, but not the depression-mania-euthymia course. Similar to Grof et al. (1983, 1993, 1999), family history of mood disorder was suggested to be associated with good response to lithium, as well as positive response to lithium in close relatives (Jefferson, 1996). Aagaard and Vestegaard (1990) suggested that bipolar patients tend to demonstrate decreased response to lithium treatment when they have a lengthy episode, they are young and of female gender. Abou-Saleh and Coppen (1990) suggested that positive prophylactic response to lithium over 6–12 months predicts further good response in the future. Patients with dysphoric and mixed mania were suggested to respond less to lithium treatment and some, but not all studies suggest the same for rapid cycling bipolar disorder (Jefferson, 1996). Grof (1993) and Goodnick et al. (1987) suggested that good level of functioning between episodes predicts good response to lithium prophylaxis. It seems that patients who have been identified as probable poor lithium responders include those with co-morbid substance abuse, a common co-morbidity with bipolar affective disorder (Goldberg, 2001).

Recently, Kleindienst, Engel and Greil (2005) conducted a study aimed at systematically integrating the available evidence on response prediction to prophylactic lithium based on clinical factors. Of 42 potential clinical predictors investigated, five variables were identified as possible response predictors of prophylactic lithium: (1) An episodic pattern of mania-depression-interval, and (2) a late age of illness onset were identified as potentially protective against a recurrence under lithium, whereas, (3) a high number of previous hospitalizations, (4) an episodic pattern of depression-mania-interval, and (5) continuous cycling were identified as potential poor predictors of lithium response.

The authors concluded "as none of the potential predictors had a very strong impact on response, prediction of lithium response should be based on a multitude of variables."

Lithium efficacy in different age groups

There is a lack of well-designed controlled studies with lithium in bipolar disorder children and adolescents. Several studies were reported suggesting a role for lithium in acute mania in adolescents and children. Youngerman and Casino (1987) reviewed the available literature, accounting for 211 cases of children and adolescents treated with lithium. In 46 cases there was enough data to assess response of which 65% responded to lithium treatment. Delong and Aldershot (1987) reported similar response (66%) to lithium in 59 children diagnosed with bipolar disorder. Papatheodorou and Kutcher (1996) reviewed the literature in this age group, and suggested that lithium was effective in adolescent mania, with a response rate of 50–66%. These authors also suggested that adolescent mania often presents itself as mixed or atypical mania, possibly resulting in lower rates of response compared with adult mania. Geller et al. (1998) conducted a double-blind controlled study of lithium administered for 6 weeks in adolescents with dual diagnosis of bipolar spectrum disorders and secondary substance dependence. Twenty-five subjects were enrolled and 21 completed the study. Lithium showed superiority for treatment of both bipolar spectrum illness and drug dependence (mainly to alcohol and marijuana). The Children's Global Assessment Scale (CGAS) was used to assess the subject's clinical status. Six out of 10 completers on lithium responded with CGAS score ≥65, whereas this was true only for one out of 11 patients treated with placebo. The mean lithium blood level for active responders was 0.9 meq/L. The results of this study should however be taken with caution since the study population was heterogenus and only a global assessment was used. There seems to be a lack of data on the use of lithium in bipolar depression and long-term prophylaxis in children. Strober et al. (1990) conducted a discontinuation study of lithium in bipolar disorder adolescents. In a follow-up of 18 months, adolescent patients treated with lithium had only 37.5% relapses compared with 92.3% of patients whose lithium was discontinued suggesting that lithium has beneficial effects in the prophylaxis of bipolar disorder in adolescents.

No placebo controlled studies of lithium have been conducted in geriatric mania. Some of the systematic studies of lithium in mania included elderly patients, but in general the effect of age and its impact on lithium response has not been extensively studied (Dunn & Rabins, 1996). Chen et al. (1999) retrospectively studied the efficacy of lithium versus valproate in the treatment of mania in 59 hospitalized manic patients, age 55 years and older. A greater proportion of patients improved on lithium versus valproate (67% vs. 38%). Higher lithium plasma levels (≥0.8 mmol/L) were associated with increased response. Further analysis showed that the superiority of lithium was associated with classic mania, while no difference between lithium and valproate was noted when mixed mania was analyzed separately. Young and Falk (1989) conducted a study of lithium, which suggested a weak negative effect of age on the response rate of lithium treatment in bipolar illness. However, elderly patients were not specifically included in this study. There is also a lack of data on the therapeutic role of lithium in prophylactic treatment for bipolar disorder in the elderly (Dunn & Rabins, 1996).

To summarize, a variety of factors seem to modify the response to lithium treatment based on age and should be considered when deciding upon lithium treatment.

Lithium in the prevention of suicidality

Long-term lithium treatment was reported to have an anti-suicidal effect in mood disorders (i.e. Baldessarini, Tondo, & Hennen, 2003; Goodwin et al., 2003). Goodwin et al. (2003) suggested that risk of death by suicide was about three times higher during treatment with divalproex than during treatment with lithium. These authors compared risk of suicide attempt and suicide death during treatment with lithium versus that of divalproex in a retrospective cohort study which examined the data in two large integrated health plans in two states in the USA. The study included a sample of over 20,000 health plan members aged 14 years or older who had at least one outpatient diagnosis of bipolar disorder and at least one filled prescription for lithium, divalproex, or carbamazepine between January 1, 1994 and December 31, 2001. Follow-up for each individual began with first qualifying prescription and ended with death, de-enrollment from the health plan, or end of the study period. The outcome measures were suicide attempt, recorded as a hospital discharge diagnosis or an emergency department diagnosis; suicide death, recorded on death certificate. After adjustment for age, sex, health plan, year of diagnosis, co-morbid medical and psychiatric conditions, and concomitant use of other psychotropic drugs, risk of suicide death was 2.7 times higher during treatment with divalproex than during treatment with lithium. Corresponding hazard ratios for nonfatal attempts were 1.7 for attempts resulting in hospitalization and 1.8 for attempts diagnosed in the emergency department. The authors concluded that patients treated for bipolar disorder, risk of suicide attempt and suicide death was lower during treatment with lithium than during treatment with divalproex.

Cipriani et al. (2005) conducted a systematic review and meta-analysis of randomized trials to investigate the effect of lithium, compared to placebo and other active treatments, on the risk of suicide, deliberate self-harm and all-cause mortality in patients with mood disorder. These authors' surveyed 32 trials where 1389 patients were assigned lithium treatment and 2069 assigned to other psychotropic drugs. Patients who received lithium were less likely to die by suicide. There were fewer deaths overall in patients who received lithium and a calculated measure of suicide and deliberate self-harm was also lower in patients receiving lithium. These authors suggest that lithium appears to decrease the risk of death and suicide by about 60% and the risk of suicide and deliberate self-harm by about 70% and that lithium is effective in the prevention of suicide, deliberate self-harm, and death from all causes in patients with mood disorders.

Baldessarini et al. (2006) recently published a meta-analytic review of 45 studies which reported rates of suicidal acts during lithium treatment. Of these 34 studies also reported rates without lithium treatment. Thirty one studies were found to be appropriate for meta-analysis (85,229 person-years of risk-exposure). The authors report that the overall risk of suicides and attempts was five times less among lithium-treated subjects than among those not treated with lithium. The incidence-ratio of attempts-to-suicides increased 2.5 times with lithium-treatment, indicating reduced lethality of suicidal acts. The authors state that "there was no indication of bias toward reporting positive findings, nor were outcomes significantly influenced by publication-year or study size". The authors concluded that risks of completed and attempted suicide were lower, by about 80%, during treatment of bipolar and other major affective disorder patients with lithium for an average of 18 months.

Thus there is substantial data to suggest a role for lithium in the prevention of suicides in bipolar and other mood disorders.

New clinical issues with lithium treatment

Point-of-care (POC) test for lithium levels

Lithium treatment requires close therapeutic monitoring due to its narrow therapeutic index. Lithium levels are monitored to prevent or recognize signs of lithium toxicity, to ensure ongoing efficacy and effectiveness, including the prevention of suicidal behavior; and, to help ensure patient adherence to the prescribed regimen.

New technologies and patient care models are driving laboratory testing to the patient's side—at the POC. POC testing is diagnostic testing or therapeutic monitoring carried out at or near the site of the patient. POC diagnostic monitoring has now been advanced in the management of diabetes mellitus, hyperlipidemia and clotting disorders, among other medical conditions.

A new instant blood test has now been developed that allows the clinician to take a finger-stick sample of whole blood and determine the plasma lithium level in a 2-minute period. Recently, the FDA approved this instant POC test for lithium blood levels (Jefferson, 2005; ReliaLab, Inc, 2005).

The test consists of three processes: (a) separation of the plasma from the whole blood by lectine-coated membrane; (b) adding the plasma to a colorimetric reagent of which the active gradient is phorphyrin (phorphyrin absorbance of light having wave length of 505 nm is reported to be increased by lithium concentration) and (c) exposing the reagent to a photometer enabling the measurement of lithium concentration between 0 and 2.5 meq/L.

The reliability of the new test was reported to be in agreement with standard laboratory values in three studies involving about 250 subjects demonstrating high reliability (>0.90).

Thus this new test seems to be reliable and to offer some advantages over the standard laboratory procedures for the measurement of lithium blood levels. Moreover, this office-based procedure may be especially useful in checking for compliance/adherence or toxicity in outpatient settings where the immediate availability of results may impact immediate clinical decision-making.

Clinical decision-making and lithium treatment

Several pharmacological algorithms were published during the last decade for the treatment of bipolar disorder, however, no one specifically addressed the variety of parameters reported to impact especially the response to lithium treatment (American Psychiatric Association, 1994b; Frances, Docherty, & Kahn, 1996; Kusumakar & Yatham, 1997; Bauer et al., 1999). In addition, these algorithms were in general of a dichotomous (each step consisting of yes or no options) qualitative nature making them less useful in complex individual cases in which a variety of patient, illness and drug related parameters have to be considered. The recommendations in Table 10.1 have tried to address the variety of parameters affecting the response to lithium treatment as well as to provide a guide for the

Table 10.1 Proposed Scoring System as to Indication for Lithium Use

Choose One Most Appropriate Score for Each of the Following Groups
(Diagnosis, Course, Family History and Treatment History)

Diagnosis	Bipolar Disorder • Manic episode (5 points) • Dysphoric mania (2 points) • Mixed episode (2 points) • Acute depressive episode (2.5 points) • In remission (5 points) Schizoaffective Disorder • Acute manic episode (4 points) • Dysphoric mania (1.5 points) • Mixed episode (1.5 points) • Acute depressive episode (0 points) • In remission (3 points) Unipolar Depression • Acute depression (1.5 points) • In remission (0 points) Schizophrenia • Acute episode (1 points) • In remission (0 points)
Course of illness:	• Depressive episodes only (0 points) • Sequence of mania-depression-euthymia (2 points) • Sequence of depression-mania-euthymia (1.5 points) • Rapid cycling (–1 points) • Missing data (0.5 point)
Family history:	• With affective disorder (2 points) • Without affective disorders (–1 points) • Missing data (0.5 point)
Previous history with lithium treatment:	• Beneficial effect in acute treatment (1 point) • Beneficial effect in acute treatment and good quality of remission (2 points) • Adequate previous acute trial with lithium therapy failed (–3 points) • Missing data (0.5 point)

Source: Developed by Joseph Levine, M.D.

clinician facing a decision as to the use of lithium in an individual patient. In the case of missing data 0.5 point is scored in order to differentiate it from a case where existing data suggests a score of zero or less. No missing data is allowed for diagnosis.

The reader should be aware that by no means is this score accurate, as it stands as a recommendation only. The clinician should take into consideration other available data before making a decision to use lithium including a detailed history of the illness and its response to previous drug therapy, the age and physical condition of the patient and available data as to side effect profile of lithium treatment and its potential for interaction with other drugs. Also, we did not include in this proposed scoring system the possible use of lithium augmentation in cases of resistant unipolar depression.

General recommendations as to indication for lithium use

If the sum of scores for diagnosis and course of illness ≥5 (maximal score is 7) and; the sum of scores for family history and previous history of lithium treatment ≥−0.5 (maximal score is 4) then: lithium treatment is probably indicated.

If the sum of scores for diagnosis and course of illness ≥3 and <5; and the sum of scores for family history and previous history of lithium treatment ≥ −0.5 (maximal score is 4) then: lithium treatment may be initiated.

If the sum of scores for diagnosis and course of illness ≥3 (maximal score is 7) and the sum of scores for family history and previous history of lithium treatment=−1 then: lithium treatment is questionable since previous trial with lithium was unfavorable.

If the sum of scores for diagnosis and course of illness <3 (minimal score is −1); and/or the sum of scores for family history and previous history of lithium treatment <−1 (minimal score is −4) then lithium treatment is probably not recommended.

References

Aagaard J, & Vestergaard P (1990). Predictors of outcome in prophylactic lithium treatment: a two year prospective study. *J. Affect. Disord.*, *18*: 259–266.

Abou-Saleh MT, & Coppen AJ (1990). Predictors of long term outcome of mood disorder on prophylactic lithium. *Lithium*, *1*: 27–35.

Akhondzadeh S, Emamian ES, Ahmadi-Abhari A, Shabestari O, & Dadgarnejad M (1999). Is it time to have another look at lithium maintenance therapy in bipolar? *Prog. Neuropsychopharmacol Biol. Psychiatry*, *23*: 1011–1017.

American Psychiatric Association (1952). *Diagnostic and Statistical Manual of Mental Disorders* (1st edn.). Washington, DC: American Psychiatric Press.

American Psychiatric Association (1968). *Diagnostic and Statistical Manual of Mental Disorders* (2nd edn.). Washington, DC: American Psychiatric Press.

American Psychiatric Association (1980). *Diagnostic and Statistical Manual of Mental Disorders* (3rd edn.). Washington, DC: American Psychiatric Press.
American Psychiatric Association (1987). *Diagnostic and Statistical Manual of Mental Disorders* (3rd, revised edn.). Washington, DC: American Psychiatric Press.
American Psychiatric Association (1994a). *Diagnostic and Statistical Manual of Mental Disorders* (4th edn.). Washington, DC: American Psychiatric Press.
American Psychiatric Association (1994b). Practice guidelines for the treatment of patients with bipolar disorder. In: *American Psychiatric Association Practice Guidelines* (pp. 135–208). Washington, DC: American Psychiatric Press.
American Psychiatric Association (2000). *Diagnostic and Statistical Manual of Mental Disorders, DSM-IV-TR.* Washington, DC: American Psychiatric Press.
Baastrup PC (1964). The use of lithium in manic depressive psychosis. *Compr. Psychiatry, 5:* 396–408.
Baastrup PC, Poulsen JC, Schou M, Thomsen K, & Amdisen A (1970). Prophylactic lithium: double-blind discontinuation in manic-depressive and recurrent-depressive disorders. *Lancet, 2:* 326–330.
Baastrup PC, & Schou M (1967). Lithium as a prophylactic agent. *Arch. Gen. Psychiatry, 16:* 162–172.
Baldessarini RJ, Tondo L, & Hennen J (2003). Lithium treatment and suicide risk in major affective disorders: update and new findings. *J. Clin. Psychiatry, 64* (Suppl 5): 44–52. Review.
Baldessarini RJ, Tondo L, Davis P, Pompili M, Goodwin FK, & Hennen J (2006). Decreased risk of suicides and attempts during long-term lithium treatment: a meta-analytic review. *Bipolar Disord., 8* (5 Pt 2): 625–639.
Baron A, Gershon ES, Rudy V, Jonas WZ, & Buchsbaum M (1975). Lithium carbonate response in depression: prediction by unipolar/bipolar illness, average-evoked response, catechol-O-methyl transferase, and family history. *Arch. Gen. Psychiatry, 32:* 1107–1111.
Bauer MS, Callahan AM, Jampala C, Petty F, Sajatovic M, & Schaefer V, et al. (1999). Clinical practice guidelines for bipolar disorder from the Department of Veterans Affairs. *J. Clin. Psychiatry, 60:* 9–21.
Berk M, Ichim L, & Brook S (1999). Olanzapine compared to lithium in mania: a double-blind randomized controlled trial. *Int. Clin. Psychopharmacol., 14* (6): 339–343.
Bowden CL, Brugger AM, Swann AC, Calabrese JR, Janicak PG, & Petty F, et al. (1994). Efficacy of divalproex vs lithium and placebo in the treatment of mania. *JAMA, 271:* 918–924.
Bowden CL, Davis J, Morris D, Swann A, Calabrese J, & Lambert M, et al. (1997). Effect size of efficacy measures comparing divalproex, lithium and placebo in acute mania. *Depression & Anxiety, 6:* 26–30.
Bowden CL, Calabrese JR, Sachs G, Yatham LN, Asghar SA, Hompland M, Montgomery P, Earl N, Smoot TM, & DeVeaugh-Geiss J (2003). Lamictal 606 Study Group. A placebo-controlled 18-month trial of lamotrigine and lithium maintenance treatment in recently manic or hypomanic patients with bipolar I disorder. *Arch. Gen. Psychiatry, 60* (4): 392–400.
Bowden CL, Grunze H, Mullen J, Brecher M, Paulsson B, Jones M, Vagero M, & Svensson K (2005). A randomized, double-blind, placebo-controlled efficacy and safety study of quetiapine or lithium as monotherapy for mania in bipolar disorder. *J. Clin. Psychiatry, 66* (1): 111–121.

Bunney WE, Goodwin FK, Davis JM, & Fawcett JA (1968). A behavioral-biochemical study of lithium treatment. *Am. J. Psychiatry, 125*: 499–512.

Burgess S, Geddes J, Hawton K, Townsend E, Jamison K, & Goodwin G (2001). Lithium for maintenance treatment of mood disorders (Cochrane Review). *The Cochrane Database of Systematic Reviews, 3*. Art. No.: CD003013. DOI:10.1002/14651858.CD003013.

Cade JFJ (1949). Lithium salts in the treatment of psychotic excitement. *Med. J. Aust., 2*: 349–352.

Cade JFJ (1970). The story of lithium. In: Ade FJ, Blackwell FB, editors. *Discoveries in Biological Psychiatry* (pp. 218–20). Philadelphia, PA: J.B. Lippincott Company.

Calabrese JR, Bowden CL, Sachs G, Yatham LN, Behnke K, Mehtonen OP, Montgomery P, Ascher J, Paska W, Earl N, & DeVeaugh-Geiss J (2003). Lamictal 605 Study Group. A placebo-controlled 18-month trial of lamotrigine and lithium maintenance treatment in recently depressed patients with bipolar I disorder. *J. Clin. Psychiatry, 64* (9): 1013–1024.

Chen ST, Altshuler LL, Melnyk KA, Erhart SM, Miller E, & Mintz J (1999). Efficacy of lithium vs. valproate in the treatment of mania in the elderly: a retrospective study. *J. Clin. Psychiatry, 60*: 181–186.

Christodoulou GN, & Lykouras EP (1982). Abrupt lithium discontinuation in manic depressive patients. *Acta Psychiatr. Scand., 65*: 310–314.

Cipriani A, Pretty H, Hawton K, & Geddes JR (2005). Lithium in the prevention of suicidal behavior and all-cause mortality in patients with mood disorders: a systematic review of randomized trials. *Am. J. Psychiatry, 162* (10): 1805–1819.

Clothier J, Swann AC, & Freeman T (1992). Dysphoric mania. *J. Clin. Psychopharmacol., 12*: 13S–16S.

Cohen S, Khan A, & Coz G (1989). Demographic and clinical features predictive of recovery in acute mania. *J. Nerv. Ment. Dis., 177*: 638–642.

Coppen A, Abou-Saleh M, Milln P, Bailey J, & Wood K (1983). Decreasing lithium dosage reduces morbidity and side effects during prophylaxis. *J. Affect. Disord., 5*: 353–362.

Coppen A, Noguera R, Bailey J, Burns BH, Swani MS, & Hare EH, et al. (1971). Prophylactic lithium in affective disorders: controlled trial. *Lancet, 2*: 275–279.

Coryell W, Solomon D, Leon AC, Akiskal HS, Keller MB, Scheftner WA, & Mueller T (1998). Lithium discontinuation and subsequent effectiveness. *Am. J. Psychiatry, 155* (7): 895–898.

Coxhead N, Silverstone T, & Cookson J (1992). Carbamazepine versus lithium in the prophylaxis of bipolar affective disorder. *Acta Psychiatr. Scand., 85*: 114–118.

Cundall RL, Brooks PW, & Murray LG (1972). A controlled evaluation of lithium prophylaxis in affective disorders. *Psychol. Med., 2*: 308–311.

Dardennes R, Even C, Bange F, & Heim A (1995). Comparison of carbamazepine and lithium in the prophylaxis of bipolar disorder [a meta-analysis]. *Br. J. Psychiatry, 166*: 378–381.

de Montigny C, Grunberg F, Mayer A, & Deschenes JP (1981). Lithium induces rapid relief of depression in tricyclic antidepressant drug non-responders. *Br. J. Psychiatry, 138*: 252–256.

Delong GR, & Aldershof AL (1987). Long-term experience with lithium treatment in childhood: correlation with clinical diagnosis. *J. Am. Acad. Child Adolesc. Psychiatry, 26*: 389–394.

Dilsaver SC, Swann AC, Shoaib AM, & Bowers TC (1993a). The manic syndrome: factors which may predict a patient's response to lithium, carbamazepine and valproate. *J. Psychiatr. Neurosci., 18*: 61–66.

Dilsaver SC, Swann AC, Shoaib AM, Bowers TC, & Halle MT (1993b). Depressive mania associated with nonresponse to antimanic agents. *Am. J. Psychiatry, 150*: 1548–1551.

Dunn KL, & Rabins PV (1996). Mania in old age. In: Shulman KI, Tohen M, Kutcher SP, editors. *Mood Disorders across the Life Span* (pp 399–406). New York, NY: John Wiley & Sons.

Dunner DL, & Fieve RR (1974). Clinical factors in lithium carbonate prophylaxis failure. *Arch. Gen. Psychiatry, 30*: 229–233.

Dunner DL, Fleiss JL, & Fieve RR (1976). Lithium carbonate prophylaxis failure. *Br. J. Psychiatry, 129*: 40–44.

Emilien G, Maloteaux JM, Seghers A, & Charles G (1996). Lithium compared to valproic acid and carbamazepine in the treatment of mania: a statistical meta-analysis. *Eur. Neuropsychopharmacol., 6*: 245–252.

Faedda GL, Baldessarini RJ, Tohen M, Strakowski SM, & Waternaux C (1991). Episode sequence in bipolar disorder and response to lithium treatment. *Am. J. Psychiatry, 148*: 1237–1239.

Fieve RR, Kumbarachi T, & Dunner DL (1976). Lithium prophylaxis of depression in bipolar I, bipolar II, and unipolar patients. *Am. J. Psychiatry, 133*: 925–929.

Fieve RR, Platman SR, & Plutchick RR (1968). The use of lithium in affective disorders: II. prophylaxis of depression in chronic recurrent affective disorder. *Am. J. Psychiatry, 125*: 492–498.

Frances AJ, Docherty JP, & Kahn DA (1996). The expert consensus guideline series: Treatment of bipolar disorder. *J. Clin. Psychiatry, 57* (Suppl 12A): 1–88.

Freeman TW, Clothier JL, Pazzaglia P, Lesem MD, & Swann AC (1992). A double-blind comparison of valproate and lithium in the treatment of acute mania. *Am. J. Psychiatry, 49*: 108–111.

Garfinkel PE, Stancer HC, & Persad E (1980). A comparison of haloperidol, lithium carbonate and their combination in the treatment of mania. *J. Affect. Disord., 2*: 279–288.

Gelenberg AL, Kane JM, Keller MB, Lavori P, Rosenbaum JF, & Cole K, et al. (1989). Comparison of standard and low serum levels of lithium for maintenance treatment of bipolar disorder. *N. Engl. J. Med., 321*: 1489–1493.

Geller B, Cooper TB, Sun K, Zimerman B, Frazier J, & Williams M, et al. (1998). Double-blind and placebo-controlled study of lithium for adolescent bipolar disorders with secondary substance dependency. *J. Am. Acad. Child Aolesc. Psychiatry, 37*: 171–178.

Gershon S, & Shopsin B (1973). *Lithium: Its Role in Psychiatric Research and Treatment.* New York, NY: Plenum Press.

Glazer WM, Sonnenberg JG, Reinstein MJ, & Akers RF (2004). A novel, point-of-care test for lithium levels: description and reliability. *J. Clin. Psychiatry, 65* (5): 652–655.

Goldberg JF (2001). Bipolar disorder with comorbid substance abuse: diagnosis, prognosis, and treatment. *J. Psychiatr. Pract., 7* (2): 109–122.

Goodnick PJ, Fieve RR, Schlegel A, & Baxter N (1987). Predictors of interepisode symptoms and relapse in affective disorder patients treated with lithium carbonate. *Am. J. Psychiatry, 144*: 367–369.

Goodwin FK, Fireman B, Simon GE, Hunkeler EM, Lee J, & Revicki D (2003). Suicide risk in bipolar disorder during treatment with lithium and divalproex. *JAMA, 290* (11): 1467–1473.

Goodwin FK, & Jamison KR (1990). *Manic-Depressive Illness*. New York, NY: Oxford University Press.

Goodwin FK, Murphy DL, & Bunney WEJ (1969). Lithium-carbonate treatment in depression and mania: a longitudinal double-blind study. *Arch. Gen. Psychiatry, 21*: 486–496.

Goodwin FK, Murphy DL, Dunner DL, & Bunney WEJ (1972). Lithium response in unipolar vs. bipolar depression. *Am. J. Psychiatry, 129*: 44–47.

Goodwin GM (1994). Recurrence of mania after lithium withdrawal. *Br. J. Psychiatry, 164*: 149–152.

Greil W, & Kleindienst N (1999a). The comparative prophylactic efficacy of lithium and carbamazepine in patients with bipolar I disorder. *Int. Clin. Psychopharmacol., 14*: 277–281.

Greil W, & Kleindienst N (1999b). Lithium versus carbamazepine in the maintenance treatment of bipolar II disorder and bipolar disorder not otherwise specified. *Int. Clin. Psychopharmacol., 14*: 283–285.

Grof P (1999). Excellent lithium responders people whose lives have been changed by lithium use. Proceeding of Symposium Lithium Lexington 99, May 6–11, Lexington, KY.

Grof P, Alda M, Grof E, Fox D, & Cameron P (1993). The challenge of predicting response to stabilizing lithium treatment. *Br. J. Psychiatry, 163* (Suppl. 21): 16–19.

Grof P, Hux M, Grof E, & Arato M (1983). Prediction of response to stabilizing lithium treatment. *Pharmacopsychiatry, 16*: 195–200.

Hartigan GP (1963). The use of lithium salts in affective disorders. *Br. J. Psychiatry, 109*: 810–814.

Heninger GR, Charney DS, & Sternberg DE (1983). Lithium carbonate augmentation of antidepressant treatment: an effective prescription for treatment–refractory depression. *Arch. Gen. Psychiatry, 40*: 1335–1342.

Himmelhoch JM, Mulla D, Neil JF, Detre TP, & Kupfer DJ (1976). Incidence and significance of mixed affective states in a bipolar population. *Arch. Gen. Psychiatry, 33*: 1062–1066.

Hirschfeld RM, Baker JD, Wozniak P, Tracy K, & Sommerville KW (2003). The safety and early efficacy of oral-loaded divalproex versus standard-titration divalproex, lithium, olanzapine, and placebo in the treatment of acute mania associated with bipolar disorder. *J. Clin. Psychiatry, 64* (7): 841–846.

Hullin RP, McDonald R, & Allsopp MNE (1972). Prophylactic lithium in recurrent affective disorders. *Lancet, 1*: 1044–1046.

Jefferson JW (1996). Lithium. In: Goodnick PJ, editor. *Predictors of Treatment Response in Mood Disorders* (pp. 95–117). Washington, DC: American Psychiatric Press.

Jefferson JW (2005). Finger-stick lithium test: in-office alternative to laboratory-based methods. *Curr. Psychiatry, 4* (10): 111–117.

Jensen HV, Davidson K, Tofteraard L, Mellerup ET, Plenge P, & Aggernaes H, et al. (1996). Double-blind comparison of the side-effect profile of daily versus alternate-day dosing schedules in lithium maintenance treatment of manic-depressive disorder. *J. Affect. Disord., 36:* 89–93.

Jensen HV, Plenge P, Mellerup ET, Davidson K, Tofteraard L, & Aggernaes H, et al. (1995). Lithium prophylaxis of manic-depressive disorder: daily dosing schedule versus second day. *Acta Psychiatr. Scand., 92:* 69–74.

Johnson G, Gershon S, Burdock EI, Floyd A, & Hekimian L (1971). Comparative effects of lithium and chlorpromazine in the treatment of acute manic states. *Br. J. Psychiatry, 119:* 267–276.

Johnson G, Gershon S, & Hekimian LJ (1968). Controlled evaluation of lithium and chlorpromazine in the treatment of manic states: an interim report. *Compr. Psychiatry, 9:* 563–567.

Keller MB, Lavori PW, Kane JM, Gelenberg AJ, Rosenbaum JF, & Walzer EA, et al. (1992). Subsyndromal symptoms in bipolar disorder: a comparison of standard and low serum levels of lithium. *Arch. Gen. Psychiatry, 49:* 371–376.

Kleindienst N, Engel R, & Greil W (2005). Which clinical factors predict response to prophylactic lithium? A systematic review for bipolar disorders. *Bipolar Disord., 7* (5): 404–17

Kukopulos A, Reginaldi D, Laddomada P, Floric G, Serra G, & Tondo L (1980). Course of the manic depressive cycle and changes caused by treatment. *Pharmacopsychiatry, 13:* 156–167.

Kulhara P, Basu D, Mattoo SK, Sharan P, & Chopra R (1999). Lithium prophylaxis of recurrent bipolar affective disorder: long-term outcome and its psychosocial correlates. *J. Affect. Disord., 54:* 87–96.

Kusumakar V, & Yatham LN (1997). The treatment of bipolar disorder: review of the literature, guidelines, and options. *Can. J. Psychiatry, 42* (Suppl. 2): 67S–100S.

Lerer B, Moore N, Meyendorff E, Cho SR, & Gershon S (1987). Carbamazepine versus lithium in the treatment of mania: a double-blind study. *J. Clin. Psychiatry, 48:* 89–93.

Lusznat RM, Murphy DP, & Nunn CMH (1988). Carbamazepine vs lithium in the treatment and prophylaxis of mania. *Br. J. Psychiatry, 153:* 198–204.

Maggs R (1963). Treatment of manic illness with lithium carbonate. *Br. J. Psychiatry, 109:* 56–65.

Maj M (1992). Clinical prediction of response to lithium prophylaxis in bipolar patients: a critical update. *Lithium, 3:* 15–21.

Maj M, Pirozzi R, Magliano L, & Bartoli L (1998). Long term outcome of lithium prophylaxis in bipolar disorder: a 5 year prospective study of 402 patients at a lithium clinic. *Am. J. Psychiatry, 155:* 30–35.

McElroy SL, Keck PE, Pope HG, Hudson JI, Faedda GL, & Swann AC (1992). Clinical and research implications of the diagnosis of dysphoric or mixed mania or hypomania. *Am. J. Psychiatry, 149:* 1633–1644.

Melia PI (1970). Prophylactic lithium: a double-blind trial in recurrent affective disorders. *Br. J. Psychiatry, 116:* 621–624.

Mendels J (1975). Lithium in the acute treatment of depressive states. In: Johnson FN, editor. *Lithium Research and Therapy* (pp. 43–62). London: Academic Press.

Murphy DL, & Beigel A (1974). Depression, elation, and lithium carbonate responses in manic patient sub-groups. *Arch. Gen. Psychiatry, 31:* 643–648.

Nemeroff CB, Evans DL, Gyulai L, Sachs GS, Bowden CL, Gergel IP, Oakes R, & Pitts CD (2001). Double-blind, placebo-controlled comparison of imipramine and paroxetine in the treatment of bipolar depression. *Am. J. Psychiatry, 158:* 906–912.

Noack CH, & Trautner EM (1951). The lithium treatment of maniacal psychosis. *Med. J. Aust., 38*: 219–222.

Noyes RJ, Dempsey GM, & Blum A (1974). Lithium treatment of depression. *Compr. Psychiatry, 15*: 187–190.

Papatheodorou G, & Kutcher SP (1996). Treatment of Bipolar in Adolescents. In: Shulman KI, Tohen M, & Kutcher SP, editors. *Mood Disorders Across the Life Span* (pp. 159–186). New York, NY: John Wiley & Sons.

Platman SR (1970). A comparison of lithium carbonate and chlorpromazine in mania. *Am. J. Psychiatry, 127*: 351–353.

Post RM, Kramlinger KG, Altschuler LL, Ketter TA, & Denicoff K (1990). Treatment of rapid cycling bipolar illness. *Psychopharmacol. Bull., 26*: 37–47.

Prien RF (1988). Maintenance treatment of depressive and manic states. In: Georgotas A, and Cancro R, editors. *Depression and Mania* (pp. 439–451). New York, NY: Elsevier.

Prien RF, Caffey EM, & Klett CJ (1972). Comparison of lithium carbonate and chlorpromazine in the treatment of mania. *Arch. Gen. Psychiatry, 26*: 146–153.

Prien RF, Caffey EM, & Klett CJ (1973a). Prophylactic efficacy of lithium in manic-depressive illness. *Arch. Gen. Psychiatry, 28*: 337–341.

Prien RF, Klett CJ, & Caffey EM (1973b). Lithium carbonate and imipramine in prevention of affective episodes. *Arch. Gen. Psychiatry, 29*: 420–425.

Prien RF, Kupfer DJ, Mansky PA, Small JG, Tuason VB, & Voss CB (1984). Drug therapy in the prevention of recurrences in unipolar and bipolar affective disorders. *Arch. Gen. Psychiatry, 41*: 1096–1104.

ReliaLab, Inc. (2005). InstaRead Lithium System. *Med. Lett. Drugs Ther., 47* (1219): 82–83.

Sachs GS, Grossman F, Ghaemi SN, Okamoto A, & Bowden CL (2002). Combination of a mood stabilizer with risperidone or haloperidol for treatment of acute mania: a double-blind, placebo-controlled comparison of efficacy and safety. *Am. J. Psychiatry, 159* (7): 1146–1154.

Sachs G, Chengappa KN, Supper T, Mullen JA, Brecher M, Devine NA, & Seitzer DE (2004). Quetiapine with lithium or divalproex for the treatment of bipolar mania: a randomized, double-blind, placebo-controlled study. *Bipolar Disord., 6* (3): 213–223.

Schou M (1959). Lithium in psychiatric therapy: stock-taking after ten years. *Psychopharmacology, 1*: 65–78.

Schou M, Juel-Nielsen N, Stromgren E, & Voldby H (1954). The treatment of manic psychoses by the administration of lithium salts. *J. Neurol. Neurosurg. Psychiatr., 17*: 250–260.

Secunda SK, Katz MM, Swann A, Koslow SH, Maas JW, & Chuang S, et al. (1985). Mania diagnosis state measurement and prediction of treatment response. *J. Affect. Disord., 8*: 113–121.

Segal J, Berk M, & Brook S (1998). Risperidone compared with both lithium and haloperidol in mania: a double-blind randomized controlled trial. *Clin. Neuropharmacol., 21*: 176–180.

Shopsin B, Gershon S, Thompson H, & Collins P (1975). Psychoactive drugs in mania: a controlled comparison of lithium carbonate, chlorpromazine, and haloperidol. *Arch. Gen. Psychiatry, 32*: 34–42.

Small JG, Klapper MH, Milstein V, Kellams JJ, Miller MJ, & Marheke JD, et al. (1991). Carbamazepine compared with lithium in the treatment of mania. *Arch. Gen. Psychiatry, 48*: 915–921.

Soares JC, & Gershon S (1998). The lithium ion: a foundation for psychopharmacological specificity. *Neuropsychopharmacology, 19*: 167–182.

Spring G, Schweid D, Gray C, Steinberg J, & Horwitz M (1970). A double-blind comparison of lithium and chlorpromazine in the treatment of manic states. *Am. J. Psychiatry, 126*: 1306–1310.

Srisurapanont M, Yatham LN, & Zis AP (1995). Treatment of acute bipolar depression: a review of the literature. *Can. J. Psychiatry, 40*: 533–544.

Stallone F, Shelley E, Mendlewicz J, & Fieve RR (1973). The use of lithium in affective disorders. III: a double-blind study of prophylaxis in bipolar illness. *Am. J. Psychiatry, 130*: 1006–1010.

Stokes PE, Shamoian CA, Stoll PM, & Patton MJ (1971). Efficacy of lithium as acute treatment of manic-depressive illness. *Lancet, 1*: 1319–1325.

Strober M, Morrell W, Lampert C, & Burroughs J (1990). Relapses following discontinuation of lithium maintenance therapy in adolescents with bipolar I illness: a naturalistic study. *Am. J. Psychiatry, 147*: 457–461.

Swann AC, Bowden CL, Morris D, Calabrese JR, Petty F, & Small J, et al. (1997). Depression during mania. Treatment response to lithium or divalproex. *Arch. Gen. Psychiatry, 54*: 37–42.

Swann AC, Secunda SK, Katz MM, Koslow SH, Maas JW, & Chuang S, et al. (1986). Lithium treatment in mania. Clinical characteristics, specificity of symptom change, and outcome. *Psychiatry Res., 18*: 127–141.

Takahashi R, Sakuma A, Itoh K, Itoh H, & Kurihara M (1975). Comparison of efficacy of lithium carbonate and chlorpromazine in mania. *Arch. Gen. Psychiatry, 32*: 1310–1318.

Tohen M, Chengappa KN, Suppes T, Zarate CA Jr, Calabrese JR, Bowden CL, Sachs GS, Kupfer DJ, Baker RW, Risser RC, Keeter EL, Feldman PD, Tollefson GD, & Breier A (2002). Efficacy of olanzapine in combination with valproate or lithium in the treatment of mania in patients partially nonresponsive to valproate or lithium monotherapy. *Arch. Gen. Psychiatry, 59* (1): 62–69.

Tohen M, Chengappa KN, Suppes T, Baker RW, Zarate CA, Bowden CL, Sachs GS, Kupfer DJ, Ghaemi SN, Feldman PD, Risser RC, Evans AR, & Calabrese JR. (2004). Relapse prevention in bipolar I disorder: 18-month comparison of olanzapine plus mood stabiliser v. mood stabiliser alone. *Br. J. Psychiatry, 184*: 337–345.

Tohen M, Greil W, Calabrese JR, Sachs GS, Yatham LN, Oerlinghausen BM, Koukopoulos A, Cassano GB, Grunze H, Licht RW, Dell'Osso L, Evans AR, Risser R, Baker RW, Crane H, Dossenbach MR, & Bowden CL (2005). Olanzapine versus lithium in the maintenance treatment of bipolar disorder: a 12-month, randomized, double-blind, controlled clinical trial. *Am. J. Psychiatry, 162* (7): 1281–1290.

Watanabe S, Ishino H, & Otsuki S (1975). Double-blind comparison of lithium carbonate and imipramine in treatment of depression. *Arch. Gen. Psychiatry, 32*(5): 659–668.

Worrall EP, Moody JP, Peet M, Dick P, Smith A, & Chambers C, et al. (1979). Controlled studies of the acute antidepressant effects of lithium. *Br. J. Psychiatry, 135*: 255–262.

Young RL, & Falk JR (1989). Age, manic psychopathology and treatment response. *Int. J. Geriatr. Psychiatry, 4*: 73–78.

Youngerman J, & Casino IA (1987). Lithium carbonate use in children and adolescents: a survey of the literature. *Arch. Gen. Psychiatry, 35*: 216–224.

chapter eleven

Antipsychotic medications in bipolar disorder: A critical review of randomized controlled trials

David J. Bond
University of British Columbia

Eduard Vieta
University of Barcelona

Mauricio Tohen
Lilly Research Laboratories

Lakshmi N. Yatham
University of British Columbia

Contents

Introduction 296
FGAs in bipolar disorder 297
   FGAs in acute bipolar I mania 297
   Depot FGAs in the maintenance treatment of
      bipolar disorder.. 299
SGAs in bipolar disorder 300
   SGAs versus placebo in acute bipolar I mania 300
      Change in the primary outcome measure........................... 308
      Onset of action.. 308
      Dosages... 309
      Response and remission rates 309
      Rates of depressive symptoms...310
   SGAs versus active comparators in acute bipolar I mania 310
      Comparisons with haloperidol 311

        Comparisons with lithium and divalproex.......................... 324
        Risperidone versus olanzapine.. 325
    Combination therapy studies in acute bipolar I mania................... 325
        Efficacy 331
        Effect on depressive symptoms 332
        Limitations.. 332
        Adverse events... 332
        Meta-analysis.. 333
    SGAs in acute bipolar I depression...................................... 333
        Placebo-controlled studies.. 341
        Olanzapine-fluoxetine combination
            versus lamotrigine 341
        Preliminary results of recent quetiapine studies.................. 342
        Adverse events.. 342
        Summary and recommendations 343
    SGAs in the maintenance treatment of bipolar I disorder 343
        Trial design and definitions.. 353
        Efficacy in preventing relapse.. 354
    Depot SGAs in the maintenance treatment of
        bipolar disorder.. 355
Conclusions 356
References.. 357

Introduction

Providing optimal pharmacotherapy for patients with bipolar disorder remains a challenge for clinicians. Bipolar patients experience symptoms in numerous domains, including mania/hypomania, depression, psychosis, and anxiety. Traditional mood stabilizing medications are ineffective or only partially effective in controlling symptoms and promoting full recovery in a substantial number of patients (Post et al., 1998), and the tolerability and acceptability to patients of mood stabilizers is frequently poor, as reflected in low rates of adherence during maintenance treatment (Lingam and Scott, 2002). Even patients who achieve symptomatic recovery from mood episodes find that functional recovery is frequently delayed or not attained (Conus et al., 2006; Tohen et al., 2003).

These facts underscore the need for medications which are effective across a broad range of symptoms in the acute and maintenance treatment of bipolar illness, and which are well tolerated by patients. In recent years the pharmacotherapeutic armamentarium for bipolar disorder has expanded dramatically (Mitchell and Malhi, 2002), and antipsychotic medications have been among the most avidly studied of the new therapies. While the clinical utility of the first-generation antipsychotics

(FGAs), such as chlorpromazine and haloperidol, has been limited by tolerability concerns, a new class of medications, the second-generation antipsychotics (SGAs), has been studied in the treatment of acute mania, bipolar depression, and in the maintenance phase of bipolar illness. They appear to be better tolerated than the FGAs, and they have become widely used in the management of bipolar disorder in North America and around the world. The purpose of this review is to critically assess data from randomized controlled trials regarding the efficacy and safety of FGAs and SGAs in all phases of bipolar disorder.

FGAs in bipolar disorder

FGAs in acute bipolar I mania

FGAs have been utilized in the treatment of bipolar patients since Delay and Deniker first demonstrated the effectiveness of chlorpromazine in controlling agitated states in 1952 (Delay, Deniker, and Harl, 1952). Until the introduction of the SGAs in the 1990s, FGAs were among the most commonly prescribed medications for bipolar patients. In fact, a meta-analysis of inpatient and outpatient studies carried out prior to the common use of SGAs reported that 74% of 2378 bipolar patients were prescribed FGAs at some point during their illness (Tohen et al., 2001).

Most of the clinical trials that assessed the efficacy of FGAs in bipolar disorder were carried out in the 1970s and early 1980s, and compared an FGA (most commonly chlorpromazine) to a mood stabilizing medication (primarily lithium). These studies suggested that while chlorpromazine has greater efficacy in reducing activity level and behavioral disturbances in manic patients, particularly early in the course of treatment (Garfinkel, Stancer, and Persad, 1980; Johnson et al., 1971; Johnson, Gershon, and Hekimian, 1968; Prien, Caffey, and Klett, 1972; Shopsin et al., 1975), lithium is more effective in decreasing core symptoms of mania (Johnson et al., 1971; Johnson, Gershon, and Hekimian, 1968; Platman, 1970; Shopsin et al., 1975; Spring et al., 1970; Takahashi et al., 1975). Two reports in which manic patients were subdivided based on psychomotor activity confirmed that chlorpromazine was more effective than lithium primarily in the "highly active" groups (Braden et al., 1982; Prien, Caffey, and Klett, 1972). Studies of comparative efficacy have generally suggested equivalence among chlorpromazine and the other FGAs in the treatment of acute mania (Cookson, Silverstone, and Wells, 1981; Janicak et al., 1988; Shopsin et al., 1975). Combination therapy trials have demonstrated that the addition of a mood stabilizing medication to an FGA was superior in efficacy compared to an FGA alone (Chou et al., 1999; Müller-Oerlinghausen et al., 2000) except when very high doses of FGAs (in the range of 30 mg/day of haloperidol equivalents) were used (Chou et al., 1999; Garfinkel, Stancer, and Persad, 1980; Klein et al., 1984), and FGA doses were consistently lower across all studies in combination therapy than monotherapy arms.

Given their previous widespread use, it is surprising that relatively few well-designed randomized controlled trials have compared FGAs to placebo in bipolar patients. Two recent placebo-controlled trials of the SGAs risperidone and quetiapine also included haloperidol arms, and reported that monotherapy with haloperidol was more effective than placebo in the treatment of acute mania (Smulevich et al., 2005; McIntyre et al., 2005). The effect was evident as early as day 4, and was maintained for the duration of both trials (21 and 84 days, respectively). Response rates at 3 weeks were 47% and 53% for haloperidol versus 33% and 35% for placebo. A single acute-phase trial comparing the addition of haloperidol or placebo to lithium or divalproex also demonstrated a significant benefit for combination therapy compared to mood stabilizer monotherapy (Sachs et al., 2002).

The utility of FGAs in bipolar disorder, particularly during maintenance treatment, must be balanced against their propensity to cause extrapyramidal symptoms and their association with exacerbation of the depressive pole of the illness. Bipolar patients are reported to have an increased liability for EPS including tardive dyskinesia, even compared to patients with schizophrenia, when treated with antipsychotic medications (Kane and Smith, 1982; Yassa, Nair, and Schwartz, 1984). Rates of EPS were 59.6% and 28% for haloperidol, versus 15.8% and 4% for placebo, in the two placebo-controlled monotherapy studies reviewed above (McIntyre et al., 2005; Smulevich et al., 2005). The depressogenic effect and poor tolerability of the FGA perphenazine was confirmed in a recent double-blind maintenance study of acutely manic patients who remitted during treatment with a mood stabilizer and perphenazine (Zarate and Tohen, 2004). Those randomized to continue perphenazine for 6 months had a shorter time to depressive relapse, higher rates of EPS, and were less likely to complete the study than those who were switched to placebo.

As a result of these concerns, the role of FGAs in bipolar patients has largely been supplanted by the SGAs since their introduction in the 1990s. Direct comparisons between FGAs and SGAs have produced mixed results. Haloperidol was found to be equivalent in efficacy to risperidone (Sachs et al., 2002; Smulevich et al., 2005) and olanzapine (Tohen et al., 2003a), superior to quetiapine on some secondary outcome measures (McIntyre et al., 2005), and inferior to aripiprazole at 12 weeks but not at 3 weeks in manic patients (Vieta et al., 2005a) in recent double blinded trials. Haloperidol was associated with more frequent treatment-emergent depression (8–18% vs 3–11% for SGAs) and markedly greater rates of EPS (24–63% vs 2–24%). Largely for tolerability reasons, the role of the FGAs in bipolar disorder today is most commonly confined to PRN use to control acute agitation, aggression, and behavioral disturbances during the early treatment of acute mania, consistent with their rapid effect in diminishing psychomotor agitation.

Depot FGAs in the maintenance treatment of bipolar disorder

The median nonadherence rate during maintenance treatment in bipolar disorder is 41%, with a range of 20–66% across studies (Lingam and Scott, 2002). The outcome of medication nonadherence is frequently dire. For example, a review of six randomized controlled trials reported that patients who discontinued lithium had a 28-fold increased risk of relapse compared to patients who were maintained on medication (Suppes, 1991). Depot medication formulations offer several advantages over oral medications in nonadherent patients (Kane, 2003). A single injection ensures an adequate supply of medication for several weeks, resulting in a reduced likelihood of rapid relapse following nonadherence. As well, injections are administered by mental health professionals, necessitating frequent contact between the patient and the treatment team, and making nonadherence immediately apparent. As no depot mood stabilizing medication has yet been developed, depot FGAs have been commonly used in bipolar patients who repeatedly relapse due to nonadherence.

Seven published studies have reported on the use of depot FGAs in bipolar disorder (Ahlfors et al., 1981; Esparon et al., 1986; Littlejohn, Leslie, and Cookson, 1994; Lowe, 1985; Lowe and Batchelor, 1986; Naylor and Scott, 1980; White, Cheung, and Silverstone, 1993). Aside from two small randomized controlled trials (RCTs) (Ahlfors et al., 1981; Esparon et al., 1986), these studies were case series or open-label trials which compared depot treatment to retrospectively-obtained information on course of illness prior to depot therapy. The preponderance of evidence suggests that depot FGAs decrease the frequency and severity of manic symptoms during maintenance treatment, but that they worsen the depressive phase of bipolar illness, particularly in patients with a significant depressive burden prior to initiating depot therapy. Depressive symptoms became more prominent during depot therapy in three of the four studies from which this information could be extracted (Ahlfors et al., 1981; Esparon et al., 1986; White, Cheung, and Silverstone, 1993), and improved marginally in only one (Littlejohn, Leslie, and Cookson, 1994). The open-label study with the largest sample size indicated that improvement in manic symptoms was outweighed by a worsening of depression (Ahlfors et al., 1981). Furthermore, depot medication did not guarantee medication adherence, as the three reports from which data could be extracted reported discontinuation rates of 20% (Naylor and Scott, 1980), 27% (Esparon et al., 1986), and 33% (Lowe and Batchelor, 1986). Based on these studies, depot FGAs can be recommended only for bipolar patients with a predominantly manic course of illness who repeatedly relapse due to nonadherence, or who fail to respond to standard therapies (Bond, Pratoomsri, and Yatham, 2007).

SGAs in bipolar disorder

The term second-generation antipsychotic, or "atypical antipsychotic", refers to a class of medications which are efficacious in treating psychosis but which have less propensity than FGAs to cause EPS (Jibson and Tandon, 1998; Kane, 1993). Pharmacodynamically, SGAs have a higher affinity for the serotonin type-2A (5HT-2A) receptor than the dopamine type-2 (D2) receptor. This may underlie their decreased liability for EPS (Kane, 1993), though that view remains controversial (Kapur and Seeman, 2001). The antimanic activity of SGAs has been repeatedly demonstrated, and is most likely related to their blockade or partial agonism of D2 receptors (Yatham, 2003), and in this respect they are similar to the FGAs. Some, but not all, of the SGAs have also been shown to have antidepressant properties, but the mechanism of this effect is less clear. It may result from their blocking 5HT-2A receptors, as 5HT-2 antagonism and down-regulation have been associated with antidepressant response (Yatham et al., 1999, 2001). Additionally, a metabolite of quetiapine, the SGA with the most convincing evidence for acute antidepressant activity, has recently been shown to inhibit the presynaptic reuptake of norepinephrine (Goldstein et al., 2007; McIntyre et al., 2007), which might confer additional antidepressant properties.

Six SGAs—risperidone, olanzapine, quetiapine, ziprasidone, aripiprazole, and clozapine—are currently commercially available in North America. Clinical trials of monotherapy and combination therapy with SGAs have been carried out in patients with acute mania, acute bipolar depression, and in the maintenance treatment of bipolar illness. The results of these studies are reviewed below.

SGAs versus placebo in acute bipolar I mania

For the treatment of acute mania, olanzapine, quetiapine, ziprasidone, and aripiprazole have each been compared to placebo in two published RCTs, and risperidone has been examined in three trials (Bowden et al., 2005; Hirschfeld et al., 2004; Keck et al., 2003a,b; Khanna et al., 2005; McIntyre et al., 2005; Potkin et al., 2005; Sachs et al., 2006; Smulevich et al., 2005; Tohen et al., 1999, 2000). In addition, preliminary results have been presented for a placebo-controlled trial of an extended release preparation of quetiapine (quetiapine XR) (Cutler et al., 2008) (Table 11.1). Change from baseline to endpoint in Young Mania Rating Scale (YMRS) score after 3 weeks of treatment (4 weeks in one olanzapine study) was the primary outcome measure in all studies except the ziprasidone trials, which utilized

Table 11.1 Randomized Placebo-Controlled Trials of SGAs in the Treatment of Acute Mania

Study	Duration	Study arms	YMRS scores	Response/ remission rates	Separation from placebo	Depression rating scale scores	Common side effects
Risperidone							
Hirschfeld et al., 2004	3 weeks	Risperidone: N=134 Range: 1–6 mg/day Mean modal dose: 4.1 mg/day Placebo: N=125	*Baseline:* R: 29.1 P: 29.2 *Change during treatment:* R: –10.6 P: –4.8 *Difference:* 5.8	*Response:* R: 43% P: 24% *Remission:* R: 38% P: 20%	3 days	The authors noted that MADRS scores decreased during the trial in the risperidone arm, but no other information was provided	*Discontinuation due to AE:* R: 8% P: 6% *Weight change:* R: 1.63 kg P: –0.25 kg EPS (measured by ESRS) were greater in risperidone arm Increased PRL in risperidone arm Other common S/E: somnolence, dyspepsia, nausea
Khanna et al., 2005	3 weeks	Risperidone: N=146 Range: 1–6 mg/day Mean modal dose: 5.6 mg/day Placebo: N=144	*Baseline:* R: 37.1 P: 37.5 *Change during treatment:* R:–23.2 P: –10.8 *Difference:* 12.4	*Response:* R: 73% P: 36% *Remission:* R: 42% P: 13%	1 week	*Baseline MADRS:* R: 5.1 P: 5.9 *Change during treatment:* R: –3.2 P: –2.5	*Discontinuation due to AE:* R: 3.4% P: 2.1% *Weight change:* R: 0.07 kg P: 0.06 kg *EPS:* R: 35% P: 6% Increased PRL in risperidone arm

(continued)

Table 11.1 Randomized Placebo-Controlled Trials of SGAs in the Treatment of Acute Mania (Continued)

Study	Duration	Study arms	YMRS scores	Response/ remission rates	Separation from placebo	Depression rating scale scores	Common side effects
Smulevich et al., 2005	3 weeks	Risperidone: N=154 Range: 1–6 mg/day Mean modal dose: 4.2 mg/day Placebo: N=140	Baseline: R: 32.1 P: 31.5 Change during treatment: R: −15.1 P: −9.4 Difference: 5.7	Response: R: 48% P: 33% Remission: R: N/A P: N/A	1 week	Baseline MADRS: R: 6.6 P: 6.3 Change during treatment: R: −3.4 P: −1.7	Discontinuation due to AE: R: 4% P: 5% Weight change: R: 0.3 kg P: 0.0 kg EPS: R: 17% P: 9%
Olanzapine							
Tohen et al., 1999	3 weeks	Olanzapine: N=70 Range: 5–20 mg/day Mean modal dose: 14.9 mg/day Placebo: N=69	Baseline: O: 28.7 P: 27.7 Change during treatment: O: −10.3 P: −4.9 Difference: 5.4	Response: O: 49% P: 24% Remission: O: N/A P: N/A	3 weeks	Baseline HAM-D: O: 12.6 P: 14.0 Change during treatment: O: −2.9 P: −3.0	Discontinuation due to AE: O: 0% P: 3% Weight change: O: 1.7 kg P: −0.4 kg EPS: no greater than PBO Other common S/E: Somnolence, dry mouth, dizziness

Tohen et al., 2000	4 weeks	Olanzapine: N=55 Range: 5–20 mg/day Mean modal dose: 16.4 mg/day Placebo: N=60	Baseline: O: 28.8 P: 29.4 Change during treatment: O: –14.8 P: –8.1 Difference: 6.7	Response: O: 65% P: 43% Remission: O: 61% P: 36%	1 week	Baseline HAM-D: O: 17.3 P: 16.2 Change during treatment: O: –7.8 P: –4.5 Patients with moderate–severe symptoms (baseline HAM-D ≥20): O: –12.3 P: –6.8	Discontinuation due to AE: O: 4% P: 2% Weight change: O: 2.1 kg P: 0.5 kg EPS: no greater than PBO. Other common S/E: Somnolence
Quetiapine McIntyre et al., 2005	3 weeks 12 week data also presented	Quetiapine: N=101 Range: 400–800 mg/day Mean modal dose: N/A Placebo: N=100	Baseline: Q: 34.0 P: 33.1 Change during treatment: 3 weeks: Q: –12.3 P: –8.3	3 weeks: Response: Q: 43% P: 35% Remission: Q: 28% P: 24% 12 weeks:	4 days	Baseline MADRS: Q: 9.1 P: 9.2 Change during treatment: 3 weeks: Q: –2.8 P: –0.9	Discontinuation due to AE: Q: 5% P: 6% Weight change (12 weeks): Q: 2.1 kg P: –0.1 kg Weight gain ≥7%: Q: 13% P: 4%

(continued)

Table 11.1 Randomized Placebo-Controlled Trials of SGAs in the Treatment of Acute Mania (*Continued*)

Study	Duration	Study arms	YMRS scores	Response/remission rates	Separation from placebo	Depression rating scale scores	Common side effects
			12 weeks: Q: −17.5 P: −9.5 *Difference:* 3 weeks: 4.0 12 weeks: 8.0	*Response:* Q: 61% P: 39% *Remission:* Q: 61% P: 35%		12 weeks: Q: −3.3 P: −0.7 *Treatment-emergent MDE:* Q: 2.9% P: 8.9%	EPS: Q: 12% P: 16% PRL decreased during treatment in quetiapine group Other common S/E: Somnolence
Bowden et al., 2005	3 weeks 12 week data also presented	Quetiapine: N=107 *Range:* 400–800 mg/day *Mean last-week dose in responders:* 3 weeks: 586 mg/day 12 weeks: 618 mg/day Placebo: N=97	*Baseline:* Q: 32.7 P: 34.0 *Change during treatment:* 3 weeks: Q: −14.6 P: −6.7 12 weeks: Q: −20.3 P: −9.0 *Difference:* 3 weeks: 7.9 12 weeks: 11.3	3 weeks: *Response:* Q: 53% P: 27% *Remission:* Q: 47% P: 22% 12 weeks: *Response:* Q: 72% P: 41% *Remission:* Q: 69% P: 34%	7 days	*Baseline MADRS:* Q: 6.1 P: 6.2 *Change during treatment:* 3 weeks: Q: −1.6 P: −0.1 12 weeks: Q: −1.5 P: 1.2	*Discontinuation due to AE:* Q: 7% P: 4% *Weight change (12 weeks):* Q: 2.6 kg P: −0.1 kg EPS: no different than PBO Other common S/E: Somnolence, dry mouth, dizziness

Cutler et al., 2008	3 weeks	Quetiapine XR: N=149 Range: 400–800 mg/day Mean dose: 604 mg/day Placebo: N=159	Baseline: N/A Change during treatment: Q: −14.3 P: −10.5 Difference: 3.8	Response: Q: 55% P: 33% Remission: Q: 42% P: 28%	4 days	Baseline MADRS: N/A Change during treatment: Q: −4.4 P: −1.9	Discontinuation due to AE: Q: 5% P: 8% Weight change: Q: 1.3 kg P: 0.1 kg EPS: Q: 7% P: 4% Other common S/E: Somnolence, dry mouth, headache, constipation, dizziness
Ziprasidone							
Keck et al., 2003	3 weeks	Ziprasidone: N=140 Range: 80–160 mg/day Mean last-week dose: 130.1 mg/day Placebo: N=70	Baseline: Z: 27.0 P: 26.7 Change during treatment: Z: −12.4 P: −7.8 Difference: 4.6	Response: Z: 50% P: 35% Remission: Z: N/A P: N/A	2 days	N/A	Discontinuation due to AE: Z: 4% P: 1% Weight change: no different than PBO; data not provided EPS: hypertonia (11% vs 3%) and akathisia (11% vs 6%) Other common S/E: Somnolence, dizziness
Potkin et al., 2005	3 weeks	Ziprasidone: N=137 Range: 80–160 mg/day	Baseline: Z: 26.2 P: 26.4	Response: Z: 46% P: 29%	7 days	MADRS and HAM-D scores derived from SADS-C	Discontinuation due to AE: Z: 6% P: 2%

(continued)

Table 11.1 Randomized Placebo-Controlled Trials of SGAs in the Treatment of Acute Mania (*Continued*)

Study	Duration	Study arms	YMRS scores	Response/remission rates	Separation from placebo	Depression rating scale scores	Common side effects
		Mean last-week dose: 126.5 mg/day; Placebo: N=65	*Change during treatment:* Z: −11.1; P: −5.6; *Difference:* 5.5	*Remission:* Z: N/A; P: N/A	(separated from PBO at 2 days, then not significantly different at 4 days)	*Baseline MADRS:* Z: 13.3; P: 11.9; *Change in MADRS during treatment:* Z: −3.7; P: −2.1; *Baseline HAM-D:* Z: 7.0; P: 6.4; *Change in HAM-D during treatment:* Z: −2.4; P: −1.4	*Weight change(median):* Z: 0 kg; P: 0 kg; *EPS:* Z: 11%; P: 2%; QTc interval increased by 10.1 ms in ziprasidone arm; no patient had QTc > 480 ms; Other common S/E: Somnolence, dizziness, headache, tremor, nausea
Aripiprazole							
Keck et al., 2003	3 weeks	*Aripiprazole:* N=130; *Range:* 15–30 mg/day	*Baseline:* A: 28.2; P: 29.7	*Response:* A: 40%; P: 19%	4 days	*CGI for depression at endpoint:*	*Discontinuation due to AE:* A: 11%; P: 10%

Study	Duration	Dose	Outcome	Response/Remission		Weight/Side effects
		Mean dose at endpoint: 27.9 mg/day Placebo: N=132	*Change during treatment:* A: −8.2 P: −3.4 *Difference:* 4.8	*Remission:* A: N/A P: N/A	A: 3.6 P: 4.4	*Weight change:* A: −0.3 kg P: −0.8 kg EPS: akathisia (11%), tremor (6%) Prolactin levels decreased with treatment in aripiprazole arm Other common S/E: Somnolence, nausea, vomiting, dyspepsia, constipation
Sachs et al., 2006	3 weeks	Aripiprazole: N=137 Range: 15–30 mg/day Mean dose at endpoint: 27.7 mg/day Placebo: N=135	*Baseline:* A: P: *Change during treatment:* A: −12.5 P: −7.2 *Difference:* 5.3	*Response:* A: 53% P: 32% *Remission:* A: N/A P: N/A		
	4 days				*Baseline MADRS:* A: N/A P: N/A *Change during treatment:* A: −4.3 P: −3.0 *Baseline CGI for depression:* A: 2.66 P: 2.59 *Change during treatment:* A: −0.6 P: −0.3	*Discontinuation due to AE:* A: 9% P: 8% *Weight change:* A: 0.5 kg P: 0.2 kg EPS: akathisia more common in aripiprazole arm (18% vs 5%) Prolactin levels decreased with treatment in aripiprazole arm Other common S/E: Somnolence, nausea, dyspepsia, constipation

the Mania Rating Scale (MRS) from the Schedule for Affective Disorders and Schizophrenia. Twelve week data were additionally presented for the two published quetiapine studies, and one risperidone study was followed by a 9-week open label extension. All trials enrolled moderately to severely manic patients (YMRS≥20 or MRS≥14) and included patients with psychotic mania. Patients with mixed episodes were enrolled in the olanzapine, ziprasidone, aripiprazole and quetiapine XR trials and one risperidone study, and patients with a rapid cycling course were included in the olanzapine, aripiprazole and quetiapine XR trials.

Change in the primary outcome measure

All placebo-controlled studies reported significantly greater improvement on the primary outcome measure in the SGA arm compared to the placebo arm. Change from baseline to week 3 in mania rating scale scores in SGA patients varied considerably between studies, from 8.2 points to 15.1 points. One risperidone study, which enrolled particularly ill patients (baseline YMRS score=37.1), demonstrated a very large improvement (23.2 points) over 3 weeks. The average differences between the medication and placebo groups, however, were remarkably similar in the trials involving olanzapine (6.05 points), quetiapine (5.94 in the two published studies), ziprasidone (5.05), and aripiprazole (5.07). The difference between medication and placebo in two of three risperidone studies also fell within this range (5.7 and 5.8), while the study with severely ill patients demonstrated a greater difference (12.4). Mean mania rating scale scores at study endpoint ranged from 13.9 to 21.7, indicating ongoing mild to moderate manic symptoms. Along with the fact that 12 week data from the two quetiapine trials demonstrated continued improvement in YMRS scores, with additional decreases of 5.2 and 5.7 points over the last 9 weeks, this suggests that 3 weeks is an insufficient duration of treatment for complete recovery in most patients.

Onset of action

Medications which are rapidly effective can shorten the duration of acute manic episodes and reduce the length of hospital stays. The first clinical trial of an SGA in bipolar disorder compared olanzapine to placebo, and assessed efficacy weekly beginning at 1 week post-baseline. It did not detect a difference between medication and placebo until week 3. The authors hypothesized that this might be related to a relatively low starting dose of olanzapine (10 mg daily), and the fact that patients experiencing their first manic episode, who might have a high placebo response rate, were included in the trial. A second olanzapine trial, which utilized a 15 mg starting dose and required patients to have experienced at least one previous manic or mixed episode detected a significant difference between medication and placebo at week 1, the first post-baseline timepoint.

All subsequent placebo-controlled SGA studies have excluded patients experiencing their first mania, and measured efficacy as early as 2–4 days after enrolment. One risperidone study demonstrated an onset of action at day 3, and the remaining two separated from placebo at week 1. The two quetiapine trials demonstrated separation of medication from placebo at day 4 and week 1, while quetiapine XR separated from placebo at day 4. Ziprasidone was superior to placebo at day 2 in two studies, but in only one trial was the difference sustained; in the second study, medication and placebo were not significantly different at the day 4 measurement, but sustained separation occurred at 1 week. In both aripiprazole trials, medication was superior to placebo beginning at day 4.

Dosages

Dose ranges and mean medication doses in trials comparing SGAs and placebo are reported in Table 11.1. As noted above, a comparison of the two olanzapine studies suggests that a starting dose of 15 mg is more effective than 10 mg. The mean modal doses of olanzapine in the two studies were 14.9 and 16.4 mg daily, respectively, suggesting that 15 mg daily will be a sufficient dose for many patients. The initial dose of risperidone was 3 mg daily in all three published reports. The mean modal doses in two of the studies were 4.1 and 4.2 mg daily, while the study that enrolled very ill patients reported a higher dose of 5.6 mg daily. Quetiapine was initiated at a dose of 100 mg daily in both studies, titrated over 4 days to 400 mg and was prescribed at 400–800 mg/day thereafter. The mean dose in responders at endpoint was reported as 586 mg daily at 3 weeks, and 618 mg daily at 12 weeks, in one study (Bowden et al., 2005). The final dose was not reported in the second study. In the quetiapine XR trial, quetiapine was initiated at 300 mg daily, increased to 600 mg daily on day 2, and prescribed at 400–800 mg daily from days 3 to 21. A final dose of 604 mg at 3 weeks was reported. The starting doses of ziprasidone and aripiprazole were 80 and 30 mg daily, respectively. Mean doses during the last week of treatment for ziprasidone were 130.1 and 126.5 mg daily, and the average doses at endpoint for aripiprazole were 27.9 and 27.7 mg daily.

Response and remission rates

The goal of treatment of bipolar disorder is full remission, not simply a reduction in the number or severity of manic symptoms. All studies reviewed here reported rates of response, defined as a reduction in YMRS score by 50% compared to baseline, while remission rates were less consistently reported. Medication response rates at 3 weeks among studies varied considerably, from 40% to 73%. The differences in response rates between medication and placebo were more consistent, ranging from 15% to 26%, with two exceptions: the risperidone study which enrolled very ill patients, which reported a difference of 37%, and one quetiapine study, with a difference of 8%.

Only two risperidone studies, one olanzapine study, two quetiapine studies, and the quetiapine XR study reported rates of remission, which was variable defined. The three quetiapine studies reported rates of remission, which was variably defined. Post-hoc reanalyses additionally reported remission rates for both olanzapine reports combined (Chengappa et al., 2005) and both quetiapine reports combined (Vieta et al., 2005). The most commonly-used definition of remission was a YMRS score ≤ 12, and remission rates using this definition are available for the above studies except one risperidone report (Khanna et al., 2005). When this definition is employed, remission rates at 3 weeks were highly variable across studies, from 28% to 61%. The difference in remission rates between medication and placebo was 18–29% with the exception of one quetiapine study (difference = 4%) and the quetiapine XR study (difference = 14%). Twelve week data from the two quetiapine studies indicates that response rates increased by a further 18–19% and remission rates by 22–33%.

Rates of depressive symptoms

Patients with mixed episodes were included in most clinical trials, including the olanzapine, ziprasidone, and aripiprazole trials, one risperidone study (Khanna et al., 2005), and the quetiapine XR trial, but were excluded from the remaining risperidone and quetiapine trials. Scores on depression rating scales were reported in most trials, even those that did not enrol patients in full mixed episodes (Table 11.1). The average severity of depressive symptoms at study entry was low in most reports. Nonetheless, depression rating scale scores declined with treatment in all studies, and improved significantly compared to placebo in the risperidone, quetiapine and quetiapine XR trials. Given the low severity of depressive symptoms and the relatively modest improvements noted, the clinical significance of these findings is uncertain.

One olanzapine trial (Tohen et al., 2000) reported on patients with moderate to severe depressive symptoms (defined as a baseline HAM-D score of ≥ 20), and found that olanzapine-treated patients experienced a greater improvement than those who received placebo (12.3 vs 6.8 HAM-D points). In the same trial, rates of treatment-emergent depression did not differ between the olanzapine and placebo arms (11.1% vs 17.9%, $p = 0.42$). Thus, the available data indicate that SGAs do not worsen depressive symptoms during the short-term treatment of acute mania, and that olanzapine improves depressive symptoms in patients with significant mixed symptomatology.

SGAs versus active comparators in acute bipolar I mania

Eleven clinical trials have compared the efficacy of SGAs to traditional mood stabilizing medications (lithium or divalproex) or the FGA haloperidol in the treatment of acute mania (Berk, Ichim, and Brook,

1999; Bowden et al., 2005; DelBello et al., 2006; McIntyre et al., 2005; Niufan et al., 2007; Segal, Berk, and Brook, 1998; Smulevich et al., 2005; Tohen et al., 2002a, 2003a; Vieta et al., 2005a; Zajecka et al., 2002) (Table 11.2). One trial (Segal, Berk, and Brook, 1998) had three study arms (risperidone vs lithium vs haloperidol), bringing the total number of comparisons against active comparators to 12. One trial comparing quetiapine and divlaproex was carried out in adolescents (DelBello et al., 2006), while all others enrolled adult patients. Study duration varied from 3 to 12 weeks, and some trials reported outcomes from more than one timepoint. In addition to comparisons with mood stabilizers and FGAs, a single trial has compared the efficacy of risperidone and olanzapine in the treatment of mania (Perlis et al., 2006).

Comparisons with haloperidol
Trials comparing risperidone, olanzapine, quetiapine, and aripiprazole to haloperidol have been reported (Table 11.2). All studies enrolled patients who were moderately to severely ill (YMRS≥20), and included patients with psychotic mania. Patients experiencing mixed episodes were eligible to be enrolled in the olanzapine and aripiprazole trials. Patients with a rapid cycling course were specifically excluded from the risperidone, quetiapine, and aripiprazole studies, and it is not clear whether they were enrolled in the olanzapine study.

Improvement in YMRS scores at 3–6 weeks was reported in all trials, and 12 week data were also included in the olanzapine, quetiapine, and aripiprazole trials. Improvement in YMRS scores at 3–6 weeks for the SGAs ranged from 12.3 to 21.3 points, over 3–6 weeks very similar to the improvement reported in placebo-controlled studies. YMRS scores in patients receiving haloperidol improved by 13.9–23.5 points. Haloperidol was equally efficacious to risperidone and aripiprazole at 3 and 4 week timepoints, but a significant difference in response and remission rates favoring aripiprazole was detected at 12 weeks. Haloperidol was associated with a significantly greater improvement in YMRS scores than quetiapine at 3 weeks, though the difference was not sustained at 12 weeks, suggesting that it may be related to a more rapid onset of action with haloperidol. Subgroup analyses revealed that haloperidol was more effective than olanzapine and quetiapine in treating psychotic mania, and this reached statistical significance in the quetiapine trial. As was the case with placebo-controlled SGA trials, those that also included 12 week data reported ongoing improvement and greater rates of response and remission with longer treatment.

Depression rating scale scores were low in all studies comparing SGAs to haloperidol (see Table 11.2). Both SGAs and haloperidol were associated with modest reductions in average depression scores with treatment, though numerically greater improvement was consistently seen in SGA-treated

Table 11.2 Active-Comparator Trials of SGAs in the Treatment of Acute Mania

Study	Duration	Study arms	YMRS scores	Response/remission rates	Separation from comparator	Depression rating scale scores	Common side effects
		Comparisons with Haloperidol					
Risperidone							
Segal et al., 1998	4 weeks	Risperidone: N=15 Dose: 6 mg daily Haloperidol: N=15 Dose: 10 mg daily	NB–Mania Rating Scale used as primary outcome *Baseline:* R: 28.6 H: 24.8 *Change during treatment:* R: −16.2 H: −18.2	N/R	No significant differences between treatments by endpoint	N/R	EPS (measured by Simpson-Angus Scale): R=H Weight change and other side effects: N/R
Smulevich et al., 2005	3 weeks	Risperidone: N=154 *Range: 1–6 mg/day Mean modal dose:* 4.2 mg/day Haloperidol: N=144 *Range: 2–12 mg/day*	*Baseline:* R: 32.1 H: 31.3 P: 31.5 *Change during treatment:* R: −15.1 H: −13.9 P: −9.4	*Response:* R: 48% H: 47% P: 33% *Remission:* N/R	*Risperidone vs placebo:* Week 1 *Haloperidol vs placebo:* Week 1	*Baseline MADRS:* R: 6.6 H: 6.8 P: 6.3 *Change during treatment:* R: −3.4 H: −2.8 P: −1.7	*Discontinuation due to A/E:* R: 4% H: 3% P: 5% *Weight change:* R: 0.3 kg H: 0.4 kg P: 0.0 kg

			Mean modal dose: 8.0 mg/day Placebo: N=140	Difference: R vs P: 5.7 H vs P: 4.5			EPS: R: 17% H: 40% P: 9%
Olanzapine							
Tohen et al., 2003	12 weeks (6 week data presented for efficacy; 12 week data presented for adverse events)	Olanzapine: N=234 Range: 5–20 mg/day Mean dose: 15.0 mg/day Haloperidol: N=219 Range: 3–15 mg/day Mean dose: 7.1 mg/day	Baseline: O: 31.1 H: 30.6 Change during treatment: O: –21.3 H: –23.5	Response (defined as ≥ 70% reduction in YMRS score): O: 55% H: 62% Remission (defined as YMRS score ≤ 12 and HAM-D ≤ 8): O: 52.1% H: 46.1%	N/R	Baseline HAM-D: O: 8.0 H: 8.1 Change during treatment: O: –2.8 H: –1.8 Change in patients with mixed symptoms: O: –7.2 H: –1.9	Discontinuation due to A/E: O: 8.1% H: 11.4% Weight change: O: 2.8 kg H: 0.0 kg Weight change ≥ 7%: O: 39.7% H: 16.1% EPS: O: 2.1% H: 23.7%

(continued)

Table 11.2 Active-Comparator Trials of SGAs in the Treatment of Acute Mania (*Continued*)

Study	Duration	Study arms	YMRS scores	Response/ remission rates	Separation from comparator	Depression rating scale scores	Common side effects
						Change in patients with severe depression (HAM-D ≥ 20): O: −8.2 H: −12.5 *Treatment-emergent MDE (by week 12):* O: 9.4% H: 16.8%	*Other common S/E:* O: somnolence, dizziness H: increased salivation
Quetiapine							
McIntyre et al., 2005	3 weeks 12 week data also presented	Quetiapine: N=101 *Range: 400–800 mg/day Mean modal dose:* Haloperidol: N=98	*Baseline:* Q: 34.0 H: 32.3 P: 33.1 *Change during treatment:*	3 weeks: *Response:* Q: 43% H: 56% P: 35% *Remission:* Q: 28% H: 37% P: 24%	Q vs P: 4 days H vs P: 4 days H vs Q: 21 days	*Baseline MADRS:* Q: 9.1 H: 8.3 P: 9.2 *Change during treatment:*	*Discontinuation due to AE:* Q: 5% H: 10% P: 6%

Range: 2–8 mg/day
Mean modal dose:
Placebo: *N*=100

3 weeks:
Q: −12.3
H: −15.7
P: −8.3

12 weeks:
Q: −17.5
H: −18.9
P: −9.5
Difference:
3 weeks:
Q vs P: 4.0
H vs P: 7.4
12 weeks:
Q vs P: 8.0
H vs P: 9.4

12 weeks:
Response:
Q: 61%
H: 70%
P: 39%
Remission:
Q: 61%
H: 63%
P: 35%

3 weeks:
Q: −2.8
H: −2.3
P: −0.9

12 weeks:
Q: −3.3
H: −1.9
P: −0.7
Treatment-emergent MDE (by week 12):
Q: 2.9%
H: 8.1%
P: 8.9%

Weight change (12 weeks):
Q: 2.1 kg
H: 0.2 kg
P: −0.1 kg
Weight gain ≥7%:
Q: 13%
H: 5%
P: 4%
EPS:
Q: 12%
H: 60%
P: 16%
PRL decreased during treatment in quetiapine and haloperidol groups
Other common S/E:
Q: Somnolence
H: Tremor

(continued)

Table 11.2 Active-Comparator Trials of SGAs in the Treatment of Acute Mania (*Continued*)

Study	Duration	Study arms	YMRS scores	Response/ remission rates	Separation from comparator	Depression rating scale scores	Common side effects
Aripiprazole							
Vieta et al., 2005	12 weeks (3 week and 12 week data presented for efficacy; 12 week data presented for adverse events)	Aripiprazole: N=175 Range: 15–30 mg/day Mean dose at endpoint: 22.6 mg/day Haloperidol: N=172 Range: 10–15 mg/day Mean dose at endpoint: 11.6 mg/day	Baseline: A: 31.1 H: 31.5 Change during treatment: 3 weeks: A: −15.7 H: −15.7 12 weeks: A: −19.9 H: −18.2	3 weeks: Response: A: 51% H: 43% Remission: A: 35% H: 31% 12 weeks: Response: A: 50% H: 28% Remission: A: 50% H: 27%	No significant difference between treatments based on change in YMRS score Response and remission rates were greater at 12 weeks in ripiprazaole arm	Baseline MADRS: A: 9.2 H: 9.8 Change during treatment: 3 weeks: A: −3.1 H: −1.6 12 weeks: A: −2.0 H: −0.7 Treatment-emergent MDE (by week 12): A: 11.0% H: 17.7%	Discontinuation due to A/E: A: 10% H: 31% Weight change (3 weeks): A: −0.1 kg H: 0.3 kg Weight change (12 weeks): A: 0.3 kg H: −0.1 kg EPS: A: 24% H: 63% PRL decreased during treatment with aripiprazole and increased (mean 7.7 mg/mL) with haloperidol

Comparisons with Lithium

Risperidone

						Other common S/E: A: insomnia H: akathisia
Segal et al., 1998	4 weeks	Risperidone: N=15 *Dose:* 6 mg daily Lithium: N=15 *Dose range:* 800–1200 mg daily *Mean serum level:* 0.64	*NB–Mania Rating Scale used as primary outcome* *Baseline:* R: 28.6 L: 28.4 *Change during treatment:* R: −16.2 L: −12.7	N/R	N/R	No significant differences between treatments by endpoint	*EPS (measured by Simpson-Angus Scale):* R>Li Weight gain and other side effects: N/R

Olanzapine

Berk et al., 1999	4 weeks	Olanzapine: N=15 *Dose:* 10 mg/day Lithium: N=15 *Dose:* 800 mg/day *Mean serum level:* 0.74	*NB–Mania Scale used as primary outcome* *Baseline:* O: 31.7 L: 31.6 *Change during treatment:* O: −18.4 L: −21.5	N/R	N/R	No significant differences between treatments by endpoint	*EPS (measure by Simpson-Angus Scale):* O=Li

(continued)

Table 11.2 Active-Comparator Trials of SGAs in the Treatment of Acute Mania (*Continued*)

Study	Duration	Study arms	YMRS scores	Response/ remission rates	Separation from comparator	Depression rating scale scores	Common side effects
Niufan et al., 2007	4 weeks	Olanzapine: N=69 Dose range: 5–20 mg/day Mean dose: 17.8 mg/day Mean dose at endpoint: 18.3 mg/day Lithium: N=71 Dose range: 600–1800 mg/day Mean dose: 1110 mg/day Mean serum level: N/R 32.8% had level < 0.8	*Baseline:* O: 34.0 L: 32.4 *Change during treatment:* O: −24.6 L: −20.2	*Response:* O: 87% L: 73% *Remission (YMRS score ≤12):* O: 83% L: 74%	Day 28 (separated at day 3, then no difference from days 7–21)	*Baseline MADRS:* O: 5.2 L: 5.0 *Change during treatment:* O: −3.3 L: −2.5	*Discontinuation due to A/E:* O: 0% L: 1% *Weight change:* O: 1.9 kg L: 0.7 kg *Weight change ≥7%:* O: 16.2% L: 2.9% *EPS:* O: 1.4% L: 2.8% *Other common A/E:* O: constipation, somnolence, nausea L: nausea

Quetiapine

Bowden et al., 2005	3 weeks 12 week data also presented	Quetiapine: N=107 Range: 400–800 mg/day Mean last-week dose in responders: 3 weeks: 586 mg/day 12 weeks: 618 mg/day Lithium: N=98 Range: at discretion of investigator Mean serum level: 3 weeks: 0.80 12 weeks: 0.80 Placebo: N=97	Baseline: Q: 32.7 L: 33.3 P: 34.0 Change during treatment: 3 weeks: Q: −14.6 L: −15.2 P: −6.7 12 weeks: Q: −20.3 L: −20.8 P: −9.0 Difference: 3 weeks: Q vs P: 7.9 L vs P: 8.5 12 weeks: Q vs P: 11.3 L vs P: 11.8	3 weeks: Response: Q: 53% L: 53% P: 27% Change during treatment: Remission: Q: 47% L: 49% P: 22% 12 weeks: Response: Q: 72% L: 76% P: 41% Remission: Q: 69% L: 72% P: 34%	Q v P: Day 7 L v P: Day 7	Baseline MADRS: Q: 6.1 L: 6.3 P: 6.2 Change during treatment: 3 weeks: Q: −1.6 L: N/R P: −0.1 12 weeks: Q: −1.5 L: −1.8 P: 1.2 Treatment-emergent depression (by 12 weeks): Q: 5.6% L: 3.1% P: 8.4%	Discontinuation due to AE: Q: 7% L: 6% P: 4% Weight change (12 weeks): Q: 2.6 kg L: 0.7 kg P: −0.1 kg EPS: Q=L=P Other common S/E: Q: Somnolence, dry mouth, dizziness L: Tremor, insomnia, headache

(continued)

Table 11.2 Active-Comparator Trials of SGAs in the Treatment of Acute Mania (*Continued*)

Study	Duration	Study arms	YMRS scores	Response/ remission rates	Separation from comparator	Depression rating scale scores	Common side effects
			Comparisons with Divalproex				
Olanzapine							
Tohen et al., 2002	3 weeks	Olanzapine: N=125 *Dose range: 5–20 mg/day Mean modal dose: 17.4 mg/day* Divalproex: N=126 *Dose range: 500–2500 mg/day Mean modal dose: 1401 mg/day Mean serum level at endpoint: 83.9 mcg/L.* 12% had blood level ≤ 50 mcg/L at endpoint	Baseline: O: 27.4 D: 27.9 Change during treatment: O: –13.4 D: –10.4	*Response:* O: 54% D: 42% *Remission (YMRS score ≤12):* O: 47% D: 34%	Day 14 (separated at day 2 but no difference at days 3 and 7)	*HAM-D score at baseline:* O: 13.4 D: 14.8 *Change during treatment:* O: –4.9 D: –3.5 *Change in patients with severe MDE (HAM-D ≥ 20):* O: –10.3 D: –8.1	*Discontinuation due to A/E:* O: 10% D: 7% *Weight change:* O: 2.5 kg D: 0.9kg EPS: O=D *Other common A/E:* O: somnolence, dry mouth, tremor D: nausea, vomiting, diarrhea

| Zajecka et al., 2002 | 3 weeks 12 week data on adverse events also presented | Olanzapine: *N=57* *Dose range: 5–25 mg/day* *Mean maximum dose: 14.7 mg/g* Divalproex: *N=63* *Dose range: 750–3250 mg/day* *Mean maximum dose: 2115 mg/day* *Mean serum level:* 10 days: 101.2 mgc/mL 12 weeks: 84.6 mcg/mL (Day 21 level not provided) | *NB–Mania Rating Scale used as primary outcome* *Baseline:* O: 32.3 D: 30.8 *Change during treatment:* O: –17.2 D: –14.8 | N/R | No significant differences between treatments by endpoint | *HAM-D score at baseline:* O: 15.1 D: 14.9 *Change during treatment:* O: –8.1 D: –6.7 | *Discontinuation due to A/E (by 12 weeks):* O: 9% D: 11% *Weight change (at 12 weeks):* O: 4.0 kg D: 2.5 kg *Other common A/E:* O: somnolence, edema, rhinitis, increased cholesterol, increased LDL D: somnolence One death due to diabetic ketoacidosis in a patient receiving O. |

(continued)

Table 11.2 Active-Comparator Trials of SGAs in the Treatment of Acute Mania (*Continued*)

Study	Duration	Study arms	YMRS scores	Response/ remission rates	Separation from comparator	Depression rating scale scores	Common side effects
Quetiapine							
DelBello el al, 2006	4 weeks	Quetiapine: *N*=25 *Dose range:* 400–600 mg/day *Mean dose at endpoint:* 412 mg/day Divalproex: *N*=25 *Dose range:* N/R; prescribed to produce a serum level of 80–120 mcg/mL *Mean serum level at endpoint:* 101 mcg/mL 96% had therapeutic serum level (≥ 80 mcg/mL) at endpoint	Baseline: Q: 35 D: 36 *Change during treatment:* Q: −23 D: −19	*Response (CGI-BP score ≤ 2)* Q: 72% D: 40% Remission (YMRS score ≤ 12): Q: 60% D: 28%	No significant changes between treatments by endpoint	*Baseline score on Childhood Depression Rating Scale – Revised:* Q: 53 D: 58 *Change during treatment:* Q: −21 D: −22	*Discontinuation due to A/E:* Q: 0% D: 0% *Weight change:* Q: 4.4 kg D: 3.6 kg Other common A/E: Q: sedation, dizziness, gi upset, dry mouth D: sedation, dizziness, gi upset, insomnia

Risperidone Versus Olanzapine

			Baseline:	Response:	No significant	Baseline	Discontinuation
Perlis et al., 2006	3 weeks	Risperidone: N=164 Dose range: 1–6 mg/day Mean modal dose: 3.9 mg/day Olanzapine: N=165 Dose range: 5–20 mg/day Mean modal dose: 14.7 mg/day	R: 26.7 O: 26.6 Change during treatment: R: −16.6 O: −15.0	R: 60% O: 62% Remission (YMRS ≤ 12 and HAM-D ≤ 8): R: 29% O: 39%	difference between treatments by endpoint	HAM-D score: R: 15.7 O: 16.0 Baseline MADRS score: R: 16.1 O: 16.6 Change during treatment: HAM-D: R: −5.2 O: −6.1 MADRS: R: −5.4 O: −6.2	due to A/E: R: 8.5% O: 5.5% Weight change: R: 1.6 kg O: 2.5 kg EPS: O=R Elevated prolactin level: R: 79.8% O: 23.4% Sexual dysfunction: R>O

patients. Haloperidol was associated with numerically greater rates of treatment-emergent depression than olanzapine (16.8% vs 9.4%), quetiapine (8.1% vs 2.9%) and aripiprazole (17.7% vs 11.0%) over 12 weeks of treatment.

Haloperidol was associated with modestly greater rates of study discontinuation due to adverse events in most trials, and a substantially greater rate compared to aripiprazole (31% vs 10%). Rates of EPS were consistently greater with haloperidol than SGAs (24–63% vs 2–24%). Weight gain was substantially greater in patients treated with olanzapine and quetiapine compared to haloperidol, but was comparable between risperidone, aripiprazole and haloperidol.

Comparisons with lithium and divalproex

The efficacy of risperidone, olanzapine, and quetiapine has been compared with lithium, and olanzapine and quetiapine have been compared with divalproex (Table 11.2). All studies enrolled moderately to severely ill patients, including those with psychotic symptoms. Patients with mixed episodes and rapid cycling were not enrolled in the lithium trials, but were included in the comparisons with divalproex.

Improvement in YMRS scores over 3–4 weeks was reported in all trials, with 12 week data also presented for the comparison of quetiapine and lithium. YMRS scores decreased by 13.4–24.6 points in SGA-treated patients, and by 10.4–21.5 points in patients receiving mood stabilizers. Olanzapine was associated with very high response (87%) and remission (83%) rates relative to previous olanzapine studies in a 4-week comparison with lithium. This might be related to the relatively high mean dose at endpoint (18.3 mg/day, compared to 15–16 mg/day in previous trials) and the absence of patients with mixed mania and rapid cycling, unlike other olanzapine studies. Quetiapine was associated with a 23 point improvement in YMRS scores over 4 weeks in children and asolescents (12–18 years of age), almost all of whom had mixed symptomatology.

These trials generally demonstrated equivalence between SGAs and mood stabilizers with respect to improvement in YMRS scores. The only study in which an SGA evidenced superiority was a 3 week comparison of olanzapine and divalproex (Tohen et al., 2002). Interestingly, a second similarly-designed comparison of these two medications did not suggest a benefit for olanzapine (Zajecka et al., 2002). Both studies actually reported numerically similar differences between treatments (3 YMRS points vs 2.4 MRS points). The study reporting equivalence between the two treatments had a smaller sample size ($N=120$) than the study suggesting superiority of olanzapine ($N=251$), and it is likely that the resulting lower power primarily accounted for the difference between the studies in statistical significance. In some studies, some secondary outcomes including response (DelBello et al., 2006; Niufan et al., 2007) and remission rates (Delbello et al., 2002; Tohen et al., 2002) favored SGAs.

The clinical trials comparing SGAs to mood stabilizers highlight the importance of proper titration and dosing of comparator medications in active comparator trials. For instance, the average lithium level in the study comparing lithium and risperidone was only 0.64, somewhat lower than levels commonly recommended for acute mania. Almost one-third of patients in the olanzapine versus lithium trial had a lithium level below the lower end of the therapeutic range, and 17% of lithium treated patients in the quetiapine trial had received lithium in the month prior to enrolment, suggesting that they were refractory to it. The degree to which these factors affected the outcomes of the trials is difficult to determine. For example, when the patients with subtherapeutic lithium levels were removed from the analysis in the olanzapine trial, the results did not change significantly. As well, it is impossible to know how many patients received subtherapeutic doses of SGAs, as serum levels are not routinely done.

With respect to side effects, only risperidone appeared to be associated with increased rates of EPS compared to mood stabilizers. Patients receiving olanzapine and quetiapine experienced greater weight gain than those taking mood stabilizers, while weight change was not measured in the single risperidone study. One patient taking olanzapine died of diabetic ketoacidosis (Zajecka et al., 2002).

Risperidone versus olanzapine

One published report has directly compared the efficacy and safety of two SGAs: a 3-week trial comparing risperidone and olanzapine (Table 11.2). Moderately to severely manic patients, including those with mixed symptoms and rapid cycling were enrolled, but interestingly, this was the only SGA study to exclude psychotic patients. The mean modal doses for both medications were relatively low compared to previous trials (risperidone: 3.9 mg/day; olanzapine: 14.7 mg/day). Risperidone and olanzapine were equivalent with respect to improvement in YMRS scores (16.6 points vs 15.0 points) and response rates (60% vs 62%), but remission rates were significantly greater in olanzapine-treated patients (39% vs 29%). Side effects were as expected, with greater weight gain in olanzapine-treated patients and higher rates of hyperprolactinemia and sexual side effects in risperidone-treated patients. The frequency of EPS was similar between treatments.

Combination therapy studies in acute bipolar I mania

Six published reports have assessed whether the combination of a mood stabilizing medication and risperidone (Sachs et al., 2002; Yatham et al., 2003), olanzapine (Tohen et al., 2002b) or quetiapine (Delbello et al., 2002; Sachs et al., 2004; Yatham et al., 2007) is more effective than mood stabilizer plus placebo in the treatment of acute mania (Table 11.3). In addition, preliminary information is available regarding the efficacy of ziprasidone

Table 11.3 Combination Therapy Studies of SGAs in Acute Mania

Study	Duration	Study arms	YMRS scores	Response/ remission rates	Separation from comparator	Depression rating scale scores	Common side effects
Risperidone							
Yatham et al., 2003	3 weeks	Mood stabilizer + risperidone: N=75 *Dose range:* 1–6 mg/day *Median modal dose:* 4.0 mg/day Mood stabilizer + placebo: N=76	*Baseline:* R: 29.3 P: 28.3 *Change during treatment:* R: –14.5 P: –10.3 *Difference:* 4.2	*Response:* R: 59% P: 41% *Remission:* N/R	No significant difference between treatments at endpoint. Separated from placebo at week 1 but not at weeks 2 or 3.	*Baseline HAM-D score:* R: 8.6 P: 8.2 *Change during treatment:* R: –4.1 P: –2.1 *Treatment-emergent depression:* R: 1.3% P: 2.6%	*Discontinuation due to A/E:* R: 1% P: 4% *Weight change:* R: 1.7 kg P: 0.5 kg *EPS:* R: 21.3% P: 7.9%
Sachs et al., 2002	3 weeks	Mood stabilizer + risperidone: N=52 *Dose range:* 1–6 mg/day *Mean modal dose:* 3.8 mg/day Mood stabilizer + haloperidol: N=53	*Baseline:* R: 28.0 H: 27.3 P: 28.0 *Change during treatment:* R: –14.3 H: –13.4 P: –8.2	*Response:* N/R *Remission:* N/R	N/R	N/R	*Discontinuation due to A/E:* R: 4% H: 2% P: 4% *Weight change:* R: 2.4 kg H: 0.1 kg P: 0.5 kg *EPS:* R: 13%

	Duration	Design	Efficacy		Adverse effects
		Dose range: 2–12 mg/day Mean modal dose: 6.2 mg/day Mood stabilizer + placebo: N=51	Difference: R vs P: 6.1 H vs P: 5.2	N/R	H: 28% P: 4% *Other common A/E:* R: somnolence, dizziness H: somnolence, dizziness, constipation, tremor
Olanzapine Tohen et al., 2002	6 weeks	Mood stabilizer + olanzapine: N=229 Dose range: 5–20 mg/day Mean modal dose: 10.4 mg/day Mood stabilizer + placebo: N=115	*Baseline:* O: 22.3 P: 22.7 *Change during treatment:* O: –13.1 P: –9.1 Difference: 4.0	*Response:* O: 68% P: 45% *Remission (YMRS ≤ 12):* O: 79% P: 66%	*Baseline HAM-D score:* O: 14.5 P: 13.5 *Change during treatment:* O: –5.0 P: –0.9 *Patients with severe depressive symptoms (HAM-D ≥ 20):* O: –10.3 P: –1.6 *Response in patients with severe depression:* O: 43% P: 10%	*Discontinuation due to A/E:* O: 10.9% P: 1.7% *Weight change:* O: 3.1 kg P: 0.2 kg EPS: O=P *Elevated prolactin level:* O: 19.1% P: 4.3% *Other common A/E:* somnolence, dry mouth, tremor, slurred speech

(continued)

Table 11.3 Combination Therapy Studies of SGAs in Acute Mania (*Continued*)

Study	Duration	Study arms	YMRS scores	Response/ remission rates	Separation from comparator	Depression rating scale scores	Common side effects
Quetiapine							
Sachs et al., 2004	3 weeks	Mood stabilizer + quetiapine (N=91) *Dose range:* 200–800 mg/day *Mean endpoint dose:* 504 mg/day *Mean endpoint dose in responders:* 584 mg/day Mood stabilizer + placebo (N=100)	*Baseline:* Q: 31.5 P: 31.1 *Change during treatment:* Q: −13.8 P: −10.0 *Difference:* 3.8	*Response:* Q: 54% P: 33% *Remission (YMRS ≤12):* Q: 46% P: 26%	N/R	*MADRS score at baseline:* Q: 13.7 P: 14.2 *Change during treatment:* Q: −3.4 P: −2.8 *Treatment emergent depression (MADRS score ≥18):* Q: 17.3% P: 13.5%	*Discontinuation due to A/E:* Q: 6% P: 6% *Weight change:* Q: 1.6 kg P: 0.4 kg *Weight gain ≥7%:* Q: 4% P: 2% *EPS:* Q=P *Other common A/E:* somnolence, dry mouth, asthenia, postural hypotension

		Baseline:	No significant	Response:	Treatment-emergent	Discontinuation
Yatham et al., 2007	3 weeks 6 week data also reported	Mood stabilizer + quetiapine (N=106) *Dose range:* 200–800 mg/day *Mean endpoint dose in responders:* Day 21: 423 mg/day Day 42: 461 mg/day Mood stabilizer + placebo (N=105)	Q: 32.3 P: 32.6 *Change during treatment:* Day 21: Q: −15.2 P: −13.2 Day 42: Q: −17.1 P: −14.3 *Difference:* Day 21: 2.0 Day 42: 2.8	differences between treatments at week 3 or week 6	Day 21: Q: 57% P: 50% Day 42: Q: 72% P: 57% *Remission (YMRS ≤ 12):* Day 21: Q: 51% P: 40% Day 42: Q: 68% P: 57%	*depression:* Q: 6.6% P: 7.8%	*due to A/E:* Q: 2.8% P: 5.8% *Weight change:* Day 21: Q: 1.6 kg P: 0.1 kg Day 42: Q: 2.2 kg P: 0.2 kg *Weight gain ≥ 7%:* Q: 21% P: 7% *EPS:* Q: 17.9% P: 28.2% *Other common A/E:* Somnolence, dry mouth, constipation

(continued)

Table 11.3 Combination Therapy Studies of SGAs in Acute Mania (*Continued*)

Study	Duration	Study arms	YMRS scores	Response/ remission rates	Separation from comparator	Depression rating scale scores	Common side effects
DelBello et al., 2002	6 weeks	Divalproex + quetiapine (N=15) *Dose:* titrated to 450 mg/day (in all but one patient) *Mean dose:* 432 mg/day Divalproex + placebo (N=15)	*Baseline:* Q: N/R P: N/R *Change during treatment:* Q: −24.5 P: −14.0 Difference: 10.5	*Response:* Q: 87% P: 53% *Remission:* N/R	Week 6 (separated from PBO at weeks 2 and 3 but not significantly different at weeks 4 and 5)	Children's Depression Rating Scale was used but scores at baseline and endpoint were not reported. There was no difference between groups in change in CDRS scores at endpoint ($p=1.0$). One Q-treated patients discontinued study due to depression.	*Discontinuation due to A/E:* Q: 0% P: 0% *Weight change:* Q: 4.2 kg P: 2.5 kg *EPS:* Q=P Other common A/E: sedation, dry mouth

versus placebo in combination with lithium (Weisler et al., 2003). Change from baseline to endpoint in YMRS score was the primary outcome in all studies, except the ziprasidone trial, which utilized the MRS. Trial duration was either 3 or 6 weeks, and two trials reported data from both timepoints. Most studies enrolled patients with moderate—severe mania (YMRS≥20), except for the olanzapine trial, which required a YMRS score≥16, and the ziprasidone study, which required a MRS score≥14. Patients with psychotic mania were included in all studies, and those with mixed episodes were included in all trials except two quetiapine studies (Sachs et al., 2004; Yatham et al., 2007). In the third quetiapine trial, which enrolled adolescent patients, 77% had mixed mania. Rapid cycling patients were excluded from two quetiapine trials (Sachs et al., 2004; Yatham et al., 2007), and it is unclear whether they were enrolled in the other studies.

Efficacy

The average SGA doses in combination therapy trials were somewhat lower than in the monotherapy studies reviewed above, with average doses for risperidone 3.8–4.0 mg/day; for olanzapine 10.4 mg/day; and for quetiapine 423–504 mg/day. Response rates with combination treatment were 18–23% greater than those observed with mood stabilizer monotherapy in trials with risperidone, olanzapine, and one quetiapine trial, but only 7% greater in a second quetiapine trial. The highest response rate, 34% greater than placebo, was observed in a third quetiapine trial which enrolled adolescent patients, though this result must be interpreted with caution, as it was based on data only from the 53% of quetiapine treated patients who completed the trial. Remission rates were reported for three trials, and were 9–20% greater with combination therapy than mood stabilizer monotherapy.

Three combination therapy trials, however, produced negative findings on the primary outcome measure (Weisler et al., 2003; Yatham et al., 2003, 2007). This is likely related to the difficulty inherent in distinguishing a treatment effect for SGAs compared to placebo when patients in both treatment arms received an active treatment (i.e., a mood stabilizing medication). Consistent with this, response rates in the mood stabilizer plus placebo arms of these studies were 10–15% greater than in the placebo arms of monotherapy studies (33–53% vs 19–43%). This shortcoming might have been eliminated by enrolling only patients who had not responded to mood stabilizer monotherapy, but most trials did not do so. Two trials did enrol some patients who had failed a trial of a mood stabilizer, and reported that the difference in YMRS improvement between SGA and placebo in these patients was 6.3–8.3 points, compared to a difference of 0.6–1.5 points in patients who initiated treatment with a mood stabilizer and SGA concurrently (Sachs et al., 2002; Yatham et al., 2003). A second factor that may have contributed to the negative outcome in one risperidone

study (Yatham et al., 2003) was the inclusion of patients prescribed carba-
mazapine. Serum risperidone concentrations in these patients were 40%
lower than in those receiving lithium or divalproex, and removal of these
patients from the analysis produced a positive result. No other combination therapy studies included carbamazepine-treated patients.

Improvement in YMRS scores was reported separately for patients
prescribed lithium and divalproex in two studies, with one study
reporting a greater difference for combination therapy compared to
mood stabilizer plus placebo in divalproex-treated patients (Tohen et al.,
2002), and the other finding the difference to be greater in lithium-treated
patients (Sachs et al., 2004). However, it is worth noting that in all three
of the combination therapy studies in which SGA did not separate from
placebo, the majority of patients were prescribed lithium (53%, 83% and
100%) (Weisler et al.,2003; Yatham et al., 2003, 2007), while in the positive
studies, the majority received divalproex (66%, 71%, and 100%) (Delbello
et al., 2002; Sachs et al., 2004; Tohen et al., 2002). This is consistent with a
greater response rate in patients receiving lithium monotherapy, and a
greater benefit for combination therapy in patients receiving divalproex.

Effect on depressive symptoms

Consistent with previous reports, combination therapy trials demonstrated that treatment with SGAs was associated with small decreases in
depressive symptoms, and that olanzapine-treated patients who entered
into combination therapy with severe depressive symptoms (HAM-D
score$\geq$20) had substantial decreases in YMRS scores (–10.3 vs –1.6 in
placebo-treated patients). Subgroup analyses did not produce consistent
results, with risperidone achieving better outcomes in patients with pure
mania (Sachs et al., 2002), and olanzapine superior in patients with mixed
symptoms (Tohen et al., 2002b). As well, risperidone was equally efficacious
in patients with and without psychosis (Sachs et al., 2002), while olanzapine was more effective in nonpsychotic patients (Tohen et al., 2002b).

Limitations

As was the case with monotherapy studies comparing SGAs to mood stabilizers, one limitation of the combination therapy trials was the use of
suboptimal doses of mood stabilizing medications. Average serum levels
of mood stabilizers were either not reported (Yatham et al., 2003, 2007)
or were near or even below the lower end of the therapeutic range (Sachs
et al., 2004; Sachs et al., 2002; Tohen et al., 2002b) in a number of studies.

Adverse events

Side effects in the combination trials were similar to those reported in the
monotherapy studies. EPS appeared to be most common with risperidone,

weight gain with olanzapine, and sedation with quetiapine. Weight gain was generally greater with combination treatment than in the monotherapy studies, though this was confounded by differences in study length.

Meta-analysis

A recently-published meta-analysis has quantified the efficacy of SGAs in the treatment of acute bipolar I mania compared to placebo, mood stabilizers, haloperidol, and in combination therapy (Scherk, Pajonk, and Leucht, 2007). When improvement in YMRS scores from baseline to endpoint in all studies was considered, SGAs were significantly more effective than placebo, with a standardized mean difference (SMD) of −0.45 (95%CI: −0.57 to −0.32). There was a trend for superiority of SGAs over mood stabilizers, which just missed statistical significance (SMD=−0.17; 95%CI=−0.33 to 0.00), and a finding of equivalence between SGAs and haloperidol (SMD=0.11; 95%CI=−0.10 to 0.32). Pooling data from all studies demonstrated a significant benefit for combination therapy with mood stabilizer plus SGA compared to mood stabilizer plus placebo (SMD=−0.35, 95%CI=−0.47 to −0.24). There were associations between SGAs and sedation (relative risk [RR] compared to placebo=2.74, 95%CI=2.03 to 3.68), and also EPS (RR=2.71, 95%CI=1.47 − 5.00). Olanzapine and quetiapine, but not the other SGAs, were significantly associated with weight gain.

SGAs in acute bipolar I depression

Olanzapine (Tohen et al., 2003c), the combination of olanzapine and the antidepressant fluoxetine (OFC) (Tohen et al., 2003c), and quetiapine (Calabrese et al., 2005; Thase et al., 2006) have all been compared to placebo in the treatment of acute bipolar I depression. OFC has also been compared to lamotrigine in a head-to-head trial (Brown et al., 2006) (Table 11.4). As well, preliminary results are available for two studies comparing quetiapine to paroxetine and placebo (McElroy et al., 2008) and lithium and placebo (Young et al., 2008), and for a placebo-controlled trial of quetiapine XR (Suppes et al., 2008a).

Trial duration was 8 weeks for the placebo-controlled studies, and 7 weeks for the comparison of OFC and lamotrigine. Change from baseline to endpoint on the MADRS was the primary outcome measure for all studies. Patients were moderately to severely depressed, with MADRS scores of ≥30. Approximately one-third had a rapid-cycling course. Patients with mixed episodes were not enrolled in these trials, and YMRS scores were low at study entry. Psychotic symptoms were present in 4.4–13.5% of olanzapine- and OFC-treated patients; rates of psychosis were not reported in the quetiapine studies.

Table 11.4 Randomized Controlled Trials of SGAs in the Treatment of Acute Bipolar I Depression

Study	Duration	Study arms	MADRS scores	Separation from comparator	Response and remission rates	Treatment-emergent mania	Side effects
Olanzapine and Olanzapine-Fluoxetine Combination							
Tohen et al., 2003	8 weeks	Olanzapine: N=370 *Dose range:* 5–20 mg/day *Mean dose:* 9.7 mg/day Olanzapine + fluoxetine: N=86 *Doses:* 6 mg/day + 25 mg/day; 6 mg/day + 50 mg/day; 12 mg/day + 50 mg/day *Mean dose:* 7.4 mg/day +39.3 mg/day PBO: N=377	*Baseline:* OLZ: 32.6 OFC: 30.8 P: 31.3 *Change during treatment:* OLZ: 15.0 OFC: 18.5 P: 11.9 *Difference vs PBO:* OLZ: 3.1 OFC: 6.6	OLZ vs P: week 1 OFC vs P: week 1	*Response:* OLZ: 39.0% OFC: 56.1% P: 30.4% *Remission:* OLZ: 32.8% OFC: 48.8% P: 24.5%	P: 6.7% OLZ: 5.7% OFC: 6.4%	*Weight gain:* P: −0.47 kg OLZ: 2.59 kg OFC: 2.79 kg *Weight gain 7% or greater:* P: 0.3% OLZ: 18.7% OFC: 19.5% OLZ and OFC associated with significant increases in cholesterol and glucose levels. OFC associated with greater GI side effects than OLZ.

| Brown et al., 2006 | 7 weeks | Olanzapine + fluoxetine: N=205 *Doses:* 6 mg/day + 25 mg/day; 6 mg/day + 50 mg/day; 12 mg/day + 25 mg/day; 12 mg/day + 50 mg/day *Mean modal dose:* 10.7 mg/day + 38.3 mg/day Lamotrigine: N=205 *Dose range:* 25–200 mg/day *Mean modal dose:* 106.4 mg/day | *Baseline:* OFC: 30.9 L: 31.4 *Change during treatment:* O: 14.9 L: 12.9 *Difference between OFC and LTG:* 2.0 | Week 1 and all subsequent study visits except week 3 | *Response:* OFC: 68.8% L: 59.7% *Remission:* OFC: 56.4% L: 49.2% | OFC: 4.0% L: 5.2% | *Weight gain:* OFC: 3.1 kg L: −0.3 kg *Weight gain 7% or greater:* OFC: 23.4% L: 0% Tremor, somnolence, sedation, increased appetite, weight gain, and increased cholesterol, triglycerides, HbA1C significantly more common in OFC group. "Suicidal and self-injurious behavior" significantly more common in LTG group. |

(continued)

Table 11.4 Randomized Controlled Trials of SGAs in the Treatment of Acute Bipolar I Depression (Continued)

Study	Duration	Study arms	MADRS scores	Separation from comparator	Response and remission rates	Treatment-emergent mania	Side effects
Quetiapine							
Calabrese et al., 2005	8 weeks	Quetiapine 300 mg/day: N=116 Quetiapine 600 mg/day: N=114 PBO: 112	*Baseline:* Q 300 mg/day: 30.4 Q 600 mg/day: 30.3 P: 30.6 *Baseline scores reported for BDI and BDII patients combined* *Change during treatment:* Q 300 mg: 16.9 Q 600 mg: 18.1 P: 9.2 *Difference vs PBO:* Q 300 mg/day: 7.8 Q 600 mg/day: 8.9	Q 300 mg: week 1 Q 600 mg: week 1	*Response:* Q 300 mg: 62.7% Q 600 mg: 66.5% P: 38.7% *Remission:* Q 300 mg: 54.4% Q 600 mg: 56.1% P: 31.5% *Data available only for Calabrese 2005 and Thase 2006 combined*	Q 300 mg: 3.6% Q 600 mg: 3.3% P: 6.8% *Data available only for Calabrese 2005 and Thase 2006 combined*	*Weight gain:* Q 300 mg: 1.0 kg Q 600 mg: 1.6 kg P: 0.2 kg *Weight gain 7% or greater:* Q 300 mg: 8.5% Q 600 mg: 9.0% P: 1.7% Sedation, somnolence, dry mouth, dizziness, constipation significantly more common in both QTP groups *(NB—side effects reported for BDI and BDII patients combined)*

| Thase et al., 2006 | 8 weeks | Quetiapine 300 mg/day: N=104 Quetiapine 600 mg/day: N=101 PBO: N=110 | Baseline: Q 300 mg/day: 31.1 Q 600 mg/day: 29.9 P: 29.6 Baseline scores reported for BDI and BDII patients combined Change during treatment: Q 300 mg: 19.7 Q 600 mg: 18.2 P: 13.7 Difference vs PBO: Q 300 mg/day: 6.0 Q 600 mg/day: 4.5 | Q 300 mg: week 1 Q 600 mg: week 1 | Response: Q 300 mg: 62.7% Q 600 mg: 66.5% P: 38.7% Remission: Q 300 mg: 54.4% Q 600 mg: 56.1% P: 31.5% Data available only for Calabrese 2005 and Thase 2006 combined | Q 300 mg: 3.6% Q 600 mg: 3.3% P: 6.8% Data available only for Calabrese 2005 and Thase 2006 combined | *Weight gain:* Q 300 mg: 1.4 kg Q 600 mg: 1.3 kg P: 0.3 kg Sedation, somnolence, dry mouth, dizziness, constipation more common in both QTP groups. *(NB—side effects reported for BDI and BDII patients combined)* |

(continued)

Table 11.4 Randomized Controlled Trials of SGAs in the Treatment of Acute Bipolar I Depression (*Continued*)

Study	Duration	Study arms	MADRS scores	Separation from comparator	Response and remission rates	Treatment-emergent mania	Side effects
Young et al., 2008	8 weeks	Quetiapine 300 mg/day: N=255 Quetiapine 600 mg/day: N=263 Lithium: N=136 Mean dose: 970 mg/day Mean serum level: 0.61 PBO: N=129	*Baseline:* Q 300 mg/day: 28.4 Q 600 mg/day: 28.5 L: 28.4 P: 28.4 *Change during treatment:* Q 300 mg/day: 14.8 Q 600 mg/day: 16.5 L: 13.7 P: 11.2 *Difference vs. placebo:* Q 300 mg/day: 3.6 Q 600 mg/day: 5.3 L: 2.5	Q 300 mg/day: week 1 Q 600 mg/day: week 1 L: did not separate *Data available for BDI and BDII patients combined only*	*Response:* Q 300 mg/day: 69% Q 600 mg/day: 70% L: 63% P: 56% *Remission:* Q 300 mg/day: 70% Q 600 mg/day: 70% L: 63% P: 55% *Data available for BDI and BDII patients combined only*	Q 300 mg/day: 4% Q 600 mg/day: 2% L: 1% P: 2% *Data available for BDI and BDII patients combined only*	*Weight gain:* Q 300 mg: 0.6 kg Q 600 mg: 0.8 kg L: 0.2 kg P: -0.7 kg *Weight gain ≥ 7%:* Q 300 mg/day: 5% Q 600 mg/day: 8% L: 2% P: 3% *EPS:* Q 300 mg/day: 5% Q 600 mg/day: 8% L: 8% P: 4% Sedation, somnolence, dry mouth, dizziness, constipation more common in both QTP groups. *Side effects reported for BDI and BDII patients combined*

| McElroy et al., 2008 | 8 weeks | Quetiapine 300 mg/day: N=229 Quetiapine 600 mg/day: N=232 Paroxetine 20 mg/day: N=118 PBO: N=121 | *Baseline:* Q 300 mg/day: 28.1 Q 600 mg/day: 27.9 PAR: 28.3 PBO: 27.9 *Change during treatment:* Q 300 mg/day: 16.1 Q 600 mg/day: 16.4 PAR: 14.9 PBO: 13.4 *Difference vs placebo:* Q 300 mg/day: 2.7 Q 600 mg/day: 3.0 PAR: 1.5 | Q 300 mg/day: week 2 Q 600 mg/day: week 2 PAR: did not separate Data available for BDI and BDII patients combined only | *Response:* Q 300 mg/day: 67% Q 600 mg/day: 67% PAR: 55% PBO: 53% *Remission:* Q 300 mg/day: 65% Q 600 mg/day: 69% PAR: 57% PBO: 55% Data available for BDI and BDII patients combined only | Q 300 mg/day: 2% Q 600 mg/day: 4% PAR: 11% PBO: 9% Data available for BDI and BDII patients combined only | *Weight gain:* Q 300 mg: 1.1 kg Q 600 mg: 1.7 kg PAR: −0.3 kg PBO: 0.5 kg *Weight gain ≥ 7%:* Q 300 mg/day: 9% Q 600 mg/day: 11% PAR: 3% PBO: 4% *EPS:* Q 300 mg/day: 8% Q 600 mg/day: 10% PAR: 4% PBO: 2% Sedation, somnolence, dry mouth, dizziness, constipation more common in both QTP groups. *Side effects reported for BDI and BDII patients combined* |

(continued)

Table 11.4 Randomized Controlled Trials of SGAs in the Treatment of Acute Bipolar I Depression (*Continued*)

Study	Duration	Study arms	MADRS scores	Separation from comparator	Response and remission rates	Treatment-emergent mania	Side effects
Suppes et al., 2008	8 weeks	Quetiapine XR 300 mg/day: N=133 Placebo: N=137	*Baseline:* N/R *Change during treatment:* Q: 20.0 P: 14.5 *Difference vs placebo:* 5.5	Week 1 *Data available for BDI and BDII patients combined only*	*Response:* Q: 65.4% P: 43.1% *Remission:* Q: 54.1% P: 39.4% *Data available for BDI and BDII patients combined only*	Q: 4.4% P: 6.4% *Data available for BDI and BDII patients combined only*	*Weight gain:* Q: 1.3 kg P: −0.2 kg *Weight gain ≥ 7%:* Q: 8.2% P: 0.8% *EPS:* Q: 4.4% P: 0.7% Dry mouth, somnolence, sedation, increased appetite more common in QTP arm *Data available for BDI and BDII patients combined only*

Placebo-controlled studies

Both olanzapine and OFC were superior to placebo at week 1 and throughout the 8 week trial, with improvements in MADRS scores of 15.0 and 18.5 points, respectively, by endpoint, compared to a change of 11.9 points in the placebo group. Additionally, OFC was superior to olanzapine monotherapy beginning at week 4 and for the remainder of the trial. Quetiapine at doses of 300 mg/day and 600 mg/day was also more efficacious than placebo in two identically-designed trials. The magnitude of the reduction in MADRS scores in the quetiapine arms was similar in both trials (300 mg dose: 16.9 and 19.7 points; 600 mg dose: 18.1 and 18.2 points), and comparable to that seen in OFC treated patients. There appeared to be little advantage to the 600 mg dose of quetiapine in MADRS scores or in secondary outcomes such as response and remission rates. The magnitude of the difference between quetiapine and placebo was substantially greater in the first study than the second (Calabrese et al., 2005; Thase et al., 2006), primarily due to a smaller response in the placebo arm in the first trial (improvement in MADRS score of 9.2 points, compared to 13.7 in the second trial).

Although the results of the olanzapine/OFC study were interpreted as indicating that both treatments were superior to placebo, the degree to which olanzapine monotherapy has a specific antidepressant effect in acute depression is difficult to assess. The difference in MADRS improvement between treatment and placebo was substantially lower for olanzapine-treated patients (3.1 points) than those who received OFC (6.6 points), quetiapine 300 mg (7.8 and 6.0 points in the two studies), and quetiapine 600 mg (8.9 and 4.5 points). As well, response and remission rates were only modestly greater in the olanzapine arm than in placebo treated patients (response: 39.0% vs 30.4%; remission: 32.8% vs 24.5%). These were also substantially lower than response and remission rates for OFC and quetiapine (response 56.1–66.5%; remission: 48.8–56.1%). Of particular note, examination of MADRS subscale scores in olanzapine-treated patients revealed significant improvements only in reduced appetite, reduced sleep, and inner tension, consistent with the known side effects of olanzapine of appetite stimulation and sedation. OFC and quetiapine, by contrast, were associated with improvements on core depressive symptoms such as apparent sadness, reported sadness, and pessimistic thoughts. It is possible that the antidepressant effect in the OFC arm was primarily from fluoxetine, and that olanzapine itself had minimal or modest antidepressant activity.

Olanzapine-fluoxetine combination versus lamotrigine

A direct comparison of OFC and lamotrigine has also been carried out. A small but statistically significant difference in favor of OFC was apparent at week 1, and was maintained throughout the study. By endpoint, MADRS scores in OFC-treated patients improved by 14.9 points, compared to an improvement of 12.9 points in patients receiving lamotrigine. The clinical importance of this difference is not clear, as a 2 point difference in YMRS scores is unlikely to be detected by clinicians, and significant differences between the two treatments were not found on a number of secondary study outcomes, including response (68.8% for olanzapine vs 59.7% for lamotrigine) and remission rates (56.4% vs 49.2%).

Preliminary results of recent quetiapine studies

Preliminary results from two 8-week studies of quetiapine and one 8-week study of quetiapine XR produced results similar to the published quetiapine studies described above (Table 11.4). A study comparing quetiapine to lithium and placebo suggested the superiority of quetiapine over placebo, with improvements in MADRS scores of 14.8 for quetiapine 300 mg/day, 16.5 for quetiapine 600 mg/day, and 11.2 for placebo. Both doses of quetiapine were also superior to lithium (improvement in MADRS score: 13.7), but this result must be interpreted with caution as the average lithium level during the trial (0.61) was subtherapeutic (Young et al., 2008). Similarly, a comparison of quetiapine, paroxetine and placebo suggested that quetiapine, but not paroxetine, was superior to placebo in the treatment of acute bipolar depression. Improvements in MADRS scores over 8 weeks of treatment in this study were 16.1 points for quetiapine 300 mg daily, 16.4 for quetiapine 600 mg daily, 14.9 for paroxetine, and 13.4 for placebo (McElroy et al., 2008). It was not reported whether quetiapine was superior to paroxetine. Finally, a study comparing quetiapine XR 300 mg daily to placebo reported that quetiapine XR was significantly better than placebo, with improvements in MADRS scores in the bipolar I patients of 20.0 points for quetiapine XR and 14.5 points for placebo (Suppes et al., 2008a).

Adverse events

Treatment-emergent manic episodes were numerically less frequent in olanzapine-, OFC-, and quetiapine-treated patients than in those who received placebo (3.3–6.4% vs 6.7–6.8%), and were comparable between OFC and lamotrigine (4.0% vs 5.2%). Weight gain of approximately 2.5–3.0 kg was observed in olanzapine- and OFC- treated patients, compared to a smaller increase of approximately 1.0–1.5 kg in quetiapine patients and a slight weight loss in those who received lamotrigine. Clinically significant weight gain, and elevations in cholesterol and glucose levels were also apparent in the OFC and olanzapine treated groups. OFC was additionally associated with increased gastrointestinal side effects.

Summary and recommendations

Based on these results, both OFC and quetiapine can be considered first-line options for the treatment of acute bipolar depression. The magnitude of the antidepressant effect may be somewhat greater for quetiapine. Whether olanzapine monotherapy has specific antidepressant activity is less clear, and based on the available data, it cannot be recommended as a first line treatment option. This raises the possibility that antidepressant effects, unlike antimanic properties, may not be common to the SGAs as a class. In this light, it is worth noting that in a randomized (but not blinded) comparison of risperidone, lamotrgine, and inositol in addition to mood stabilizing medications and antidepressants in a mixed sample of depressed bipolar I and bipolar II patients (Nierenberg et al., 2006) risperidone was not superior to the other two medications, and in fact was associated with the lowest recovery rate (4.6% vs 23.8% for lamotrigine and 17.4% for inositol). Another study demonstrated only modest benefit when risperidone, alone or in combination with paroxetine, was added to mood stabilizing medication in the depressed phase of bipolar I or II disorders (Shelton and Stahl, 2004), though it is difficult to interpret due to its small sample size ($N=30$). Finally, preliminary unpublished results from two clinical trials comparing aripiprazole and placebo in the treatment of acute bipolar depression failed to demonstrate superiority of medication over placebo (Marcus et al., 2007). Clearly further research is needed to clarify the degree to which individual SGAs are effective in the treatment of bipolar depression.

SGAs in the maintenance treatment of bipolar I disorder

For the purposes of this review, we will consider studies which enrolled remitted bipolar patients and assessed the efficacy of treatment in preventing relapse to constitute maintenance studies. Using this definition, five published randomized double-blind trials have assessed the efficacy of SGAs in the maintenance treatment of bipolar I disorder (Keck et al., 2007; Tohen et al., 2003b, 2004, 2005, 2006) (Table 11.5). Olanzapine is the best-studied of the SGAs in maintenance therapy, having been compared to placebo, lithium, and divalproex in monotherapy trials, and to placebo in a combination therapy trial with mood stabilizers. Aripiprazole has evidence from a single published placebo-controlled monotherapy trial. Finally, preliminary results are available from a placebo-controlled trial assessing the maintenance efficacy of quetiapine monotherapy (Nolen, 2008) and from two placebo-controlled trials reporting on the efficacy of quetiapine in combination with lithium or divalproex (Suppes et al., 2008b; Vieta et al., 2008).

Table 11.5 Randomized Controlled Trials of SGAs in the Maintenance Treatment of Bipolar I Disorder

Study	Design	Study arms	Sample	% with relapse	% discontinuing trial for any reason	Median time to discontinuation	Side effects
Olanzapine							
Tohen et al., 2006	48 weeks	Olanzapine: N=225 *Dose range:* 5–20 mg/day *Mean dose:* 12.5 mg/day Placebo: N=136	Patients in symptomatic remission (YMRS ≤ 12 and HAM-D ≤8) from a recent manic or mixed episode that was treated with open-label OLZ 5–20 mg/day. Patients had at least two other manic/mixed episodes in the previous 6 years.	*Any mood episode:* O: 47% P: 80% *Manic episode:* O: 12% P: 32% *Mixed episode:* O: 4% P: 9% *Depressive episode:* O: 30% P: 39%	O: 79.7% P: 93.4%	For any reason: O: 83 days P: 26 days For any mood episode: O: 174 days P: 22 days	*Weight gain (open-label + double-blind phases):* O: 4.0 kg P: 1.0 kg Increased appetite, somnolence, sedation, dry mouth more common in OLZ arm
Tohen et al., 2005	52- weeks	Olanzapine: N=217 *Dose range:* 5–20 mg/day *Mean dose:* 11.9 mg/day Lithium: N=214	Patients in symptomatic remission (YMRS ≤ 12 and HAM-D ≤ 8) from a recent manic or mixed episode that was treatedwith open-label OLZ 5–20 mg/day and	*Any mood episode:* O: 30% L: 39% *Manic episode:* O: 14% L: 23%	O: 53.5% L: 67.3%	For any reason: O: 303 days L: 207 days	*Weight gain (open-label + double-blind phases):* O: 4.5 kg L: 1.3 kg

		Dose	Inclusion criteria				Side effects
		Mean dose: 1102.7 mg/day Mean serum level: 0.76 mEq/L	lithium. Patients had at least two other manic/mixed episodes in the previous 6 years.	*Mixed episode:* O: 1% L: 5% *Depressive episode:* O: 16% L: 11%			
Tohen et al., 2003	47 weeks	Olanzapine: N=125 *Dose range:* 5–20 mg/day *Mean dose:* 16.2 mg/day Divalproex: N=126 *Dose range:* 500–2500 mg/day *Mean dose:* 1584.7 mg/day *Mean serum level:* 58.2 mcg/mL at endpoint	Patients experiencing a manic or mixed episode with a YMRS score of ≥ 20. Patients in remission after 3 weeks of treatment were then assessed for relapse over 44 weeks of follow-up. Remission was defined in two ways: syndromal (no more than "mild" DSM symptoms of mania or depression) and symptomatic (YMRS ≤ 12 and HAM-D ≤ 8)	*Any mood episode:* O: 42% D: 57% *Manic episode:* O: 15% D: 17% *Mixed episode:* O: 3% D: 13% *Depressive episode:* O: 24% D: 26% *Calculated based on 33 O patients and 23 D patients who met remission criteria and were entered in the maintenance phase*	O: 84.8% D: 84.1% *Calculated based on entire sample of 125 O patients and 126 D patients*	*For any reason:* O: 62 days D: 49 days *Calculated based on entire sample of 125 O patients and 126 D patients*	*Weight gain:* O: 2.79 kg D: 1.22 kg *Weight gain ≥ 7%:* O: 26.3% D: 17.9% Greater increase in cholesterol but not glucose with OLZ. Low platelet levels more common with DVP. Somnolence and increased appetite more common with OLZ. There was no difference in rates of EPS between OLZ and DVP.

(continued)

Table 11.5 Randomized Controlled Trials of SGAs in the Maintenance Treatment of Bipolar I Disorder (*Continued*)

Study	Design	Study arms	Sample	% with relapse	% discontinuing trial for any reason	Median time to discontinuation	Side effects
Tohen et al., 2004	18 months	Olanzapine + mood stabilizer: *N*=51 *Dose range:* 5–20 mg/day *Mean modal dose:* 8.6 mg/day PBO + mood stabilizer: *N*=48	Patients in syndromic remission from a recent manic/mixed episode (i.e., no more than "mild" DSM symptoms of mania or depression) that was treated with OLZ 5–20 mg/day and lithium or divalproex. Sixty eight patients also met criteria for symptomatic remission (YMRS ≤ 12 and HAM-D ≤ 8) and were analyzed separately. Patients had at least two other mood episodes (depressed/manic/mixed) prior to enrolment episode.	*For those in syndromic remission: Any mood episode:* O + MS: 29% P + MS: 31% *For 68 patients in symptomatic remission: Any mood episode:* O + MS: 37% P + MS: 55% *Manic episode:* O + MS: 20% P + MS: 29% *Depressive episode:* O + MS: 23% P + MS: 40%	*For those in syndromic remission:* O + MS: 69% P + MS: 90% *For 68 patients in symptomatic remission:* N/R	*For those in syndromic remission: For any reason:* O + MS: 111 days P + MS: 82 days *Any mood episode:* O + MS: 94 days P + MS: 41 days *For 68 patients in symptomatic remission: Any mood episode:* O + MS: 163 days	*Weight gain (open-label + double-blind phases):* O + MS: 5.1 kg P + MS: 0.2 kg No significant difference between treatments in EPS, or increase in cholesterol or glucose.

Quetiapine

Study	Duration	Drug/dose	Population	Hazard Ratio		Time to relapse		Weight gain
Nolen 2008	104 weeks	Quetiapine: N=404 *Dose range:* 300–800 mg/day *Mean median dose:* 546 mg/day	Patients in remission (YMRS ≤12 and MADRS ≤12 for at least 4 weeks) from a recent manic, mixed, or depressed episode that was treated with open-label quetiapine 300–800 mg/day	*Any mood episode:* Q vs P: 0.29 L vs P: 0.46 Q vs L: 0.66 *Manic episode:* Q vs P: 0.29 L vs P: 0.37 Q vs L: 0.78	N/R	P + MS: 42 days Manic episode: O + MS: 172 days P + MS: 59 days *Depressive episode:* O + MS: 163 days P + MS: 55 days	N/R	*Weight gain:* Q: 3.6 kg (open label plus double-blind phases) L: 0.3 kg (reported for double-blind phase only) P: −5.0 kg (reported for double-blind phase only)

(continued)

Table 11.5 Randomized Controlled Trials of SGAs in the Maintenance Treatment of Bipolar I Disorder (*Continued*)

Study	Design	Study arms	Sample	% with relapse	% discontinuing trial for any reason	Median time to discontinuation	Side effects
		Lithium: N=364 Dose range: 600–1800 mg/day Mean median serum level: 0.63 mEq/L Placebo: N=404		*Depressive episode:* Q vs P: 0.30 L vs P: 0.59 Q vs L: 0.54 *NB—only hazard ratios, and not percentages experiencing relapse, were reported*			*Weight gain ≥ 7%:* Q: 41% L: 17% P: 0% *EPS:* Q: 4% L: N/R P: 5% Somnolence more common with QTP Headache, nausea, tremor, vomiting more common with Li
Vieta et al., 2008	104 weeks	Quetiapine + mood stabilizer: N=336 Dose range: 400–800 mg/day	Patients in remission (YMRS ≤12 and MADRS ≤12 for at least 4 weeks) from a recent manic, mixed, or depressed episode that was	*Any mood episode:* Q: 19% P: 49% *Manic episode:* Q: 11% P: 26%	Q: 62% P: 80%	N/R	*Weight gain:* Q: 2.0 kg (open label plus double-blind phases) P: −6.2 kg (reported for double-blind phase only)

		Mean median dose: 496 mg/day Placebo + mood stabilizer: N=367	treated with open-label quetiapine 400–800 mg/day and lithium or divalproex for ≥12 weeks	*Depressive episode:* Q: 8% P: 23%	N/R	*Weight gain ≥ 7%:* Q: 18% P: 0% *EPS:* Q: 5% P: 5% Somnolence more common with QTP
Suppes et al., 2008	104 weeks	Quetiapine + mood stabilizer: N=310 *Dose range:* 400–800 mg/day *Mean median dose:* 519 mg/day Placebo + mood stabilizer: N=313	Patients in remission (YMRS ≤12 and MADRS ≤12 for at least 4 weeks) from a recent manic, mixed, or depressed episode that was treated with open-label quetiapine 400–800 mg/day and lithium or divalproex for ≥12 weeks	*Any mood episode:* Q: 20% P: 52% *Manic episode:* Q: 7% P: 19% *Depressive episode:* Q: 13% P: 33%	Q: 81% P: 86%	*Weight gain (open label plus double-blind phases):* Q: 4.1 kg P: 0.2 kg (reported for double-blind phase only) *Weight gain ≥ 7%:* Q: 21% P: 9% EPS: Q: 11% P: 10% Somnolence and hypothyroidism more common with QTP

(continued)

Table 11.5 Randomized Controlled Trials of SGAs in the Maintenance Treatment of Bipolar I Disorder (*Continued*)

Study	Design	Study arms	Sample	% with relapse	% discontinuing trial for any reason	Median time to discontinuation	Side effects
Aripiprazole							
Keck et al., 2007	100-weeks	Aripiprazole: *N*=78 *Dose range:* 15–30 mg/day *Mean dose:* 24.1 mg/day Placebo: *N*=83	Patients in remission (YMRS ≤10 and MADRS ≤13 for at least 6 weeks) from a recent manic or mixed episode that was treated with open-label aripiprazole 15–30 mg/day for 6–18 weeks	*Any mood episode:* A: 33% P: 52% *Manic episode:* A: 12% P: 28% *Mixed episode:* A: 5% P: 6% *Depressive episode:* A: 14% P: 16% *Unknown episode:* A: 1% P: 2%	A: 91% P: 94%	N/R	*Weight gain (provided for double-blind phase only):* A: 0.4 kg P: –1.9 kg *Weight gain ≥ 7%:* A: 20% P: 5% EPS more common with ARI No significant differences in glucose, cholesterol between A and P

Risperidone Long-Acting Injectable

| Yatham, 2008 | 104 weeks | Risperidone long-acting injectable (RLAI): N=143 *Dose range:* 25–50 mg Q 2 weeks *Mean modal dose:* 27.2 mg Q 2 weeks Placebo: N=138 | Patients in remission (CGI-S ≤ 3) after 3 weeks of open-label treatment with oral risperidone followed by 26 weeks of open-label treatment with RLAI 25–50 mg Q 2 weeks. Patients may have entered the open-label treatment phase during an acute manic episode or while in remission | *Any mood episode:* R: 29% P: 57% *Manic episode:* R: 15% P: 46% *Depressive episode:* R: 14% P: 10% | N/R | N/R | *Weight gain in open-label phase:* R: 15% *Weight gain in double-blind phase:* R: 12% P: 3% 10% of patients developed above-normal fastring glucose during open-label period. |

(continued)

Table 11.5 Randomized Controlled Trials of SGAs in the Maintenance Treatment of Bipolar I Disorder (*Continued*)

Study	Design	Study arms	Sample	% with relapse	% discontinuing trial for any reason	Median time to discontinuation	Side effects
Alphs et al., 2008	52 weeks	RLAI: *N*=72 *Dose range:* 25–50 mg Q 2 weeks *Mean modal dose:* 27.9 mg Q 2 weeks Placebo: *N*=67	BDI or BDII patients with frequently-relapsing bipolar disorder (≥ 4 mood episodes in the previous year) who were in remission (YMRS and MADRS scores ≤10 and CGI-BP-S score ≤3) after 16 weeks of treatment as usual (mood stabilizers, antidepressant, and/or benzodiazepines) plus RLAI 25–50 mg Q 2 weeks	*Any mood episode:* R: 22% P: 48% *Manic episode:* R: 7% P: 21% *Depressive episode:* R: 13% P: 21% *Mixed episode:* R:3% P: 6% *Results reported for BDI and BDII patients combined*	R: 40% P: 57% *Results reported for BDI and BDII patients combined*	*Any mood episode:* R: N/A P: 307 days *Results reported for BDI and BDII patients combined*	*Weight gain in double-blind phase:* R: 7% P: 2% EPS: R:32% P: 22% *Elevated prolactin:* R: 6% P: 3% *Results reported for BDI and BDII patients combined*

The olanzapine and aripipraole studies reviewed here enrolled patients who were recently remitted from a manic episode. They also included patients with mixed symptoms, psychosis, and a rapid-cycling course, though the percentages of these patients varied markedly between trials (mixed mania: 6.3–49.5% of patients; psychotic symptoms: 18.3–73.7%; rapid cycling course: 3.0–57.4%). The quetiapine trials enrolled patients who were remitted from a recent manic, mixed, or depressed episode, and also included patients with psychosis and a rapid-cycling course of illness. The trial comparing olanzapine and divalproex, which was the first maintenance study carried out, recruited actively manic or mixed patients, and followed them during 47 weeks of treatment. Those who were in remission at 3 weeks were assessed regarding the effectiveness of medication in preventing relapse for the remainder of the trial. As only 22% (56/251) of patients met remission criteria at 3 weeks, the size of the sample for this comparison was markedly reduced. The subsequent olanzapine, aripiprazole, and quetiapine trials enrolled patients who had already remitted from a manic or mixed episode during open label treatment with the medication(s) under study, and followed them for periods of 26 weeks to 18 months.

Trial design and definitions

The term "remission" was not defined consistently between studies. The olanzapine studies considered patients with a YMRS score≤12 and a HAM-D score≤8 for at least 2 weeks to be in remission, while the aripiprazole study required a YMRS score≤10 and a MADRS score≤13 for a minimum of 6 weeks and the quetiapine studies required a YMRS score≤12 and a MADRS score≤12 for 4 weeks. As the OLZ studies had demonstrated that patients with longer periods of remission were less likely to relapse, the requirement for a longer duration of remission in the aripiprazole trial and the quetiapine trials may have resulted in the inclusion of patients with a greater likelihood of maintaining remission compared to the olanzapine studies. The definition of "recurrence" varied somewhat between reports as well. The initial olanzapine studies (comparing olanzapine to divalproex, and olanzapine plus mood stabilizer to monotherapy with a mood stabilizer) determined that olanzapine was superior in preventing "symptomatic" relapse (into *either* a full mood episode or subsyndromal episodes) but not "syndromal" relapse (into full mood episodes only). Symptomatic relapse was the definition employed in subsequent olanzapine studies. The aripiprazole versus placebo trial defined relapse as hospitalization or any change in pharmacotherapy due to depressive or manic symptoms, also a definition sensitive to mild symptoms. Thus, the published SGA maintenance studies reviewed here measure efficacy of in preventing the development of both mild and syndromal mood symptoms, and not simply relapse into full mania or depression. The definition of relapse was not explicitly stated in the preliminary information from the quetiapine studies, but they appear to assess relapse into full mania and depression.

Efficacy in preventing relapse

Due to the differences between studies, and the considerable variability in duration of follow-up, direct comparisons between maintenance trials are not as straightforward as comparisons between the acute mania studies. Nonetheless, some general observations can be made. In placebo-controlled monotherapy trials, olanzapine, aripiprazole, and quetiapine were superior to placebo in preventing relapse into any mood episode and manic episodes during maintenance treatment. The magnitude of the difference between medication and placebo in preventing relapse into any mood episode was greater for olanzapine (relapse rates: olanzapine 47% vs placebo 80%; aripiprazole 33% vs placebo 52%; quetiapine 23% vs placebo 51%). Olanzapine and quetiapine were also superior to placebo in preventing relapse into depressive episodes, while aripiprazole was not. Olanzapine, but not aripiprazole, was superior in preventing relapse into mixed episodes, while data were not provided for quetiapine.

In a head-to-head trial comparing olanzapine to divalproex, which enrolled actively manic and mixed patients, olanzapine was superior in mean improvement in YMRS score, with an average difference of 2.38 points over 47 weeks, and in median time to remission (14 days vs 62 days for divalproex). Among the patients who remitted by 3 weeks and were monitored for relapse, olanzapine demonstrated a numerical, but not statistically significant, advantage over divalproex in preventing relapse into any mood episode (42.3% of patients vs 56.5%), mania (15.2% vs 17.4%), mixed episodes (3.0% vs 13.0%), and depression (24.2% vs 26.1%). When compared to lithium in a second head-to-head trial with a larger sample size, olanzapine had a numerical advantage in preventing relapse into any mood episode (30.0% vs 38.8%), and a significant advantage in prevention of manic (13.8% vs 23.4%) and mixed (0.5% vs 4.7%) episodes. Depressive relapse occurred nonsignificantly more frequently in the olanzapine arm (15.7% vs 10.7%). A degree of caution is warranted in assessing the results of the direct comparisons of olanzapine to mood stabilizers, as in the lithium study, 37% (80/214) of the lithium patients had a documented history of poor response to lithium, while in the divalproex trial, 39% of divalproex patients had serum levels below the therapeutic range at endpoint.

The trial comparing mood stabilizer plus olanzapine to mood stabilizer plus placebo demonstrated that the combination therapy arm was superior in delaying symptomatic but not full syndromal relapse into any mood episode. Median time to relapse in the combination therapy patients was 163 days, compared to 42 days for monotherapy patients. Thirty-seven percent of combination therapy patients and 55% of monotherapy patients experienced a relapse during the follow-up period. The two trials comparing mood stabilizer plus quetiapine to mood stabilizer plus placebo demonstrated that combination therapy was superior in delaying relapse into any mood episode, mania, and depression. Relapse rates and median time to relapse was not reported.

As noted above, all of the above trials enrolled patients who had recently remitted from an index manic or mixed episode with the exception of the quetiapine trials, which enrolled patients remitted from mania, depression, or mixed episodes. As the polarity of the most recent episode has been shown to predict the polarity of relapse, patients with a recent depressive episode are at substantially elevated risk of depressive relapse (Keck et al., 2006), and the placebo arms of the three quetiapine trials confirmed this. In the trial comparing quetiapine monotherapy to placebo, quetiapine was superior in preventing relapse into any mood episode, mania and depression in both recently depressed and recently manic patients. In the two trials comparing quetiapine plus mood stabilizer to placebo plus mood stabilizer, combination therapy was superior in preventing relapse into any mood episode, mania, and depression in recently manic patients, and superior in preventing relapse into any mood episode and depression in recently depressed patients. The apparent lack of efficacy of quetiapine in preventing manic relapse in recently depressed patients was likely due to a low manic relapse rate in both the placebo and quetiapine arms. Clearly, however, further studies are needed regarding the efficacy of maintenance therapy with SGAs in recently depressed bipolar patients.

Depot SGAs in the maintenance treatment of bipolar disorder

Depot formulations of risperidone and olanzapine have been studied in bipolar patients, though only information on risperidone has been made publicly available. To date, six published reports provide data on the efficacy and safety of depot risperidone 25–50 mg IM every 2 weeks in patients with bipolar disorder (Bain et al., 2005; Han et al., 2007; Malempati, Bond, and Yatham, 2008; Medori, Braunig, and Sacchetti, 2005; Savas, Yumru, and Ozen, 2006; Yatham, Fallu, and Binder, 2007). Aside from one randomized open-label trial which compared depot risperidone to oral SGAs (Yatham, Fallu, and Binder, 2007), these studies were retrospective chart reviews or nonrandomized open-label studies. Adjunctive mood stabilizers and other medications were permitted in all studies but one (Han et al., 2007). Taken together, the results presented in these reports suggest that depot risperidone is efficacious in preventing both manic and depressive relapses during maintenance therapy in bipolar disorder, and is at least as effective and well-tolerated as oral SGAs (Yatham, Fallu, and Binder, 2007). In contrast to depot FGAs, depressive episodes were rare during treatment with depot risperidone, even in patients with a predominantly depressive course of illness (Malempati, Bond, and Yatham, 2008), and in fact depression rating scale scores decreased modestly during treatment (Bain et al., 2005; Han et al., 2007) Functional outcomes also improved during depot therapy (Han et al., 2007; Malempati, Bond, and Yatham, 2008). Weight change was modest, ranging from a loss of 0.83 kg over 1 year (Han et al., 2007) to a gain of 2 kg over 2 years (Malempati, Bond, and Yatham, 2008). Rates of EPS were also modest, with decreased scores on extrapyramidal symptom rating scales compared to the pre-depot period in most trials. In assessing weight change and EPS, it is important to note that most patients received multiple medications, often including antipsychotics, prior to initiating depot treatment.

Preliminary results have also been presented from two double-blind placebo-controlled maintenance studies of depot risperidone (Alphs et al., 2008; Yatham, 2008) (Table 11.5). A 2 year study in which euthymic patients were randomized to treatment with depot risperidone 25–50 mg Q 2 weeks or placebo demonstrated that placebo-treated patients were significantly more likely to suffer a relapse into a mood episode than risperidone-treated patients (57% vs 29%). Patients treated with placebo were especially likely to relapse into a manic episode (46% vs 15%), while the rate of depressive relapse was more similar between treatments (10% for placebo and 14% for risperidone). A 1 year study in which depot risperidone or placebo was added to treatment as usual (mood stabilizers, antidepressants, and/or benzodiazepines) also demonstrated a significant benefit for risperidone. Relapse into any mood episode occurred in 22% of risperidone treated patients and 48% who received placebo. Relapses into mania (7% vs 21%), depression (13% vs 21%), and mixed episodes (3% vs 6%) were all less frequent in risperidone treated patients.

Conclusions

While FGAs have clear anti-manic activity, their usefulness is limited by high rates of EPS and depressive symptoms, and they have therefore largely been supplanted by the SGAs in the treatment of bipolar disorder. Since their commercial introduction in the 1990s, the SGAs have been among the most exhaustively studied medications in the management of bipolar illness. The available data from randomized controlled trials demonstrates that the SGAs as a class are clearly superior to placebo in the treatment of acute mania, and that their efficacy is equivalent to that of mood stabilizing medications and FGAs. However, side effects vary between the SGAs, with olanzapine most likely to be implicated in weight gain, risperidone in causing EPS and hyperprolactinemia, and quetiapine in sedation.

The evidence also indicates that the combination of an SGA and a mood stabilizing medication is more effective than a mood stabilizer alone in the management of manic episodes, with response and remission rates 10–20% greater with combination therapy than monotherapy. However, the fact that three combination therapy trials did not separate from placebo on their primary outcome measure, and the finding in two trials that the magnitude of the effect of combination therapy was greatest in patients who had not responded to mood stabilizer monotherapy, suggests that further studies are needed to determine whether combination therapy is best targeted toward certain patient subgroups.

In contrast to their efficacy in mania, the evidence for a class effect of SGAs in bipolar depression is less compelling. Quetiapine is clearly superior to placebo in the treatment of acute depression, but the available evidence does not support the use of risperidone or aripiprazole, and studies of ziprasidone are lacking. While olanzapine reduces depressive symptoms in patients with mixed episodes, and the combination of olanzapine and fluoxetine (OFC) is efficacious in depressed patients, the acute antidepressant effect of olanzapine monotherapy appears to be relatively modest. Currently, only quetiapine and OFC can be recommended as first-line therapies for acute bipolar depression.

SGAs are also effective in preventing mood episodes during the maintenance phase of bipolar disorder. Olanzapine, quetiapine, and aripiprazole have demonstrated long-term antimanic activity during in placebo-controlled maintenance trials, and olanzapine and quetiapine are significantly more effective than placebo in preventing depression. Olanzapine has also been shown to be at least as effective as lithium and divalproex during maintenance therapy, and the combination of olanzapine plus mood stabilizer appears to offer some preventative benefits over mood stabilizer alone. The depot formulation of risperidone is also efficacious in preventing mood episodes, though the data are currently unclear as to whether it is more effective in preventing mania than depression. Maintenance studies of ziprasidone are lacking.

References

Ahlfors UG, Baastrup PC, Dencker SJ, Elgen K, Lingjaerde O, Pedersen V, Schou M, Aaskoven O. (1981). Flupenthixol decanoate in recurrent manic-depressive illness: A comparison with lithium. *Acta Psychiatr. Scand.*, 64, 226–237.

Alphs L, Haskins J, Turkoz I, et al. (2008). Adjunctive long-acting risperidone delays mood episode relapse in patients with frequently relapsing bipolar disorder [abstract P.3.c.066]. *J. Eur. Coll. of Neuropsychopharmacol., 8 (Suppl. 4)*, S441.

Bain E, Gharabawi G, Locklear J, Turkos I, Yurgelin-Todd D. (2005). A study of long-acting injectable risperidone in frequently-relapsing bipolar disorder (FRBD): Preliminary findings. Presented at the 44th Annual Meeting of the American College of Neuropsychopharmacology, Waikoloa, Hawaii.

Berk M, Ichim L, Brook S. (1999). Olanzapine compared to lithium in mania: A double-blind randomized controlled trial. *Int. Clin. Psychopharmacol., 14*, 339–343.

Bond, DJ, Pratoomsri W, Yatham LN. (2007). Depot antipsychotic medications in bipolar disorder: A review of the literature. *Acta Psychiatr. Scand., 116*, 3–16.

Bowden CL, Grunze H, Mullen J, Brecher M, Paulsson B, Jones M, Vågerö M, Svensson K. (2005). A randomized, double-blind, placebo-controlled efficacy and safety study of quetiapine or lithium as monotherapy for mania in bipolar disorder. *J. Clin. Psychiatry, 66*, 111–121.

Braden W, Fink EB, Qualls CB, Ho CK, Samuels WO. (1982). Lithium and chlorpromazine in psychotic inpatients. *Psychiatr. Res., 7*, 69–81.

Brown EB, McElroy SL, Keck PE, Deldar A, Adams DH, Tohen M, Williamson DJ. (2006). A 7-week, double-blind trial of olanzapine/fluoxetine combination versus lamotrigine in the treatment of bipolar I depression. *J. Clin. Psychiatry, 67*, 1025–1033.

Calabrese JR, Keck PE, Macfadden W, Minkwitz M, Ketter TA, Weisler RH, Cutler AJ, McCoy R, Wilson E, Mullen J. (2005). A randomized, double-blind, placebo-controlled trial of quetiapine in the treatment of bipolar I or II depression. *Am. J. Psychiatry, 162*, 1351–1360.

Chengappa KN, Hennen J, Baldessarini RJ, Kupfer DJ, Yatham LN, Gershon S, Baker RW, Tohen M. (2005). Recovery and functional outcomes following olanzapine treatment for bipolar I mania. *Bipolar Disord., 7*, 68–76.

Chou JC, Czobor P, Charles O, Tuma I, Winsberg B, Allen MH, Trujillo M, Volavka J. (1999). Acute mania: Haloperidol dose and augmentation with lithium or lorazepam. *J. Clin. Psychopharmacol., 19*, 500–505.

Conus P, Cotton S, Abdel-Baki A, Lambert M, Berk M, McGorry PD. (2006). Symptomatic and functional outcome 12 months after a first episode of psychotic mania: Barriers to recovery in a catchment area sample. *Bipolar Disord., 8*, 221–231.

Cookson J, Silverstone T, Wells B. (1981). Double-blind comparative clinical trial of pimozide and chlorpromazine in mania. A test of the dopamine hypothesis. *Acta Psychiatr. Scand., 64*, 381–397

Cutler A, Datto C, Nordenhem A, et al. (2008). Effectiveness of extended-release formulation of quetiapine as monotherapy for the treatment of acute bipolar mania (trial D144CC00004). Presented at the Annual Meeting of the American Psychiatric Association, Washington, DC.

Delay J, Deniker P, Harl JM. (1952). Therapeutic use in psychiatry of phenothiazine of central elective action (4560 RP). *Annales Medico Psychologiques, 100*, 112–117.

DelBello MP, Kowatch RA, Adler CM, Stanford KE, Welge JA, Barzman DH, Nelson E, Strakowski SM. (2006). A double-blind randomized pilot study comparing quetiapine and divalproex for adolescent mania. *J. Am. Acad. Child Adol. Psychiatry, 45*, 305–313.

Delbello MP, Schwiers ML, Rosenberg HL, Strakowski SM. (2002). A double-blind, randomized, placebo-controlled study of quetiapine as adjunctive treatment for adolescent mania. *J. Am. Acad. Child Adol. Psychiatry, 41,* 1216–1223.

Esparon J, Kolloori J, Naylor GJ, McHarg AM, Smith AH, Hopwood SE. (1986). Comparison of the prophylactic action of flupenthixol with placebo in lithium treated manic-depressive patients. *Br. J. Psychiatry, 148,* 723–725.

Garfinkel PE, Stancer HC, Persad E. (1980). A comparison of haloperidol, lithium carbonate and their combination in the treatment of mania. *J. Affect. Disord.,* 2, 279–288.

Goldstein JM, Christoph G, Grimm S, Liu JW, Widzowski D, Brecher M. (2007). Unique mechanism of action for the antidepressant properties of the atypical antipsychotic quetiapine. Presented at the 160th Annual Meeting of the American Psychiatric Association, San Diego, CA, May 19–24, 2007.

Han C, Lee MS, Pae CU, Ko YH, Patkar AA, Jung IK. (2007). Usefulness of long-acting injectable risperidone during 12-month maintenance therapy of bipolar disorder. *Prog. Neuropsychopharmacol. Biol. Psychiatry, 31,* 1219–1223.

Hirschfeld RM, Keck PE, Kramer M, Karcher K, Canuso C, Eerdekens M, Grossman F. (2004). Rapid antimanic effect of risperidone monotherapy: A 3-week multicenter, double-blind, placebo-controlled trial. *Am. J. Psychiatry,* 161, 1057–1065.

Janicak PG, Bresnahan DB, Sharma R, Davis JM, Comaty JE, Malinick C. (1988). A comparison of thiothixene with chlorpromazine in the treatment of mania. *J. Clin. Psychopharmacol.,* 8, 33–37.

Jibson MD, Tandon R. (1998). New atypical antipsychotic medications. *J. Psychiatr. Res.,* 32, 215–228.

Johnson G, Gershon S, Burdock EI, Floyd A, Hekimian L. (1971). Comparative effects of lithium and chlorpromazine in the treatment of acute manic states. *Br. J. Psychiatry, 119,* 267–276.

Johnson G, Gershon S, Hekimian LJ. (1968). Controlled evaluation of lithium and chlorpromazine in the treatment of manic states: An interim report. *Compr. Psychiatry, 9,* 563–567.

Kane JM, Smith JM. (1982). Tardive dyskinesia: Prevalence and risk factors, 1959 to 1979. *Arch. Gen. Psychiatry 39,* 473–481.

Kane JM. (1993). Newer antipsychotic drugs. A review of their pharmacology and therapeutic potential. *Drugs, 46,* 585–593.

Kane JM. (2003). Strategies for improving compliance in treatment of schizophrenia by using a long-acting formulation of an antipsychotic: Clinical studies. *J. Clin. Psychiatry, 64 (Suppl. 16),* 34–40.

Kapur S, Seeman P. (2001). Does fast dissociation from the dopamine d(2) receptor explain the action of atypical antipsychotics?: A new hypothesis. *Am. J. Psychiatry, 158,* 360–369.

Keck PE, Calabrese JR, McIntyre RS, McQuade RD, Carson WH, Eudicone JM, Carlson BX, Marcus RN. (2007). Aripiprazole monotherapy for maintenance therapy in bipolar I disorder: A 100-week, double-blind study versus placebo. *J. Clin. Psychiatry, 68,* 1480–1491.

Keck PE, Marcus R, Tourkodimitris S, Ali M, Liebeskind A, Saha A, Ingenito G. (2003a). A placebo-controlled, double-blind study of the efficacy and safety of aripiprazole in patients with acute bipolar mania. *Am. J. Psychiatry, 160,* 1651–1658.

Keck PE, Versiani M, Potkin S, West SA, Giller E, Ice K. (2003b). Ziprasidone in the treatment of acute bipolar mania: A three-week, placebo-controlled, double-blind, randomized trial. *Am. J. Psychiatry, 160,* 741–748.

Khanna S, Vieta E, Lyons B, Grossman F, Eerdekens M, Kramer M. (2005). Risperidone in the treatment of acute mania: Double-blind, placebo-controlled study. *Br. J. Psychiatry, 187,* 229–234.

Klein E, Bental E, Lerer B, Belmaker RH. (1984). Carbamazepine and haloperidol v placebo and haloperidol in excited psychoses: A controlled study. *Arch. Gen. Psychiatry, 41,* 165–170.

Lingam R, Scott J. (2002). Treatment nonadherence in affective disorders. *Acta Psychiatr. Scand., 105,* 164–172.

Littlejohn R, Leslie F, Cookson J. (1994). Depot antipsychotics in the prophylaxis of bipolar affective disorder. *Br. J. Psychiatry, 165,* 827–829.

Lowe MR, Batchelor DH. (1986). Depot neuroleptics and manic depressive psychosis. *Int. Clin. Psychopharmacol., 1 (Suppl. 1),* 53–62.

Lowe MR. (1985). Treatment of rapid cycling affective illness. *Br. J. Psychiatry, 146,* 558.

Malempati RN, Bond DJ, Yatham LN. (2008). Depot risperidone in the outpatient management of bipolar disorder: A 2-year study of 10 patients. *Int. Clin. Psychopharmacol., 23,* 88–94.

Marcus RN, Owen R, Swanink R, McQuade RD, Carson WH, Iwamoto T. (2007). Two studies to evaluate the safety and efficacy of aripiprazole monotherapy in outpatients with bipolar I disorder with a major depressive episode without psychotic features (studies CN138-096 and CN138-146). Presented at the 160th Annual Meeting of the American Psychiatric Association, San Diego, CA.

McElroy S, Young A, Carlsson A, Olausson B, Nordenhem A, Paulsson B, Brecher M. (2008). A double-blind, placebo-controlled study with acute and continuation phases of quetiapine and paroxetine in adults with bipolar depression (EMBOLDEN II). Presented at the 3rd Biennial Conference of the International Society for Bipolar Disorders, Delhi, India.

McIntyre RS, Brecher M, Paulsson B, Huizar K, Mullen J. (2005). Quetiapine or haloperidol as monotherapy for bipolar mania—A 12-week, double-blind, randomised, parallel-group, placebo-controlled trial. *European Neuropsychopharmacol., 15,* 573–585.

McIntyre RS, Scozynska JK, Woldeyohannes HO, Alsuwaidan M, Konarski JK. (2007). A preclinical and clinical rationale for quetiapine in mood syndromes. *Exp. Opin. Pharmacother., 8,* 1211–1219.

Medori R, Braunig P, Sacchetti E. (2005). Bipolar diorder: 6-months efficacy of risperidone injectable. *World J. Biol. Psychiatry, 6 (Suppl. 1),* 192–193.

Mitchell PB, Malhi GS. (2002). The expanding pharmacopoeia for bipolar disorder. *Ann. Rev. Med., 53,* 173–188.

Müller-Oerlinghausen B, Retzow A, Henn FA, Giedke H, Walden J. (2000). Valproate as an adjunct to neuroleptic medication for the treatment of acute episodes of mania: A prospective, randomized, double-blind, placebo-controlled, multicenter study. *J. Clin. Psychopharmacol., 20,* 195–203.

Naylor GJ, Scott CR. (1980). Depot injections for affective disorders. *Br. J. Psychiatry, 136,* 105.

Nierenberg AA, Ostacher MJ, Calabrese JR, Ketter TA, Marangell LB, Miklowitz DJ, Miyahara S, Bauer MS, Thase ME, Wisniewski SR, Sachs GS. (2006). Treatment-resistant bipolar depression: A STEP-BD equipoise randomized effectiveness trial of antidepressant augmentation with lamotrigine, inositol, or risperidone. *Am. J. Psychiatry, 163,* 210–216.

Niufan G, Tohen M, Qiuqing A, Fude Y, Pope E, McElroy H, Ming L, Gaohua W, Xinbao Z, Huichun L, Liang S. (2007). Olanzapine versus lithium in the acute treatment of bipolar mania: A double-blind, randomized, controlled trial. *J. Affect. Disord., 105,* 101–108.

Nolen W. (2008). New clinical data in the maintenance treatment of bipolar disorder. Presented at the 21st ECNP Congress, Barcelona, Spain.

Perlis RH, Baker RW, Zarate CA, Brown EB, Schuh LM, Jamal HH, Tohen M. (2006). Olanzapine versus risperidone in the treatment of manic or mixed states in bipolar I disorder: A randomized, double-blind trial. *J. Clin. Psychiatry, 67,* 1747–1753.

Platman SR. (1970). A comparison of lithium carbonate and chlorpromazine in mania. *Am. J. Psychiatry, 127,* 351–353.

Post RM, Frye MA, Denicoff KD, Leverich GS, Kimbrell TA, Dunn RT. (1998). Beyond lithium in the treatment of bipolar illness. *Neuropsychopharmacol., 19,* 206–219.

Potkin SG, Keck PE, Segal S, Ice K, English P. (2005). Ziprasidone in acute bipolar mania: A 21-day randomized, double-blind, placebo-controlled replication trial. *J. Clin. Psychopharmacol., 25,* 301–310.

Prien RF, Caffey EM, Klett CJ. (1972). Comparison of lithium carbonate and chlorpromazine in the treatment of mania. Report of the Veterans Administration and National Institute of Mental Health Collaborative Study Group. *Arch. Gen. Psychiatry, 26,* 146–153.

Sachs G, Chengappa KN, Suppes T, Mullen JA, Brecher M, Devine NA, Sweitzer DE. (2004). Quetiapine with lithium or divalproex for the treatment of bipolar mania: A randomized, double-blind, placebo-controlled study. *Bipolar Disord., 6,* 213.

Sachs G, Sanchez R, Marcus R, Stock E, McQuade R, Carson W, Abou-Gharbia N, Impellizzeri C, Kaplita S, Rollin L, Iwamoto T. (2006). Aripiprazole in the treatment of acute manic or mixed episodes in patients with bipolar I disorder: A 3-week placebo-controlled study. *J. Psychopharmacol., 20,* 536–546.

Sachs GS, Grossman F, Ghaemi SN, Okamoto A, Bowden CL. (2002). Combination of a mood stabilizer with risperidone or haloperidol for treatment of acute mania: A double-blind, placebo-controlled comparison of efficacy and safety. *Am. J. Psychiatry, 159,* 1146–1154.

Savas HA, Yumru M, Ozen ME. (2006). Use of long-acting risperidone in the treatment of bipolar patients. *J. Clin. Psychopharmacol., 26,* 530–531.

Scherk H, Pajonk FG, Leucht S. (2007). Second-generation antipsychotic agents in the treatment of acute mania: A systematic review and meta-analysis of randomized controlled trials. *Arch. Gen. Psychiatry, 64,* 442–455.

Segal J, Berk M, Brook S. (1998). Risperidone compared with both lithium and haloperidol in mania: A double-blind randomized controlled trial. *Clin. Neuropharmacol., 21,* 176–180.

Shelton RC, Stahl SM. (2004). Risperidone and paroxetine given singly and in combination for bipolar depression. *J. Clin. Psychiatry, 65,* 1715–1719.

Shopsin B, Gershon S, Thompson H, Collins P. (1975). Psychoactive drugs in mania. A controlled comparison of lithium carbonate, chlorpromazine, and haloperidol. *Arch. Gen. Psychiatry, 32*, 34–42.

Smulevich AB, Khanna S, Eerdekens M, Karcher K, Kramer M, Grossman F. (2005). Acute and continuation risperidone monotherapy in bipolar mania: A 3-week placebo-controlled trial followed by a 9-week double-blind trial of risperidone and haloperidol. *Eur. Neuropsychopharmacol., 15*, 75–84.

Spring G, Schweid D, Gray C, Steinberg J, Horwitz M. (1970). A double-blind comparison of lithium and chlorpromazine in the treatment of manic states. *Am. J. Psychiatry, 126*, 1306–1310.

Suppes T, Datto C, Minkwitz M, et al. (2008a). Effectiveness of the new extended-release formulation of quetiapine as monotherapy for the treatment of acute bipolar depression (trial D144CC00002). Presented at the Annual Meeting of the American Psychiatric Association, Washington, DC.

Suppes T, Liu S, Brecher M, Paulsson B, Lazarus A. (2008b). Maintenance treatment in bipolar I disorder with quetiapine concomitant with lithium or divalproex: A placebo-controlled, randomized multicentre trial (trial D1447C00127). Presented at the 3rd Biennial Conference of the International Society for Bipolar Disorders, Delhi, India, January 27–30, 2008.

Suppes, T. (1991). Risk of recurrence following discontinuation of lithium treatment in bipolar disorder. *Arch. Gen. Psychiatry, 48*, 1082–1088.

Takahashi R, Sakuma A, Itoh K, Itoh H, Kurihara M. (1975). Comparison of efficacy of lithium carbonate and chlorpromazine in mania. report of collaborative study group on treatment of mania in Japan. *Arch. Gen. Psychiatry, 32*, 1310–1318.

Thase ME, Macfadden W, Weisler RH, Chang W, Paulsson B, Khan A, Calabrese JR. (2006). Efficacy of quetiapine monotherapy in bipolar I and II depression: A double-blind, placebo-controlled study (the BOLDER II study). *J. Clin. Psychopharmacol., 26*, 600–609.

Tohen M, Baker RW, Altshuler LL, Zarate CA, Suppes T, Ketter TA, Milton DR, Risser R, Gilmore JA, Breier A, Tollefson GA. (2002a). Olanzapine versus divalproex in the treatment of acute mania. *Am. J. Psychiatry, 159*, 1011–1017.

Tohen M, Calabrese JR, Sachs GS, Banov MD, Detke HC, Risser R, Baker RW, Chou JC, Bowden CL. (2006). Randomized, placebo-controlled trial of olanzapine as maintenance therapy in patients with bipolar I disorder responding to acute treatment with olanzapine. *Am. J. Psychiatry, 163*, 247–256.

Tohen M, Chengappa KN, Suppes T, Baker RW, Zarate CA, Bowden CL, Sachs GS, Kupfer DJ, Ghaemi SN, Feldman PD, Risser RC, Evans AR, Calabrese JR. (2004). Relapse prevention in bipolar I disorder: 18-month comparison of olanzapine plus mood stabiliser v. mood stabiliser alone. *Br. J. Psychiatry, 184*, 337–345.

Tohen M, Chengappa KN, Suppes T, Zarate CA Jr, Calabrese JR, Bowden CL, Sachs GS, Kupfer DJ, Baker RW, Risser RC, Keeter EL, Feldman PD, Tollefson GD, Breier A. (2002b). Efficacy of olanzapine in combination with valproate or lithium in the treatment of mania in patients partially nonresponsive to valproate or lithium monotherapy. *Arch. Gen. Psychiatry, 59*, 62–69.

Tohen M, Goldberg JF, Gonzalez-Pinto Arrillaga AM, Azorin JM, Vieta E, Hardy-Bayle M-C, Lawson WB, Emsley RA, Zhang F, Baker RW, Risser RC, Namjoshi, MA, Evans AR, Breier A. (2003a). A 12-week, double-blind comparison of olanzapine vs haloperidol in the treatment of acute mania. *Arch. Gen. Psychiatry, 60,* 1218–1226.

Tohen M, Greil W, Calabrese JR, Sachs GS, Yatham LN, Oerlinghausen BM, Koukopoulos A, Cassano GB, Grunze H, Licht RW, Dell'Osso L, Evans AR, Risser R, Baker RW, Crane H, Dossenbach MR, Bowden CL. (2005). Olanzapine versus lithium in the maintenance treatment of bipolar disorder: A 12-month, randomized, double-blind, controlled clinical trial. *Am. J. Psychiatry, 162,* 1281–1290.

Tohen M, Jacobs TG, Grundy SL, McElroy SL, Banov MC, Janicak PG, Sanger T, Risser R, Zhang F, Toma V, Francis J, Tollefson GD, Breier A. (2000). Efficacy of olanzapine in acute bipolar mania: A double-blind, placebo-controlled study. *Arch. Gen. Psychiatry, 57,* 841–849.

Tohen M, Ketter TA, Zarate CA, Suppes T, Frye M, Altshuler L, Zajecka J, Schuh LM, Risser RC, Brown E, Baker RW. (2003b). Olanzapine versus divalproex sodium for the treatment of acute mania and maintenance of remission: A 47-week study. *Am. J. Psychiatry, 160,* 1263–1271.

Tohen M, Sanger TM, McElroy SL, Tollefson GD, Chengappa KN, Daniel DG, Petty F, Centorrino F, Wang R, Grundy SL, Greaney MG, Jacobs TG, David SR, Toma V. (1999). Olanzapine versus placebo in the treatment of acute mania. *Am. J. Psychiatry, 156,* 702–709.

Tohen M, Vieta E, Calabrese J, Ketter TA, Sachs G, Bowden C, Mitchell PB, Centorrino F, Risser R, Baker RW, Evans AR, Beymer K, Dube S, Tollefson GD, Breier A. (2003c). Efficacy of olanzapine and olanzapine-fluoxetine combination in the treatment of bipolar I depression. *Arch. Gen. Psychiatry, 60,* 1079–1088.

Tohen M, Zarate CA Jr, Hennen J, Khalsa HM, Strakowski SM, Gebre-Medhin P, Salvatore P, Baldessarini RJ. (2003d). The McLean-Harvard first-episode mania study: Prediction of recovery and first recurrence. *Am. J. Psychiatry, 160,* 2099–2107.

Tohen M, Zhang F, Taylor CC, Burns P, Zarate C, Sanger T, Tollefson G. (2001). A meta-analysis of the use of typical antipsychotic agents in bipolar disorder. *J. Affect. Disord., 65,* 85–93.

Vieta E, Bourin M, Sanchez R, Marcus R, Stock E, McQuade R, Carson W, Abou-Gharbia N, Swanink R, Iwamoto T. (2005a). Effectiveness of aripiprazole v. haloperidol in acute bipolar mania: Double-blind, randomised, comparative 12-week trial. *Br. J. Psychiatry, 187,* 235–242.

Vieta E, Eggens I, Persson I, Paulsson B, Brecher M. (2008). Efficacy and safety of quetiapine in combination with lithium/divalproex as maintenance treatment for bipolar I disorder. *Bipolar Disord., 10 (Suppl. 1),* 57.

Vieta E, Mullen J, Brecher M, Paulsson B, Jones M. (2005b). Quetiapine monotherapy for mania associated with bipolar disorder: Combined analysis of two international, double-blind, randomised, placebo-controlled studies. *Curr. Med. Res. Opin., 21,* 923–934.

Weisler R, Dunn J, English P. (2003). Adjunctive ziprasidone for acute bipolar mania: Randomized, placebo-controlled trial. Presented at the 4th International Forum on Mood and Anxiety Disorders, Monte Carlo, Monaco.

White E, Cheung P, Silverstone T. (1993). Depot antipsychotics in bipolar affective disorder. *Int. Clin. Psychopharmacol., 8*, 119–122.

Yassa R, Nair V, Schwartz G. (1984). Tardive dyskinesia and the primary psychiatric diagnosis. *Psychosomatics, 25*, 135–138.

Yatham LN. (2003). Brain imaging investigations of dopaminergic pathways in mood disorders. In Soares JC (Ed.), *Brain Imaging in Affective Disorders*. New York: Marcel Dekker.

Yatham LN. (2008). Current maintenance treatments for bipolar disorder. Presented at the XVII CINP, Munich, Germany.

Yatham LN, Fallu A, Binder CE. (2007). A 6-month randomized open-label comparison of continuation of oral atypical antipsychotic therapy or switch to long acting injectable risperidone in patients with bipolar disorder. *Acta Psychiatr. Scand., 116*, 50–56.

Yatham LN, Grossman F, Augustyns I, Vieta E, Ravindran A. (2003). Mood stabilisers plus risperidone or placebo in the treatment of acute mania. international, double-blind, randomised controlled trial. *Br. J. Psychiatry, 182*, 141–147.

Yatham LN, Liddle PF, Dennie J, Shiah IS, Adam MJ, Lane CJ, Lam RW, Ruth TJ. (1999). Decrease in brain serotonin 2 receptor binding in patients with major depression following desipramine treatment: A positron emission tomography study with fluorine-18-labeled setoperone. *Arch. Gen. Psychiatry, 56*, 705–711.

Yatham LN, Liddle PF, Shiah IS, Lam RW, Adam MJ, Zis AP, Ruth TJ. (2001). Effects of rapid tryptophan depletion on brain 5-HT(2) receptors: A PET study. *Br. J. Psychiatry, 178*, 448–453.

Yatham LN, Vieta E, Young AH, Möller HJ, Paulsson B, Vågerö M. (2007). A double blind, randomized, placebo-controlled trial of quetiapine as an add-on therapy to lithium or divalproex for the treatment of bipolar mania. *Int. Clin. Psychopharmacol., 22*, 212–220.

Young AH, McElroy S, Chang W, Olausson B, Paulsson B, Brecher M. (2008). A double-blind, placebo-controlled study with acute and continuation phase in adults with bipolar depression (EMBOLDEN I). Presented at the 3rd Biennial Conference of the International Society for Bipolar Disorders, Delhi, India.

Zajecka JM, Weisler R, Sachs G, Swann AC, Wozniak P, Sommerville KW. (2002). A comparison of the efficacy, safety, and tolerability of divalproex sodium and olanzapine in the treatment of bipolar disorder. *J. Clin. Psychiatry, 63*, 1148–1155.

Zarate CA, Tohen M. (2004). Double-blind comparison of the continued use of antipsychotic treatment versus its discontinuation in remitted manic patients. *Am. J. Psychiatry, 161*, 169–171.

chapter twelve

Antidepressants for bipolar disorder: A review of efficacy

Harm J. Gijsman
University Medical Centre Nijmegen

Willem A. Nolen
University of Groningen

Contents

Introduction 366
Efficacy of various classes of antidepressants 367
    Randomized studies 367
        Tricyclic antidepressants 367
        Monoamine oxidase inhibitors (MAOI) 367
        Selective serotonin re-uptake inhibitors (SSRIs) 368
        Venlafaxine 369
        Bupropion 369
        Other antidepressants 369
Systematic review 370
Maintenance treatment 370
    Randomized studies 370
    Systematic review 372
Adverse effects 372
    Switch to (hypo)mania during acute treatment 372
        Naturalistic studies 372
        Randomized studies 373
        Reviews 373
    Conclusions 374
    (Hypo)mania during maintenance treatment 374
        Rapid cycling 375
        Retrospective studies 375
        Prospective study 375

Randomized studies 376
Conclusion 376
Withdrawing antidepressants 376
Naturalistic studies 376
Conclusion 377
Epilogue 377
References 377

Introduction

A switch from severe depression to severe mania is arguably one of the most impressive courses of illness that a patient and his or her psychiatrist can encounter. Many such patients will have been on antidepressants at the time of this switch; in these patients there is always the question and even an ongoing debate about whether the antidepressant has caused the switch, or whether the natural course of the illness has contributed to this switch. As a consequence of this debate however, over the past decades, the place of antidepressants in the treatment of bipolar disorder has switched almost as dramatically from first choice (even in maintenance treatment) to no place at all, in some guidelines not even in the acute treatment of bipolar depression.

The first antidepressants were discovered 50 years ago serendipitously because they improved depressive symptoms in patients who were prescribed the medications for other reasons. From that moment on, antidepressants have become a standard treatment for unipolar depression, based on evidence from hundreds of clinical trials. In bipolar depression, few randomized placebo controlled exist. Hence, in the absence of firm evidence, there has been much room for expert opinion, and as a consequence the role of antidepressants in bipolar depression has been much debated for two main reasons: one related to doubts about antidepressants actual efficacy; and the second is in relation to concerns about their propensity to induce switch to mania and destabilize the course of bipolar disorder.

This latter concern originally seems to have been based on either case reports (Bunney, 1978) or on much smaller body of evidence such as naturalistic studies (Wehr & Goodwin, 1987). This has however not prevented a rather restricted recommendation for the use of antidepressants in several guidelines. Only more recently, these guidelines have been challenged on this point (Möller & Grunze, 2000; Gijsman et al., 2004).

In this chapter, we will try to summarize the results of the limited number of studies that reported on the efficacy and/or on potential harmful effects of antidepressants in bipolar disorder, in the acute treatment of bipolar depression as well as maintenance treatment of bipolar disorder.

Efficacy of various classes of antidepressants

Randomized studies

Tricyclic antidepressants

One 6-week RCT compared imipramine ($n=30$) with placebo ($n=29$) (Cohn et al., 1989). The proportion of patients completing the study between the imipramine group (47%) and placebo group (34%) was not significantly different. Similarly, there was no significant difference in clinical response between imipramine and placebo groups. However, the reduction in Hamilton Depression Rating Scale (HDRS) score was significantly greater (6 points) for imipramine than for placebo.

One 10-week RCT compared imipramine ($n=39$) up to 300 mg per day (average 166 mg per day) with placebo ($n=43$) (Nemeroff et al., 2001). Almost 60% of patients completed the study. There was no significant difference in clinical response. All patients were on lithium as well. In an *a priori* defined sub-group of patients with lithium levels under 0.8 meq/L, the reduction in HDRS score was on average 5 points less in the placebo group. This suggests that the main treatment effect was due to higher lithium levels and not to antidepressants. The authors suggested that antidepressants should only be used in patients who cannot tolerate high lithium levels or who do not respond to lithium.

Monoamine oxidase inhibitors (MAOI)

One 6-week RCT compared the irreversible non-selective MAOI tranylcypromine ($n=28$; doses not given) with placebo ($n=31$) in patients with anergic depression (Himmelhoch et al., 1982). About 50% of patients had bipolar depression and none used a mood-stabilizer. Thirty-nine patients (66%) completed the study. Significantly more (20/28) patients in the tranylcypromine group had a clinical response compared to those on placebo (4/31).

Another 6-week RCT from the same group compared tranylcypromine ($n=28$; up to 60 mg per day, average dose 37 mg per day) monotherapy with imipramine ($n=28$; up to 300 mg per day, average dose 245 mg per day) alone in patients with "anergic" bipolar depression (Himmelhoch et al., 1991). On average 70% of patients completed the study: 60% in the imipramine group and 80% in the tranylcypromine group. Tranylcypromine was significantly more effective than imipramine.

A study from the Stanley Foundation Bipolar Network (SFBN) compared tranylcypromine with lamotrigine, as add-on to a mood stabilizer in patients not responding to conventional antidepressants (Nolen et al., 2007). In this failed study (only 20 of 70 planned patients were included), 5/8 patients (63%) on tranylcypromine responded without mania versus only 4/11 patients (36%) on lamotrigine (difference not statistically significant).

There are no studies comparing the reversible, selective MAO-A inhibitor (RIMA) moclobemide with placebo.

One 8-week RCT compared moclobemide ($n=81$; up to 750 mg per day) with imipramine ($n=75$; up to 150 mg per day) add-on to lithium. 69% of patients completed the study. There was no difference in efficacy between the two groups. There was however a striking, but not statistically significant difference in mania induction: two patients on moclobemide and six on imipramine had a manic switch.

Selective serotonin re-uptake inhibitors (SSRIs)

In the study by Cohn et al. (1989), there also was a comparison between fluoxetine up to 80 mg (average dose 66 mg) and placebo. 57% of patients on fluoxetine completed the study versus 34% on placebo. It is unclear what the primary efficacy measure was in this study but on all efficacy variables, the improvement in fluoxetine group was numerically greater than the placebo group. On the HDRS, the reduction in the fluoxetine group was significantly greater (10 points) than the placebo group. The clinical response for fluoxetine was better than placebo (and than imipramine).

In the study by Nemeroff et al. (2001), there also was a comparison between paroxetine up to 50 mg per day (average dose 32 mg per day) and placebo. There was no difference between the two groups in the intent-to-treat population on the primary efficacy measure, but in the sub-group of patients with lithium levels below 0.8 meq/L, paroxetine was more effective than placebo add-on to lithium.

One large 8-week RCT allowed for a comparison between fluoxetine ($n=86$) and placebo ($n=370$) (Tohen et al., 2003), both given in combination with olanzapine (average dose 7–10 mg per day). These data were extracted from a large study comparing fluoxetine plus olanzapine with olanzapine alone and with placebo (total $n=833$). Fluoxetine was given up to 50 mg per day with an average dose of 39 mg per day. Only 51% of patients completed this study. The clinical response and remission rates for the fluoxetine group were with 56% and 49%, significantly higher than for the placebo group (39% and 33%).

One small 6-week RCT among non-responders to either lithium or valproate compared addition of paroxetine (average dose 36 mg per day) with addition of a second (i.e. other) mood-stabilizer (Young et al., 2000). In the paroxetine group ($n=11$) there were no drop-outs, while in the other group ($n=16$) six patients dropped out. In all completers, there was a 9 point average reduction in HDRS score with no difference between groups. Based on the higher drop out in the second mood stabilizer group, the authors concluded that adding an antidepressant seems more suitable than adding a second mood-stabilizer.

Venlafaxine

There are no double blind studies comparing venlafaxine with placebo.

A 6-week single-blind RCT compared venlafaxine ($n=30$; average dose 179 mg per day) with paroxetine ($n=30$; average dose 32 mg per day) (Vieta et al., 2002) add-on to a mood stabilizer. Seventy-seven % of patients completed the study. There was no difference in clinical response. Four patients on venlafaxine switched to mania while only one patient did so on paroxetine.

A large 10-week RCT trial from the SFBN ($n=174$) compared venlafaxine, sertraline and bupropion, added to ongoing treatment with a mood stabilizer and/or an atypical antipsychotic (Post et al., 2006). Drop-out ranged from 20 to 40%. All three antidepressants were associated with a similar range of acute response (49–53%) and remission (34–41%). The switch to mania was greater in the venlafaxine group.

Bupropion

There are no studies that have randomized bipolar patients between monotherapy with bupropion and placebo. Two studies often included in reviews on bipolar depression have actually included only unipolar patients (Fabre et al., 1983; Merideth & Feighner, 1983; Gijsman et al., 2004).

One small 8-week RCT compared bupropion ($n=8$; average dose 358 mg per day) with desipramine ($n=7$; average dose 140 mg per day) (Sachs et al., 1994). There was no difference in treatment effect. Two patients developed mania on desipramine and one on bupropion. In a following cross-over study and a maintenance phase of one year, a further three patients developed (hypo)mania on desipramine and none on bupropion. The authors concluded that bupropion is less likely to induce mania.

In a recent large placebo-controlled study by the Systematic Treatment Enhancement Program for Bipolar Disorder (STEP-BD), 366 patients were randomized to double-blind treatment with an antidepressant (bupropion or paroxetine) or placebo as add-on to ongoing treatment with a mood stabilizer (lithium, valproate or carbamazepine) and/or an atypical antipsychotic for 26 weeks (Sachs et al., 2007). Around 34% of patients dropped out and around 66% reached a study outcome, but with only 34% completing 16 weeks of treatment. Only 24% of patients who received an antidepressant had a durable recovery (8 weeks of euthymia) compared to 27% on placebo. There were no significant differences between both groups, neither in sustained recovery, nor in response or switch to (hypo)mania.

Other antidepressants

There are no studies available with noradrenergic and specific serotonergic antidepressants such as mirtazapine in bipolar disorder.

Systematic review

We included in a systematic review and meta-analysis 12 randomized controlled trials with a total of 1088 patients (Gijsman et al., 2004). The maximum follow-up of these trials was 10 weeks. The percentage of patients per trial who used a concurrent mood-stabilizer (lithium, valproate, carbamazepine, atypical antipsychotic) varied widely from none to all. Clinical response as an outcome measure was available for 662 patients, most often the cut-off was 50% reduction compared to baseline of the total score on the HDRS.

Only four trials compared an antidepressant with placebo. These trials were somewhat heterogeneous in design, but the results all pointed in the same direction: The difference in response between antidepressants and placebo was 16%, resulting in a combined relative risk of 1.86 in favor of antidepressants (95% CI 1.49–2.30). The number needed to treat (NNT) was six, indicating that six patients need to be treated to get one more responder on the antidepressant compared to placebo. This suggests that antidepressants are about equally effective for bipolar depression as for unipolar depression. It must be noted, however, that the majority of the patients in this meta-analysis came from the Olanzapine plus fluoxetine trial.

Maintenance treatment

Randomized studies

Three older studies have examined the efficacy of antidepressant monotherapy in maintenance treatment:

One RCT randomized 130 patients with recurrent affective episodes (at least two hospitalizations in the past 5 years), and the double blind study duration was 2 years (Prien, Klett & Caffey, 1973). All patients were admitted for treatment of an index depressive episode with antidepressants and/or ECT. After response they were maintained on either lithium (median dose 1250 mg/day and median blood level 0.8 meq/L; range 0.5–1.4) or imipramine (median dose 125 mg/day, range 50–200 mg/day). At discharge from hospital they were randomized to either their maintenance medication or to placebo. Reviews on bipolar disorder usually focus on the 44 bipolar patients in this sample. The general conclusion is that imipramine was less effective than lithium: During months 5–24 relapses occurred in 3/17 patients or 18% (lithium), 6/9 patients or 67% (imipramine) and 6/9 patients or 67% (placebo). However, this is based on very small numbers of only nine patients per group. This study, however, has some methodological limitations. First, the bipolar patients were not randomized separately, making it less valid to look at these patients separately. Second, for eight patients who dropped-out directly after randomization the diagnosis was not given. This means that no intention to treat analysis was possible for these patients. Third, from the paper one gets the strong impression that the unipolar/bipolar distinction was made post-hoc. Fourth, there is a suggestion of a strong bipolar component in the unipolar sample in this pre-bipolar era when diagnosis may be was not as thorough as today: Interestingly, 15% of relapse in the unipolar group was due to a manic episode (this was numerically less frequently in the imipramine group!). And finally, the major outcome measures are only available for the whole group: All cause drop-out after 4 months was 37% in the lithium versus 51% in the imipramine versus 67% in the placebo group. Sustained remission over the full 2 years occurred in 41% (lithium) versus 32% (imipramine) versus 7% (placebo). These data suggest that imipramine monotherapy was an acceptable maintenance treatment for a large proportion of patients that included a unipolar sample, with no large differences between lithium and imipramine.

In a second RCT, 216 bipolar patients were included after successful treatment of an index manic or depressive episode (Prien et al., 1984). Half of these patients had been inpatients and all were severely ill with a median of seven previous episodes. In a preliminary phase they had to be stable for at least two months on both lithium (0.6–0.9 meq/L) and imipramine (75–150 mg per day). After this phase 117 patients were randomized to either imipramine ($n=36$), lithium ($n=44$), or both ($n=37$), and followed for up to 2 years. About 16% of patients withdrew from the study in euthymic condition. Three patients were—in our view unjustly—removed from the analysis because they were rapid cyclers (two in the lithium group and one in the combination group). If we do a sensitivity analysis and assume them to have had a depressive relapse, the resulting relapse risks for depression would be: imipramine 28%, lithium 32% and both 24%. If we assume these three to have had a manic relapse the risks for manic relapse would be: imipramine 53%, lithium 31% and both 31%. A post-hoc sub-group analysis showed that this latter striking effect was caused by patients with an index manic episode and absent for patients with an index depressive episode. This suggests that this trial was probably invalidated by the relapse of mania after stopping lithium, because patients in the imipramine arm had had to stop the lithium they were initially on. This effect became even more clearly in a re-analysis using a survival model, showing that most manic relapses on imipramine occurred in the first few months after randomization (Shapiro, Quitkin & Fleiss, 1989). As a consequence, this study shows no proof that antidepressants induce mania during long-term monotherapy.

A third small RCT randomized 22 bipolar II patients to imipramine, lithium, the combination, and placebo, and tried to follow them for 2 years (Kane, Quitkin & Rifkin, 1982). With 22 patients randomized over four groups, and half the patients leaving the study in euthymic state, numbers unfortunately were too small to draw any conclusions.

One RCT looked at the effect of an antidepressant added to lithium: patients with bipolar I disorder who were euthymic on lithium for at least 6 weeks were randomized to either imipramine ($n=37$; 100–150 mg per day) or placebo ($n=38$) (Quitkin et al., 1981). The lithium was maintained at blood levels between 0.8 and 1.2 meq/L. Patients were followed for up to 4 years until relapse or withdrawal. In both groups about half the patients withdrew euthymic after on average 18 months. There was no significant difference in depressive relapses between groups (three vs four patients), but a trend towards more mania in the imipramine group: nine versus four patients. Against expectation, manic relapses occurred on average 3 months later in the imipramine group and depressive relapses on average 8 months earlier in the imipramine group.

Systematic review

Ghaemi, Lenox and Baldessarini (2001) included seven trials with a total of 358 patients in a systematic review of the long-term effects of antidepressants in bipolar disorder. These studies did not yield enough comparable data to allow for meta-analysis. The authors concluded that there is too little information to conclude that antidepressants are either effective or safe during long-term use.

Adverse effects

Switch to (hypo)mania during acute treatment

Naturalistic studies

Lewis and Winokur (1982) in an early attempt to look into this issue studied 87 bipolar patients who were not on antidepressant when admitted to hospital. Twenty five (29%) of these patients became manic within 6 months of admission. The risk for mania was 41% in the 27 patients receiving no treatment, 15% in the patients on lithium or neuroleptics, and around 20% for the patients on TCA. The authors concluded that TCA do not induce mania in bipolar patients.

Boerlin et al. (1998) in a naturalistic study of 29 bipolar depressed patients compared those treated with moodstabilizers only to those treated with antidepressants as well. There was no difference between the groups for manic switches, but switches did occur more frequently in patients treated with TCAs or MAOIs.

Randomized studies

In an open randomized study (n=40) treatment with venlafaxine was associated with more switches than paroxetine (13% vs 3%) (Vieta et al., 2002). This was confirmed in the SFBN trial comparing sertraline, bupropion and venlafaxine, finding a significantly increased risk of switches into hypomania or mania in participants treated with venlafaxine compared with bupropion or sertraline (Post et al., 2006). In both studies venlafaxine was not more effective against depression.

It is unclear to what degree MAOIs have a higher risk of mania. In the original trial comparing imipramine with tranylcypromine the risks of mania were 18% and 11%, respectively. These are high rates for both antidepressants, but it should be realized that both were given as monotherapy, i.e. without the protection of a concurrent mood stabilizer (Himmelhoch et al., 1991).

The recent STEP-BD trial comparing bupropion or paroxetine as add-on to a mood stabilizer or an atypical antipsychotic did not find any significant difference in switch rates between the antidepressant and placebo groups (Sachs et al., 2007).

It is uncertain whether mood stabilizers differ in their (presumed) protective effect. One small study suggested that lithium protects better against switches than an anticonvulsant, but the study size was small and the probability of the effect close to chance (Henry et al., 2001).

Reviews

A review of databases of several pharmaceutical industries concluded that patients with unipolar depression participating in placebo-controlled trials more often showed a switch to mania on antidepressants than on placebo (Peet, 1994). Patients with bipolar depression did not switch more often on SSRIs (3.7%; 9/242) than on placebo (4.2%; 2/48), but they did switch more often on tricyclic antidepressants (11.2%; 14/125). However, this review suffered from two major limitations: Firstly, the criteria for manic switch differed substantially between databases. Secondly, there was no weighted analysis of the databases, taking into account numbers of patients in each database.

In our meta-analysis, the risk of switch also was not higher with antidepressants (3.8%) compared to placebo (4.7%) (Gijsman et al., 2004). However, the number of switches was low: 5/86 for antidepressants and 19/370 for placebo. This resulted in a wide confidence interval of the risk ratio, which happened to be exactly 1.00: 0.47–2.13. This means that a doubling of switches by antidepressants compared to placebo cannot be excluded on the basis of the five included trials. More trials with large sample sizes will be needed to exclude or confirm this.

Despite the fact that there is no proof—from placebo controlled studies—for an increased switch rate of antidepressants overall, there are indications that some antidepressants have a higher risk than others. In a post-hoc analysis of our meta-analysis comparing different classes of antidepressants we showed that TCAs are more likely to induce mania than the other classes of antidepressants combined (SSRI, MAOI or bupropion) ($n = 370$, RR 2.92, 95% CI 1.28–6.71). Possibly this is explained by the fact that TCAs inhibit the reuptake of both serotonin and noradrenalin, suggesting that also the novel serotonin and noradrenaline reuptake inhibitors (SNRIs) may be associated with an increased switch rate. Indeed this was the finding in two trials mentioned above with the SNRI venlafaxine.

Conclusions

In conclusion, on the basis of evidence from naturalistic studies, randomized studies, and reviews, there is on the one hand little evidence for antidepressants causing manic switches, but on the other hand the recurring finding that adrenergic antidepressants may carry such a risk. On the basis of this we conclude that SSRI probably should be the first, second and third choice of antidepressant in bipolar depression, and that TCA should be rarely used and reserved for treatment resistant patients.

It is uncertain to what extend mood stabilizers protect against a manic switch. Only in the older trials the patients have no added mood stabilizers and in those studies manic symptoms were often monitored poorly or not at all. We are not aware of any study in which patients were randomized to mono-therapy with antidepressants versus antidepressants plus a mood stabilizer or plus an atypical antipsychotic.

(Hypo)mania during maintenance treatment

Few studies have addressed the occurrence of (hypo)mania during long term treatment with a concurrent mood stabilizer.

In the study by Prien, Klett and Caffey (1973) the authors report that over 2 years in the imipramine group, six out of nine (67%) bipolar patients had a manic episode compared to three out of nine (33%) in the placebo group and two out of 17 (12%) in the lithium group.

In a follow-up during year 1, of the responders ($n = 87$) of the described SFBN trial comparing bupropion, venlafaxine and sertraline, 18.4% met criteria for "sub-threshold" hypomania, 21.8% for hypomania and 14.9% for mania (Leverich et al., 2006). In agreement with the results of the acute study, venlafaxine was associated with more switches and (hypo)manic recurrences than the other two antidepressants.

Rapid cycling

It has been suggested in a case-report of five patients that the use of antidepressants could lead to an increased frequency of episodes over time (Wehr & Goodwin, 1979). In response, others have challenged this pointing to evidence of similar changes in episode frequency that have been present before the psychopharmacological era (Angst, 1985).

Retrospective studies

There are some retrospective naturalistic studies, which have addressed this issue. It should be noted that these studies by design suffer from selection bias towards patients with a chronic rapid cycling pattern and from recall and assessment bias towards a causal link between antidepressants and mania.

Wehr et al. (1988) reported that 37 out of 51 patients (73%) with rapid cycling were taking antidepressants at the time of onset of rapid cycling. Altshuler et al. (1995) in a retrospective life-chart study of up to 30 years of 35 patients with at least 6 months treatment with antidepressants, nine patients (26%) were judged to have had cycle acceleration. Eight out of these nine were female and four of these patients had bipolar II disorder. Four of these patients were taking a mood-stabilizer as well. In eight out of nine the cycling decelerated after stopping the antidepressant.

Ghaemi, Boiman and Goodwin (2000) reviewed the charts of 85 bipolar and unipolar patients and concluded that 23% of them experienced a rapid-cycling course that could have been attributed to the use of antidepressants. Koukopoulos et al. (2003) in a cohort of 109 patients with rapid cycling reported that in only 12% rapid cycling had emerged spontaneously and in the other 88% it was related to the use of antidepressants. Kupka et al. (2005) followed 539 patients with bipolar disorder for 1 year with life charts and diagnosed rapid cycling in 206 of them. This latter group had a greater number of lifetime depressive episodes. Although in itself not surprising, this does point us in the direction of a confounder: both rapid cycling and use of antidepressants may be related to a high number of depressive episodes, rather than antidepressants causing rapid cycling (see below). The patients with rapid cycling also more often had a history of childhood physical or sexual abuse and of drug abuse. This suggests that etiological factors other than the use of antidepressants may play a role in cycle acceleration.

Prospective study

Of the greatest relevance is one prospective study, which followed 345 patients with bipolar I or bipolar II disorder for more than 5 years (Coryell et al., 2003). Eighty-nine patients (25.8%) at some stage fulfilled criteria for rapid cycling. These patients were more likely to have an illness onset before 17 years of age and they were more likely to make serious suicide attempts. They also experienced more depressive morbidity, especially when no antidepressants were taken. The use of antidepressants was not more likely before shifts from depression to mania. Patients with and without rapid cycling had similar earlier exposure to lithium as well as to antidepressants, predominantly TCAs. Patients with rapid cycling had greater exposure to the combination of lithium plus TCA, probably reflecting more severe depression rather than a causal relationship. This study suggests that the occurrence of rapid cycling is not caused by the use of antidepressants, but that both phenomena may be related to the high prevalence of depressive morbidity in this group. The authors advised against restricted use of antidepressants in bipolar disorder.

Randomized studies

There are no RCTs comparing the occurrence of cycle acceleration between antidepressants and other drugs or placebo. The RCTs reviewed above under maintenance treatment come closest, but they have not specifically looked into this issue. However, there are some possibly relevant findings: In the study by Prien, Klett and Caffey (1973) the percentage of patients having more than one relapse was similar in the imipramine (7%) and lithium (8%) group and much lower than the placebo group (27%), suggesting no increased frequency on imipramine. In the study by Quitkin et al. (1981) the 13 patients who became manic (nine on imipramine and four on placebo) were followed for another 2.5 years: Nine of them were symptomatic less than 10% of the time; the other four had a poor outcome. Although information on treatment-group is not given, this is not suggestive of a high risk of poor outcome after mania on imipramine.

Conclusion

These studies suggest that there is no conclusive evidence that antidepressants can induce rapid cycling. In our view it should not be a reason to avoid antidepressants. If in individual cases a rapid cycling pattern seems to be linked to the use of antidepressants this might be a reason to stop using antidepressants.

Withdrawing antidepressants

Naturalistic studies

In a naturalistic study of 1078 patients with bipolar disorder from the SFBN, 549 patients were treated with an antidepressant, of whom 189 patients at least two months, and 84 patients with good result. Of these latter 84, 43 patients decided to stop the antidepressant after 6 months, while 41 continued using it (Altshuler et al., 2003). At 1 year follow-up the relapse/recurrence risk for depression was 70% in the discontinuation group and 36% in the continuation group. The risk for mania was 21% in the discontinuation group and 7.3% in the continuation group. This means that patients who discontinue their antidepressants may have a higher risk of not only depression but also of mania. However, it might have been the case that these patients decided to stop their antidepressants in the prodromal phase of a (hypo)manic episode (Soldani et al., 2004).

Another naturalistic study followed 59 patients one year after remission of depression (Joffe et al., 2005). Twenty patients stopped the antidepressant within 6 months, 12 did so within one year, and 27 continued up to 1 year. The relapse rates for depression for these three groups were 90%, 75% and 44%, respectively. For manic relapses, the percentages were 20% for the first group and 13% for the latter two groups combined.

Conclusion

These two studies suggest that patients for whom antidepressants have been effective may stay on them, at least as far as they are tolerated. They may also be stopped, but there is no evidence that it is better or safer to do so. This is not in line with several current guidelines advising to stop antidepressants 6 months after remission.

Epilogue

The bottom line may be that in bipolar disorder antidepressants should not be avoided when the depression is severe or enduring; they should be stopped when they are ineffective, when a manic episode occurs or when they cause side-effects, but they may also be continued when the depression has come into remission without a switch into (hypo)mania and with good tolerance

References

Altshuler LL, Post RM, Leverich GS, Mikalauskas K, Rosoff A, & Ackerman L. (1995). Antidepressant-induced mania and cycle acceleration: A controversy revisited. *Am. J. Psychiatry, 152*: 1130–38.

Altshuler L, Suppes T, Black D, Nolen WA., Keck PE, Frye MA, McElroy S, Kupka R, Grunze H, Walden J, Leverich G., Denicoff K, Luckenbaugh D, & Post R. (2003). Impact of antidepressant discontinuation after acute bipolar depression remission on rates of depressive relapses after 1-year follow-up. *Am. J. Psychiatry, 160*: 1252–62.

Angst J. (1985) Switch from depression to mania – a record study over decades between 1920 and 1982. *Psychopathology, 18*: 140–54.

Boerlin HL, Gitlin MJ, Zoellner LA, & Hammen CL. (1998) Bipolar depression and antidepressant induced mania: a naturalistic study. *J. Clin. Psychiatry*, 59: 374–9.

Bunney WE. (1978). Psychopharmacology of the switch process in affective illness. In: *Psychopharmacology: A Generation of Progress*, MA Lipton, A DiMascio, & KF Killam (Eds). Raven Press, New York.

Cohn JB, Collins G, Ashbrook E, & Wernicke JF. (1989). A comparison of fluoxetine imipramine and placebo in patients with bipolar depressive disorder. *Int. Clin. Psychopharmacol.*, 4: 313–22

Coryell W, Solomon D, Turvey C, Keller M, Leon AC, Endicott J, Schettler P, Judd L, & Mueller T. (2003). The long-term course of rapid-cycling bipolar disorder. *Arch. Gen. Psychiatry*, 60: 914–20.

Fabre LF, Brodie KH, Garver D, & Zung WWK. (1983). A multicenter evaluation of bupropion versus placebo in hospitalized depressed patients. *J. Clin. Psychiatry*, 44: 88–94.

Ghaemi SN, Lenox MS, & Baldessarini RJ. (2001). Effectiveness and safety of long-term antidepressant treatment in bipolar disorder. *J. Clin. Psychiatry*, 62: 565–69.

Ghaemi SN, Boiman EE, & Goodwin FK. (2000). Diagnosing bipolar disorder and the effect of antidepressants: a naturalistic study. *J. Clin. Psychiatry*, 61: 804–8.

Gijsman HJ, Geddes JR, Rendell JM, Nolen WA, & Goodwin, GM. (2004). Antidepressants for bipolar depression: a systematic review of randomized, controlled trials. *Am. J. Psychiatry*, 161: 1537–47.

Henry C, Sorbara F, Lacoste J, Gindre C, & Leboyer M. (2001). Antidepressant-induced mania in bipolar patients: identification of risk factors. *J. Clin. Psychiatry*, 62: 249–55.

Himmelhoch JM, Thase ME, Mallinger AG, & Houck P. (1991). Tranylcypromine versus imipramine in anergic bipolar depression. *Am. J. Psychiatry*, 148: 910–6.

Himmelhoch JM, Fuchs CZ, & Symons BJ (1982). A double-blind study of tranylcypromine treatment of major anergic depression. *J. Nerv. Ment. Dis.*, 170: 628–34.

Joffe RT, MacQueen GM, Marriott M, & Young LT. (2005). One-year outcome with antidepressant-treatment of bipolar disorder. *Acta Psychiatr. Scand.*, 112: 105–9.

Kane JM, Quitkin FM, & Rifkin A. (1982) Lithium carbonate and imipramine in the prophylaxis of unipolar and bipolar II illness: a prospective placebo-controlled comparison. *Arch. Gen. Psychiatry*, 39: 1065–9.

Koukopoulos A, Sani G, Koukopoulos AE, Minnai GP, Pani L, Albert MJ, & Reginaldi D. (2003) Duration and stability of the rapid-cycling course: a long-term personal follow-up of 109 patients. *J. Affect. Disord.*, 73: 75–85.

Kupka RW, Luckenbaugh DA, Post RM, Suppes T, Altshuler LL, Keck PE, Frye MA, Denicoff KD, Grunze H, Leverich GS, McElroy SL, Walden J, & Nolen WA. (2005) Comparison of rapid-cycling and non-rapid-cycling bipolar disorder based on prospective mood ratings in 539 outpatients. *Am. J. Psychiatry*, 162: 1273–80.

Leverich GS, Altshuler LL, Frye MA, Suppes T, McElroy SL, Keck PE, Kupka RW, Denicoff KD, Nolen WA, Grunze H, Martinez MI, & Post RM. (2006) Risk of switch in mood polarity to hypomania or mania in patients with bipolar depression during acute and continuation trials of venlafaxine, sertraline, and bupropion as adjuncts to mood stabilizers. *Am. J. Psychiatry*, 163: 232–39.

Lewis J, & Winokur G. (1982). The induction of mania: a natural history study with controls. *Arch. Gen. Psychiatry, 39*: 303–306.

Merideth CH, & Feighner JP. (1983). The use of bupropion in hospitalized depressed patients. *J. Clin. Psychiatry, 44*: 85–87.

Möller H-J, & Grunze H. (2000). Have some guidelines for the treatment of acute bipolar depression gone too far in the restriction of antidepressants? *Eur. Arch. Psychiat. Clin. Neurosci., 250* (2): 57–68.

Nemeroff CB, Evans DL, Gyulai L, Sachs GS, Bowden CL, Gergel IP, Oakes R, & Pitts CD. (2001). Double-blind, placebo-controlled comparison of imipramine and paroxetine in the treatment of bipolar depression. *Am. J. Psychiatry, 158*: 906–12.

Nolen WA, Kupka RW, Hellemann G, Frye MA, Altshuler LL, Leverich GS, Suppes T, Keck PE, McElroy S, Grunze H, Mintz J, & Post RM. (2007). Tranylcypromine vs lamotrigine in the treatment of refractory bipolar depression: a failed but clinically useful study. *Acta Psychiatr. Scand., 115*: 360–5.

Peet M. (1994) Induction of mania with selective serotonin re-uptake inhibitors and tricyclic antidepressants. *Br. J. Psychiatry, 164*: 549–50.

Post RM, Altshuler LL, Leverich GS, Frye MA, Nolen WA, Kupka RW, Suppes T, McElroy S, Keck PE, Denicoff KD, Grunze H, Walden J, Kitchen CMR, & Mintz J. (2006). Mood switch in bipolar depression: comparison of adjunctive venlafaxine, bupropion and sertraline. *Br. J. Psychiatry, 189*: 124–31.

Prien RF, Klett CJ, & Caffey EM. (1973). Lithium carbonate and imipramine in prevention of affective episodes. *Arch. Gen. Psychiatry, 29*: 420–25.

Prien RF, Kupfer DJ, Mansky PA, Small JG, Tuason VB, Voss CB, & Johnson WE. (1984). Drug therapy in the prevention of recurrences in unipolar and bipolar affective disorders: a report of the NIMH Collaborative Study Group comparing lithium carbonate, imipramine, and a lithium carbonate-imipramine combination. *Arch. Gen. Psychiatry, 41*: 1096–1104.

Quitkin FM, Kane J, Rifkin A, Ramoz Lorenzi JR, & Nayak DV. (1981). Prophylactic lithium carbonate with and without imipramine for bipolar I patients. *Arch. Gen. Psychiatry, 38*: 902–7.

Sachs GS, Lafer B, Stoll AL, Banov M, Thibault AB, Tohen M, & Rosenbaum JF. (1994). A double-blind trial of bupropion versus desipramine for bipolar depression. *J. Clin. Psychiatry, 55*: 391–93.

Sachs GS, Nierenberg AA, Calabrese JR, Marangell LB, Wisniewski SR, Gyulai L, Friedman ES, Bowden CL, Fossey MD, Ostacher MJ, Ketter TA, Patel J, Hauser P, Rapport D, Martinez JM, Allen MH, Miklowitz DJ, Otto MW, Dennehy EB, & Thase ME. (2007). Effectiveness of adjunctive antidepressant treatment for bipolar depression. *N Engl. J. Med., 356*: 1711–22.

Shapiro DR, Quitkin FM, & Fleiss JL. (1989) Response to maintenance therapy in bipolar illness. Effect of index episode. *Arch. Gen. Psychiatry, 46*: 401–5.

Soldani F, Ghaemi SN, Tondo L, Akiskal HS, & Goodwin FK. (2004) Relapse after antidepressant discontinuation. *Am. J. Psychiatry, 161*: 1312–3.

Tohen M, Vieta E, Calabrese J, Ketter TA, Sachs G, Bowden C, Mitchell PB, Centrorrino F, Risser R, Baker RW, Evans AR, Beymer K, Dube S, Tollefson GD, & Breier A. (2003). Efficacy of olanzapine and olanzapine-fluoxetine combination in the treatment of bipolar I depression. *Arch. Gen. Psychiatry, 60*: 1079–1088; Correction, 2004; *61*: 176.

Vieta E, Martinez-Aran A, Goikolea JM, Torrent C, Colom F, Benabarre A, & Reinares M. (2002). A randomized trial comparing paroxetine and venlafaxine in the treatment of bipolar depressed patients taking mood stabilizers. *J. Clin. Psychiatry,* 63 (6): 508–12.

Wehr TA, & Goodwin FK. (1979). Rapid cycling in manic-depressives induced by tricyclic antidepressants. *Arch. Gen. Psychiatry,* 36: 555–59.

Wehr TA, & Goodwin FK. (1987). Can antidepressants cause mania and worsen the course of affective illness? *Am. J. Psychiatry,* 144: 1403–11.

Wehr TA, Sack DA, Rosenthal NE, & Cowdry RW. (1988). Rapid cycling affective disorder: contributing factors and treatment responses in 51 patients. *Am. J. Psychiatry,* 145: 179–84.

Young LT, Joffe RT, Robb JC, MacQueen GM, Marriott M, & Patelis SI. (2000). Double-blind comparison of addition of a second mood stabilizer versus an antidepressant to an initial mood stabilizer for treatment of patients with bipolar depression. *Am. J. Psychiatry,* 157: 124–26.

chapter thirteen

Anticonvulsants in treatment of bipolar disorder: A review of efficacy

Lakshmi N. Yatham
University of British Columbia

Vivek Kusumakar
Dalhousie University
Johnson & Johnson Pharmaceutical Research and Development

Contents

Introduction 382
Carbamazepine 383
    Acute mania 383
    Acute bipolar depression 384
    Prophylaxis of bipolar disorder 384
Extended release (ER) carbamazepine 385
    Acute mania 385
    Acute bipolar depression and prophylaxis of bipolar disorder 386
Oxcarbazepine 386
    Acute mania 386
    Acute bipolar depression and prophylaxis of bipolar disorder 387
Valproate 387
    Acute mania 387
    Acute bipolar depression 389
    Prophylaxis of bipolar disorder 390
Lamotrigine 392
    Double-blind studies 392
        Acute mania 392
        Acute bipolar depression 393
        Prophylaxis 395

Gabapentin.. 397
   Acute mania and acute bipolar depression........................ 397
      Double-blind studies.. 397
   Prophylaxis of bipolar disorder... 398
Topiramate 398
   Double-blind studies... 399
      Acute mania... 399
      Acute bipolar depression.. 399
      Prophylaxis of bipolar disorder.............................. 399
Clonazepam 399
   Acute mania... 400
   Acute bipolar depression.. 400
   Prophylaxis 401
Tiagabine 401
Felbamate 401
Levatiracetam 402
Conclusions... 402
References... 402

Introduction

The first report of the use of an anticonvulsant (i.e. valpromide, the amide prodrug of valproate) for manic depressive illness was published by Lambert and colleagues (1966). Dalby (1971) reported mood altering properties of carbamazepine in patients with epilepsy; Takezaki and Hanaoka (1971) around the same time described the use of cabamazepine in 10 acute manic patients with seven of these showing marked to moderate improvement in symptoms. Ballenger and Post (1978) conducted and reported the results of the first double-blind study that examined the efficacy of an anticonvulsant in bipolar disorder. The interest in studying of anticonvulsants was to some extent fueled by increasing recognition and awareness of the limitations of lithium for treating bipolar disorder.

In the last two decades, a number of studies have appeared in the literature supporting the efficacy of both carbamazepine and valproate in the treatment of bipolar disorder. A number of other newer anticonvulsants such as lamotrigine, gabapentin, and topiramate have also been studied for their efficacy in bipolar disorder. In this chapter, we will review the controlled studies that have examined the efficacy of anticonvulsants in acute mania, acute bipolar depression, and prophylaxis of bipolar disorder. Where controlled studies are not available, we will provide a brief overview of the relevant data from open studies.

Carbamazepine

Carbamazepine is an iminostilbene derivative and has a structure that is similar to the tricyclic antidepressant imipramine. It was developed in the late 1950s, and its antiepileptic properties were first reported in the early 1960s. It was approved as an antiepileptic in the USA in 1974 and has been used for treatment of generalized and partial complex seizure disorders and paroxysmal pain syndromes. We will provide below an overview of controlled studies of carbamazepine in acute mania, acute bipolar depression and prophylaxis of bipolar disorder.

Acute mania

Antimanic efficacy of carbamazepine was examined in fifteen double-blind studies. Of these, one compared carbamazepine with placebo in an off-on-off-on design (Post et al., 1984a), five with placebo in a parallel design (Klein et al., 1984; Gonclaves & Stoll, 1985; Desai et al., 1987; Okuma et al., 1988; Moller et al., 1989), four with neuroleptics (Okuma et al., 1979; Grossi et al., 1984; Stoll et al., 1986; Brown, Silverstone, & Cookson, 1989), and another five with lithium (Lenzi et al., 1986; Lerer et al., 1987; Lusznat, Murphy, & Nunn, 1988; Okuma et al., 1990; Small et al., 1991).

The study that used an off-on-off-on double-blind design did not permit concurrent use of neuroleptics. Carbamazepine led to improvement in symptoms in 12 out of 19 patients and most of these patients relapsed with placebo substitution providing fairly convincing evidence for antimanic efficacy of carbamazepine (Post et al., 1984a). All the studies that compared carbamazepine with antipsychotics reported equal efficacy with one study reporting fewer side effects with carbamazepine (Brown, Silverstone, & Cookson, 1989). Only two out of five studies that compared carbamazepine with lithium did not permit concurrent neuroleptic use (Lerer et al., 1987; Small et al., 1991), and both these studies reported equal efficacy. In the largest study to date ($n=100$), Okuma et al. (1990) reported that 62% of the carbamazepine group and 59% of the lithium group responded, again confirming equal efficacy of carbamazepine with lithium.

In the above described 15 double-blind studies to date, a total of 703 patients with bipolar disorder were studied and, of these, 355 received carbamazepine, 69 neuroleptics, 122 lithium and 157 placebo. The data in terms of number of responders for each medication were provided in only some studies. The data are available for 203 patients on carbamazepine and of these 123 (61%) have been reported to improve with this medication. The available evidence, therefore, clearly supports antimanic efficacy of carbamazepine.

Some studies have reported that several factors associated with non-response to lithium might predict response to carbamazepine. These include dysphoric mania, greater severity of mania, a negative family history of bipolar disorder, and those with greater decrements in T4 during treatment (Roy-Byrne et al., 1984; Post et al., 1984a, 1986a, 1987). Although it was initially thought that rapid cycling might predict a response to carbamazepine, more recent data seem to suggest that it predicts poor response to both lithium and carbamazepine, and that in such patients a combination of these two agents might offer better efficacy (Okuma, 1993; Denicoff et al., 1997).

Acute bipolar depression

The efficacy of carbamazepine was examined in a total of 40 bipolar depressed patients in three double-blind placebo cross over studies (Ballenger & Post, 1980; Post et al., 1983, 1986b). Twenty-seven out of 40 (68%) responded while on carbamazepine and 50% relapsed with placebo substitution. In the largest of these three studies, which had a total of 24 bipolar depressed patients (Post et al., 1986b), 62% had mild improvement as defined by a reduction of one point or more on Bunney–Hamburg scale with carbamazepine. When a stricter two point criterion was used for improvement, about 42% of bipolar depressed patients met criteria for response.

In summary, the available evidence suggests that carbamazepine has at least modest antidepressant properties in bipolar depressed patients.

Prophylaxis of bipolar disorder

In the only double-blind placebo controlled study of prophylaxis to date (carbamazepine $n=12$, placebo $n=10$), Okuma et al. (1981) reported that 60% of patients randomized to carbamazepine and 22% randomized to placebo were stable during the 1 year study period. A number of other controlled studies compared carbamazepine with lithium and reported that up to two-thirds of patients respond to carbamazepine (Placidi et al., 1986; Watkins et al., 1987; Bellaire, Demisch, & Stoll, 1988; Lusznat, Murphy, & Nunn, 1988; Coxhead, Silverstone, & Cookson, 1992; Simhandl, Denk, & Thau, 1993; Greil et al., 1997; Wolf, Berky, & Kovacs, 1997; Hartong et al., 2003).

Greil et al. (1998) reported that there was a negative association between hospitalization rate and the number of non-classical bipolar features in their study population. Furthermore, there was a trend in favor of carbamazepine in the non-classical bipolar group compared to lithium, in terms of lower hospitalization rates. Simhandl, Denk, & Thau (1993) in their 2 year study that compared carbamazepine with lithium noted that variations in blood levels of carbamazepine had no impact on prophylactic efficacy. Hartong et al. (2003) noted that carbamazepine carried a 40% risk of an episode per year. Post et al. (1990) reported that a substantial number of bipolar patients develop tolerance to prophylactic efficacy of carbamazepine. This raises questions about the wisdom of using carbamazepine as a monotherapy for prophylaxis of bipolar disorder.

Extended release (ER) carbamazepine

Acute mania

ER formulations of carbamazepine (carbamazepine ER) have been developed to reduce administration frequency, to improve tolerability as they are less likely to cause peaks in levels, and to improve patient adherence.

Two double-blind parallel design placebo controlled trials examined the efficacy of carbamazepine ER in acute mania (Weisler et al., 2004, 2005), and the design of these two trials was identical. After a single blind placebo lead-in for 5–7 days, patients with manic or mixed episode who had a score of 20 or more on Young Mania Rating Scale (YMRS) were randomized to monotherapy with carbamazepine ER or placebo for 3 weeks. A total of 443 were recruited and of these 223 received carbamazepine ER and 220 received placebo (Weisler et al., 2006). Carbamazepine ER was started at 200 mg bid per day and titrated by 200 mg/day to a final dose between 200 mg/day and 1600 mg/day as clinically indicated and tolerated. The primary outcome measure was a change in the YMRS from baseline to endpoint.

The mean dose of carbamazepine ER was 707 ± 386 mg/day. Carbamazepine ER group had a greater reduction in YMRS scores compared with placebo at end point in both studies. The separation from placebo began at week 1 in one study (Weisler et al., 2005) and at week 2 in the other (Weisler et al., 2004). Combined analysis of two studies showed that the mean reduction in YMRS scores was 6.1 points greater in the carbamazepine ER group compared with the placebo group. Response rates were significantly greater in the carbamazepine ER group (52%) compared with the placebo group (26%). A sub-analysis showed that improvements were significantly greater for carbamazepine ER group for both manic and mixed patients compared with the placebo group.

As to adverse events, 90% of carbamazepine ER group experienced an adverse event compared with 64% of those in the placebo group. The most commonly reported events included dizziness, somnolence, nausea, vomiting and ataxia.

These studies clearly suggest that carbamazepine ER is effective in acute manic and mixed episodes in patients with bipolar disorder.

Acute bipolar depression and prophylaxis of bipolar disorder

No controlled trials of carbamazepine ER yet for these indications.

Oxcarbazepine

Acute mania

A total of five double-blind trials and a single blind trial examined the efficacy of oxcarbazepine for acute mania. Of these, two were placebo controlled trials (Emrich, Dose, & von Zerssen, 1985; Wagner et al., 2006), two compared oxcarbazepine with haloperidol (Muller & Stoll, 1984; Emrich, 1990), one compared oxcarbazepine with lithium (Emrich, 1990) and in the single blind trial, the comparator was valproate (Suppes et al., 2007).

In the only placebo trial in adults, which assessed a small number of patients (oxcarbazepine 7, and placebo 5), six out of seven patients on oxcarbazepine improved based on scores on Inpatient Multidimension Psychophathology Scale (Emrich, Dose, & von Zerssen, 1985). However, in a larger double-blind parallel design placebo controlled trial in children and adolescents that compared oxcarbazepine ($n=59$) with placebo ($n=57$), the changes on the primary endpoint (i.e. changes in YMRS scores relative to baseline) were not greater in the oxcarbazepine group (−10.90 points) compared with the placebo group (−9.79). Further, the incidence of adverse events was twice as common in the oxcarbazepine group compared with the placebo group (Wagner et al., 2006).

In the active comparator trials, oxcarbamazepine 900–1200 mg/day was compared with 15–20 mg/day of haloperidol in 20 patients with acute mania over a 2 week period in one trial (Muller & Stoll, 1984) and oxcarbazepine (mean dose 2400 mg/day) with haloperidol (mean dose 42 mg/day) in 38 patients in another trial (Emrich, 1990). The efficacy as measured by changes in Bech-Raefelson Mania Rating Scale (BRMS) was similar for both groups. The onset of action was reported to be faster (Muller & Stoll, 1984) and the incidence of side effects fewer (Emrich, 1990) for oxcarbazepine compared with the haloperidol group.

Emrich (1990) reported that oxcarbazepine ($n=28$; mean dose 1400 mg/day) was as effective as lithium ($n=24$; mean dose 1100 mg/day) in a double-blind trial of 2 weeks duration using BRMS. In a single blind trial, oxcarbazepine add-on therapy was as effective as valproate add-on therapy in treating hypomanic symptoms (Suppes et al., 2007).

In summary, oxcarbazepine appears to be effective for acute mania in adult population and its efficacy appears to be comparable to haloperidol, lithium and valproate. However, oxcarbazepine is not effective in children and adolescents with acute mania.

Acute bipolar depression and prophylaxis of bipolar disorder

No controlled trials of oxcarbazepine yet for these indications.

Valproate

Valproic acid is a simple branched-chain carbosylic acid. It was approved for use as an antiepileptic in the USA in 1978. It is now FDA approved for use as an antimanic agent. It is available in the USA and several other countries in various oral preparations such as valproic acid, sodium valproate, and divalproex sodium.

Acute mania

Five double-blind placebo controlled trials assessed the efficacy of valproate/divalproex/divalproex ER in acute mania. Of these, two used a cross-over design (Emrich, Dose, & von Zerssen, 1985; Brennan, Sandyk, & Borsook, 1984) while three more recent studies used a parallel design (Pope et al., 1991; Bowden et al., 1994, 2006). One double-blind trial assessed the efficacy of divalproex in symptomatic youth at high risk of developing bipolar disorder (Findling et al., 2007), and another compared divalproex with quetiapine for acute mania in adolescents.

Emrich, Dose, & von Zerssen (1985) were the first to document the evidence for antimanic efficacy of valproate in a controlled study. Using a double-blind placebo cross-over A-B-A design, they reported that four out of five manic patients had marked response to valproate. Brennan, Sandyk, & Borsook (1984) using a similar design found that six out of eight manic patients responded to valproate.

Pope et al. (1991) conducted the first double-blind, placebo controlled, parallel group study with valproate in 36 acute manic patients for 1–3 weeks. Patients were not allowed to receive any concurrent psychotropic medication with the exception of lorazepam (for agitation/insomnia for the first 10 days). Valproate was significantly superior to placebo on all measures. Nine out of 17 (53%) valproate treated patients and two out of 19 (11%) placebo treated patients improved as defined by a 50% or greater reduction in mania rating scale (MRS) scores. In a second study that led to FDA approval of divalproex for acute mania, Bowden et al. (1994) assessed the efficacy in 179 acute manic patients in comparison to placebo and lithium. About 48% of patients in the valproate group, 49% in the lithium group, and 25% in the placebo group achieved significant clinical improvement by the end of the study as defined by a reduction in MRS scores of 50% or more. The percentage of responders using 30%, 40% or 50% reduction in MRS scores was significantly higher in the valproate group compared with the placebo group. Improvement in symptoms was evident by the end of one week, particularly in patients that had serum valproate levels of 45 ug/L or greater (Bowden et al., 1996). In a more recent study of 3 weeks duration, divalproex ER ($n=192$) was compared with placebo ($n=185$) in bipolar I patients with a manic/mixed episodes. Divalproex was commenced at 25 mg/kg and dose adjusted to serum levels of 85–125 ug/ml. The improvement as measured by mean reductions in MRS scores at endpoint relative to baseline was significantly greater in the divalproex ER group compared with the placebo group. The response rates of 48% in the divalproex ER group were significantly greater compared with 34% in the placebo group (Bowden et al., 2006).

Children and adolescents between the ages of 5 and 17 who met criteria for bipolar disorder NOS or cyclothymia and had at least one biological parent with bipolar I disorder were randomized to treatment with divalproex ($n=29$) or placebo ($n=27$) for up to 5 years. There was no significant difference between the two groups in efficacy as measured by discontinuation due to mood event or discontinuation due to any reason (Findling et al., 2007).

In the two studies that compared valproate/divalproex with lithium (Freeman et al., 1992; Bowden et al., 1994), valproate/divalproex was found to be as effective as lithium in acute mania. Presence of depressive symptoms predicted better response to valproate in both studies. Response also was seen in 50% of rapid cyclers (Bowden et al., 1994), and the response in manic symptoms was unrelated to previous history of response to lithium.

Two studies compared divalproex with olanzapine for acute mania. Tohen and colleagues (2002) randomized 126 patients to divalproex and 125 patients to olanzapine for 3 weeks. Olanzapine group had significantly greater reductions in YMRS scores (13.4 points) compared with the divalproex group (10.4 points). Response rates were 54.4% for the olanzapine group and 42.3% for the valproate group, and this difference was not significant. Nausea was more frequent in the divalproex group while increased appetite, dry mouth and somnolence were more frequent in the olanzapine group. In a second study, Zajecka and colleagues (2002) randomized 63 patients to divalproex and 57 patients to olanzapine. No significant differences were observed between the two groups on any efficacy variables in this study.

Divalproex was compared with quetiapine in 50 adolescents with acute mania in a 4 week study. Repeated measures analysis of variance using the LOCF showed no differences between the two groups in YMRS scores while mixed regression analysis showed improvements were more rapid in quetiapine group. Response and remission rates, however, are greater for the quetiapine group compared with the divalproex group (Delbello et al., 2006).

Valproate oral loading has been reported to be safe and rapidly effective in treating manic symptoms (Oluboka et al., 2002); the speed of response has been reported to be similar to the onset of action with haloperidol (Keck et al., 1993; McElroy et al., 1996; Hirschfeld et al., 1999) and olanzapine (Hirschfeld et al., 2003). A recent report suggested that intravenous valproate loading is also well tolerated and led to improvement in six out of seven patients including one patient who was nonresponsive to previous oral loading (Grunze et al., 1999b). A linear relationship between serum valproate levels and therapeutic efficacy in acute mania has been reported with efficacy significantly greater beginning at 71.4–85 ug/ml and the higher levels being more effective than lower levels. Serum valproate levels in the lowest effective range were 60% more effective than placebo while higher ranges were 120% more effective than placebo. This would suggest that valproate should be titrated to the highest tolerable dose for best efficacy (Allen et al., 2006).

Acute bipolar depression

McElroy et al. (1992) reviewed open studies of valproate in bipolar depression and concluded that 30% (58 out of 195) of depressed patients respond to valproate. Since then, Davis et al. (1996) published another open-label prospective study of the efficacy of valproate in major depression and reported that 66% had a response based on intent to treat analysis.

A total of 4 small double-blind placebo controlled trials assessed the efficacy of valproate monotherapy vs placebo monotherapy in acute bipolar depression. Of these, three reported that valproate was significantly superior to placebo (Davis et al., 2005; Ghaemi et al., 2007; Mizuna et al., 2008) while the fourth study showed only numerical but not statistical superiority (Sachs et al., unpublished observation). In an unpublished 8 week double-blind trial, although numerically greater reduction in Hamilton Depression Rating Scale scores were oberved in the divalproex monotherapy ($n=21$) group compared with the placebo monotherapy ($n=22$), the difference was not significant (Sachs et al., unpublished observation). In a second trial, Davis, Bartolucci, & Petty (2005) randomized 25 patients with acute bipolar depression (12 patients to placebo and 13 patients to divalproex) over 8 weeks. Using a LOCF, they reported significantly greater reductions in depressive symptoms on HAM-D 17 item scale in the divalproex group compared with the placebo group. Ghaemi and colleagues (2007) reported that divalproex monotherapy ($n=9$) was superior to placebo therapy ($n=9$) in acute bipolar depressed patients as measured by greater improvement in MADRS scores over a six week study period with a 13.6 points reduction in divalproex group vs 1.4 points improvement in the placebo group. Finally, in a more recent larger trial of divalproex ER versus placebo in mood stabilizer naive and newly diagnosed bipolar I or II acute depression ($n=54$), divalproex ER monotherapy showed significantly greater improvements in MADRS scores than placebo group with improvement beginning at week 3 and maintained throughout the remainder of the 6 week study (Muzina et al., 2008). Similarly, response rates in the divalproex ER group were significantly greater but not the remission rates compared with the placebo group. The improvement was significant in the bipolar I but not in bipolar II groups.

In conclusion, the results of these studies support the efficacy of divalproex monotherapy for acute bipolar depression, particularly in those that are non-refractory and mood stabilizer naive bipolar I patients. However, further larger studies and meta-analysis might clarify it's utility in managing bipolar depression.

Prophylaxis of bipolar disorder

A number of open studies suggest that valproate is effective in reducing the frequency and severity of both manic and depressive episodes (Semadeni, 1967; Lambert, 1984; Brennan, Sandyk, & Borsook, 1984; Emrich, Dose, & von Zerssen, 1985; Vencovsky, Peterova, & Kabes, 1987; Zapletalek, Hanus, & Kindernayova, 1988; Hayes 1989; Lambert & Venaud, 1992). However, it appears to have a better efficacy in preventing manic compared to depressive episodes. Lambert and Venaud (1992) conducted the best published prospective study to date on the efficacy of valproate. They randomly assigned 150 patients (121 bipolar and 29 unipolar) to lithium or valproate for a two year maintenance treatment. If a patient did not tolerate the drug, or if the outcome was poor, a switch to an alternative drug was allowed. The number of episodes decreased from 4.12 during 2 years prior to the study to 0.51 during the study period for the valproate group and from 3.92 to 0.61 for the lithium group. This study clearly showed that the efficacy for valproate was similar to lithium. In addition, there were fewer drop-outs in the valproate (10%) group compared to the lithium group (25%).

The only prospective double-blind study placebo controlled trial to date compared the efficacy of divalproex with lithium and placebo over a 12 month period (Bowden et al., 2000). In this study, 372 patients who met recovery criteria within three months of an index manic episode were randomized to maintenance treatment with divalproex, lithium, or placebo in a 2:1:1 ratio. Psychotropic medications were discontinued before randomization, except for open-label divalproex or lithium, which were gradually tapered over the first two weeks of maintenance treatment. The divalproex group did not differ significantly from the placebo group in time to any mood episode, which was the primary outcome measure. Divalproex, however, was superior to placebo in terms of lower rates of discontinuation for either a recurrent mood episode or depressive episode. Divalproex was also superior to lithium in longer duration of successful prophylaxis in the study and less deterioration in depressive symptomatology and GAS scores. In patients who were stabilized on divalproex monotherapy for mania in the open label phase and subsequently randomized to either divalproex or placebo, divalproex was significantly superior to placebo in time to mood episode. This would suggest that divalproex may be most appropriate for maintenance therapy in those patients that had been stabilized with divalproex for acute mania. Further, patients in the placebo group in this study had surprisingly good outcomes that may have been due to the inclusion of patients with milder forms of illness and patients receiving highly supportive care by study personnel during the study. These and other factors led to a lower proportion of manic relapses in the placebo group than projected, yielding inadequate power to test the primary outcome variable, i.e. 0.3 rather than the planned power of greater than 0.8.

Calabrese and colleagues (2005) assessed the efficacy of divalproex in comparison to lithium in 60 patients with rapid cycling bipolar disorder who recently had an acute manic/hypomanic episode and were stabilized with lithium and divalproex combination. During the 20 month double-blind period, 56% of patients on lithium and 50% of patients randomized to divalproex relapsed with no significant differences between the two groups. Similarly, rates of relapse into manic or depressive episodes did not differ between the two groups.

In another study with a similar design, 60 children and adolescents between the ages of 5 and 17 years with bipolar I or bipolar II disorder who were initially treated with divalproex and lithium combination and meeting remission criteria were randomized to divalproex or lithium monotherapy for 76 weeks (Findling et al., 2005). There were no significant differences between the two groups for time to mood episode or time to discontinuation for any reason.

Salloum and colleagues (2005) in a double-blind trial of 24 weeks duration assessed the efficacy of divalproex vs placebo add-on to lithium in 59 patients with bipolar disorder with co-morbid alcohol abuse. Divalproex group had significantly lower proportion of heavy drinking days and a trend for fewer drinks per heavy drinking day compared with the placebo group. Mood symptoms improved equally with no difference between the two groups.

In summary, the results of open studies suggest efficacy of valproate in prophylaxis of bipolar disorder. Although there was no difference in the primary outcome measure between valproate and placebo groups in the double-blind study, valproate was superior to placebo and lithium on various secondary measures supporting the efficacy of this medication. Further, studies that compared divalproex with lithium in younger subjects with bipolar disorder or those with rapid cycling reported equal efficacy. As well, divalproex appears to provide additional benefit in reducing the frequency of drinking in bipolar patients with co-morbid alcohol abuse.

Lamotrigine

Lamotrigine (3,5,-diamino-6(2,3-dichlorophenly)-1,2,4-triazine) is a phenyltriazine that acts at voltage sensitive sodium channels and stabilizes neuronal membranes. It is approved for treatment of refractory seizures as adjunctive therapy.

Double-blind studies

Acute mania

Two Glaxo Smith Kline sponsored studies assessed the efficacy of lamotrigine monotherapy or add-on therapy in acute mania (Bowden et al., 2000). In one study (study 609), lamotrigine monotherapy (n=84) was compared with placebo (n=95) or lithium monotherapy (n=36) over a 3 week period. Lamotrigine was dosed at 25 mg/day for the first 2 weeks and 50 mg/day during the third week. The primary outcome measure was change in MRS score relative to baseline using LOCF. There were no significant differences between the three groups either on the primary efficacy measure or changes in CGI-severity or improvement scales. This study was likely underpowered to test the efficacy of lithium, and it is likely lamotrigine was underdosed.

In the second study (study 610), lamotrigine (n=74) was compared with placebo (n=77) or lithium (n=78) over a 6 week period. Lamotrigine was dosed at 25 mg/day for the first 2 weeks, 50 mg/day for weeks 3 and 4, 100 mg/day during week 5, and 200 mg/day during week 6. Haloperidol and droperidol were allowed during the first 20 days of the study. Lithium was significantly better than placebo on MRS change scores, CGI severity change scores as well as proportion of responders on CGI but lamotrigine was no different from placebo.

Lamotrigine monotherapy or add-on versus placebo monotherapy or add-on was assessed in an 8-week double-blind study in 16 lithium-refractory manic or hypomanic patients (Anand et al., 1999). Of the 16 patients who participated in the study, half were randomized to lamotrigine up to 200 mg/day while the other eight received placebo. The primary efficacy measure was a 50% or greater reduction on YMRS scores. Five of the eight patients who were given lamotrigine either adjunctively with lithium or as monotherapy responded while four of the eight patients assigned to placebo also responded. The difference between the two groups in terms of percentage of responders was not significant.

In an active comparator trial, Berk (1999) examined the efficacy of lamotrigine ($n=15$) up to 100 mg/day in acute mania in comparison to olanzapine ($n=15$) and lithium ($n=15$) using a 4-week double-blind randomized design in 45 patients. The YMRS scores declined significantly in all the groups with no significant difference in the magnitude of change in scores between three groups. The results of this study suggest that lamotrigine may have some antimanic efficacy. However, the interpretation of this study's results is markedly confounded because the study was not properly powered to show equivalence.

In summary, three out of four studies did not support the efficacy of lamotrigine in acute mania and in the one study showing positive results design issues complicated the interpretation of the data. The consensus is that there is no compelling evidence for the efficacy of lamotrigine in acute mania.

Acute bipolar depression

A total of five Glaxo Smith Kline sponsored double-blind parallel design placebo controlled trials examined the efficacy of lamotrigine monotherapy in comparison to placebo in acute bipolar depression. Of these one has been published (Calabrese et al., 1999), and a pooled analysis of the five trials is currently in press (Beynon et al., in press).

In the published trial (study 602), 195 patients with bipolar depression were randomized to receive monotherapy with lamotrigine 50 mg ($n=66$), lamotrigine 200 mg ($n=63$), or placebo ($n=66$) for 7 weeks (Calabrese et al., 1999). Patients in the lamotrigine groups received lamotrigine 25 mg at randomization that was increased to 50 mg at the end of 2 weeks. Those in the 200 mg group had the dose increased to 100 mg at the end of week 3 and to 200 mg at the end of week 4. Entry criteria included a score of 18 or more on 17 item Hamilton Rating Scale for Depression (HAM-D), and the changes in clinical status were assessed using 31 item HAM-D, Montgomerry Asberg Depression Rating Scale (MADRS), Clinical Global Impression (CGI)-Severity and improvement scales. The improvement in the lamotrigine group was not significantly greater compared to the placebo group on the primary efficacy measure of changes in HAM-D scores from baseline using last observation carried forward analysis (LOCF). However, it has since been agreed that

changes in HAM-D are not as sensitive as changes in MADRS in sepa-
rating active drug from placebo in bipolar depression. Interestingly, on
MADRS, both the 50 mg and 200 mg groups were significantly better
compared to the placebo group using LOCF. The lamotrigine 200 mg
group did better on both CGI-Severity and Improvement scales whereas
the 50 mg group did better only on the CGI-Severity scale compared
to the placebo group. A significantly higher number of patients had a
50% or more decrease in MADRS scores in both the lamotrigine groups
compared to the placebo group, but the differences were not significant
on HAM-D. Lamotrigine was well tolerated, and headache was the only
adverse event that was more common in the lamotrigine groups compared to the placebo group. The incidence of manic episodes was not
significantly different between lamotrigine and placebo groups. The
results of this study clearly suggest that lamotrigine is effective in treating bipolar depression and that it does not appear to have a propensity
to induce a manic switch.

Of the four other trials, two included only bipolar I depressed
(SCA40910, and SCA30924) while the other two (GW 603, and SCA100223)
included both bipolar I and bipolar II depressed patients (Calabrese
et al., 2007). The GW 603 was 10 weeks in duration and included HAM-D
change as the primary efficacy measure while the other three studies
were 8 weeks in duration and included MADRS change scores as a primary efficacy measure. All four studies failed to superiority of lamotrigine over placebo on the primary efficacy measure.

Recently, a meta-analysis of 5 GSK sponsored studies has been conducted to assess the efficacy (Beynon et al., in press). The results showed
that patients treated with lamotrigine were more likely to respond compared with those treated with placebo on both MADRS (pooled relative
risk, RR 1.21, 95% CI 1.05–1.39, p=.005) and HAM-D (RR 1.27, CI=1.09, 1.47,
p=.002) (Beynon et al., in press). This meta-analysis suggests a mild to
moderate antidepressant effects for lamotrigine.

In a Lilly sponsored study, Lamotrigine monotherapy (n=205) was
compared with olanzpine/fluoxetine combination (OFC) (n=205) in a 7
week double-blind trial (Brown et al., 2006) in patients with acute bipolar I depression. The OFC group had significantly greater improvements
on CGI-Severity, MADRS, and YMRS change scores relative to baseline
compared with the lamotrigine group but the response rates were not significantly different between the two groups. Similarly, the study completion rates were also similar between the two groups while the side effect
profile was different for the two groups.

Two double-blind trials examined the efficacy of lamotrigine add-on
to a mood stabilizer. In a larger trial supported by GSK, patients with
bipolar I or II depression who had been taking lithium and had a score

of 18 or more on MADRS were randomized to the addition of lamotrigine (n=64) or placebo (n=60) for 8 weeks. Lamotrigine group had greater reduction (–15.38) in MADRS scores compared with the placebo (–11.03) group (p=.024) (van der Loos et al., 2007). More patients met criteria for response on MADRS in the lamotrigine group (51.6%) compared with the placebo (31.7%) group (p=.03). In a smaller trial double-blind trial that compared lamotrigine add-on with citalopram add-on to lithium or valproate in acute bipolar depression. Lamotrigine add-on (n=10) was as effective as citalopram add-on (n=10) as measured by changes in MADRS scores in a 12 week double-blind trial (Schaffer, Zuker, & Levitt, 2006). Similarly, no significant differences were noted in response/remission or switch rates into mania/hypomania between the two groups.

One double-blind trial and two randomized open studies assessed the efficacy of lamotrigine in treatment refractory mood disorders. Frye et al. (2000) examined the efficacy of lamotrigine or gabapentin monotherapy in comparison to placebo in 31 patients (11 with bipolar I, 14 with bipolar II, and six with unipolar depression) with treatment resistant (primarily rapid cycling bipolar) mood disorder (of the 25 bipolars, 23 had rapid cycling) using a randomized double-blind crossover design. Each monotherapy trial lasted for 6 weeks. The overall response rate of much or very much improvement based on the CGI-I scale was 52% (16 out of 31) for the lamotrigine group, 26% (eight out of 31) for the gabapentin group, and 23% (seven out of 31) for the placebo group. Post-hoc analysis showed that the lamotrigine group did significantly better than the gabapentin and placebo groups. Lamotrigine was effective in treating depressive symptoms in 45% of patients in comparison to 19% efficacy for placebo against depression. No significant differences were noted on the primary efficacy between lamotrigine, inositol or risperidone in a randomized open study. The recovery rates, however, were numerically greater for lamotrigine group (23.8%) compared with risperidone (4.6%) or inositol (17.4%) groups (Nierenberg et al., 2006). In another trial, lamotrigine add-on was as effective as tranylcypromine add-on but this study may have been underpowered to show significant differences (Nolen et al., 2007).

In summary, overall, there is reasonable evidence to support the efficacy of lamotrigine for acute bipolar depression both in monotherapy and in combination therapy with lithium or valproate.

Prophylaxis
Two randomized double-blind placebo controlled trials examined the efficacy of lamotrigine in comparison to placebo or lithium over an 18 month period (Bowden et al., 2003; Calabrese et al., 2003). One of these trials recruited patients with bipolar I disorder (n=326) who were or recently

had manic or hypomanic episode (Bowden et al., 2003) while the other recruited bipolar I patients who were or recently had a depressive episode (Calabrese et al., 2003). All patients entered an open label phase during which they were treated with addition of lamotrigine for 8–16 weeks. Those meeting stabilization criteria in each study were randomized to treatment with lamotrigine or lithium or palcebo for upto 18 months. Both studies showed that lamotrigine and lithium were superior to placebo in time to intervention for a mood episode, and that lamotrigine was superior to placebo in time to intervention for a depressive episode but not manic episode. A combined analysis of both studies showed that lamotrigine was superior to placebo for both depressive as well as manic episodes (Goodwin et al., 2004). Further, lamotrigine and lithium were also superior to placebo for time to intervention for any mood episode when relapses occurring in the first 90 days were excluded but they were similar when relapses occurring within the first 180 days were excluded (Calabrese et al., 2006).

In a double-blind trial, lamotrigine was compared to placebo during a 26-week period in patients with rapid cycling bipolar disorder (Calabrese, 2000). Patients with bipolar I or bipolar II rapid cycling in manic, hypomanic, mixed or depressed phases ($n=324$) entered a preliminary open label phase and were treated with the addition of lamotrigine 100–300 mg/day. Concomitant medications were tapered off and those who met criteria for response ($n=182$, 130 BP 1 and 52 BP 2) were randomized to double-blind treatment with either placebo ($n=89$) or lamotrigine monotherapy ($n=93$) for 26 weeks. The primary efficacy measure was time to additional pharmacotherapy for a mood episode or emerging mood symptoms. Fifty six percent of the placebo ($n=49$) and 50% ($n=45$) of the lamotrigine treated patients met criteria for "time to intervention" and the difference between the groups was not significant ($p=.177$). There were also no significant differences between median survival times between the two groups. However, when survival is defined as any premature discontinuation including requiring additional pharmacotherapy, the median survival time was 8 weeks for the placebo group and 14 weeks for the lamotrigine group, a difference that was significant statistically ($p=.036$). When subtype analysis was performed for "time to intervention", there was a trend towards a significant difference ($p=.073$) favoring lamotrigine for the bipolar II subtype but not in those with the bipolar I subtype. There was also a significant difference ($p=.015$) favoring lamotrigine for overall survival in the study for bipolar II patients. The percentage of patients who were stable without relapse for the entire study period on monotherapy was significantly greater ($p=.03$) for the lamotrigine group (41% for lamotrigine vs 26% for placebo) compared with the placebo group. The latter finding was primarily due to those patients with bipolar II; 46% on lamotrigine remained stable for the entire study as opposed to only 18% on placebo.

Although the findings did not reach significance on a primary efficacy measure, patients randomized to lamotrigine, particularly those with bipolar II subtype did significantly better on a number of other efficacy measures supporting the efficacy of lamotrigine.

Lamotrigine was compared with OFC in a double-blind trial over 25 weeks in patients with acute bipolar I depression (Brown et al., 2006; Brown et al., personal communication) and the results at 7 weeks for this study are reviewed in the section on acute bipolar depression. Over 25 weeks, the improvements were greater for the OFC group compared with lamotrigine on CGI-S ($p = .008$), MADRS ($p = .005$), and YMRS ($p < .001$) scores. However, there was no signficiant difference in relapse rates between the two groups in those that had met criteria for remission at 7 weeks).

In summary, lamotrigine monotherapy is clearly effective in preventing depressive relapse but it's efficacy in preventing manic relapse is modest. There is also some support for the efficacy of lamotrigine in rapid cycling bipolar II patients.

Gabapentin

Gabapentin has a chemical structure similar to that of the branched chain amino acids leucine and valine and also the aromatic amino acid phenylalanine. It was developed as a structural analog of the inhibitory neurotransmitter, GABA, and was initially thought to act via GABAergic mechanisms. However, it was found that gabapentin does not interact with GABA receptors, nor does it interfere with GABA uptake or degradation. Gabapentin may increase the GABA content of some brain regions, and unlike carbamazepine, gabapentin does not interact with sodium channels, nor does it appear to have any significant effects on receptors for benzodiazepines, NMDA, catecholamines, or acetylcholine. The mechanism of action of gabapentin remains unknown. It is approved for use as add on therapy in management of refractory epilepsy.

Acute mania and acute bipolar depression

Double-blind studies
A randomized, double-blind, placebo controlled trial examined the efficacy of gabapentin add on vs placebo add on to lithium or valproate in acute mania (Pande, 1999). Patients who met DSM-IV criteria for bipolar manic/hympomanic/mixed episode and scored 12 or more on YMRS were optimized on either lithium or valproate for 2 weeks. Patients who continued to be symptomatic and scored eight or more on YMRS were randomized to adjunctive treatment with placebo ($n = 59$) or gabapentin ($n = 58$) for 10 weeks. Both treatment groups had a decrease in YMRS scores from baseline to endpoint but the decrease was significantly greater in the

placebo group (–8.9) than the gabapentin group (–5.8) ($p<.05$). There were no significant differences between the groups on HAM-D, the Internal States Scale, or National Institute of Mental Health-Life Chart Method (NIMH-LCM) scale scores. The results of this double-blind study suggest that gabapentin is not superior to placebo in treating acute manic symptoms.

In another small double-blind randomized trial, patients received gabapentin, lamotrigine or placebo monotherapy for six weeks with two subsequent crossovers so that by the end of the study, each patient would have received all three agents, each for six weeks (Frye et al., 1998). For treatment of mania, the response rates for gabapentin were 20% in comparison to 44% for lamotrigine and 32% for placebo and the differences between the three groups were not significant. For depression, the response rates were 26% for gabapentin, 45% for lamotrigine and 19% for placebo. Again, the differences were not significant between the three groups.

In summary, gabapentin does not appear to have efficacy in treating acute mania or bipolar depression.

Prophylaxis of bipolar disorder

Bipolar I or II patients who were euthymic and taking either lithium, valproate, carbamazepine or any combination of these medications were randomly assigned to gabapentin ($n=13$) or placebo ($n=12$) add-on for 1 year (Vieta et al., 2006). The primary efficacy measure was change in CGI-S from baseline to endpoint which was significant in favor of gabapentin and gabapentin was well tolerated. These results support the efficacy of gabapentin for long term treatment as an add-on to a mood stabilizer. However, given that this is a very small trial and that gabapentin has not shown efficacy for acute mania or depression, further studies are needed before it can be recommended for long term treatment of bipolar disorder.

Topiramate

Topiramate is a sulfamate substitued monosaccharide. This novel anticonvulsant has multiple mechanisms of action, including the potentiation of γ-aminobutyric acid (GABA) at GABA receptors, state dependent blockade of voltage sensitive sodium channels, and antagonism of the ability of kainate to activate the kainate/AMPA subtype of glutamate receptor but not NMDA receptor subtype. It is approved for treatment of refractory epilepsy as adjunctive therapy.

Double-blind studies

Acute mania

Four double-blind trials examined the efficacy of topiramate in comparison to placebo and two of these trials had lithium as an active comparator (Kushner et al., 2006). All four studies recruited acute manic patients with bipolar I disorder who had at least one previous manic episode and scored 20 or more on YMRS at entry. They were randomized to treatment with topiramate 400 mg/day of topiramate in two studies, 400 or 600 mg/day in the third study, and 200 or 400 mg/day in the fourth study for 3 weeks. There were no significant differences between topiramate or placebo in any of the studies on the primary efficacy measure of mean change in YMRS from baseline to endpoint but lithium was superior to both placebo and topiramate in both studies. Weight loss was more common with topiramate.

Topiramate adjunctive therapy was assessed in a double-blind trial in comparison to placebo (Roy Chengappa et al., 2006) and again, no differences were noted between the two groups on the primary efficacy measure of mean change in YMRS scores.

In summary, these data thus clearly suggest that topiramate monotherapy or adjunctive therapy is ineffective in acute mania.

Acute bipolar depression

A single blind trial compared topiramate add-on ($n=18$) versus bupropion SR add-on ($n=18$) in acute bipolar I and II patients over an 8 week period (McIntyre et al., 2002). There was a significant reduction in HAM-D scores in both groups from baseline to end point. Response rates were 56% in the topiramate group and 59% in the bupropion SR group. There were no significant differences between the two groups on any efficacy measures. However, in the absence of other placebo controlled trials, firm conclusions can not be drawn about the efficacy of topiramate in acute bipolar depression from this single blind trial.

Prophylaxis of bipolar disorder

No double-blind or single blind trials have been conducted.

Clonazepam

Clonazepam is a high potency benzodiazepine anticonvulsant. It is approved for treatment of myoclonic and petit mal seizures. First reports of usefulness of clonazepam for treatment of bipolar disorder appeared in the early 1980s (Chouinard, Young, & Annable, 1983; Victor et al., 1984; Lechin & van der Dijs, 1983).

Acute mania

In a 5 day double-blind trial, Edwards, Stephenson, & Flewett (1991) compared the efficacy of clonazepam with placebo for treatment of acute mania (n=40). The group receiving clonazepam was significantly better in their manic symptoms but not in psychotic symptoms compared to the placebo group. Patients, in this study, however, were allowed to receive chlorpromazine on an as needed basis which might have confounded the results.

Clonazepam was also compared with lithium for treatment of acute mania. In a double-blind, crossover design, twelve acutely manic patients, newly admitted from the emergency room, were treated with clonazepam or lithium carbonate (Chouinard, Young, & Annable, 1983). Half the patients (chosen randomly) received 10 days of treatment with clonazepam followed immediately by 10 days of treatment with lithium, while the others received the same treatments in reverse order. Improvement occurred with both treatments and, overall, there was no significant difference on the clinical global impression scale between the two treatments.

Clonazepam was less effective than lorazepam or haloperidol in other double-blind trials. Bradwejn et al. (1990) examined the efficacy of clonazepam versus lorazepam in 24 patients with acute mania using a double-blind randomized design. In the lorazepam group, 61% of patients responded to treatment, with 38.5% achieving remission, as compared to an 18.2% response rate and 0% remission rate in patients treated with clonazepam. In another double-blind trial of 16 acutely agitated psychotic patients with manic/manic-like symptoms who required rapid tranquilization, subjects were randomized to receive intramuscular preparations of clonazepam (1–2 mg) or haloperidol (5–10 mg) at 0, 0.5, and 1.0 hours (Chouinard et al., 1993). Both medications produced significant reduction of manic symptoms within two hours of initial treatment. Haloperidol, however, produced beneficial results more rapidly than clonazepam. This study concluded that I.M. clonazepam was an effective, safe, but slower acting alternative to I.M. haloperidol for treatment of agitated psychiatric patients.

In summary, clonazepam appears to have some utility at least as an adjunct in treating acute manic symptoms. It should, however, be noted that behavioral disinhibition with clonazepam has also been reported and that clinicians should be wary of this possible complication, especially in manic patients (Binder, 1987; Kubacki, 1987; Amiel, Bryan, & Herjanic, 1987).

Acute bipolar depression

Clonazepam has also been reported to have antidepressant properties (Alvarez & Freinhar, 1987). Of the 27 patients (major depression=18, bipolar disorder=9) treated with 1.5–6.0 mg (mean 3.4 mg) of clonazepam, 21 (84%) had marked to moderate improvement (Kishimoto et al., 1988). The onset of the antidepressive effect of clonazepam was noted within one week in the majority of cases who responded to the therapy. Scores on the Hamilton Depression Rating Scale and the Beck Self-Rating Scale were significantly reduced after treatment. Side effects occurred in 14 patients, and two dropped out of the study in the early stages. There are no double-blind studies that examined the antidepressant effect of clonazepam in bipolar depression.

Prophylaxis

Aronson, Shukla, & Hirschowitz (1989) examined the efficacy of clonazepam as a substitute to neuroleptics in the maintenance treatment of lithium-refractory bipolar disorder. Five patients who were euthymic on a combination of lithium and neuroleptics were switched from neuroleptics to clonazepam and followed prospectively. All five patients relapsed quickly after taking clonazepam (one within 2 weeks, and the other four within 10–15 weeks) leading to premature termination of the study. Further studies are needed to determine if clonazepam has any utility in the maintenance treatment of bipolar disorder There are also concerns about the risks of tolerance, abuse and dependence with this medication.

Tiagabine

Tiagabine is a nipecotic acid linked to an aliphatic chain and a lipophilic anchor. It is a selective inhibitor of GABA uptake and is currently FDA approved as adjunctive treatment for refractory partial seizures. In a case report on three patients, two with bipolar disorder and one with schizoaffective disorder-bipolar type, tiagabine as an adjunct was reported to be effective with few side effects (Kaufman, 1998). In a more recent case report, Schaffer, Schaffer, & Hughes (1999) found a similar positive response to adjunctive tiagabine in two patients with refractory bipolar disorder. However, Grunze et al. (1999b) in an open study systematically evaluated the efficacy of tiagabine using Bech-Rafaelsen MRS in acute mania. Two patients received tiagabine monotherapy and six others received tiagabine as an adjunct to previously insufficient mood stabilizing medication. None of the patients showed significant improvement over the two week study period. Hence, it is currently unknown if tiagabine has any role in treatment of bipolar disorder. Further studies are clearly warranted.

Felbamate

There are no published clinical reports regarding felbamate therapy for bipolar disorder. However, like some other anticonvulsants, secondary mania has been noted to result from felbamate treatment (Hill, Stagno, & Tesar, 1995).

Levatiracetam

In an open label add-on study with an on-off-on design, Grunze and colleagues (2003) reported that YMRS scores decreased during the "on" phase, worsened during the "off" phase and improved again during the "on" phase. The mean dose of levatiracetam in the study was 3125 mg/day and the medication was well tolerated. These data are promising but controlled trials are clearly needed.

Conclusions

It has become increasingly clear that lithium alone, or in combination with antidepressants or neuroleptics, is inadequate for a significant proportion of bipolar patients. The recognition of the efficacy of anticonvulsants in bipolar disorder has offered some new hope for patients with this devastating medical illness. Carbamazepine, oxcarbazepine divalproex are clearly effective in acute mania while lamotrigine is effective in acute bipolar depression and prophylaxis but not useful in treating acute mania or prevention of mania. Topirmate and gabapentin do not appear to provide any benefit in treating core manic or depressive symptoms. The role of these medications in prophylaxis requires further study. Levatiracetam is promising but clearly further studies are needed.

There are also many unanswered questions such as what medication or what combination of medications is best for which patient. This is largely because predictors of response to medications are still unknown and response (or nonresponse) to one anticonvulsant is not predictive of response to another (Calabrese et al., 1992; Schaff, Fawcett, & Zajecka, 1993). Hence, systematic clinical trials are needed to uncover the optimal treatment algorithm for acute phase of the illness. Trials regarding the prophylactic efficacy of the newer treatments are also required. Unlike the situation 20 years ago when lithium was the sole option, these effective alternatives/adjuncts to lithium are being effectively utilized by clinicians to ameliorate the effects of a debilitating illness.

References

Allen MH, Hirschfeld RM, Wozniak PJ, Baker JD, & Bowden CL (2006): Linear relationship of valproate serum concentration to response and optimal serum levels for acute mania. *Am. J. Psychiatry, 163*: 272–75.

Alvarez WA, & Freinhar JP (1987): Clonazepam: an antidepressant? [letter]. *Am. J. Psychiatry, 144*: 536–37.

Amiel M, Bryan S, & Herjanic M (1987): Clonazepam in the treatment of bipolar disorder in patients with non- lithium-induced renal insufficiency [letter]. *J. Clin. Psychiatry, 48*: 424.

Anand A, Oren D, Berman R, Cappliello A, & Charney D (1999): Lamotrigine treatment of lithium failure outpatient mania-a double blind placebo controlled trial. In: Soares J, Gershon S (eds), *Third International Conference on Bipolar Disorder* (Vol 1, pp. 23). Pittsbugh, PA: Munksgaard.

Aronson TA, Shukla S, & Hirschowitz J (1989): Clonazepam treatment of five lithium-refractory patients with bipolar disorder. *Am. J. Psychiatry, 146*: 77–80.

Ballenger JC, & Post RM (1980): Carbamazepine in manic depressive illness: a new treatment. *Am. J. Psychiatry, 137*: 782–90.

Ballenger JC, & Post RM (1978): Therapeutic effects of carbamazepine in affective illness: a preliminary report. *Commun. Psychopharmacol., 2*: 159–75.

Bellaire W, Demisch, K, & Stoll KD (1988): Carbamazepine versus lithium in prophylaxis of recurrent affective disorders. *Psychopharmacology, 96*: 287.

Berk M (1999): Lamotrigine and the treatment of mania in bipolar disorder. *Eur. Neuropsychopharmacology*, Aug. 9 (Suppl 4): S119–23.

Beynon S, Soares-Weiser K, Woolacott N, Duffy S, & Geddes JR (in press): Pharmacological interventions for the prevention of relapse in bipolar disorder: a systematic review of controlled trials. *J. Psychopharmocol.*

Binder RL (1987): Three case reports of behavioral disinhibition with clonazepam. *Gen. Hosp. Psychiatry, 9*: 151–53.

Bowden C, Brugger A, & Swann A, et al. (1994): Efficacy of divalproex vs lithium and placebo in the treatment of mania. The Depakote Mania Study Group. *JAMA, 271*: 918–24.

Bowden C, Calabrese JR, & McElroy S, et al. (2000): A randomized placebo controlled 12 month trial of divalproex and lithium in the treatment of outpatients with bipolar 1 disorder. *Arch. Gen. Psychiatry, 57*: 481–89.

Bowden CL, Calabrese JR, Sachs G, Yatham LN, Asghar SA, Hompland M, Montgomery P, Earl N, Smoot TM, & DeVeaugh-Geiss J (2003): A placebo-controlled 18-month trial of lamotringine and lithium maintenance treatment in recently manic or hypomanic patients with bipolar I disorder. *Arch. Gen. Psychiatry, 60*: 392–400.

Bowden CL, Janicak PG, & Orsulak P, et al. (1996): Relation of serum valproate concentration to response in mania. *Am. J. Psychiatry, 153*: 765–70.

Bowden C, Calabrese JR, & Asher J, et al. (2000). Spectrum of efficacy of lamotrigine in bipolar disorder: overview of double blind placebo controlled studies. Presented at the American College of Neuropsychopharmacology, 39th Annual Meeting, San Juan, Puerto Rico, December.

Bowden CL, Swann AC, Calabrese JR, Rubenfaer LM, Wozniak PJ, Collins MA, Abi-Saab W, Slatarelli M, Depakote ER & Mania Study Group (2006): A randomized, placebo-controlled, multicenter study of divalproex sodium extended release in the treatment of acute mania. *J. Clin. Psychiatry, 67* (10): 1501–10.

Bradwejn J, Shriqui C, Koszycki D, & Meterissian G (1990): Double-blind comparison of the effects of clonazepam and lorazepam in acute mania. *J. Clin. Psychopharmacol., 10*: 403–8.

Brennan MJW, Sandyk R, & Borsook D (1984): Use of sodium valproate in the management of affective disorders: basic and clinical aspects. In: Emrich HM, Okuma T, Muller AA (eds), *Anticonvulsants in Affective Disorders*. Amsterdam: Excerpta Medica.

Brown D, Silverstone T, & Cookson J (1989): Carbamazepine compared to halo-peridol in acute mania. *Int. Clin. Psychopharmacol., 4:* 229–38.

Brown EB, McElroy SL, Keck PE Jr, Deldar A, Adams DH, Tohen M, & Williamson DJ (2006): A 7-week, randomized, double-blind trial of olanzapine/fluox-etine combination versus lamotrigine in the treatment of bipolar I depres-sion. *J. Clin. Psychiatry, 67* (7): 1025–33.

Calabrese JR, Markovitz PJ, Kimmel SE, & Wagner SC (1992): Spectrum of efficacy of valproate in 78 rapid-cycling bipolar patients. *J. Clin. Psychopharmacol., 12* (Suppl 1): 53S–56S.

Calabrese JR, Bowden CL, Sachs GS, Ascher JA, Monaghan E, & Rudd GD (1999): A double-blind placebo-controlled study of lamotrigine monotherapy in outpatients with bipolar I depression. Lamictal 602 Study Group. *J. Clin. Psychiatry, 60:* 79–88.

Calabrese JR (2000): Update on the use of topiramate in bipolar disorder. *American Psychiatric Association Annual Meeting.* Chicago, IL, May.

Calabrese JR, Bowden CL, Sachs G, Yatham LN, Behnke K, Mehtonen OP, Montgomery P, Ascher J, Paska W, Earl N, & DeVeaugh-Geiss J (2003): A placebo-controlled 18-month trial of lamotrigine and lithium maintenance treatment in recently depressed patients with bipolar I disorder. *J. Clin. Psychiatry, 64* (9): 1013–24.

Calabrese JR, Goldberg JF, Ketter TA, Suppes T, Frye M, White R, DeVeaugh, Geiss A, & Thompson TR (2006): Recurrence in bipolar I disorder: a post hoc analysis excluding relapses in two double-blind maintenance studies. *J. Biol. Psychiatry, 59:* 1061–64.

Calabrese JR, Human RF, White RL, Edwards S, Thompson TR, Ascher JA, Monaghan ET, & Leadbetter RA (2007): Lamotrigine in the acute treatment of bipolar depression: results of five double-blind, placebo-controlled clinical trials. *Bipolar Disorders, 9:* 1–11.

Calabrese JR, Shelton MD, Rapport DJ, Youngstrom EA, Jackson K, Balali S, Ganocy SJ, & Findling RL (2005): A 20-month, double-blind, maintenance trial of lithium versus divalproex in rapid-cycling bipolar disorder. *Am. J. Psychiatry, 162:* 2152–61.

Calabrese JR, Suppes T, Bowden C, Sachs G, Swann A, MCElroy S, Kusamakar V, Ascher J, Earl N, Greene P, & Monaghan E (2000): A double-blind, placebo-controlled, prophylaxis study of lamotrigine in rapid-cycling bipolar disorder. Lamictal 614 Study Group. *J. Clin. Psychiatry, 61* (11): 841–50.

Chouinard G, Annable L, Turnier L, Holobow N, & Szkrumelak N (1993): A double-blind randomized clinical trial of rapid tranquilization with I.M. clonazepam and I.M. haloperidol in agitated psychotic patients with manic symptoms [see comments]. *Can. J. Psychiatry, 38* (Suppl 4): S114–21.

Chouinard G, Young SN, & Annable L (1983): Antimanic effect of clonazepam. *Biol. Psychiatry, 18:* 451–66.

Coxhead N, Silverstone T, & Cookson J (1992): Carbamazepine versus lithium in the prophylaxis of bipolar affective disorder. *Acta Psychiatr. Scand., 85:* 114–18.

Dalby MA (1971): Antiepileptic and psychotropic effect of carbamazepine (Tegretol) in the treatment of psychomotor epilepsy. *Epilepsia, 12:* 325–34.

Davis LL, Kabel D, Patel D, Choate AD, Fosliennash C, Gurguis GNM, Kramer GL, & Petty F. (1996): Valproate as an antidepressant in major depressive disorder. *Psychopharmacol. Bull., 32:* 647–52.

Davis LL, Bartolucci A, & Petty F (2005): Divalproex in the treatment of acute bipolar depression: A placebo controlled study. *J. Affect. Disord., 85* (3): 259–66.

DelBello MP, Kowatch RA, Adler CM, Stanford KE, Welge JA, Barzman DH, Nelson E, & Strakowski SM. (2006): A double-blind randomized pilot study comparing quetiapine and divalproex for adolescent mania. *J. Am. Acad. Child Adolesc. Psychiatry, 45* (3): 305–13.

Denicoff KD, Smith-Jackson EE, Disney ER, Ali SO, Leverich GS, & Post RM (1997): Comparative prophylactic efficacy of lithium, carbamazepine, and the combination in bipolar disorder. *J. Clin. Psychiatry, 58*: 470–78.

Desai NG, Gangadhas BN, & Channabasavanna SM, et al. (1987): Carbamazepine hastens therapeutic action of lithium in mania. In: *Proceedings of the International Conference on New Directions in Affective Disorders.* Jerusalem, April 5–9, 97 (abst).

Edwards R, Stephenson U, & Flewett T (1991): Clonazepam in acute mania: a double blind trial [see comments]. *Aust. N Z J. Psychiatry, 25*: 238–42.

Emrich HM, Dose M, & von Zerssen D (1985): The use of sodium valproate, carbamazepine and oxcarbazepine in patients with affective disorders. *J. Affect. Disord., 8*: 243–50.

Emrich HM (1990): Studies with oxcarbazepine (Trileptal) in acute mania. *Int. Clin. Psychopharmacol., 5* (Suppl): 83–88.

Findling RL, Frazier TW, Youngstrom EA, McNamara NK, Stansbrey RJ, Gracious BL, Reed MD, Demeter CA, & Calabrese JR (2007): Double-blind, placebo-controlled trial of divalproex monotherapy in the treatment of symptomatic youth at high risk for developing bipolar disorder. *J. Clin. Psychiatry, 68* (5): 781–8.

Findling RL, McNamara NK, Youngstrom EA, Stansbrey R, Gracious BL, Reed MD, & Calabrese JR (2005): Double-blind 18-month trial of lithium versus divalproex maintenance treatment in pediatric bipolar disorder. *J. Am. Acad. Child Adolesc. Psychiatry, 44* (5): 409–17.

Freeman TW, Clothier JL, Pazzaglia P, Lesem MD, & Swann AC (1992): A double-blind comparison of valproate and lithium in the treatment of acute mania. *Am. J. Psychiatry, 149*: 108–11.

Frye M, Ketter T, & Kimbrell T, et al. (1998): Gabapentin and lamotrigine monotherapy in mood disorder. *American Psychiatric Association Meeting*, pp. 150. Washington, DC.

Frye MA, Ketter TA, Kimbrell TA, Dunn RT, Speer AM, Osuch EA, Luckenbaugh DA, Corá-Locatelli G, Leverich GS, & Post RM (2000): A placebo-controlled study of lamotrigine and gabapentin monotherapy in refractory mood disorders. *J. Clin. Psychopharmacology, 20* (6): 607–614.

Ghaemi SN, Gilmer WS, Goldberg JF, et al. (2007): Divalproex in the treatment of acute bipolar depression: a preliminary double-blind, randomized, placebo-controlled pilot study. *J. Clin. Psychiatry, 68* (12): 1840–44.

Gonclaves N, & Stoll KD (1985): Carbamazepine in manic syndromes. A controlled double-blind study. *Nervenarzt, 56*: 43–47.

Goodwin GM, Bowden CL, Calabrese JR, Grunze H, Kasper S, White R, Greene P, & Leadbetter R (2004): A pooled analysis of 2 placebo-controlled 18-month trials of lamotrigine and lithium maintenance in bipolar I disorder. *J. Clin. Psychiatry, 65* (3): 432–41.

Greil W, Kleindienst N, Erazo N, & Muller-Oerlinghausen B (1998): Differential response to lithium and carbamazepine in the prophylaxis of bipolar disorder. *J. Clin. Psychopharmacol., 18*: 455–60.

Greil W, Ludwig-Mayerhofer W, & Erazo N, et al. (1997): Lithium versus carbamazepine in the maintenance treatment of bipolar disorders—a randomised study. *J. Affect. Disord., 43*: 151–61.

Grossi E, Sacchetti E, & Vita A, et al. (1984): Carbamazepine vs chlorpromazine in mania: a double blind trial. In: Emrich HM, Okuma T, Muller AA (eds.), *Anticonvulsants in Affective Disorders* (pp. 177–187). Amsterdam: Excerpta Medica.

Grunze H, Erfurth A, Amann B, Giupponi G, Kammerer C, & Walden J (1999a): Intravenous valproate loading in acutely manic and depressed bipolar I patients. *J. Clin. Psychopharmacol., 19*: 303–9.

Grunze H, Erfurth A, Marcuse A, Amann B, Normann C, Walden J (1999b): Tiagabine appears not to be efficacious in the treatment of acute mania. *J. Clin. Psychiatry, 60* (11): 759–62.

Grunze H, Langosch J, Born C, Schaub G, & Walden J (2003): Levetiracetam in the treatment of acute mania: an open add-on study with an on-off-on design. *J. Clin. Psychiatry, 64* (7): 781–84.

Hartong EG, Moleman P, Hoogduin CA, Broekman TG, & Nolen WA (2003): Prophylactic efficacy of lithium versus carbamazepine in treatment naïve bipolar patients. *J. Clin. Psychiatry, 64* (2): 144–51.

Hayes SG (1989): Long-term use of valproate in primary psychiatric disorders. *J. Clin. Psychiatry, 50* (Suppl): 35–9.

Hill RR, Stagno SJ, & Tesar GE (1995): Secondary mania associated with the use of felbamate. *Psychosomatics, 36* (4): 404–406.

Hirschfeld RM, Allen MH, McEvoy JP, Keck PE, Jr., & Russell JM (1999): Safety and tolerability of oral loading divalproex sodium in acutely manic bipolar patients. *J. Clin. Psychiatry, 60*: 815–18.

Hirschfeld RM, Baker JD, Wozniak P, Tracy K, & Sommerville KW (2003): The safety and early efficacy of oral-loaded divalproex versus standard-titration divalproex, lithium, olanzapine, and placebo in the treatment of acute mania associated with bipolar disorder. *J. Clin. Psychiatry, 64* (7): 841–46.

Kaufman KR (1998): Adjunctive tiagabine treatment of psychiatric disorders: three cases. *Ann. Clin. Psychiatry, 10*: 181–84.

Keck PE, Jr., McElroy SL, Tugrul KC, & Bennett JA (1993): Valproate oral loading in the treatment of acute mania. *J. Clin. Psychiatry, 54*: 305–8.

Kishimoto A, Kamata K, & Sugihara T, et al. (1988): Treatment of depression with clonazepam. *Acta Psychiatr. Scand., 77*: 81–6.

Klein E, Bental E, Lerer B, & Belmaker RH (1984): Carbamazepine and haloperidol v placebo and haloperidol in excited psychoses. A controlled study. *Arch. Gen. Psychiatry, 41*: 165–70.

Kubacki A (1987): Sexual disinhibition on clonazepam [letter]. *Can. J. Psychiatry, 32*: 643–45.

Kushner SF, Khan A, Lane R, & Olson WH (2006): Topiramate monotherapy in the management of acute mania: results of four double-blind placebo-controlled trials. *Bipolar Disorders, 8*: 15–27.

Lambert P, Cavaz G, Borselli S, et al. (1966): Action neuropsychotrope d'un nouvel anti-epileptique: le depamide. *Ann. Med. Psychol., 1*: 707–10.

Lambert PA (1984): Acute and prophylactic therapies of patients with affective disorders using valpromide (Dipropylacetamide). In: Emrich HM, Okuma T, Muller AA (eds.), *Anticonvulsants in Affective Disorders* (pp. 33–44). Amsterdam: Excerpta Medica.

Lambert PA, & Venaud G (1992): Comparative study of valpromide versus Li in treatment of affective disorders. *Nervure, 5* (2): 57–65.

Lechin F, & van der Dijs B (1983): Antimanic effect of clonazepam [letter]. *Biol. Psychiatry, 18*: 1511.

Lenzi A, Lazzerine F, Grossi E, Massimetti G, & Placidi GF (1986): Use of carbamazepine in acute psychosis: a controlled study. *J. Int. Med. Res., 14*: 78–84.

Lerer B, Moore N, Meyendorff E, Cho SR, & Gershon S (1987): Carbamazepine versus lithium in mania: a double-blind study. *J. Clin. Psychiatry, 48*: 89–93.

Lusznat RM, Murphy DP, & Nunn CMH (1988): Carbamazepine vs lithium in the treatment and prophylaxis of mania. *Br. J. Psychiatry, 153*: 198–204.

McIntyre RS, Mancini DA, McCann S, Srinivasan J, Sagman D, & Kennedy SH (2002): Topiramate versus Bupropion SR when added to mood stabilizer therapy for the depressive phase of bipolar disorder: a preliminary single-blind study. *Bipolar Disorders, 4*: 207–213.

McElroy S, Keck P, Stanton SP, Tugrul KC, Bennett JA, & Strakowski S (1996): A randomized comparison of divalproex oral loading versus haloperidol in the initial treatment of acute psychotic mania. *J. Clin. Psychiatry, 57*: 142–46.

McElroy SL, Keck PE, Jr., Pope HG, Jr., & Hudson JI (1992): Valproate in the treatment of bipolar disorder: literature review and clinical guidelines. *J. Clin. Psychopharmacol., 12*: 42S–52S.

Moller HJ, Kissling W, Riehl T, Bauml J, Binz U, & Wendt G (1989): Doubleblind evaluation of the antimanic properties of carbamazepine as a comedication to haloperidol. *Prog. Neuropsychopharmacol. Biol. Psychiatry, 13*: 127–36.

Muller AA, & Stoll K-D (1984): Carbamazepine and oxcarbazepine in the treatment of manic syndromes—studies in Germany. In: Emrich HM, Okuma T, Muller AA (eds.), *Anticonvulsants in Affective Disorders* (pp. 139–147). Amsterdam: Excerpta Medica.

Muzina DJ, Ganocy S, Khalife S, et al. (2008). A double-blind placebo-controlled study of divalproex extended-release in newly diagnosed mood stabilizer naïve patients with acute bipolar I or II depression. Presented at American Psychiatric Association Annual Meeting, 5 May 2008, Washington, DC.

Nierenberg AA, Ostacher MJ, Calabrese JR, Ketter TA, Marangell LB, Miklowitz DJ, Miyahara S, Bauer MS, Thase ME, Wisniewski SR, & Sachs GS (2006): Treatment-resistant bipolar depression: A STEP-BD equipoise randomized effectiveness trial of antidepressant augmentation with lamotrigine, inositol, or risperidone. *Am. J. Psychiatry, 163*: 210–16.

Nolen WA, Kupka RW, Hellemann G, Frye MA, Altshuler LL, Leverich GS, Suppes T, Keck PE Jr, McElroy S, Grunze H, Mintz J, & Post RM (2007): Tranylcypromine vs. lamotrigine in the treatment of refractory bipolar depression: a failed but clinically useful study. *Acta Psychiatr. Scand., 115*: 360–65.

Okuma T (1993): Effects of carbamazepine and lithium on affective disorders. *Neuropsychobiology 27*: 138–45.

Okuma T, Inanaga K, & Otsuki S, et al. (1979): Comparison of the antimanic efficacy of carbamazepine and chlorpromazine: a double-blind controlled study. *Psychopharmacology, 66*: 211–17.

Okuma T, Yamashita I, Takahashi R, Itoh H, Kurihara M, Otsuki S, Watanabe S, Sarai K, Hazama H, & Inangana K (1988): Double-blind controlled studies on the therapeutic efficacy of carbamazepine in affective and schizophrenic patients. *Psychopharmaxology, 96*: 102 (abstract#TH18.05).

Okuma T, Inanaga K, & Otsuki S, et al. (1981): A preliminary double-blind study on the efficacy of carbamazepine in prophylaxis of manic-depressive illness. *Psychopharmacology, 73*: 95–6.

Okuma T, Yamashita I, & Takahashi R, et al. (1990): Comparison of the antimanic efficacy of carbamazepine and lithium carbonate by double-blind controlled study. *Pharmacopsychiatry, 23*: 143–50.

Oluboka OJ, Bird DC, Kutcher S, & Kusumaker V (2002): A pilot study of loading versus titration of valproate in the treatment of acute mania. *Bipolar Disorder, 4* (5): 341–45.

Pande A (1999): Combination treatment in bipolar disorder. *Third International Conference on Bipolar Disorder*, Pittsburgh, PA, June 17–19.

Placidi GF, Lenzi A, Lazzerine F, Cassano GB, & Akiskal HS (1986): The comparative efficacy and safety of carbamazepine versus lithium: a randomized, double-blind 3-year trial in 83 patients. *J. Clin. Psychiatry, 47*: 490–94.

Pope H, McElroy S, & Keck P, et al. (1991): Valproate in the treatment of acute mania. *Arch. Gen. Psychiatry, 48*: 62–68.

Post RM, Ballenger JC, & Uhde TW, et al. (1984a): Efficacy of carbamazepine in manic depressive illness: implications for underlying mechanisms. In: Post R, Ballanger J (eds.), *Neurobiology of Mood Disorders*. Baltimore, MD: Williams & Wilkens.

Post RM, Uhde T, Kramlinger K, & Rubinow D (1986a): Carbamazepine treatment of mania: clinical and biochemical aspects. *Clin. Neuropharmacol., 9*: 547–9.

Post RM, Uhde TW, Ballenger JC, Chatterji DC, Green RF, & Bunney WE (1983): Carbamazepine and its 10,11-epoxide metabolite in plasma and CSF: relationship to antidepressant response. *Arch. Gen. Psychiatry, 40*: 673–76.

Post RM, Leverich GS, Rosoff AS, & Altshuler LL (1990): Carbamazepine prophylaxis in refractory affective disorders: a focus on long-term follow-up. *J. Clin. Psychopharmacol., 10*: 318–27.

Post RM, Uhde TW, Roy-Byrne PP, & Joffe RT (1986b): Antidepressant effects of carbamazepine. *Am. J. Psychiatry, 143*: 29–34.

Post RM, Uhde TW, Roy-Byrne PP, & Joffe RT (1987): Correlates of antimanic response to carbamazepine. *Psychiatry Res., 21*: 71–83.

Roy-Byrne PP, Joffe RT, Uhde TW, & Post RM (1984): Approaches to the evaluation and treatment of rapid-cycling affective illness. *Br. J. Psychiatry, 145*: 543–50.

Roy Chengappa K, Schwarzman L, Hulihan J, Xiang J, Rosenthal N, & Clinical Affairs Product Support Study-168 Investigators (2006): Adjunctive topiramate therapy in patients receiving a mood stabilizer for bipolar I disorder: a randomized, placebo-controlled trial. *J. Clin. Psychiatry, 67* (11): 1698–706.

Salloum IM, Cornelius JR, Daley DC, Kirisci L, Himmelhoch JM, & Thase ME (2005): Efficacy of valproate maintenance in patients with bipolar disorder and alcoholism. A double-blind placebo-controlled study. *Arch. Gen. Psychiatry, 62*: 37–45.

Schaff M, Fawcett J, & Zajecka J (1993): Divalproex sodium in the treatment of refractory affective disorders. *J. Clin. Psychiat., 54*: 380–84.

Schaffer A, Zuker P, & Levitt A (2006): Randomized, double-blind pilot trial comparing lamotrigine versus citalopram for the treatment of bipolar depression. *J. Affect. Disorders, 96*: 95–99.

Schaffer L, Schaffer C, & Hughes T (1999): Tiagabine and the treatment of refractory bipolar disorder. In: Soares J, Gershon S (eds), *Third International Conference on Bipolar Disorder* (Vol 1, pp. 49). Pittsburgh, PA: Munksgaard.

Semadeni GW (1967): Study of the clinical efficacy of dipropylacetamide in mood disorders. *Acta Psychiatr. Belg., 76*: 458–66.

Simhandl CH, Denk E, & Thau K (1993): The comparative efficacy of carbamazepine low and high serum level and lithium carbonate in the prophylaxis of affective disorders. *J. Affect. Disord., 28*: 221–31.

Small J, Klapper M, & Milstein V, et al. (1991): Carbamazepine compared with lithium in the treatment of mania. *Arch. Gen. Psychiatry, 48*: 915–21.

Stoll KD, Bisson HE, & Fischer E, et al. (1986): Carbamazepine versus haloperidol in manic syndromes — first report of a multicentric study in Germany. In: Shagass C, Josiassen RC, Bridger WH, et al. (eds.), *Biological Psychiatry 1985: Proceedings of the IVth World Congress of Biological Psychiatry Sept. 8–13 Philadelphia, PA* (pp. 332–334). New York: Elsevier.

Suppes T, Brown ES, & McElroy SL, et al. (1999): Lamotrigine for the treatment of bipolar disorder: a clinical case series. *J. Affect. Disord., 53*: 95–8.

Suppes T, Kelly DI, Hynan LS, et al. (2007): Comparison of two anticonvulsants in a randomized, single-blind treatment of hypomanic symptoms in patients with bipolar disorder. *Aust. NZ. J. Psychiatry, 41* (5): 397–402.

Takezaki H, & Hanaoka M (1971): The use of carbamazepine (Tegretol) in the control of manic-depressive psychosis and other manic, depressive states. *Seishin-igaku (Clinical Psychiatry) 13*: 173–83.

Tohen M, Baker RW, Altshuler LL, Zarate CA, Suppes T, Ketter TA, Milton DR, Risser R, Gilmore JA, Breier A, & Tollefson GA (2002): Olanzpine versus divalproex in the treatment of acute mania. *Am. J. Psychiatry, 159*: 1011–17.

van der Loos ML, Kölling P, Knoppert-van der Klein EA, & Nolen WA (2007): Lamotrigine in the treatment of bipolar disorder, a review. *Tijdschr Psychiatr., 49* (2): 95–103.

Vencovsky E, Peterova E, & Kabes J (1987): [Preventive effect of dipropylacetamide in bipolar manic-depressive psychoses]. *Psychiatr. Neurol. Med. Psychol. (Leipz), 39*: 362–4.

Vieta E, Manuel Goikolea J, Martínez-Arán A, Comes M, Verger K, Masramon X, Sanchez-Moreno J, & Colom F (2006): A double-blind, randomized, placebo-controlled, prophylaxis study of adjunctive gabapentin for bipolar disorder. *J. Clin. Psychiatry, 67* (3): 473–7.

Victor BS, Link NA, Binder RL, & Bell IR (1984): Use of clonazepam in mania and schizoaffective disorders. *Am. J. Psychiatry, 141*: 1111–112.

Wagner KD, Kowatch RA, Emslie GJ, Findling RL, Wilens TE, McCague K, D'Souza J, Wamil A, Lehman RB, Berv D, & Linden D (2006): A double blind randomized placebo controlled trial of oxcarbazepine in the treatment of bipolar disorder in children and adolescents. *Am. J. Psychiatry, 163*: 1179–86.

Watkins SE, Callender K, Thomas DR, Tidmarsh SF, & Shaw DM (1987): The effect of carbamazepine and lithium on remission from affective illness. *Br. J. Psychiatry, 150*: 180–82.

Weisler RH, Kalali AH, Ketter TA, & SPD417 Study group (2004): A multicenter randomized double blind placebo controlled trial of extended release carbamazepine capsules as monotherapy for bipolar disorder patients with manic or mixed episodes. *J. Clin. Psychiatry, 65* (4): 478–84.

Weisler RH, Keck PE Jr, Swann AC, Cutler AJ, Ketter TA, Kalali AH, & SPD417 Study group (2005): Extended release carbamazepine capsules as monotherapy for acute mania in bipolar disorder: a multicenter randomized double blind placebo controlled trial. *J. Clin. Psychiatry, 66* (3): 323–30.

Weisler RH, Hirschfeld R, Cutler AJ, Gazda T, Ketter TA, Keck PE Jr, Swann AC, Kalali AH, & SPD417 Study group (2006): Extended release carbamazepine capsules as monotherapy for acute mania in bipolar disorder: pooled results from two randomized double blind placebo controlled trials. *CNS Drugs, 20* (3): 219–31.

Wolf C, Berky M, & Kovacs G (1997): Carbamazepine versus lithium in the prophylaxis of bipolar affective disorders: A randomised, double-blind 1-year study in 168 patients (abstract). *Eur. Neuropsychopharmacol., 7* (Suppl. 2): S176.

Zajecka JM, Weisler R, Sachs G, Swann AC, Wozniak P, & Sommerville KW (2002): A comparison of the efficacy, safety, and tolerability of divalproex sodium and olanzapine in the treatment of bipolar disorder. *J. Clin. Psychiatry, 63* (12): 1148–55.

Zapletalek M, Hanus H, & Kindernayova H (1988): [Personal experience with the prophylactic effect of dipropylacetamide]. *Cesk Psychiatr., 84*: 7–10.

chapter fourteen

Somatic treatments for bipolar disorder

Raymond W. Lam, Peter Chan, and Andrew Howard
University of British Columbia

Contents

Introduction 411
Electroconvulsive therapy 412
    ECT for bipolar disorder 413
    Concomitant medications during ECT 414
    ECT-emergent euphoria, hypomania, and mania 415
    Maintenance ECT 416
Light therapy 417
    Light therapy for BD 418
    Light therapy for bipolar depression: Special considerations 420
Wake therapy (sleep deprivation) 420
    Wake therapy for bipolar depression 421
Transcranial magnetic stimulation 422
    rTMS for bipolar disorder 423
Neurosurgical treatments 424
    Ablative neurosurgical procedures 424
    Vagus nerve stimulation 426
    VNS and bipolar disorder 426
    Deep brain stimulation 427
Conclusions 428
References 428

Introduction

The biological revolution in our understanding of psychiatric conditions has produced an unparalleled number of treatments for bipolar disorder (BD). Much of the attention has been focused on psychopharmacology, where the medication armamentarium for treating BD grows steadily. However, electroconvulsive therapy (ECT) was among the first somatic treatments used for mental illness, and it remains one of the most effective treatments today.

In the past two decades, a large number of studies have shown that other somatic treatments, including light therapy, sleep deprivation (wake therapy), and repetitive transcranial magnetic stimulation, can be effective for treating depression and BD. Additionally, there has been renewed interest in neurosurgical approaches to refractory mood disorders, including vagus nerve stimulation, ablative limbic neurosurgery, and deep brain stimulation (DBS).

Unfortunately, unlike psychopharmacology, the resources of the pharmaceutical industry do not back research into these somatic treatments. The evidence for these treatments is therefore not as substantial as that for medications because it is more difficult to design suitable "placebo" conditions and there is scarce funding for large-scale randomized controlled trials (RCTs). Hence, evaluation of somatic treatments for clinical use often depends on independent replication of small-sample studies. Even when somatic treatments have demonstrated evidence-based efficacy, it remains a challenge to educate busy clinicians about these treatments and to promote their use in clinical settings.

In this chapter, we review the evidence for the use of these somatic treatments for BD, and focus on how the clinician can apply these tools as primary or adjunctive treatments for their patients with BD.

Electroconvulsive therapy

The ECT is a safe and effective treatment for a variety of psychiatric conditions, including BD, and even some medical conditions (American Psychiatric Association Task Force on Electroconvulsive Therapy, 2001). It has proven superiority in prospective studies comparing ECT with "sham" ECT and with standard antidepressant treatment in "medication-resistant" patients (UK ECT Group, 2003). The efficacy and rapidity of response can reduce the length of stay and hospital costs, especially when patients are identified early in the course of hospitalization and offered ECT as a treatment option (Olfson et al., 1998).

In unipolar major depressive disorder (MDD), response rates for acute treatment with ECT are reported as 80–90% overall, and somewhat lower at 60–70% for patients with treatment resistant depression (TRD) (Prudic et al., 1996). However, relapse rates after an acute course of ECT are high (greater than 50%) without continuation or maintenance pharmacotherapy (Sackeim et al., 2001) and/or maintenance ECT. Clinical experience suggests similar outcomes in those with bipolar depression.

ECT for bipolar disorder

Many clinical guidelines for treatment of BD have included ECT. Table 14.1 summarizes the indications for ECT during depressive episodes. Earlier retrospective studies indicated similar responses to ECT in unipolar and bipolar depressive episodes (e.g., Black, Winokur, & Nasrallah, 1986) but patients with BD may show faster onset of response. This view is supported by a study combining data from three RCTs comparing ECT in depressed patients with BD I and II ($n=66$) and unipolar MDD ($n=162$) (Daly et al., 2001). Both groups had similar overall response and remission rates, but patients with BD responded sooner and required fewer treatments. The median number of ECT treatments to achieve a 60% reduction in Ham-D scores was four for BD and six for MDD. The evidence supports the observation that bipolar depression may respond quickly with ECT, and that careful monitoring for switching is required.

ECT is also effective in acute mania with response rates as high as 80% (Mukherjee, Sackeim, & Schnur, 1994), although it is generally used only for patients not responding to standard pharmacotherapy. Older, retrospective studies found that response to ECT was comparable to, or better than, chlorpromazine or lithium treatment (e.g., Black, Winokur, & Nasrallah, 1987; Thomas & Reddy, 1982). These findings were also supported by small-sample RCTs. In a sham-controlled

Table 14.1 Indications for ECT in Bipolar Disorder

For unipolar or bipolar depressive episodes:
- Acute suicidality with high risk of acting on suicidal thoughts
- Psychotic features
- Catatonia
- Rapidly deteriorating physical status due to complications from the depression, such as poor oral intake
- History of poor response to medications
- History of good response to ECT
- The risks of standard antidepressant treatment outweigh the risks of ECT, particularly in medically frail or elderly patients
- Patient preference

For other types of bipolar episodes:
- Manic delirium
- Acute mania, unresponsive to medications
- Mixed states and rapid cycling, unresponsive to medications

Source: Adapted from American Psychiatric Association Task Force on Electroconvulsive Therapy, 2001.

study ($n = 30$ manic patients), ECT with chlorpromazine was superior to chlorpromazine alone (Sikdar et al., 1994). Bilateral ECT was also superior to lithium carbonate over an 8-week period in 34 manic inpatients (Small et al., 1988), while recurrence rates in the two groups were comparable after a 2-year follow up while on maintenance treatment with lithium. In 20 patients with treatment-resistant mania randomized to unilateral or bilateral ECT or lithium plus haloperidol, 59% responded within the ECT groups compared to none in the medication group (Mukherjee, Sackeim, & Lee, 1988).

ECT is especially useful in the presence of extreme and sustained agitation, such as found in "manic delirium". In this condition, ECT can be rapidly therapeutic (within one to two treatments rather than the average of eight to nine treatments with depression) and can avoid the risk of neuroleptic malignant syndrome with antipsychotic medications (Fink, 1999). Since it may be difficult to differentiate manic delirium from an organic delirium, a full medical work-up needs to be done before initiating ECT. Patients with rapid-cycling (Koukopoulos et al., 2003) and mixed-state (Devanand et al., 2000; Gruber et al., 2000; Ciapparelli et al., 2001) bipolar episodes can also benefit from ECT.

For patients with BD undergoing a course of ECT, clinical factors such as use of concomitant medications and risk of switching to hypomania/mania with ECT should be considered.

Concomitant medications during ECT

Antidepressants and antipsychotics. Antidepressants and antipsychotics, including atypicals, can lower seizure thresholds but can be safely given during ECT. Some agents such as bupropion, chlorpromazine, clomipramine, clozapine, and maprotiline (Pisani et al., 2002) are especially prone to reducing seizure threshold, and careful consideration is warranted when these medications are used with ECT.

Benzodiazepines. Benzodiazepines can increase seizure threshold (sometimes to a point when a seizure cannot be triggered with the maximum energy output from the ECT device), decrease seizure duration, and theoretically reduce the efficacy of ECT (Boylan et al., 2000). Strategies to counter this include holding the benzodiazepine dose the night before and morning of the ECT, switching to a short half-life agent, or giving the intravenous benzodiazepine antagonist, flumazenil (Krystal et al., 1998), immediately prior to the ECT stimulus (with use of intravenous midazolam after ECT to prevent withdrawal). The risks (prolonging seizures or nonconvulsive status epilepticus) and benefits (preventing increased seizure threshold) of tapering high-dose benzodiazepines before ECT need to be weighed, especially when the medications have been used long term.

Lithium. Early reports raised concern about lithium causing acute confusional states that lingered post-ECT and contributed to persistent cognitive dysfunction (e.g., Remick, 1978), or causing anaethestic complications including prolonged recovery of breathing and time to awakening by potentiating neuromuscular blocking agents (Hill, Wong, & Hodges, 1976). Additionally, lithium can induce sinus node dysfunction (Roose et al., 1979), which could be of theoretical concern if bradycardia is induced by the ECT stimulus. However, later reviews (Dolenc & Rasmussen, 2005) have not shown these risks to be as high as previously considered or clinically significant. Regardless, there is no consensus amongst ECT practitioners about whether to stop lithium, reduce the dose, or maintain usual doses during ECT. If lithium initiation or continuation is considered during ECT, it would be prudent to adjust the dosage to achieve serum levels in the lower therapeutic range (e.g., 0.6–0.8 mEq/L in younger adults; 0.3–0.5 mEq/L in the elderly), and then to hold the dose the night before and morning of the ECT.

Anticonvulsants. Like benzodiazepines, the seizure-modifying properties of anticonvulsants can theoretically reduce efficacy of ECT. Although there are no prospective RCTs, studies have shown that concomitant use of anticonvulsants, whether for epilepsy or a psychiatric condition, does not affect ECT outcomes (Sienaert & Peuskens, 2007). Therefore, anticonvulsants can be safely prescribed during ECT. In nonepileptic older adults, in whom higher seizure thresholds are more likely, holding the anticonvulsant dose the night before and morning of the ECT can be helpful. This may also be helpful during the course of ECT as seizure threshold may successively increase. Carbamazepine can prolong the action of succinylcholine, but this effect is likely not clinically relevant.

ECT-emergent euphoria, hypomania, and mania

ECT can precipitate euphoric mood states and hypomanic or manic episodes. In a retrospective study of 1057 patients, some of whom were treated with ECT, hypomanic or manic switches occurred in 12% of those diagnosed as endogenous depression and 10% in psychotic depression (Angst et al., 1992). Switches occurred more often in those with bipolar depression (especially when psychotic; 32% of these patients switched) or with a family history of BD. Other studies suggest the risk is as low as 7% (Beyer, Weiner, & Glick, 1998). These data must be considered preliminary, as these were retrospective and observational studies that did not include control groups.

ECT-emergent hypomania should be differentiated from the delirium with euphoria, or "organic euphoria" (Devanand et al., 1988), that can occur during ECT. Organic euphoria is usually a transient state lasting a few hours to days, characterized by confusion, disorientation and cognitive impairment. There is an associated silly, inappropriate quality to the mood. The disorientation and cognitive changes differentiates this from hypomania or mania.

There are few data about treatment for ECT-emergent hypomania/ mania. Some clinicians opt to stop ECT and observe with or without the introduction of a mood stabilizer. Others, given the effectiveness of ECT for manic episodes, would continue the ECT (American Psychiatric Association Task Force on Electroconvulsive Therapy, 2001). Factors to consider for this treatment decision include severity of emergent symptoms, whether they occur early or later in the course of ECT, and severity of past episodes of mania.

Maintenance ECT

Given the high relapse rate after ECT, maintenance ECT (in which a single treatment is given every 1–8 weeks or longer) has been used in selected patients to maintain response. A recent prospective RCT compared continuation ECT, beginning weekly then tapering to monthly, with continuation pharmacotherapy in patients with unipolar depression who remitted following an index course of bifrontotemporal ECT (Kellner et al., 2006). The six-month relapse rates were comparable for continuation ECT (37%) and pharmacotherapy (32%), suggesting that continuation ECT can be considered for some patients. For BD, a number of case reports indicate benefits of maintenance ECT in pharmacotherapy-resistant cases (e.g., Gagne et al., 2000; Nascimento et al., 2006; Vaidya, Mahableshwarkar, & Shahid, 2003) with demonstration of cost savings by avoiding re-hospitalizations (Bonds et al., 1998).

There is no evidence to indicate that maintenance ECT contributes to cognitive impairment (Abraham et al., 2006). Even patients with ECT-related cognitive changes during acute treatment may experience significant cognitive improvement during maintenance ECT. However, a recent neuropsychological study suggests that patients with BD with a remote (more than 6 months) history of receiving ECT have poorer performance on certain anterograde memory and verbal learning tests compared to those never receiving ECT (MacQueen et al., 2007). These results conflict with studies in unipolar depression showing that anterograde memory and learning deficits usually resolve quickly post-ECT and do not persist by 6 months following ECT (Reisner, 2003; Sackeim et al., 2007). Therefore, further study of ECT and cognition is required in BD.

Light therapy

Light therapy (also called phototherapy) consists of daily exposure to bright artificial light. Light treatment has been shown to be effective for seasonal affective disorder (SAD, also known as winter depression). In DSM-IV, SAD is characterized as a "seasonal pattern" qualifier for MDD or BD, with recurrent major depressive episodes that occur during the fall and winter, with natural remissions occurring during spring and summer (Westrin & Lam, 2007). For patients with BD, the offset of depressive episodes may be heralded by hypomanic or manic episodes in the spring.

Initially, SAD was considered to be primarily a subtype of BD, with clinical reports indicating that up to 95% of patients had hypomanic or manic responses in the springtime (Rosenthal et al., 1984). The atypical depressive features (hypersomnia, hyperphagia, weight gain) found in SAD also seemed consistent with those described in bipolar depression. Subsequent studies, however, have placed the rate of BD in SAD to be much lower, in the order of 11–15% (White et al., 1990; Lam, 1998).

Since 1984, dozens of controlled studies, including larger-sample RCTs comparing light therapy against plausible placebo conditions (Terman, Terman, & Ross, 1998; Eastman et al., 1998), have shown that light therapy is effective for SAD with an overall response rate of about 65%. Additionally, several systematic reviews and meta-analyses have also confirmed that bright light therapy is effective in SAD (Thompson, 2001; Golden et al., 2005). Consequently, light therapy is now included in major clinical guidelines for the treatment of depression.

For clinical use, the 10,000 lux fluorescent light box is the "gold standard" light device, although newer devices such as the Litebook, a portable device that uses light emitting diodes (LED) are also effective (Desan et al., 2007) (see Figure 14.1). Commercial light devices are now readily available at local medical supply shops or by mail order at a cost of between US$100 and US$300. The method is quite straight forward, with patients using the light device at home for 30 minutes per day, as soon as possible upon arising in the morning (Westrin & Lam, 2007). The response to light therapy usually occurs rapidly and is often noticeable within a week of starting light therapy. However, relapse of symptoms also occurs within the same time period when light therapy is stopped, so daily treatment needs to continue throughout the winter season, until the time of usual spring remission.

Side effects to light therapy are relatively mild, with headache, eyestrain, agitation, and nausea the most common effects reported (Westrin & Lam, 2007). Most side effects subside with regular use of light therapy, or can be

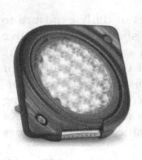
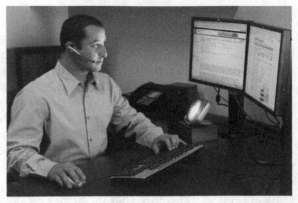

Figure 14.1 An example of an LED light device.

managed by reducing the "dose" of light, either by reducing the duration of daily exposure or by reducing the intensity (e.g., sitting slightly farther back from the light source). There are no absolute contraindications to using light therapy. The 10,000 lux light schedule should be safe for most patients, and no adverse retinal effects were found after 5 year follow-up of patients treated with light therapy (Gallin et al., 1995).

The mechanism of action of light therapy for SAD remains unclear (for review, see Lam & Levitan, 2000 and Sohn & Lam, 2005). There is evidence that bright light corrects dysregulated circadian rhythms in depression, and that light therapy has effects on the serotonergic and catecholaminergic dysfunction found in SAD. It is well recognized that light is the strongest synchronizer of human circadian rhythms, and timed bright light exposure can reliably shift human circadian rhythms in the same predictable manner as in animals. Circadian rhythm dysregulation hypotheses have also been proposed for nonseasonal BD (Kripke et al., 1978; Wirz-Justice, 1995). Light therapy is also useful in treating circadian disorders such as phase-delayed sleep disorder, shift work, and jet lag (Terman, 2007).

Light therapy for BD

Many studies of SAD, including treatment studies of light therapy, have included mixed samples of unipolar and bipolar patients. In fact, the first SAD patient to receive light therapy had a BD (Lewy et al., 1982). Most of the studies, however, involve drug-free patients, so patients with BD II are more likely to be included while BD I are more likely excluded. There are no published controlled studies directly comparing the response of unipolar and bipolar SAD patients to light therapy (Sohn & Lam, 2004).

Although much of the research on light therapy has been done in SAD, light was first investigated as a treatment for nonseasonal depression (Kripke, 1981). Since then, there have been several controlled studies of light therapy for nonseasonal MDD. Results have been inconsistent, in part because of small sample sizes, short durations (one to two weeks), and differences in light treatment parameters. However, a Cochrane systematic review found that light therapy had significant effects in patients with nonseasonal depression (Tuunainen, Kripke, & Endo, 2004), suggesting that further investigation is certainly warranted.

There are only limited, pilot studies of light therapy for nonseasonal BD. In one study, bipolar patients had better responses to light therapy than unipolar patients, but the bipolar patients responded to both bright (2500 lux) and dim (400 lux) light (Deltito et al., 1991). In another study, light therapy (10,000 lux for 45 minutes, twice a day for 4 weeks) was used in a small sample of young patients with BD who had subsyndromal depressive symptoms during the winter (Papatheodorou & Kutcher, 1995). Moderate or marked response was found in five of the seven patients. The effects of morning, midday, or evening light therapy were studied over a period of 3 months each in nine patients with rapid cycling BD who were on stable doses of medications, and compared to 3 months without light therapy (Leibenluft et al., 1995). Only midday light exposure had beneficial effects, in three of five patients; morning light exposure worsened symptoms in three patients. In this study, the light therapy was better tolerated when patients discontinued the light treatment on days when they were hypomanic.

A recent pilot study examined the use of bright light therapy in nine women with bipolar depression (seven with BD I, two with BD II) (Sit et al., 2007). Again, morning light exposure induced mixed states in three of the first four patients treated, so midday timing was used for the rest. The optimum response appeared to be 7000 lux x 45–60 minutes at midday. Four of the nine patients had a sustained response to light therapy, either with midday or morning exposure, while two others had partial responses.

In summary, although the evidence is still limited, there is a strong suggestion that light therapy is beneficial in nonseasonal bipolar and unipolar depression. Given the mild side effects of light therapy, and the fact that light can be combined with other medications without worrying about drug–drug interactions, some investigators have recommended wider use of light therapy as an adjunctive treatment for nonseasonal depression (Kripke, 1998).

Light therapy for bipolar depression: Special considerations

Like other effective antidepressant treatments, light therapy can precipitate hypomanic or manic responses in susceptible patients (Chan, Lam, & Perry, 1994; Kripke, 1991). Feeling agitated or "revved up" can be part of an immediate, energizing effect of bright light exposure, even in normal subjects (Bauer et al., 1994). There has also been some suggestion that bipolar patients are more sensitive to light than unipolar patients or normal subjects (Lewy, Sack, & Singer, 1985). In our experience, patients with BD, Type I (with previous manic episodes) are more likely to experience some agitation with light therapy and usually require dosage adjustment (e.g., reducing the time spent under the lights or sitting farther away from the light source). We also recommend that patients with BD I be on a mood stabilizer when treated with light therapy.

Medications used to treat BD may also require special attention when prescribing light therapy. Lithium can affect the retina, although clinical studies have not shown any adverse retinal effects of long term lithium use by ophthalmological examination or by electrophysiological tests of retinal function (Lam et al., 1997). However, data from animal studies suggest that bright light exposure may potentiate some of the lithium-induced retinal changes (Reme et al., 1996). Similarly, other drugs that may potentially have photosensitizing effects include phenothiazine antipsychotics (e.g., thioridazine), melatonin and St. John's Wort (hypericum). Ophthalmological consultation prior to light therapy and regular monitoring (e.g., annually) are recommended for patients taking these medications.

Wake therapy (sleep deprivation)

Disturbances in the sleep–wake cycle are cardinal symptoms of BD. Patients have reduced need for sleep during manic episodes, while insomnia or hypersomnia is experienced during bipolar depression. It is well recognized that disruption of the sleep–wake cycle can precipitate mania. Hence, manipulation of the sleep–wake cycle has been investigated as a treatment for BD.

The most studied sleep manipulation for depression is that of total sleep deprivation (TSD), now known as wake therapy. When patients are kept awake all night, they often show an improvement in mood that continues through the next day (Pflug & Tolle, 1971). The mood changes can be dramatic, and many patients feel that their mood returns to baseline. Although it is difficult to design placebo-controlled studies, the fact that TSD is so counterintuitive to patients (most of whom think they will feel better if only they had *more* sleep) makes a placebo response less likely.

Unfortunately, the mood improvement after TSD is not long lived. The majority of patients relapse after a recovery sleep the next day after TSD. Several reviews of sleep deprivation studies found the clinical response rate to TSD averaged about 60%, but 80–85% of patients relapsed the next day after the recovery sleep (Wu & Bunney, 1992; Wirz-Justice & van den Hoofdakker RH, 1999). Relapse can occur even after brief naps. However, it is intriguing that up to 15% of patients appear to have sustained responses to TSD even after a recovery sleep.

Various strategies have been studied to prolong the antidepressant effect after wake therapy. Some have used partial sleep deprivation, particularly in the second half of the night (Leibenluft et al., 1993). Other strategies include use of bright light (Neumeister et al., 1996), lithium and pindolol (see following section).

Wake therapy for bipolar depression

Although early studies found that diurnal variation predicted response to TSD while unipolar/bipolar diagnoses did not (Elsenga & Van den Hoofdakker, 1987), other studies suggest that bipolar patients have better responses to wake therapy than unipolar patients (Barbini et al., 1998). Rapid cycling patients had the best responses in a study of 16 patients treated with TSD twice a week for 4 weeks (Papadimitriou et al., 1993). Bipolar I patients also had the best responses to late sleep deprivation (sleep time set at 21:00 to 02:00 hrs) (Szuba et al., 1991). Bipolar patients do not necessarily switch into hypomania or mania after TSD. The "switch rate" of bipolar patients to TSD was 5–6% in a sample of 206 bipolar patients, a switch rate similar to that of antidepressants (Colombo et al., 1999).

Lithium treatment in bipolar patients can also maintain the antidepressant response to wake therapy. Forty depressed patients with BD were treated with a TSD conducted three times over 1 week with a recovery night between TSD sessions. Thirteen of 20 patients responded to lithium plus TSD compared to two of 12 patients with TSD alone (Benedetti et al., 1999). In a placebo-controlled study of 40 patients with bipolar depression, the addition of pindolol (a beta-blocker that in low doses is a specific 5-HT1A autoreceptor antagonist) prevented relapse after three cycles of TSD in 9 days; 15 of 20 patients on pindolol continued to be well, compared to three of 20 patients on placebo (Smeraldi et al., 1999). Following wake therapy, patients were maintained on lithium alone, and 65% of the pindolol+TSD cases sustained the response for 6 months (Smeraldi et al., 1999).

Given the evidence for the favorable clinical responses to wake therapy, which bipolar patients could be considered for wake therapy? We would consider wake therapy for patients who need a rapid response, e.g., acutely suicidal patients or patients starting on an antidepressant. Patients with variability of mood within the day and/or with melancholic symptoms may be more likely to respond.

How can wake therapy be used in a clinical setting? In our experience, it is very difficult to conduct TSD as an outpatient without significant help from a family member. Even partial sleep deprivation protocols are difficult to initiate and maintain. We find that wake therapy is more feasible to conduct in an inpatient setting. Patients can watch television and/or videos through the night and the hospital staff can periodically monitor patients to ensure that they are awake. Given the current economic climate, any simple intervention that can improve mood quickly and reduce the number of days in hospital should generate significant interest. A regimen of three repeated TSD sessions over the course of one week is well tolerated by patients who respond to wake therapy. On days one, three, and five, patients undergo TSD by staying awake for 36 hours from 07:00 hrs to 19:00 hrs the next day. On days two, four, and six, patients have a recovery sleep from 19:00 hrs to 07:00 hrs the next day (adapted from Smeraldi et al., 1999).

If patients respond to wake therapy, efforts should focus on maintaining their response. This will likely include medications (lithium or antidepressants), or alternatively bright light exposure. Mood stabilizing medication can be continued while wake therapy is conducted, especially given the studies showing that lithium can maintain the antidepressant effect of wake therapy. Unfortunately, there are no data about whether other mood stabilizers also share this effect.

Transcranial magnetic stimulation

Transcranial magnetic stimulation (TMS) is a noninvasive technique in which a high intensity magnetic field is generated and used to stimulate cortical neurons. When directed over the motor cortex, TMS can induce neuronal depolarization and result in observable involuntary movements of the contralateral hand and fingers. For therapeutic applications TMS has been modified to incorporate a "train" of sequential magnetic pulses, termed repetitive TMS (rTMS). Parameters of the magnetic pulse which can be varied include pulse frequency ("fast" distinguished from "slow" when the frequency is greater than one per second) and intensity (as a percentage of the energy required for observable motor movements, called the motor threshold). rTMS studies in depression have generally applied 20–40 trains of 2–10 seconds each, with daily sessions over 5 days of the week.

Since the mid-1990s, dozens of sham-controlled studies have examined rTMS for depressive conditions while varying the treatment parameters, including location of brain areas for stimulation. There is increasing consensus that antidepressant effects are associated with fast frequency rTMS to the left dorsolateral prefrontal cortex (DLPFC) or slow frequency rTMS to the right DLPFC, using stimulus intensity of at least 80% motor threshold (George et al., 1995). A large scale ($n=301$), sham-controlled, 4-week RCT using these left DLPFC parameters showed efficacy in a mixed group of depressed patients who had not responded to at least one antidepressant (O'Reardon et al., 2007).

Several meta-analyses of rTMS studies in depression have been done, showing conflicting results depending on the selection criteria for studies. Most have concluded that there is a significant benefit of active rTMS over sham. However, the response and remission rates have been disappointingly low, perhaps because the studies are all of very short duration (1–4 weeks, median 2 weeks) and included heterogeneous samples of patients. We recently conducted a meta-analysis of 24 rTMS studies for TRD, which arguably is a more important population to study, given the time and resource constraints (daily treatment conducted in a hospital or clinic setting) required (Lam et al., 2008). We found a significant superiority of active rTMS over sham treatment in response (25% vs 9%, respectively) and remission (17% vs 6%). However, the same limitations applied to these studies, as the treatment durations were short (all 4 weeks or less) and there has been no attention to maintenance of effects once a course of rTMS is completed.

rTMS for bipolar disorder

Only smaller, less controlled studies have examined rTMS specifically for patients with BD. A pilot study randomized 23 patients with BD I and II depression to active rTMS (5Hz, 110% motor threshold, left DLPFC) or sham for 2 weeks (Nahas et al., 2003). No differences were found between conditions in depression scores or response rates. However, rTMS was well tolerated with no manic switches.

It is not surprising that rTMS, as do other effective antidepressant treatments, can induce mania. A recent systematic review identified ten of 53 rTMS trials that reported on treatment emergent mania and found low rates with no differences between active and sham conditions (Xia et al., 2008). Including case reports, there were ten cases of rTMS-emergent mania reported in the literature, with all cases responding to discontinuation of rTMS and/or use of anti-manic medications. There were no obvious treatment parameters associated with rTMS-emergent mania.

In contrast to these reports of rTMS-emergent mania, rTMS has also been studied as a treatment for mania. Given the lateralizing effects of rTMS in both depressed patients and in healthy controls, the effects of high frequency rTMS over the right DLPFC would be predicted to have antimanic effects. Open studies supported this hypothesis (Saba et al., 2004; Michael & Erfurth, 2004). An RCT of left versus right DLPFC rTMS in 16 patients with acute mania also treated with medications (Grisaru et al., 1998). The right-sided rTMS led to greater improvement compared to left-sided. In a follow-up study of right DLPFC using the same parameters ($n = 19$), however, there were no differences between active rTMS and the sham condition (Kaptsan et al., 2003). While it is possible that the antidepressant effects of rTMS were obscured by the higher number of patients with psychosis in the rTMS condition (since rTMS has been reported less effective in psychosis associated with depression), it is also possible that the apparent benefits of right rTMS in the previous study were because of worsening of mania in the left-sided condition.

In summary, the clinical utility of rTMS for either unipolar or bipolar depression (or mania) is still to be determined, in part due to very limited data on sustained and maintenance effects of rTMS. However, given the advantages of rTMS (its noninvasive nature, lack of cognitive and other side effects, no need for anaesthesia, etc.), it will be important to investigate further rTMS as a treatment for depression.

Neurosurgical treatments

Ablative neurosurgical procedures

Since the 1949 Nobel Prize in medicine and physiology was awarded to Egas Moniz, a Portuguese neurologist, and his neurosurgical colleague, Almeida Lima, for pioneering neurosurgery for psychiatric disorders, the field has been severely criticized for its lack of objective and systematic evaluation of outcomes, its uncritical selection of patients, and its unrefined techniques (Diering & Bell, 1991). Despite the suggested benefits of early psychosurgery, significant complications and morbidity accompanied many of the procedures, such as devastating effects on cognition and personality (Malizia, 1997). Today, there is still considerable negative public opinion about psychosurgery.

Despite this questionable history, modern neurosurgical procedures with better evidence for effectiveness are still performed for psychiatric conditions in a small number of tertiary centers around the world. The morbidity and mortality of these newer procedures are greatly reduced due to introduction of stereotactic techniques, brain imaging guidance for lesion location, smaller and more precise lesions, increased surgical proficiency and more careful selection of appropriate patients with highly refractory illness (Spangler et al., 1996).

Cingulotomy, the most common historically performed neurosurgery for mental disorders, severs the supracallosal fibers of the anterior cingulate with a thermocoagulative lesion (Greenberg et al., 2003). Cingulotomy was reported to have a 42% rate of recovery and only 1 suicide in a case series of 400 patients with difficult to treat affective and anxiety disorders (Greenberg et al., 2003). No deaths or permanent cognitive or personality changes were seen. Complications of seizures, hemorrhage, and hydrocephalus were rare. A report of a series of 34 patients undergoing cingulotomy included five patients with BD; two patients responded, two experienced partial response, and one did not respond (Spangler et al., 1996). Side effects included transient ataxia, urinary retention, and confusion. In another cohort, four of 13 patients (including two with BD) responded to cingulotomy (Dougherty et al., 2003).

Subcaudate tractotomy uses radiofrequency thermocoagulation to produce a lesion of the white matter beneath the caudate head bilaterally (Greenberg et al., 2003). In the most recent case series, 32% of 249 patients with OCD or severe mood disorders, including 44 with BD, were recovered or well after one year, and 38% were improved (Hodgkiss et al., 1995). In nine patients with longstanding severe BD, post-surgery follow-up for up to 6 years revealed excellent improvement in three patients, with reduction of frequency and severity of illness episodes seen in all patients. Complications included necessary extension of the lesions due to inadequate results in two patients and focal seizures in one patient. Rarely have personality changes been reported in the literature since 1975 and adverse events typically include transient headache, confusion, lethargy, and urinary incontinence (Skidmore et al., 2006).

Capsulotomy (ablation of the ventral aspect of the anterior limb of the internal capsule) and limbic leucotomy (combined cingulotomy and subcaudate tractotomy) are the two other neurosurgical procedures still used in patients with mood and anxiety disorders. Although the evidence is variable in quality, both are reported to have similar response rates (e.g., 48–78% for capsulotomy (Greenberg et al., 2003); 40–50% for limbic leucotomy (Montoya et al., 2002)). No specific data on patients with BD are available for either procedure.

In summary, after 50 years of ablative surgery for severe psychiatric disorders including OCD, depression, and BD, an impressive response rate of 35–70% is reported in a highly refractory population. However, the outcome data are all retrospective and uncontrolled, and there is much variability in the literature in the inclusion criteria of patients for surgery, the definition of their illnesses, and the outcome measures used. The benefits, even in these severely and chronically ill patients, must be weighed against the uncommon but serious risks of neurosurgery, including stroke, seizures, infections and personality or cognitive changes.

Vagus nerve stimulation

In vagus nerve stimulation (VNS), a small incision is made on the left side of the neck and an electrode is placed around the vagus nerve and connected to a pulse generator (similar to a pacemaker) that is implanted superficially over the left chest wall (Andrews, 2003). An external magnetic device is used to adjust stimulation parameters including current intensity, pulse width, frequency, and duration of on/off periods (Eitan & Lerer, 2006). The electrical stimulation is usually set at a continuous cycle of 30 seconds on and 5 minutes off. VNS is safe and well-tolerated with few complications. Common but mild side effects include voice alteration and hoarseness, dyspnea, paraesthesiae, dysphagia, neck pain, headache, and cough (Carpenter et al., 2006).

In the 1990s, VNS was approved in Europe and North America for use in patients with medication-resistant epilepsy. Since then, approximately 32,000 patients with epilepsy have undergone VNS. Benefits in this group appear to increase over time; 43% reported at least 50% reduction in seizure frequency, 15% obtained effective seizure control, and 10% were able to discontinue medications (Nemeroff et al., 2006).

Interest in VNS as a possible therapy for depression was sparked by the observation of mood improvement seen in patients with epilepsy regardless of improvement in seizures (Holtzheimer & Nemeroff, 2006). VNS reportedly has antidepressant-like effects on sleep architecture in patients with epilepsy and depression, shows similar effects to ECT and desipramine in animal models of depression, and results in changes in neurochemical, functional imaging, neuroimmune and neuroendocrine markers similar to those seen during antidepressant treatment (Nemeroff et al., 2006).

VNS and bipolar disorder

A 10-week pilot study of VNS in 60 patients with chronic, treatment-refractory depression (including lithium-resistant or intolerant patients with BD I and II) found a clinical response (50% or greater reduction in depression scores) in 30% (Goodnicket al., 2001). After 2-year naturalistic follow-up, response improved to 42% while remission was seen in 22% (Nahas et al., 2005). Moreover, 56% of patients endorsed improvement in social functioning, emotional role, vitality, and overall mental health. Side effects were minimal and no serious adverse effects were related to the device.

Subsequently, a sham-controlled RCT was conducted in 235 patients with unipolar or bipolar depression (excluding rapid-cycling) (Nemeroff et al., 2006). All patients were implanted with the VNS device, but only half were turned on for the first 10 weeks. At the end of acute treatment, there was a nonsignificant difference in response (15% for the treatment group versus 10% for the sham group). All devices were then turned on. Patients after 1 year with naturalistic VNS treatment ($n=205$) were compared with a control group of patients with TRD ($n=124$) treated with usual care consisting of pharmacotherapy, psychotherapy and ECT (George et al., 2005). Despite greater severity and treatment resistance at baseline, the VNS group demonstrated greater improvement than the usual care group in response rates (27% vs 13%, respectively) and remission rates (13% vs 3%). Of the bipolar patients, five of 17 (29%) responded to VNS versus one of 15 (7%) to usual care. While the study lacked a placebo control, the authors argued that a placebo response rate of > 10% would not be likely in such a treatment-refractory population, nor would a placebo response tend to increase over time.

VNS now has regulatory approval in Canada, the United States, and Europe for treatment-resistant unipolar and bipolar major depressive episodes. Dosing trials are ongoing, as are investigations to identify the population of responders and the neurochemical and functional imaging correlates of response (George et al., 2007).

Deep brain stimulation

DBS involves introducing electrodes into specific brain regions using stereotactic surgery guided by computerized navigation programs and intraoperative neurophysiological mapping. The leads are looped under the scalp, tunneled into the neck and connected to a pulse generator, similar to that of VNS, implanted in the left chest wall. The pulse generator can be magnetically programmed to deliver a repetitive and continuous train of electrical pulses of variable intensity, frequency, and duration. Complications include the possibility of hardware-related malfunction, seizures, and neurological deficits depending on the target chosen and nearby structures that may be injured, especially if several passes of the electrode are required.

There are various explanations proposed for the mechanism of action of DBS, e.g., it appears to mimic an ablative lesion when a frequency of greater than 100 pulses per second is applied (Skidmore et al., 2006). Regardless, DBS is now an approved treatment for medication-refractory Parkinson's disease, dystonia and essential tremor (Schupbach et al., 2005).

There are currently only two published studies describing the use of DBS in treatment-refractory depression, in a total of 11 patients, one of whom was diagnosed with BD II. In one study, five patients underwent 3 months of DBS of the ventral anterior limb of the internal capsule and adjacent dorsal ventral striatum (Carpenter, 2006). Three of the five demonstrated clinical response and the other two showed 23% and 17% reduction in HDRS scores, with improvement in social and occupational functioning. In the second study, the DBS target was the subgenual gyrus (Brodmann area 25), in the area of the ventromedial orbitofrontal cortex (Mayberg et al., 2005). This region was chosen because of convergence of data from connectivity and histopathological reports, functional imaging analyses, and anatomical involvement of this area in previous successful ablative lesions. In addition, brain activity in this area is suppressed nonspecifically with a variety of antidepressant treatments (Mayberg et al., 2000). A robust and persistent response was demonstrated for up to 6 months in four of six patients with TRD, and two were in remission at follow-up. While this initial study had small numbers, the investigators systematically tested parameters of stimulation, examined patients clinically and with PET imaging at baseline and at follow-up, and demonstrated a lack of response to sham stimulation.

In summary, further controlled studies are needed to identify the magnitude of the effect of VNS and DBS, but there is a cautious optimism that surgical methods of neuromodulation will be effective for treatment-refractory psychiatric illness (Kopell, Greenberg, & Rezai, 2004; Schlaepfer & Lieb, 2005).

Conclusions

Somatic treatments are among the oldest and the newest of therapies for depression. Minimally invasive treatments, such as light therapy, wake therapy and rTMS, have sufficient evidence to recommend judicious use as adjunctive treatments for patients with BD. ECT, while more invasive and negatively perceived by the public, is still widely used for severe and treatment-resistant depression and mania, but more study is required in BD, particularly in respect to cognitive effects. Newer surgical techniques that incorporate neuromodulation, such as VNS and DBS, may achieve increasing prominence for patients with BD unresponsive to pharmacotherapy, given their advantages of 100% adherence and the long term nature of the condition.

References

Abraham, G., Milev, R., Delva, N., & Zaheer, J. (2006). Clinical outcome and memory function with maintenance electroconvulsive therapy: a retrospective study. *J. ECT, 22*, 43–45.

American Psychiatric Association Task Force on Electroconvulsive Therapy. (2001). *The Practice of Electroconvulsive Therapy* (2nd edition). Washington DC: American Psychiatric Association.

Andrews, R. J. (2003). Neuroprotection trek—the next generation: neuromodulation I. Techniques–deep brain stimulation, vagus nerve stimulation, and transcranial magnetic stimulation. *Ann. N. Y. Acad. Sci., 993*, 1–13.

Angst, J., Angst, K., Baruffol, I., & Meinherz-Surbeck, R. (1992). ECT-induced and drug-induced hypomania. *Convuls. Ther., 8,* 179–185.

Barbini, B., Colombo, C., Benedetti, F., Campori, E., Bellodi, L., & Smeraldi, E. (1998). The unipolar-bipolar dichotomy and the response to sleep deprivation. *Psychiatry Res., 79,* 43–50.

Bauer, M. S., Kurtz, J. W., Rubin, L. B., & Marcus, J. G. (1994). Mood and behavioral effects of four-week light treatment in winter depressives and controls. *J. Psychiatr. Res., 28,* 135–145.

Benedetti, F., Colombo, C., Barbini, B., Campori, E., & Smeraldi, E. (1999). Ongoing lithium treatment prevents relapse after total sleep deprivation. *J. Clin. Psychopharmacol., 19,* 240–245.

Beyer, J., Weiner, R. D., & Glick, M. D. (1998). *Electroconvulsive Therapy. A Programmed Text.* Washington DC: American Psychiatric Press.

Black, D. W., Winokur, G., & Nasrallah, A. (1986). ECT in unipolar and bipolar disorders: A naturalistic evaluation of 460 patients. *Convuls. Ther., 2,* 231–237.

Black, D. W., Winokur, G., & Nasrallah, A. (1987). Treatment of mania: a naturalistic study of electroconvulsive therapy versus lithium in 438 patients. *J. Clin. Psychiatry, 48,* 132–139.

Bonds, C., Frye, M. A., Coudreaut, M. F., Cunningham, M., Spearing, M., McGuire, M., et al. (1998). Cost reduction with maintenance ECT in refractory bipolar disorder. *J. ECT, 14,* 36–41.

Boylan, L. S., Haskett, R. F., Mulsant, B. H., Greenberg, R. M., Prudic, J., Spicknall, K., et al. (2000). Determinants of seizure threshold in ECT: benzodiazepine use, anesthetic dosage, and other factors. *J. ECT, 16,* 3–18.

Carpenter, L. L. (2006). Neurostimulation in resistant depression. *J. Psychopharmacol., 20,* 35–40.

Carpenter, L. L., Friehs, G. M., Tyrka, A. R., Rasmussen, S., Price, L. H., & Greenberg, B. D. (2006). Vagus nerve stimulation and deep brain stimulation for treatment resistant depression. *Med. Health R. I., 89,* 137, 140–137, 141.

Chan, P. K., Lam, R. W., & Perry, K. F. (1994). Mania precipitated by light therapy for patients with SAD. *J. Clin. Psychiatry, 55,* 454.

Ciapparelli, A., Dell'Osso, L., Tundo, A., Pini, S., Chiavacci, M. C., Di, S. I., et al. (2001). Electroconvulsive therapy in medication-nonresponsive patients with mixed mania and bipolar depression. *J. Clin. Psychiatry, 62,* 552–555.

Colombo, C., Benedetti, F., Barbini, B., Campori, E., & Smeraldi, E. (1999). Rate of switch from depression into mania after therapeutic sleep deprivation in bipolar depression. *Psychiatry Res., 86,* 267–270.

Daly, J. J., Prudic, J., Devanand, D. P., Nobler, M. S., Lisanby, S. H., Peyser, S., et al. (2001). ECT in bipolar and unipolar depression: differences in speed of response. *Bipolar Disord., 3,* 95–104.

Deltito, J. A., Moline, M., Pollak, C., Martin, L. Y., & Maremmani, I. (1991). Effects of phototherapy on nonseasonal unipolar and bipolar depressive spectrum disorders. *J. Affect. Disord., 23,* 231–237.

Desan, P. H., Weinstein, A. J., Michalak, E. E., Tam, E. M., Meesters, Y., Ruiter, M. J., et al. (2007). A controlled trial of the Litebook light-emitting diode (LED) light therapy device for treatment of Seasonal Affective Disorder (SAD). *BMC Psychiatry, 7,* 38.

Devanand, D. P., Polanco, P., Cruz, R., Shah, S., Paykina, N., Singh, K., et al. (2000). The efficacy of ECT in mixed affective states. *J. ECT, 16,* 32–37.

Devanand, D. P., Sackeim, H. A., Decina, P., & Prudic, J. (1988). The development of mania and organic euphoria during ECT. *J. Clin. Psychiatry, 49*, 69–71.

Diering, S. L. & Bell, W. O. (1991). Functional neurosurgery for psychiatric disorders: a historical perspective. *Stereotact. Funct. Neurosurg., 57*, 175–194.

Dolenc, T. J. & Rasmussen, K. G. (2005). The safety of electroconvulsive therapy and lithium in combination: a case series and review of the literature. *J. ECT, 21*, 165–170.

Dougherty, D. D., Weiss, A. P., Cosgrove, G. R., Alpert, N. M., Cassem, E. H., Nierenberg, A. A., et al. (2003). Cerebral metabolic correlates as potential predictors of response to anterior cingulotomy for treatment of major depression. *J. Neurosurg., 99*, 1010–1017.

Eastman, C. I., Young, M. A., Fogg, L. F., Liu, L., & Meaden, P. M. (1998). Bright light treatment of winter depression: a placebo-controlled trial. *Arch. Gen. Psychiatry, 55*, 883–889.

Eitan, R. & Lerer, B. (2006). Nonpharmacological, somatic treatments of depression: electroconvulsive therapy and novel brain stimulation modalities. *Dialogues Clin. Neurosci., 8*, 241–258.

Elsenga, S. & Van den Hoofdakker, R. H. (1987). Response to total sleep deprivation and clomipramine in endogenous depression. *J. Psychiatric Res., 21*, 151–161.

Fink, M. (1999). ECT in delirious states. *J. ECT, 15*, 175–177.

Gagne, G. G., Jr., Furman, M. J., Carpenter, L. L., & Price, L. H. (2000). Efficacy of continuation ECT and antidepressant drugs compared to long-term antidepressants alone in depressed patients. *Am. J. Psychiatry, 157*, 1960–1965.

Gallin, P. F., Terman, M., Reme, C. E., Rafferty, B., Terman, J. S., & Burde, R. M. (1995). Ophthalmologic examination of patients with seasonal affective disorder, before and after bright light therapy. *Am. J. Ophthalmol., 119*, 202–210.

George, M. S., Nahas, Z., Borckardt, J. J., Anderson, B., Burns, C., Kose, S., et al. (2007). Vagus nerve stimulation for the treatment of depression and other neuropsychiatric disorders. *Expert. Rev. Neurother., 7*, 63–74.

George, M. S., Rush, A. J., Marangell, L. B., Sackeim, H. A., Brannan, S. K., Davis, S. M., et al. (2005). A one-year comparison of vagus nerve stimulation with treatment as usual for treatment-resistant depression. *Biol. Psychiatry, 58*, 364–373.

George, M. S., Wassermann, E. M., Williams, W. A., Callahan, A., Ketter, T. A., Basser, P., et al. (1995). Daily repetitive transcranial magnetic stimulation (rTMS) improves mood in depression. *Neuroreport, 6*, 1853–1856.

Golden, R. N., Gaynes, B. N., Ekstrom, R. D., Hamer, R. M., Jacobsen, F. M., Suppes, T., et al. (2005). The efficacy of light therapy in the treatment of mood disorders: a review and meta-analysis of the evidence. *Am. J. Psychiatry, 162*, 656–662.

Goodnick, P. J., Rush, A. J., George, M. S., Marangell, L. B., & Sackeim, H. A. (2001). Vagus nerve stimulation in depression. *Expert. Opin. Pharmacother., 2*, 1061–1063.

Greenberg, B. D., Price, L. H., Rauch, S. L., Friehs, G., Noren, G., Malone, D., et al. (2003). Neurosurgery for intractable obsessive-compulsive disorder and depression: critical issues. *Neurosurg. Clin. N. Am., 14*, 199–212.

Grisaru, N., Chudakov, B., Yaroslavsky, Y., & Belmaker, R. H. (1998). Transcranial magnetic stimulation in mania: a controlled study. *Am. J. Psychiatry, 155*, 1608–1610.

Gruber, N. P., Dilsaver, S. C., Shoaib, A. M., & Swann, A. C. (2000). ECT in mixed affective states: a case series. *J. ECT, 16,* 183–188.

Hill, G. E., Wong, K. C., & Hodges, M. R. (1976). Potentiation of succinylcholine neuromuscular blockade by lithium carbonate. *Anesthesiology, 44,* 439–442.

Hodgkiss, A. D., Malizia, A. L., Bartlett, J. R., & Bridges, P. K. (1995). Outcome after the psychosurgical operation of stereotactic subcaudate tractotomy, 1979–1991. *J. Neuropsychiatry Clin. Neurosci., 7,* 230–234.

Holtzheimer, P. E. & Nemeroff, C. B. (2006). Emerging treatments for depression. *Expert. Opin. Pharmacother., 7,* 2323–2339.

Kaptsan, A., Yaroslavsky, Y., Applebaum, J., Belmaker, R. H., & Grisaru, N. (2003). Right prefrontal TMS versus sham treatment of mania: a controlled study. *Bipolar Disord., 5,* 36–39.

Kellner, C. H., Knapp, R. G., Petrides, G., Rummans, T. A., Husain, M. M., Rasmussen, K., et al. (2006). Continuation electroconvulsive therapy vs pharmacotherapy for relapse prevention in major depression: a multisite study from the Consortium for Research in Electroconvulsive Therapy (CORE). *Arch. Gen. Psychiatry, 63,* 1337–1344.

Kopell, B. H., Greenberg, B., & Rezai, A. R. (2004). Deep brain stimulation for psychiatric disorders. *J. Clin. Neurophysiol., 21,* 51–67.

Koukopoulos, A., Sani, G., Koukopoulos, A. E., Minnai, G. P., Girardi, P., Pani, L. et al. (2003). Duration and stability of the rapid-cycling course: a long-term personal follow-up of 109 patients. *J. Affect. Disord., 73,* 75–85.

Kripke, D. F. (1981). Photoperiodic mechanisms for depression and its treatment. In C. Perris, G. Struwe, & B. Janson (Eds.), *Biological Psychiatry* (pp. 1248–1252). Amsterdam: Elsevier Press.

Kripke, D. F. (1991). Timing of phototherapy and occurrence of mania [letter; comment]. *Biol. Psychiatry, 29,* 1156–1157.

Kripke, D. F. (1998). Light treatment for nonseasonal depression: speed, efficacy, and combined treatment. *J. Affect. Disord., 49,* 109–117.

Kripke, D. F., Mullaney, D. J., Atkinson, M. L., & Wolf, S. (1978). Circadian rhythm disorders in manic-depressives. *Biol. Psychiatry, 13,* 335–351.

Krystal, A. D., Watts, B. V., Weiner, R. D., Moore, S., Steffens, D. C., & Lindahl, V. (1998). The use of flumazenil in the anxious and benzodiazepine-dependent ECT patient. *J. ECT, 14,* 5–14.

Lam, R. W. (1998). *Seasonal Affective Disorder and Beyond. Light Treatment for SAD and NonSAD Conditions.* Washington, DC: American Psychiatric Press.

Lam, R. W., Allain, S., Sullivan, K., Beattie, C. W., Remick, R. A., & Zis, A. P. (1997). Effects of chronic lithium treatment on retinal electrophysiologic function. *Biol. Psychiatry, 41,* 737–742.

Lam, R. W., Chan, P. K., Wilkins-Ho, M., & Yatham, L. N. (2008). Repetitive transcranial magnetic stimulation for treatment-resistant depression: A systematic review and meta-analysis. *Can. J. Psychiatry, 53*(9), 621–631.

Lam, R. W. & Levitan, R. D. (2000). Pathophysiology of seasonal affective disorder: a review. *J. Psychiatry Neurosci., 25,* 469–480.

Leibenluft, E., Moul, D. E., Schwartz, P. J., Madden, P. A., & Wehr, T. A. (1993). A clinical trial of sleep deprivation in combination with antidepressant medication. *Psychiatry Res., 46,* 213–227.

Leibenluft, E., Turner, E. H., Feldman-Naim, S., Schwartz, P. J., Wehr, T. A., & Rosenthal, N. E. (1995). Light therapy in patients with rapid cycling bipolar disorder: preliminary results. *Psychopharmacol. Bull., 31*, 705–710.

Lewy, A. J., Kern, H. A., Rosenthal, N. E., & Wehr, T. A. (1982). Bright artificial light treatment of a manic-depressive patient with a seasonal mood cycle. *Am. J. Psychiatry, 139*, 1496–1498.

Lewy, A. J., Sack, R. L., & Singer, C. M. (1985). Treating phase typed chronobiologic sleep and mood disorders using appropriately timed bright artificial light. *Psychopharmacol. Bull., 21*, 368–372.

MacQueen, G., Parkin, C., Marriott, M., Begin, H., & Hasey, G. (2007). The long-term impact of treatment with electroconvulsive therapy on discrete memory systems in patients with bipolar disorder. *J. Psychiatry Neurosci., 32*, 241–249.

Malizia, A. L. (1997). The frontal lobes and neurosurgery for psychiatric disorders. *J. Psychopharmacol., 11*, 179–187.

Mayberg, H. S., Brannan, S. K., Tekell, J. L., Silva, J. A., Mahurin, R. K., McGinnis, S., et al. (2000). Regional metabolic effects of fluoxetine in major depression: serial changes and relationship to clinical response. *Biol. Psychiatry, 48*, 830–843.

Mayberg, H. S., Lozano, A. M., Voon, V., McNeely, H. E., Seminowicz, D., Hamani, C., et al. (2005). Deep brain stimulation for treatment-resistant depression. *Neuron, 45*, 651–660.

Michael, N. & Erfurth, A. (2004). Treatment of bipolar mania with right prefrontal rapid transcranial magnetic stimulation. *J. Affect. Disord., 78*, 253–257.

Montoya, A., Weiss, A. P., Price, B. H., Cassem, E. H., Dougherty, D. D., Nierenberg, A. A., et al. (2002). Magnetic resonance imaging-guided stereotactic limbic leukotomy for treatment of intractable psychiatric disease. *Neurosurgery, 50*, 1043–1049.

Mukherjee, S., Sackeim, H. A., & Lee, C. (1988). Unilateral ECT in the treatment of manic episodes. *Convuls. Ther., 4*, 74–80.

Mukherjee, S., Sackeim, H. A., & Schnur, D. B. (1994). Electroconvulsive therapy of acute manic episodes: a review of 50 years' experience. *Am. J. Psychiatry, 151*, 169–176.

Nahas, Z., Kozel, F. A., Li, X., Anderson, B., & George, M. S. (2003). Left prefrontal transcranial magnetic stimulation (TMS) treatment of depression in bipolar affective disorder: a pilot study of acute safety and efficacy. *Bipolar Disord., 5*, 40–47.

Nahas, Z., Marangell, L. B., Husain, M. M., Rush, A. J., Sackeim, H. A., Lisanby, S. H., et al. (2005). Two-year outcome of vagus nerve stimulation (VNS) for treatment of major depressive episodes. *J. Clin. Psychiatry, 66*, 1097–1104.

Nascimento, A. L., Appolinario, J. C., Segenreich, D., Cavalcanti, M. T., & Brasil, M. A. (2006). Maintenance electroconvulsive therapy for recurrent refractory mania. *Bipolar Disord., 8*, 301–303.

Nemeroff, C. B., Mayberg, H. S., Krahl, S. E., McNamara, J., Frazer, A., Henry, T. R., et al. (2006). VNS therapy in treatment-resistant depression: clinical evidence and putative neurobiological mechanisms. *Neuropsychopharmacology, 31*, 1345–1355.

Neumeister, A., Goessler, R., Lucht, M., Kapitany, T., Bamas, C., & Kasper, S. (1996). Bright light therapy stabilizes the antidepressant effect of partial sleep deprivation. *Biol. Psychiatry, 39*, 16–21.

O'Reardon, J. P., Solvason, H. B., Janicak, P. G., Sampson, S., Isenberg, K. E., Nahas, Z., et al. (2007). Efficacy and safety of transcranial magnetic stimulation in the acute treatment of major depression: a multisite randomized controlled trial. *Biol. Psychiatry, 62,* 1208–1216.

Olfson, M., Marcus, S., Sackeim, H. A., Thompson, J., & Pincus, H. A. (1998). Use of ECT for the inpatient treatment of recurrent major depression. *Am. J. Psychiatry, 155,* 22–29.

Papadimitriou, G. N., Christodoulou, G. N., Katsouyanni, K., & Stefanis, C. N. (1993). Therapy and prevention of affective illness by total sleep deprivation. *J. Affect. Disord., 27,* 107–116.

Papatheodorou, G. & Kutcher, S. (1995). The effect of adjunctive light therapy on ameliorating breakthrough depressive symptoms in adolescent-onset bipolar disorder. *J. Psychiatry Neurosci., 20,* 226–232.

Pflug, B. & Tolle, R. (1971). Disturbance of the 24-hour rhythm in endogenous depression and the treatment of endogenous depression by sleep deprivation. *Int. Pharmacopsychiatry, 6,* 187–196.

Pisani, F., Oteri, G., Costa, C., Di Raimondo, G., & Di Perri, R. (2002). Effects of psychotropic drugs on seizure threshold. *Drug Saf., 25,* 91–110.

Prudic, J., Haskett, R. F., Mulsant, B., Malone, K. M., Pettinati, H. M., Stephens, S., et al. (1996). Resistance to antidepressant medications and short-term clinical response to ECT. *Am. J. Psychiatry, 153,* 985–992.

Reisner, A. D. (2003). The electroconvulsive therapy controversy: evidence and ethics. *Neuropsychol. Rev., 13,* 199–219.

Reme, C. E., Rol, P., Grothmann, K., Kaase, H., & Terman, M. (1996). Bright light therapy in focus: lamp emission spectra and ocular safety. *Technol. Health Care, 4,* 403–413.

Remick, R. A. (1978). Acute brain syndrome associated with ECT and lithium. *Can. J. Psychiatry, 23,* 129–130.

Roose, S. P., Nurnberger, J. I., Dunner, D. L., Blood, D. K., & Fieve, R. R. (1979). Cardiac sinus node dysfunction during lithium treatment. *Am. J. Psychiatry, 136,* 804–806.

Rosenthal, N. E., Sack, D. A., Gillin, J. C., Lewy, A. J., Goodwin, F. K., Davenport, Y., et al. (1984). Seasonal affective disorder: a description of the syndrome and preliminary findings with light therapy. *Arch. Gen. Psychiatry, 41,* 72–80.

Saba, G., Rocamora, J. F., Kalalou, K., Benadhira, R., Plaze, M., Lipski, H., et al. (2004). Repetitive transcranial magnetic stimulation as an add-on therapy in the treatment of mania: a case series of eight patients. *Psychiatry Res., 128,* 199–202.

Sackeim, H. A., Haskett, R. F., Mulsant, B. H., Thase, M. E., Mann, J. J., Pettinati, H. M., et al. (2001). Continuation pharmacotherapy in the prevention of relapse following electroconvulsive therapy: a randomized controlled trial. *JAMA, 285,* 1299–1307.

Sackeim, H. A., Prudic, J., Fuller, R., Keilp, J., Lavori, P. W., & Olfson, M. (2007). The cognitive effects of electroconvulsive therapy in community settings. *Neuropsychopharmacology, 32,* 244–254.

Schlaepfer, T. E. & Lieb, K. (2005). Deep brain stimulation for treatment of refractory depression. *Lancet, 366,* 1420–1422.

Schupbach, W. M., Chastan, N., Welter, M. L., Houeto, J. L., Mesnage, V., Bonnet, A. M., et al. (2005). Stimulation of the subthalamic nucleus in Parkinson's disease: a 5 year follow up. *J. Neurol. Neurosurg. Psychiatry, 76,* 1640–1644.

Sienaert, P. & Peuskens, J. (2007). Anticonvulsants during electroconvulsive therapy: review and recommendations. *J. ECT, 23,* 120–123.

Sikdar, S., Kulhara, P., Avasthi, A., & Singh, H. (1994). Combined chlorpromazine and electroconvulsive therapy in mania. *Br. J. Psychiatry, 164,* 806–810.

Sit, D., Wisner, K. L., Hanusa, B. H., Stull, S., & Terman, M. (2007). Light therapy for bipolar disorder: a case series in women. *Bipolar Disord., 9,* 918–927.

Skidmore, F. M., Rodriguez, R. L., Fernandez, H. H., Goodman, W. K., Foote, K. D., & Okun, M. S. (2006). Lessons learned in deep brain stimulation for movement and neuropsychiatric disorders. *CNS Spectr., 11,* 521–536.

Small, J. G., Klapper, M. H., Kellams, J. J., Miller, M. J., Milstein, V., Sharpley, P. H., et al. (1988). Electroconvulsive treatment compared with lithium in the management of manic states. *Arch. Gen. Psychiatry, 45,* 727–732.

Smeraldi, E., Benedetti, F., Barbini, B., Campori, E., & Colombo, C. (1999). Sustained antidepressant effect of sleep deprivation combined with pindolol in bipolar depression. A placebo-controlled trial. *Neuropsychopharmacology, 20,* 380–385.

Sohn, C. H. & Lam, R. W. (2004). Treatment of seasonal affective disorder: unipolar versus bipolar differences. *Curr. Psychiatry Rep., 6,* 478–485.

Sohn, C. H. & Lam, R. W. (2005). Update on the biology of seasonal affective disorder. *CNS Spectr., 10,* 635–646.

Spangler, W. J., Cosgrove, G. R., Ballantine, H. T., Jr., Cassem, E. H., Rauch, S. L., Nierenberg, A., et al. (1996). Magnetic resonance image-guided stereotactic cingulotomy for intractable psychiatric disease. *Neurosurgery, 38,* 1071–1076.

Szuba, M. P., Baxter, L. R. J., Fairbanks, L. A., Guze, B. H., & Schwartz, J. M. (1991). Effects of partial sleep deprivation on the diurnal variation of mood and motor activity in major depression. *Biol. Psychiatry, 30,* 817–829.

Terman, M. (2007). Evolving applications of light therapy. *Sleep Med. Rev., 11,* 497–507.

Terman, M., Terman, J. S., & Ross, D. C. (1998). A controlled trial of timed bright light and negative air ionization for treatment of winter depression. *Arch. Gen. Psychiatry, 55,* 875–882.

Thomas, J. & Reddy, B. (1982). The treatment of mania. A retrospective evaluation of the effects of ECT, chlorpromazine, and lithium. *J. Affect. Disord., 4,* 85–92.

Thompson, C. (2001). Evidence-based treatment. In Partonen T, Magnusson A (Eds), *Seasonal Affective Disorder: Practice and Research* (pp. 151–158). New York: Oxford University Press.

Tuunainen, A., Kripke, D. F., & Endo, T. (2004). Light therapy for nonseasonal depression. *Cochrane Syst. Rev., 2,* CD004050.

UK ECT Group (2003). Efficacy and safety of electroconvulsive therapy in depressive disorders: a systematic review and meta-analysis. *Lancet, 361,* 799–808.

Vaidya, N. A., Mahableshwarkar, A. R., & Shahid, R. (2003). Continuation and maintenance ECT in treatment-resistant bipolar disorder. *J. Electroconvulsive Therapy, 19,* 10–16.

Westrin, A. & Lam, R. W. (2007). Seasonal affective disorder: a clinical update. *Ann. Clin. Psychiatry, 19,* 239–246.

White, D. M., Lewy, A. J., Sack, R. L., Blood, M. L., & Wesche, D. L. (1990). Is winter depression a bipolar disorder? *Compr. Psychiatry, 31,* 196–204.

Wirz-Justice, A. (1995). Biological rhythms in mood disorders. In F.E.Bloom & D. J. Kupfer (Eds.), *Psychopharmacology: the Fourth Generation of Progress* (pp. 999–1017). New York: Raven Press.

Wirz-Justice, A. & van den Hoofdakker, R. H. (1999). Sleep deprivation in depression: what do we know, where do we go? *Biol. Psychiatry, 46,* 445–453.

Wu, J. C. & Bunney, W. E. (1992). The biological basis of an antidepressant response to sleep derivation and relapse: review and hypothesis. *Am. J. Psychiatry, 147,* 14–21.

Xia, G., Gajwani, P., Muzina, D. J., Kemp, D. E., Gao, K., Ganocy, S. J., et al. (2008). Treatment-emergent mania in unipolar and bipolar depression: focus on repetitive transcranial magnetic stimulation. *Int. J. Neuropsychopharmacol., 11*(1), 119–130.

chapter fifteen

Psychotropic medications in bipolar disorder: Pharmacodynamics, pharmacokinetics, drug interactions, adverse effects and their management

Terence A. Ketter and Po W. Wang
Stanford University School of Medicine

Contents

Introduction 438
Mood stabilizers 441
    Lithium 442
        Adverse events and their management 449
        Dosing strategies 453
        Clinical recommendations 454
    Valproate 455
        Adverse events and their management 459
        Dosing strategies 461
        Clinical recommendations 462
    Carbamazepine 462
        Adverse events and their management 474
        Dosing strategies 475
        Clinical recommendations 476
    Lamotrigine 477
        Adverse events and their management 479
        Dosing strategies 481
        Clinical recommendations 481

Antipsychotics 482
    Traditional antipsychotics 482
    Atypical antipsychotics 485
        Clozapine 485
        Risperidone 489
        Olanzapine 492
        Quetiapine 495
        Ziprasidone 497
        Aripiprazole 500
Adjunctive antidepressants 503
    Selective serotonin reuptake inhibitors 504
    Serotonin-norepinephrine reuptake inhibitors 505
    Bupropion and atypical antidepressants 506
    Monoamine oxidase inhibitors 508
    Tricyclic antidepressants 510
Benzodiazepines and mechanistically related drugs 511
Newer anticonvulsants 512
    Felbamate 513
    Gabapentin 513
    Topiramate 515
    Tiagabine 517
    Oxcarbazepine 518
        Dosing strategies 520
    Levetiracetam 520
    Zonisamide 522
    Pregabalin 523
Conclusion 525
References 525

Introduction

Pharmacotherapy of bipolar disorders is a complex and rapidly evolving field. The development of new treatments has helped refine concepts of illness subtypes and generated important new management options. Although the mood stabilizers lithium, carbamazepine (CBZ), valproate (VPA), and lamotrigine (LTG) are the primary medications for bipolar disorders, antipsychotics, antidepressants, anxiolytic/hypnotics, and other anticonvulsants are commonly combined with mood stabilizers in clinical settings. These diverse medications have varying pharmacodynamics, pharmacokinetics, drug-drug interactions, and adverse effects; thus offering not only new therapeutic opportunities, but also a variety of new potential pitfalls. Therefore, clinicians are challenged with integrating the complex data regarding efficacy spectra, described elsewhere in this volume, with the pharmacological properties described in this chapter, in efforts to provide safe, effective, state-of-the-art pharmacotherapy for patients with bipolar disorders.

Pharmacodynamic interactions occur at the site(s) of action of drugs to yield similar or opposing therapeutic and adverse effects. For example, combination of lithium with valproate may yield additive therapeutic (mood stabilization) and adverse (tremor) effects. Pharmacokinetic interactions alter drug absorption (in the digestive tract), distribution (in the blood), metabolism (in the liver), and excretion (in the kidney) to change the amount of drug or metabolite that reaches the site(s) of action for therapeutic and adverse effects. Although drug interactions involving absorption (e.g. food doubles ziprasidone absorption), distribution (e.g. valproate increases free fraction of carbamazepine), and excretion (e.g. hydrochlorothiazide decreases the renal excretion of lithium) can occur in the management of patients with bipolar disorder, hepatic metabolic mechanisms are the most common sources of clinically significant pharmacokinetic drug interactions in patients with bipolar disorder. For example, combination of lamotrigine with valproate inhibits lamotrigine metabolism to increase serum lamotrigine concentrations by approximately 100%, whereas combination of lamotrigine with carbamazepine induces lamotrigine metabolism to decrease serum lamotrigine concentration by approximately 50%.

Understanding of the molecular mechanisms of drug metabolism and related drug interactions has advanced substantially in the last decade (Anderson, 1998; Ketter et al., 1995; Murray, 2006). Many drugs are initially metabolized by phase I reactions, which introduce functional groups by oxidation, reduction, or hydrolysis to yield active or inactive metabolites (Shen, 1997). Oxidative reactions involving cytochrome P450 monooxygenase (CYP) isozymes constitute the most important group of phase I reactions. Nomenclature for the gene superfamily encoding CYP isoenzymes includes the root symbol "CYP" followed by a number representing the family, a letter designating the subfamily, and a number denoting the individual gene within the family or subfamily (e.g. CYP1A2, CYP2D6, CYP3A4) (Nelson et al., 1996; Wilkinson, 2005). For some CYPs (e.g. CYP2C9, CYP2C19, CYP2D6), a significant (>1%) proportion of the population has a mutated allele with increased or decreased activity, referred to as a genetic polymorphism (Meyer, 1994). Thus, extensive as compared to normal or poor metabolizers of CYP2D6 have lower serum concentrations of the CYP2D6 substrate paroxetine (Sindrup, Brosen, & Gram, 1992).

Many substances, psychotropic drugs, and non-psychotropic medications relevant to the management of bipolar disorder are metabolized by three particularly important CYP isoforms, namely CYP1A2 (e.g. caffeine, clozapine, olanzapine, propranolol), CYP2D6 (e.g. risperidone, airpiprazole, codeine), and CYP3A4 (e.g. carbamazepine, quetiapine, hormonal contraceptives). Various substances, psychotropic drugs, and non-psychotropic medications can inhibit CYP1A2 (e.g. fluvoxamine, ciprofloxacin), CYP2D6 (e.g. fluoxetine, paroxetine, quinidine), and CYP3A4 (e.g. grapefruit juice, nefazodone, ketoconazole, erythromycin), while diverse substances, psychotropic drugs, and non-psychotropic medications can induce CYP1A2 (e.g. tobacco smoking, charbroiled meats, omeprazole), and CYP3A4 (e.g. Saint John's Wort, carbamazepine, rifampin). These observations are clinically relevant. For example, CYP2D6 and CYP3A4 inhibitors are frequently co-prescribed with CYP2D6 and CYP3A4 substrates in medical practice (Molden et al., 2005).

Following phase I reactions, many drugs are subsequently metabolized by phase II reactions such as glucuronidation, sulfation, methylation, or acetylation to yield less active derivatives that are more water soluble and hence can be excreted by the kidney (Shen, 1997). However, some drugs such as valproate, lamotrigine, and olanzapine undergo direct conjugation reactions. Glucuronidation reactions constitute the most important group of phase II reactions. Nomenclature for the gene superfamily encoding enzymes mediating phase II conjugation reactions involving uridine diphosphate glycosyltransferase (UGT) isozymes includes the root symbol "UGT" followed by a number representing the family, a letter designating the subfamily, and a number denoting the individual gene within the family or subfamily (e.g. UGT1A4, UGT2B7) (Mackenzie et al., 1997). Substances, psychotropic drugs, and non-psychotropic medications relevant to the management of bipolar disorder are metabolized by two particularly important UGT isoforms, namely UGT1A4 (e.g. pregnanediol, lamotrigine, olanzapine, imipramine, amitriptyline, doxepin, clomipramine, cyproheptadine, promethazine) and UGT2B7 (e.g. estrogens, lamotrigine, valproate, propranolol, morphine, codeine). Although more limited than for CYPs, knowledge regarding inducers and inhibitors of UGTs is emerging (De Leon, 2003).

Thus, many substances and medications relevant to the management of bipolar disorder are metabolized by isozymes in the CYP and UGT superfamilies. Knowledge of the specific CYP and UGT isozymes mediating metabolism of individual drugs and the ability of individual drugs to gradually induce or rapidly inhibit activity of these isozymes can help explain and predict drug interactions (Anderson, 1998; Ketter et al., 1995; Lin & Lu, 1998; Rendic & Di Carlo, 1997), as described below.

Mood stabilizers

The mood stabilizers lithium, carbamazepine (carbamazepine), valproate (VPA), and lamotrigine (LTG) have varying structures (Figure 15.1), efficacy spectra, pharmacodynamics, pharmacokinetics, drug–drug interactions, and adverse effects, indicating the need to appreciate both the commonalities and difference between these agents. Mood stabilizers are available in immediate release formulations, also lithium, carbamazepine, and valproate are available in suspension and extended release formulations, and valproate is available in an intravenous formulation. Unfortunately, intramuscular and depot formulations have not been feasible, as these agents can cause necrosis when in direct contact with muscle tissue.

Baseline evaluation of bipolar disorder patients includes not only psychosocial assessment, but also general medical evaluation, in view of the risk of medical processes, which could confound diagnosis or influence management decisions, and the risk of adverse effects that may occur with treatment. Assessment commonly includes history, physical examination,

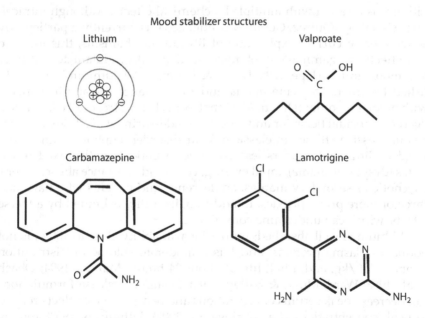

Figure 15.1 Mood stabilizer structures. The mood stabilizers have dramatically different structures. Lithium (top left) is an ion, valproate (top right) is a branched chain fatty acid, carbamazepine (bottom) is a tricyclic molecule with a carbamyl side chain, and lamotrigine is a phenyltriazine. Not illustrated to scale, as the lithium ion is much smaller than carbamazepine, valproate, and lamotrigine. (Adapted from Yatham, Kusumakar, & Kutcher, eds., *Bipolar Disorder: A Clinician's Guide to Biological Treatments,* Routledge, New York, 2002.)

complete blood count with differential and platelets, renal, hepatic and thyroid function, toxicology, and pregnancy tests, as well as other chemistries and electrocardiogram as clinically indicated (American Psychiatric Association, 2002; Yatham et al., 2005). Such evaluation provides baseline values for parameters which influence decisions regarding choice of medication and intensity of clinical and laboratory monitoring.

In view of the relative complexity of mood stabilizer therapy, patient education regarding common and serious adverse events is crucial. Information sheets or booklets describing clinical monitoring for problems such as neurotoxicity with lithium, hematologic reactions and drug interactions with carbamazepine, hepatic and pancreatic reactions and teratogenicity with valproate, and dermatologic reactions with lamotrigine, can aid in prevention and early detection of adverse events to enhance tolerability and safety.

Lithium

Lithium is a cation with multiple biochemical effects. Although intracellular signaling (Quiroz, Gould, & Manji, 2004) is currently a particularly active area of current exploration of lithium mechanisms, this ion also has effects on gamma-aminobutyric acid (GABA), glutamate, calcium, and monoamines (Jope, 1999; Lenox & Hahn, 2000). Lithium is an established treatment for acute mania and maintenance therapy in patients with bipolar disorder (Dinan, 2002) that with chronic treatment appears to decrease suicidal behavior and suicide (Baldessarini et al., 2006). Lithium has impressive efficacy in classic bipolar disorder (euphoric manias, not rapid cycling), but appears less effective in patients with mixed mood states (dysphoric mania), rapid cycling, comorbid substance abuse, severe, psychotic or secondary manias, adolescents, and patients who have had three or more prior episodes. In addition, its utility is limited by adverse effects, which can undermine compliance.

Lithium is well absorbed, with a bioavailability close to 100%, is not bound to plasma proteins, and has a moderate volume of distribution of about 1 L/kg, and a half-life of about 24 hours (Marcus, 1994; Obach et al., 1988; Ward, Musa, & Bailey, 1994). Sustained release formulations can decrease peak serum concentrations and hence adverse effects related to peak concentrations (Castrogiovanni, 2002). Lithium is >95% renally excreted unchanged with a clearance about one fourth that of creatinine (generally ranging from 10 to 40 mL/min), so that dosage may need to be decreased in patients with decreased renal function. This, taken together with evidence suggesting adverse renal effects of lithium, suggests patients with decreased renal function may not be good candidates for lithium therapy.

Due to its near-exclusive renal excretion unchanged, lithium has renally mediated rather than hepatically mediated pharmacokinetic drug-drug interactions (Amdisen, 1982; Finley, Warner, & Peabody, 1995; Jefferson et al., 1987; Jefferson, Greist, & Baudhuin, 1981). Thus, as described below, certain non-psychotropic medications with prominent effects on renal function can have clinically significant pharmacokinetic interactions with lithium. Medications with near-exclusive (>95%, gabapentin, pregabalin) and prominent (>50%, topiramate, levetiracetam) renal excretion unchanged could, in theory, also have clinically significant pharmacokinetic interactions with lithium—but systematic studies are needed to assess if such putative interactions occur. In contrast, most psychotropic and anticonvulsant medications encountered in the management of bipolar disorder have minimal (<5%, e.g. valproate, carbamazepine, lamotrigine, atypical antipsychotics, tiagabine, and oxcarbazepine) or minor (30%, e.g. zonisamide) renal excretion unchanged and lack prominent effects on renal function, and are thus not generally expected to have clinically significant pharmacokinetic interactions with lithium—but again, systematic studies are needed to confirm the lack of such interactions.

As expected, lithium and the mood stabilizer valproate appear to lack clinically significant pharmacokinetic interactions with one another (Granneman et al., 1996). Although carbamazepine and lithium are not expected to have significant pharmacokinetic interactions with one another, systematic studies to confirm the absence of such interactions remain to be performed. A few case reports suggest that occasional individuals may experience neurotoxicity with the carbamazepine plus lithium combination, despite having serum concentrations of both drugs within the therapeutic range, presumably related to a pharmacodynamic interaction. As expected, lamotrigine does not yield clinically significant changes in the pharmacokinetics of lithium (Chen, Veronese, & Yin, 2000). Although lithium is not expected to influence the pharmacokinetics of lamotrigine, the absence of such an interaction remains to be confirmed.

Based on case reports, concerns have been raised regarding development of an encephalopathic syndrome (weakness, lethargy, fever, tremulousness, confusion, extrapryamidal symptoms, leukocytosis, elevated serum enzymes, blood urea nitrogen, and fasting blood sugar) that may overlap neuroleptic malignant syndrome when combining lithium with typical antipsychotics. Cases reporting problems with the lithium plus haloperidol combination have been prominent in this literature. However, systematic efforts to assess such risks in larger numbers of patients, and clinical trials have suggested that combining lithium with typical antipsychotics does not generally yield more than merely additive adverse effects. The absence of compelling consistent evidence of clinically significant pharmacokinetic interactions between lithium and typical antipsychotics suggests that sporadic cases in which problems occur during combination therapy may be due to pharmacodynamic interactions.

In a fashion similar to that seen with typical antipsychotics, case reports suggest that occasional individuals could develop serious adverse effects such as neuroleptic malignant syndrome when lithium is combined with atypical antipsychotics such as clozapine, risperidone, olanzapine, ziprasidone, and aripiprazole. However, observational and controlled clinical trials suggest that combining lithium with atypical antipsychotics such as clozapine, risperidone, olanzapine, quetiapine, ziprasidone, and aripiprazole does not generally yield more than merely additive adverse effects. Indeed, risperidone, olanzapine, and quetiapine have received FDA approval for combination with lithium (or valproate) for the treatment of acute mania. As expected, lithium does not appear to generally yield clinically significant alterations in the pharmacokinetics of the atypical antipsychotics olanzapine, risperidone, quetiapine, and aripiprazole. Although lithium is also expected to not influence the pharmacokinetics of clozapine, risperidone, and ziprasidone, the absence of such interactions remains to be confirmed. As expected, olanzapine, quetiapine, and ziprasidone do not appear to yield clinically significant alterations in lithium pharmacokinetics. One study found that changing patients from typical antipsychotics plus lithium to risperidone plus lithium did not yield clinically significant alterations in lithium pharmacokinetics. Although clozapine and aripiprazole are expected to not influence lithium pharmacokinetics, the absence of such interactions remains to be confirmed. Taken together, the above evidence suggests that lithium combined with atypical antipsychotics is generally well tolerated, and lacks clinically significant pharmacokinetic interactions, raising the possibility that sporadic instances of serious adverse effects with such combinations could be mediated by pharmacodynamic mechanisms.

Lithium combined with antidepressants is commonly administered and well tolerated in both bipolar disorder and major depressive disorder patients. Systematic assessments of lithium combined with tricyclic antidepressants and monoamine oxidase inhibitors are limited, and fail to provide compelling consistent evidence of changes in lithium pharmacokinetics. As expected, systematic assessments suggest that lithium does not have clinically significant pharmacokinetic interactions with newer antidepressants such as citalopram, venlafaxine, nefazodone, or mirtazapine, or cause clinically significant changes in fluvoxamine pharmacokinetics, and fluoxetine, paroxetine and sertraline do not yield generally clinically significant changes in lithium pharmacokinetics. However, there are case reports suggesting that some individuals may experience substantive adverse events while taking lithium combined with antidepressants, in most instances presumably related to pharmacodynamic rather than pharmacokinetic mechanisms.

Similarly, given their differential elimination, pharmacokinetic interactions between lithium and benzodiazepines are not expected. Lithium is commonly administered along with benzodiazepines in patients with bipolar disorder, with merely additive central nervous system (e.g. sedation, ataxia) adverse effects. Indeed, contemporary controlled lithium trials routinely permit some adjunctive benzodiazepine (e.g. lorazepam) administration. However, limited data suggest that for at least some patients, caution is indicated with such combinations. Thus, occasional patients may experience problematic additive neurotoxicity, presumably related to pharmacodynamic mechanisms. Unfortunately, there are sparse systematic data to confirm the absence of pharmacokinetic interactions between lithium and benzodiazepines, although one study found that alprazolam did not yield clinically significant changes in lithium pharmacokinetics.

There are limited data regarding interactions between lithium and newer anticonvulsants. Gabapentin and topiramate have near-exclusive (>95%) and prominent (50–70%) renal excretion unchanged, respectively, but do not appear to generally yield clinically significant changes in lithium kinetics. However, case reports have raised the possibility that topiramate cause clinically significant increases in serum lithium concentrations in some individuals. Pregabalin and levetiracetam also have near-exclusive (>95%) and prominent (66%) renal excretion unchanged, respectively, but systematic data are lacking regarding their effects upon lithium pharmacokinetics. In addition, data are lacking regarding the effects of lithium upon the pharmacokinetics of gabapentin, topiramate, pregabalin, and levetiracetam. Although tiagabine, oxcarbazepine, and zonisamide are expected to not have clinically significant pharmacokinetic interactions with lithium, the absence of such interactions remains to be confirmed.

Taken together, the above evidence suggests that for most patients, lithium generally lacks clinically significant pharmacokinetic interactions with psychotropic and anticonvulsant medications encountered in the management of patients with bipolar disorder. However, case reports suggest that occasional patients receiving lithium combined with some of these agents (particularly antipsychotics) can experience serious adverse effects, in most instances presumably related to pharmacodynamic interactions.

In contrast, several agents with prominent renal effects that are commonly used in general medical practice have been clearly implicated in altering lithium pharmacokinetics (Finley, Warner, & Peabody, 1995; Harvey & Merriman, 1994). For example, thiazide diuretics, certain nonsteroidal anti-inflammatory drugs (NSAIDs), angiotensin I converting enzyme inhibitors (ACEIs), and angiotensin II receptor type-1 (AT_1) antagonists can increase lithium reabsorption in the proximal tubule yielding increased serum lithium concentrations and lithium toxicity (Table 15.1). Although case reports suggest that in some individuals use of antibiotics such as levofloxacin, trimethoprim, metronidazole, tetracycline, and doxycycline could be associated with lithium intoxication, such phenomena could also be related to fever, dehydration, and the underlying infection.

Table 15.1 Factors Affecting Lithium Clearance

Decreased by	Not changed by	Increased by
Diuretics	**Diuretics**	**Diuretics**
Thiazides	Amiloride	Acetazolamide
	Furosemide	Mannitol
Older NSAIDs	**Analgesics**	
Diclofenac	±ASA (conflicting	
±Ibuprofen (less	data)	
consistent effect)	Acetaminophen	
Indomethacin		
Ketoprofen		
Mefenamic acid		
Meloxicam		
Naproxen (smaller effect		
with OTC dose)		
Piroxicam		
± Sulindac (conflicting data)		
COX-2 Inhibitors		
Celecoxib		
Rofecoxib		
ACEIs		**Methylxanthines**
Captopril		Aminophylline
Enalapril		±Caffeine (conflicting
Fosinopril		data)
Lisinopril		Theophylline
Perindopril		
AT₁ Antagonists		
Candesartan		
Losartan		
Valsartan		
Physiologic/ Disease States		**Physiologic/Disease States**
Advanced age		Pregnancy
Dehydration		±Mania (conflicting data)
Renal disease		
Sodium depletion		

Diuretics are commonly prescribed for patients with bipolar disorder, not only for hypertension, but also to help attenuate lithium-induced nephrogenic diabetes insipidus. Certain diuretics can induce sodium depletion, resulting in increased proximal tubule sodium and lithium reabsorption. Thus, thiazide diuretics, but not furosemide or amiloride, yield clinically significant decreases in lithium excretion. Due to lithium's relatively low therapeutic index, addition of thiazide diuretics can result in clinical lithium toxicity, unless a dosage adjustment is made. Amiloride has been suggested to be a particularly attractive option for lithium-induced nephrogenic diabetes insipidus as it has less effect on lithium clearance, and does not cause hypokalemia or require sodium restriction. In contrast, other diuretics such as acetazolamide and mannitol may increase lithium excretion, potentially yielding clinical inefficacy, if serum lithium concentrations fall below the therapeutic range.

Analgesics are commonly administered to patients with bipolar disorders. Certain NSAIDs inhibit prostaglandin synthesis, decreasing glomerular filtration rate and lithium clearance, potentially yielding lithium toxicity. Thus, lithium clearance is decreased with indomethacin, piroxicam, diclofenac, naproxen, mefenamic acid, meloxicam, and ketoprofen, perhaps less consistently so with ibuprofen, and perhaps to a lesser extent with sulindac (although there are conflicting data), and not with aspirin (although there are conflicting data), or with over-the-counter doses of naproxen and acetaminophen. The newer cyclooxygenase-2 (COX-2) inhibitor NSAIDs celecoxib and rofecoxib have also been implicated in increasing serum lithium concentrations. A recent review concluded that most NSAIDs can increase serum lithium concentrations, but acknowledged differences between drugs in the class, and emphasized patient interindividual variability. Thus, addition of certain NSAIDs in certain individuals can result in clinical lithium toxicity, unless a dosage adjustment is made. Clinically problematic adverse effects will likely be more of a concern for patients with lithium concentrations in the upper part of the therapeutic range before the addition of an NSAID.

Antihypertensives are commonly administered to patients with bipolar disorders. Certain angiotensin I converting enzyme inhibitors (ACEIs) and angiotensin II receptor type-1 (AT_1) antagonists can induce volume depletion and hence decrease glomerular filtration rate and lithium clearance, potentially yielding lithium toxicity. Case reports have described an average 35% increase in lithium levels with various ACEIs. Such reports have most often implicated lisinopril and enalapril in yielding adverse effects with increased serum lithium concentrations. However, in a systematic assessment of nine healthy volunteers, enalapril did not significantly alter serum lithium concentrations. Case reports have also implicated captopril, perindopril, and fosinopril. A case report of lithium toxicity when switching from fosinopril to lisinopril suggested that different ACEIs may have varying effects on lithium pharmacokinetics. Case reports also suggest that the newer AT_1 antagonists candesartan, losartan, and valsartan can decrease lithium clearance, yielding clinical lithium toxicity.

Methylxanthines such as aminophylline, theophylline, and caffeine are commonly encountered in the management of patients with bipolar disorder. These adenosine antagonists have renal effects that can increase lithium clearance, potentially yielding inefficacy. Thus, the bronchodilators aminophylline and theophylline appear to increase renal lithium clearance. Caffeine may also increase renal lithium clearance, although one study failed to detect this effect.

Lithium may prolong the effects of neuromuscular blocking agents, but the clinical significance of this potential interaction for patients receiving anesthesia for electroconvulsive therapy has been questioned. Although alkalinizing agents such as sodium bicarbonate may increase lithium clearance in some individuals, in 10 healthy controls the mean increase was less than 1% (as compared to 51% with theophylline).

There are varying reports of potential interactions between lithium and calcium channel blockers. Neurotoxicity, including nausea, weakness, tremor, ataxia, parkinsonian symptoms, and choreoathetosis has been reported when combining lithium with verapamil, diltiazem, and nifedipine. One patient experienced this with lithium plus verapamil, but not with lithium plus nifedipine. Two elderly manic patients taking lithium with verapamil developed profound bradycardia that was followed by a fatal myocardial infarction in one of them. In two patients verapamil decreased serum lithium concentrations. Two reports suggested nifedipine may decrease lithium clearance. In a single case report, the lithium plus nimodipine combination was well tolerated with no changes in serum lithium concentrations. It has been pointed out that calcium channel blockers are very commonly used, and post-marketing surveillance has failed to provide systematic evidence that problems commonly occur when combining these agents with lithium. Taken together, the above suggest the need for some caution when combining lithium and calcium channel blockers, as occasional individuals may have problems.

Different physiologic and disease states can have varying effects on lithium clearance. Increasing age is associated with decreased renal clearance and increased sensitivity to adverse effects, yielding the need for (on average approximately 40–50%) lower lithium doses and serum concentrations in older adults. Dehydration, renal disease, and sodium depletion also decrease renal lithium clearance, increasing the risk of toxicity. In contrast, lithium clearance increases during pregnancy, and may also increase during strenuous exercise. Patients who become manic or hypomanic often have dramatic increases in physical activity which may yield increased cardiac output and perhaps increased renal lithium filtration and excretion, and decreased serum lithium concentrations at the very time when this medication is needed most in some individuals. However, there do not appear to be statistically significant mean changes in lithium clearance in groups of patients with mania.

Adverse events and their management

Common, dose-related adverse effects with lithium include renal (polyuria, polydipsia), metabolic (weight gain), central nervous system (sedation, tremor, ataxia, lethargy, decreased coordination, and cognitive problems), gastrointestinal (nausea, vomiting, diarrhea), and dermatological (hair loss, acne) problems, and edema (Table 15.2) (Gelenberg, 1988). Lithium-induced central nervous system adverse effects can be important reasons for poor adherence (Gitlin, Cochran, & Jamison, 1989). Lithium can compromise memory and information processing speed, even without subjective complaints or awareness of mental slowness.

The United States lithium prescribing information includes a boxed warning regarding the risk of lithium toxicity that can occur at doses close to therapeutic levels (Bell et al., 1993). Lithium intoxication can present with central nervous system, cardiovascular, renal, and gastrointestinal symptoms (Delva & Hawken, 2001; Hansen & Amdisen, 1978; Livingstone & Rampes, 2006; Timmer & Sands, 1999; Vestergaard, Amdisen, & Schou,

Table 15.2 Common and Serious Adverse Effects of Mood Stabilizers

Lithium	Valproate	Carbamazepine	Lamotrigine
Gastrointestinal	Gastrointestinal	Gastrointestinal	Gastrointestinal
Weight gain	Weight gain	Rash	Rash
Neurotoxicity	Tremor	Neurotoxicity	Headache
Renal toxicity	Hepatotoxicity	Hepatotoxicity	Dizziness
Thyroid toxicity	Thrombocytopenia	Thyroid changes	Pruritus
Hair Loss	Hair Loss	Blood dyscrasia	Dream abnormality
Cardiac toxicity	Pancreatitis	Cardiac toxicity	
Acne, Psoriasis	Polycystic ovarian syndrome	Hyponatremia	
Teratogen	Teratogen	Teratogen	Teratogen

Underlined adverse effects have a boxed warning in the United States Prescribing Information.

Frequencies of common or serious adverse effects are provided in the text.

1980). In severe cases lithium intoxication can yield irreversible central nervous system, cardiac, or renal problems, and even death. The risk of lithium toxicity is high in patients with significant renal or cardiovascular disease, severe debilitation, dehydration, sodium depletion, or taking diuretics or angiotensin converting enzyme (ACE) inhibitors. However, in medically healthy individuals, at doses of 900 mg/day or less, lithium is usually well tolerated, and even with low serum levels may yield benefit in milder forms of bipolar disorders or when used as an adjunct to other mood stabilizers or antidepressants.

Other warnings include the risks of renal problems such as nephrogenic diabetes insipidus, morphological changes with glomerular and interstitial fibrosis and nephron atrophy with chronic therapy (as described below), as well as drug interactions (as described above), such as encephalopathic syndrome with neuroleptics. Patients need to maintain adequate fluid and sodium intake, and caution is indicated in the setting of protracted sweating, diarrhea, infection, and fever. Lithium can also yield thyroid problems, as described below.

Lithium can cause digestive tract disturbances, with the lithium citrate solution having more proximal absorption and thus exacerbating upper (nausea and vomiting), or attenuating lower (diarrhea) gastrointestinal adverse effects (Table 15.3). The reverse holds for sustained release preparations. Administration of divided doses and with food can help attenuate gastrointestinal adverse effects. Although lithium is often given in divided doses to decrease peak serum levels and thus minimize adverse effects, doses can also be weighted towards bedtime, and patients receiving low to moderate doses may tolerate a single daily dose at bedtime. The latter regimen may aid sleep, attenuate daytime neurotoxicity, and possibly even decrease polyuria. Beta blocking agents can attenuate lithium-induced tremor.

Lithium has endocrine adverse effects, and can yield hypothyroidism in up to one-third of patients, and women and patients with rapid cycling may be at particular risk (Amdisen & Andersen, 1982; Bocchetta et al., 2001; Henry, 2002; Livingstone & Rampes, 2006). Moreover, lower serum levothyroxine concentrations appear to be associated with more frequent affective episodes and more depression in patients with mood disorders. Patients with hypothyroidism (increased thyroid stimulating hormone (TSH) and decreased free thyroxine) need levothyroxine replacement therapy. However, there is controversy regarding the management of subclinical hypothyroidism (increased TSH and normal free thyroxine). One proposed approach entails instituting levothyroxine if TSH exceeds 10 mU/L, even in the absence of clinical symptoms, in view of the risk of progression of thyroid disease, and increasing laboratory monitoring and considering levothyroxine if TSH is between 5 and 10 mU/L (Kleiner

Table 15.3 Treatment of Mood Stabilizer Adverse Effects

Adverse effect	Management options
General	Decrease/divide dose.
	Change mood stabilizer.
Gastrointestinal	Give with food.
	Change to extended release if nausea or vomiting.
	Change to suspension or immediate release if diarrhea.
	Symptomatic relief with gastrointestinal agents.
Weight gain	Prior warning; diet; exercise.
	Aggressively treat hyperphagic, anergic depression
	(e.g. add bupropion, thyroid)
	Add topiramate, zonisamide, or atomoxetine.
Neurotoxicity	Dose at bedtime.
	Gradual initiation to improve tolerance
	(with Li and carbamazepine).
Tremor	Add propranolol; atenolol; pindolol.
Hair loss	Add selenium 25–100 mcg/day, zinc 10–50 mg/day.
Polyuria	Single daily dose.
	Add amiloride; thiazide; indomethacin.
Thyroid	Thyroid replacement.
Hepatic	Discontinue carbamazepine/VPA if hepatic indices
	>3 × upper limit of normal.
Rash	Gradual initiation.
	Limit other new antigens during initiation?
	Dermatology consultation regarding desensitization.
	Discontinue carbamazepine, LTG if another explanation for
	rash is not evident.
Leukopenia	Add lithium.
	Discontinue carbamazepine if WBC <3000 or
	neutrophils <1000.
Hyponatremia	Add lithium, demeclocycline, doxycycline?

et al., 1999). Hyperthyroidism, although far less common, can also occur with lithium therapy. Hypercalcemia and hyperparathyroidism can also be seen with lithium. Thus, if hypercalcemia is detected on electrolyte screening, serum parathyroid hormone needs to be assessed.

As noted above, lithium has significant interactions with renal function, as lithium clearance is by renal excretion, and lithium can cause common benign as well as rare serious renal adverse effects (Livingstone & Rampes, 2006; Vestergaard & Amdisen, 1981; Vestergaard et al., 1979). Nephrogenic diabetes insipidus may occur in as many as 10% of patients with chronic lithium therapy. Polyuria and polydipsia (greater than 3 L 24-hour urine volume) can be attenuated by lithium dosage reduction or single daily dosage, and by administration of diuretics, but as noted above, care must be taken as such agents can influence lithium clearance. Hence, hydrochlorothiazide 50 mg/day may attenuate polyuria, but using this agent requires decreasing lithium dose and replacing potassium. Indomethacin has also been considered, but this agent also decreases lithium clearance, and could yield renal problems. Amiloride 5–10 mg twice a day has been suggested to be a preferable option for lithium-induced nephrogenic diabetes insipidus. Chronic lithium less commonly yields more longstanding and serious renal complications that are apparently more prevalent in cases with repeated lithium toxicity, advanced age, and concurrent NSAID therapy or chronic medical illness. Clinical and laboratory monitoring may help detect problems early, thus allowing interventions to attenuate adverse effects.

Weight gain can occur with lithium therapy (Baptista et al., 1995; Bowden et al., 2006, 2000; Peselow et al., 1980; Sachs et al., 2006; Vendsborg, Bech, & Rafaelsen, 1976), and can be a significant contributor to compliance problems. Weight gain appears to be more of an issue with lithium than with lamotrigine, particularly in patients who are already obese, but less of an problem than with valproate or olanzapine. Thus, in 12-month maintenance trials, the incidence of weight gain was 13% with lithium, 21% with valproate, and 7% with placebo (Bowden et al., 2000), and 10% with lithium and 30% with olanzapine (Tohen et al., 2005).

Many of the agents used in treating bipolar disorder patients can yield weight gain, as can residual hyperphagia, hypersomnia, and anergy of bipolar depression, or lithium-induced hypothyroidism. Counseling regarding weight gain early in the maintenance phase of treatment may allow early attention to diet and exercise to attenuate this effect. In some cases, early detection of a rising high normal or modestly elevated TSH can allow crossing over to another mood stabilizer, thus avoiding the need for chronic replacement thyroid hormones, which is necessary in more advanced cases of lithium-induced hypothyroidism. Even in some euthyroid patients, addition of thyroid hormones may offer adjunctive antidepressant effects, increasing energy and activity, and thus attenuating weight gain. Another important approach is to minimize the number of concurrent medications that also yield weight gain, thus avoiding potential synergistic weight increases. Classical prescription weight loss agents and stimulants are most often avoided, as they can destabilize mood and result in abuse or dependence. Adjunctive anticonvulsants such as topiramate and zonisamide and the norepinephrine reuptake inhibitor atomoxetine may allow patients to lose weight without systematically destabilizing mood, provided there is adequate concurrent antimanic therapy.

Acneiform and maculopapular eruptions, psoriasis, and folliculitis can occur with lithium. In some patients, symptomatic treatment of dermatological adverse effects with topical agents or retinoic acid can yield enough improvement to allow continuation of therapy, whereas in others switching to or adding another mood stabilizer to allow lithium dosage decrease or discontinuation is necessary.

Lithium can have adverse cardiac effects, ranging from benign eletrocardiographic T wave morphologic changes to clinically significant sinus node dysfunction or sinoatrial block, and onset or aggravation of ventricular irritability.

Lithium, like the other mood stabilizers, is a teratogen (FDA pregnancy category D) (Gentile, 2006), yielding cardiac malformations at a rate of 0.1–1.0% (Cohen et al., 1994). Ultrasound may allow early detection of such malformations. In patients with milder illness, a medication-free interval during pregnancy may be feasible. As rapid discontinuation of lithium may yield rebound episodes (Baldessarini et al., 1996), gradual tapering off of medication is a preferable strategy. Some patients have sufficiently severe illness to merit continuing lithium during pregnancy. Frank counseling and discussion of the risks and benefits of this approach is crucial in the management of such cases. Lithium and other mood stabilizers generally ought to be restarted immediately postpartum in view of the risk of relapse which may be as high as 60% (Cohen et al., 1995). As lithium and other mood stabilizers are excreted to varying degrees in breast milk, the most cautious approach is to not breastfeed while taking mood stabilizers. The FDA recommends "a decision should be made whether to discontinue nursing or to discontinue the drug, taking into account the importance of the drug to the mother". However, recent data suggesting that lithium concentrations fall 50% from maternal serum to milk, and another 50% from milk to infant serum, yielding adequate tolerability in infants, suggest that recommendations against lithium during breastfeeding may need to be reassessed (Viguera et al., 2007).

Dosing strategies

In acute settings, such as the inpatient treatment of mania, lithium therapy is commonly initiated at 600–1200 mg/day in two or three divided doses, and increased as necessary and tolerated every 2–4 days by 300 mg/day, with final doses commonly not exceeding 1800 mg/day. Some patients may better tolerate weighting the dose towards bedtime or even taking the entire daily dose at bedtime. Euthymic or depressed patients tend to tolerate aggressive initiation less well than manic patients. Thus, in less acute situations, such as the initiation of prophylaxis or adjunctive use, lithium can be started at 300–600 mg/day, and increased as necessary and tolerated, by 300 mg/day every 4–7 days. Thus, target doses are commonly between 900 and 1800 mg/day, yielding serum levels from 0.6 to 1.2 mEq/L (0.6–1.2 mM/L), with the higher portion of the range used acutely, and lower doses used in adjunctive therapy or prophylaxis (Sproule, 2002). In acute mania studies of the adjunctive atypical antipsychotics risperidone, olanzapine, and quetiapine, target serum lithium concentrations ranged from 0.60 to 1.4 mEq/L, yet mean serum lithium concentrations ranged between 0.70 and 0.76 mEq/L (Sachs et al., 2002; Tohen et al., 2002; Yatham et al., 2004). Older data suggest that during maintenance treatment, serum lithium concentrations maintained at 0.4–0.6 (median average 0.54) mEq/L compared to 0.8–1.0 (median average 0.83) mEq/L were better tolerated but less effective (Gelenberg et al., 1989). However, in a European lithium versus carbamazepine maintenance study, serum trough lithium concentrations were maintained at 0.6–0.8 mEq/L, with a mean of 0.63 mEq/L (Greil et al., 1997). In an American lithium versus carbamazepine maintenance study, serum trough lithium concentrations were maintained at 0.5–1.2 mEq/L, with a mean of 0.84 mEq/L (Denicoff et al., 1997). In a lithium versus valproate versus placebo maintenance study, serum trough lithium concentrations were maintained at 0.8–1.2 mEq/L, with a mean of 1.0 mEq/L at day 30 of randomized treatment (Bowden et al., 2000). In a lithium versus lamotrigine versus placebo maintenance study, serum trough lithium concentrations were maintained at 0.8–1.1 mEq/L, with a steady state mean of 0.8 mEq/L during randomized treatment (Calabrese et al., 2003). In a lithium versus olanzapine maintenance study, serum trough lithium concentrations were maintained at 0.6–1.2 mEq/L, with a mean of 0.76 mEq/L during randomized treatment (Tohen et al., 2005).

Clinical recommendations

Patients need to be advised of lithium adverse effects, drug interactions, and the importance of adequate hydration. Clinical assessments with lithium therapy includes a baseline physical examination, and routinely querying patients regarding central nervous system (sedation, tremor, ataxia), gastrointestinal (nausea, vomiting, diarrhea), metabolic (weight gain), and renal (polyuria, polydipsia) disorders and adverse effects at baseline and during treatment. Laboratory monitoring includes baseline pregnancy test, electrocardiogram (in patients over 40 years of age), and renal (blood urea nitrogen, serum creatinine and electrolytes) and thyroid (thyroid stimulation hormone) indices, with re-evaluation of renal and thyroid indices at 3 and 6 months, and then every 6–12 months thereafter, and as clinically indicated (American Psychiatric Association, 2002). Serum lithium concentrations are commonly assessed at steady state, which occurs at about 5 days after a dosage change, and then as indicated by inefficacy or adverse effects. More frequent laboratory monitoring is prudent in the medically ill and in patients with abnormal indices. Titrating lithium to the maximum dose that is well tolerated (commonly 0.8–1.2 mEq/L in acute mania and 0.6–1.0 mEq/L in bipolar depression and maintenance), and promptly addressing adverse effect concerns can help enhance adherence.

Valproate

Valproate (VPA) is a fatty acid with a variety of biochemical actions, including effects on sodium channels, gamma-aminobutyric acid (GABA), glutamate, dopamine, and intracellular signaling (Chapman et al., 1982; Chen et al., 1994; Li, Ketter, & Frye, 2002; Vayer, Cash, & Maitre, 1988). Valproate appears to have a wide efficacy spectrum, which includes benefiting some bipolar disorder patients who are refractory to lithium. Controlled trials have demonstrated that valproate is effective for acute manic and mixed episodes (Bowden et al., 1994, 2006; Pope et al., 1991). A controlled trial of valproate maintenance therapy failed, as neither valproate nor lithium separated from placebo on the primary outcome measure, perhaps due to methodological limitations (Bowden et al., 2000). Nevertheless, valproate is commonly recommended for longer-term therapy in patients with bipolar disorder (American Psychiatric Association, 2002; Suppes et al., 2005). Valproate is also effective for prevention of migraine headaches, a common comorbid problem encountered in patients with bipolar disorder.

Valproate is well absorbed, with bioavailability close to 100% (DeVane, 2003). It is 80–90% bound to plasma proteins. This binding is saturable, so that at higher doses a greater percentage of the drug may be in the free form. Valproate is quite hydrophilic with a low volume of distribution of about 0.1 L/kg. At higher doses, the increased free fraction may remain in the blood compartment (rather than escaping into the tissues) and thus be cleared by the liver. This may yield "sublinear" kinetics, so that with higher serum concentrations, greater increases in dose may be required to yield the desired increase in serum level (Graves, 1995).

In monotherapy valproate has a half-life of about 12 hours, and clearance of about 10 mL/min. Combined with enzyme inducers such as carbamazepine, phenytoin, or phenobarbital, valproate's half-life falls 50% to approximately 6 hours and clearance doubles to about 20 mL/min. Valproate is available as valproic acid and as divalproex delayed release, with the latter having better gastrointestinal tolerability (Zarate et al., 1999). Recently, the United States Food and Drug Administration (FDA) approved an extended release divalproex formulation for the treatment of acute manic and mixed episodes (Bowden et al., 2006), and this formulation has potentially even better tolerability than the divalproex delayed release formulation (Smith et al., 2004).

Valproate is extensively metabolized, with less than three percent being excreted unchanged in the urine. There are three principal routes of elimination (Aly & Abdel-Latif, 1980; Baillie, 1992) (Figure 15.2). Conjugations to inactive glucuronides and other inactive metabolites account for 50% of valproate disposition, and appear to be mediated primarily by UGT1A6, UGT1A9, and UGT2B7 (Ethell, Anderson, & Burchell, 2003). In addition, about 40% undergoes beta-oxidation in the mitochondria to several metabolites, including the desaturation product 2-ene-valproate that may contribute to the therapeutic effects of valproate. Preliminary evidence suggests that patients who experience weight gain on valproate may have higher levels of 2-ene-valproate, suggesting that dysfunction of the beta-oxidation pathway (which metabolizes endogenous lipids) could play a role in this adverse effect (Gidal et al., 1994). About 10% of valproate undergoes cytochrome P450 oxidation reactions that appear to be mediated primarily by CYP2C9, CYP2A6, and CYP2B6, whereas other CYPs relevant to psychopharmacology, such as CYP1A2, CYP2C19, CYP2D6, and CYP2E1, do not appear to provide substantial contributions to valproate metabolism (Kiang et al., 2006). P450 oxidation reactions yield a variety

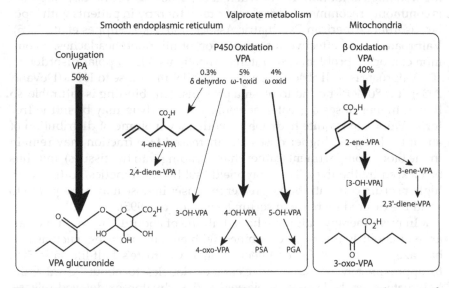

Figure 15.2 Metabolism of valproate (VPA) via microsomes on the smooth endoplasmic reticulum and via mitochondrial β oxidation. The thickness of the arrows and percentage figures roughly indicate relative proportions going through various pathways. (From Potter, W. Z., & Ketter T. A., *Can. J. Psychiatry, 38*, S51–56, 1993.)

of metabolites including hydroxylation (3-OH-valproate, 4-OH-valproate, 5-OH-valproate), and subsequent ketone (4-oxo-valproate) and dicarboxylic acid {propylsuccinic acid (PSA) and propylglutaric acid (PGA)} products. In addition, the desaturation product, 4-ene-valproate, may be hepatotoxic and teratogenic. Induction of formation of this metabolite by enzyme inducing anticonvulsants could explain why these problems are a greater concern in combination therapies compared to valproate monotherapy.

Valproate has a somewhat more favorable therapeutic index than lithium or carbamazepine, with a lower incidence of neurotoxicity being an important advantage. This favorable therapeutic index, along with the existence of three principal metabolic pathways (Figure 15.2), may account for the fact that clinical drug–drug interactions yielding valproate toxicity appear less prominent than with lithium or carbamazepine.

However, valproate has metabolic interactions with some drugs (Bourgeois, 1988) (Table 15.4). Valproate is an inhibitor of hepatic metabolism, including epoxide hydrolase, some glycosyltransferase(s), and some P450 isoforms (Ethell, Anderson, & Burchell, 2003; Svinarov & Pippenger, 1995; Wen et al., 2001). In human liver microsomes, valproate inhibits UGT2B7 (Rowland et al., 2006) and CYP2C9 (Wen et al., 2001), but only tends to inhibit CYP2C19, CYP3A4, and CYP2A6, and has minimal effects on CYP1A2, CYP2D6 and CYP2E1.

Thus, valproate can yield increased serum concentrations of carbamazepine-E by inhibiting epoxide hydrolase, and can inhibit glucuronidation of carbamazepine-10,11-trans-diol. In addition, carbamazepine induces valproate metabolism, yielding decreased serum valproate concentrations. Carbamazepine appears to induce valproate metabolism by increasing clearance via both the conjugation and cytochrome P450 oxidation routes. Valproate doubles serum lamotrigine concentrations,

Table 15.4 ValproateMetabolicDrug Interactions

VPA→↑Drug	Drug→↑VPA	Drug→↓VPA
Amitriptyline	Aspirin	CBZ
CBZ-E	Felbamate	±Lamotrigine
Ethosuximide		Meropenem
Lamotrigine		Phenobarbital
Nortriptyline		Phenytoin
Phenobarbital		Rifampin
Phenytoin		
Zidovudine		

presumably mediated by inhibition of UGT2B7, and thus increases the risk of rash with lamotrigine, so that it is particularly important to take care to introduce lamotrigine even more conservatively (halving lamotrigine doses) in patients who are taking valproate, as noted below. Lamotrigine may only yield modest (25%) clinically insignificant decreases in valproate levels. Valproate and lithium lack clinically significant pharmacokinetic interactions with one another.

Valproate does not appear to yield clinically significant changes in serum concentrations of haloperidol, risperidone, or aripiprazole. Although some evidence suggests that valproate does not yield clinically significant changes in serum clozapine concentrations, limited data suggest valproate might decrease clozapine levels. Valproate decreased dose-corrected olanzapine concentrations in four patients, and this potential interaction needs to be confirmed in a larger sample. Valproate may or may not increase quetiapine serum concentrations, and the clinical significance of this potential interaction remains to be established. Quetiapine does not appear to yield clinically significant changes in serum valproate concentrations. Case reports suggest that in occasional patients risperidone may yield increased or decreased serum valproate concentrations, although case series and a systematic 22-patient study failed to demonstrate such an interaction. Haloperidol, chlorpromazine, and quetiapine do not appear to yield clinically significant changes in serum valproate concentrations, while the effects of clozapine, olanzapine, ziprasidone, and aripiprazole on valproate pharmacokinetics remain to be established.

There are varying reports regarding the effect of valproate on tricyclic antidepressant pharmacokinetics, as valproate may increase serum amitriptyline/nortriptyline and clomipramine concentrations, yet decrease desipramine concentrations. In contrast to carbamazepine, valproate fails to alter serum bupropion concentrations. Fluoxetine may increase or decrease valproate serum concentrations. In one patient, sertraline increased valproate levels. Paroxetine does not generally yield clinically significant changes in valproate kinetics.

Valproate is commonly administered along with benzodiazepines in patients with bipolar disorder, with merely additive central nervous system (e.g. sedation, ataxia) adverse effects. Indeed, contemporary controlled valproate trials routinely permit some adjunctive benzodiazepine (e.g. lorazepam) administration. Valproate modestly decreases diazepam and lorazepam clearance, while lorazepam does not alter valproate pharmacokinetics. A pharmacoepidemiologic study suggested that valproate and clonazepam only modestly affect one another's metabolism. However, limited data suggest that for at least some patients, caution is indicated when combining valproate with benzodiazepines. Occasional patients might experience serious central nervous system depression when valproate is combined with lorazepam. Valproate combined with clonazepam may induce absence status in patients with a history of absence status. A single case report described somnambulism when valproate was combined with zolpidem.

Valproate can yield increased serum concentrations of ethosuximide, felbamate, obarbital, and phenytoin, with the latter presumably mediated by valproate inhibition of CYP2C9. Valproate does not yield clinically significant changes in serum total tiagabine concentrations, but can increase the free fraction of tiagabine, while tiagabine does not generally yield clinically significant changes in the pharmacokinetics of valproate. Felbamate can yield increased, and phenobarbital and phenytoin can yield decreased serum valproate concentrations. Valproate does not appear to have clinically significant pharmacokinetic interactions with the anticonvulsants gabapentin, topiramate, oxcarbazepine, levetiracetam, zonisamide, and pregabalin in patients with epilepsy.

Aspirin can yield decreased valproate clearance, presumably by inhibiting beta-oxidation, as well as decreased valproate protein binding. The antimicrobials rifampin and meropenem can yield decreased serum valproate concentrations. Valproate can yield increased serum concentrations of zidovudine. In contrast to carbamazepine, valproate does not yield clinically significant decreases in serum concentrations of hormonal contraceptives.

Binding interactions can also occur, so that valproate can increase free fractions of diazepam (but not lorazepam), carbamazepine, phenytoin, tiagabine, tolbutamide, and warfarin. In contrast, the NSAIDs aspirin, diflunisal, tolmetin, mefenamic acid, fenoprofen, ibuprofen, and naproxen can increase the free fraction of valproate.

Adverse events and their management

Common, dose-related adverse effects with valproate include gastrointestinal (nausea, vomiting, dyspepsia, diarrhea), hepatic (transaminase elevations), central nervous system (tremor, sedation, dizziness), and metabolic (weight gain, osteoporosis) problems, and hair loss (Dreifuss & Langer, 1988). As valproate can cause gastrointestinal disturbances (Schmidt, 1984), the divalproex extended release formulation is preferred since it yields such problems less often than the divalproex delayed release formulation (Smith et al., 2004), which in turn appears better tolerated than valproic acid (Zarate et al., 1999). Central nervous system adverse effects may be attenuated by weighting valproate dosage toward bedtime or dosage reduction. Beta blockers may attenuate valproate-induced tremor. Valproate can cause weight gain, which appears to be more of an problem than with lithium, but less of an issue than with olanzapine.

Thus, in a 12-month maintenance trial, the incidence of weight gain was 21% with valproate, 13% with lithium, and 7% with placebo (Bowden et al., 2000), and in a 47-week maintenance trial was 18% with valproate and 24% with olanzapine (Tohen et al., 2003). Valproate-related weight gain can be approached in a fashion similar to that described above for lithium. Limited data suggest that valproate-induced hair loss may be avoided or attenuated by the addition of selenium 25–100 mcg/day, or zinc 10–50 mg/day, presumably by counteracting valproate-induced depletion of these elements.

The United States valproate prescribing information includes boxed warnings regarding the risks of: (1) hepatotoxicity; (2) teratogenicity; and (3) pancreatitis. Hepatic fatalities are of concern in infants receiving valproate along with enzyme-inducing agents, but rates for patients over 10 years of age are about 1/609,000 with valproate monotherapy, and about 1/28,000 when valproate is given with enzyme inducers (Bryant & Dreifuss, 1996). Valproate, like carbamazepine, is generally discontinued if hepatic indices rise above three times the upper limit of normal. Recent data suggest that rates of major congenital malformations with valproate exposure could be higher compared to rates with lamotrigine exposure or compared to rates with no anticonvulsant exposure (Alsdorf et al., 2004; Cunnington, 2004; Vajda et al., 2004). Valproate-induced pancreatitis may occur in as many as one in 1000 patients, and is detectable by assessing serum amylase in patients with persistent or severe gastrointestinal problems. Other warnings include the risks of hyperammonemic encephalopathy in patients with urea cycle disorders, somnolence in the elderly, and thrombocytopenia. The latter appears to be dose-related, particularly if serum valproate concentrations are above 100 mcg/mL (700 μM/L).

For over a decade, there have been varying reports regarding a possible association between valproate therapy and polycystic ovarian syndrome (PCOS) in women with epilepsy (Isojarvi et al., 1993; Rasgon, 2004). Two recent studies in bipolar disorder patients consistent with the possibility of a modest (6–10%) risk of PCOS with valproate in women with bipolar disorder (Joffe et al., 2006; Rasgon et al., 2005) have indicated the need for prospective trials to systematically assess this issue.

Valproate, like the other mood stabilizers, is a teratogen (FDA pregnancy category D) (Gentile, 2006). As noted above, recent data suggest that rates of major congenital malformations with valproate exposure could be higher compared to rates with lamotrigine exposure or compared to rates with no anticonvulsant exposure (Alsdorf et al., 2004; Cunnington, 2004; Vajda et al., 2004). Folate supplementation may attenuate the risk of spina bifida, and ultrasound may allow early detection. In view of these recent findings, the issue of valproate therapy in pregnancy appears to be more problematic than for other mood stabilizers, so that careful assessments of the risks and benefits of treatment are particularly crucial for patients who are taking valproate. Although valproate concentrations in breast milk and infant serum are low (less than 10% of maternal serum levels), the FDA recommends "consideration should be given to discontinuing nursing when [valproate] is administered to a nursing woman."

Dosing strategies

In acute settings, such as the inpatient treatment of mania, valproate therapy is commonly initiated at 750–2000 mg/day, and increased as necessary and tolerated, by 250 mg/day every 1–2 days. Over the last decade, studies have described more aggressive valproate initiation in acute mania utilizing divalproex formulations. Thus, with the divalproex delayed release formulation, initiating at 10 mg/lb (20 mg/kg) or even loading with 30 mg/kg per day for 1 or 2 days, followed by 20 mg/kg per day appears generally well tolerated in acute mania (Lima et al., 1999; McElroy et al., 1996). Due to lower bioavailability, doses with the divalproex extended release formulation may need to be 6–20% higher than with the divalproex direct release formulation. In a recent acute mania study, the divalproex extended release formulation was started at 25 mg/kg per day rounded up to the nearest 500 mg, increased by 500 mg on day 3, and intermittently adjusted based on clinical effects targeting serum levels from 85 to 125 mcg/mL (600–850 µM/L) (Bowden et al., 2006). However, euthymic or depressed patients tend to tolerate aggressive initiation less well than manic patients. Thus, in less acute situations, such as the initiation of prophylaxis or adjunctive use, valproate is often started at 250–500 mg/day, and increased as necessary and tolerated, by 250 mg/day every 4–7 days. Target doses in the past have commonly between 750 and 2500 mg/day, yielding serum levels from 50 to 125 mcg/mL (350–850 µM/L) (Bowden et al., 1996), with the higher portion of the range used acutely, and lower doses used in adjunctive therapy or prophylaxis. The divalproex extended release formulation (Bowden et al., 2006), and in some cases, all or the majority of the divalproex delayed release formulation (Winsberg et al., 2001) can be given in a single dose at bedtime. In a recent meta-analysis of controlled acute mania studies, therapeutic effect size increased linearly with serum valproate concentrations (Allen et al., 2006). As noted above, in a recent acute mania study with divalproex extended release formulation, target serum levels ranged from 85 to 125 mcg/mL (600–850 µM/L) (Bowden et al., 2006). In acute mania studies of the adjunctive atypical antipsychotics risperidone, olanzapine, and quetiapine, target serum valproate concentrations have ranged from 50 to 125 ug/mL, and mean serum valproate concentrations have ranged between 64 and 70 ug/mL (Sachs et al., 2002; Tohen et al., 2002; Yatham et al., 2004). In a divalproex delayed release versus lithium versus placebo maintenance study, serum trough valproate concentrations were maintained at 71–125 ug/mL, with a mean of 85 ug/mL at day 30 of randomized treatment (Bowden et al., 2000).

Clinical recommendations

Patients need to be advised of valproate adverse effects and drug interactions. Clinical assessments with valproate therapy include a baseline physical examination, and routinely querying patients regarding hepatic and hematologic disorders and adverse effects at baseline and during treatment. Laboratory monitoring during valproate therapy commonly includes baseline complete blood count, differential, platelets, and hepatic indices, and re-evaluation every 6–12 months, and as clinically indicated (American Psychiatric Association, 2002). As with carbamazepine, most of the concerning hematological reactions occur in the first 3 months of therapy (Tohen et al., 1995). Serum valproate concentrations are typically assessed at steady state, and then as clinically indicated by inefficacy or adverse effects. Titrating valproate to the maximum dose that is well tolerated (commonly 85–125 mcg/mL in acute mania and 50–100 mcg/mL in bipolar depression and maintenance), and promptly addressing adverse effect concerns can help enhance adherence.

Carbamazepine

Carbamazepine (CBZ) has a tricyclic structure, and a wide array of biochemical effects including effects on sodium channels, GABA, glutamate, somatostatin, adenosine, and intracellular signaling (Li, Ketter, & Frye, 2002; Post et al., 1994). Unlike tricyclic antidepressants, carbamazepine does *not* block reuptake of monoamines. Carbamazepine has an efficacy spectrum similar to valproate, and to some extent complementary to lithium. Controlled trials studies have confirmed the efficacy of a proprietary beaded, extended-release capsule formulation of carbamazepine in acute mania (Weisler, Kalali, & Ketter, 2004; Weisler et al., 2005).

Carbamazepine has erratic absorption and a bioavailability of about 80% (Bertilsson, 1978; Bertilsson & Tomson, 1986; Graves et al., 1998). It is about 75% bound to plasma proteins and has a moderate volume of distribution of about 1 L/kg. Carbamazepine is extensively metabolized with less than 1% excreted unchanged in the urine. Before auto-induction of the epoxide pathway (presumably via induction of CYP3A3/4), the half-life of carbamazepine is about 24 hours, and the clearance is about 25 mL/min. However, after auto-induction (2–4 weeks into therapy), the half-life falls to about 8 hours, and clearance rises to about 75 mL/min. This may require dose adjustment to maintain adequate blood levels and therapeutic effects. The active carbamazepine-10,11-epoxide (CBZ-E) metabolite has a half-life of about 6 hours. Two sustained release carbamazepine formulations have been approved for the treatment of epilepsy in the United States. These formulations given twice a day yield steady state carbamazepine levels similar to those seen with the immediate release formulation given four times a day (Garnett et al., 1998; Thakker et al., 1992), and potentially fewer adverse effects related to lower peak serum concentrations (Aldenkamp et al., 1987; Persson et al., 1990). One of these, an extended release capsule formulation, has been approved for the treatment of acute mania in the United States (Weisler, Kalali, & Ketter, 2004; Weisler et al., 2005).

The pharmacokinetic properties of carbamazepine are atypical among medications prescribed by psychiatrists, and necessitate special care when treating patients concurrently with other medications (Ketter, Post, & Worthington, 1991a, 1991b). Carbamazepine is extensively metabolized with only about three percent being excreted unchanged in the urine. The main metabolic pathway of carbamazepine (to its active 10,11-epoxide, CBZ-E) appears to be mediated primarily by CYP3A3/4 (Figure 15.3), with a minor contribution by CYP2C8. This epoxide pathway accounts for about 40% of carbamazepine disposition, and even more in patients with induced epoxide pathway metabolism (presumably via CYP3A3/4 induction). Although a genetic polymorphism has been observed for CYP2C8, this probably does *not* account for the variability observed in carbamazepine disposition, in view of the minor role of this isoform. The frequency distribution of carbamazepine kinetic parameters is unimodal, consistent with CYP3A3/4 (which lacks genetic polymorphism) being the crucial isoform. With enzyme induction (of the epoxide pathway, presumably via CYP3A3/4 induction), formation of carbamazepine-epoxide triples, its subsequent transformation to the inactive diol doubles, and thus the carbamazepine-epoxide/carbamazepine ratio increases. Other pathways include aromatic hydroxylation (25%), which is apparently mediated by CYP1A2 and not induced concurrently with the epoxide pathway, and glucuronide conjugation of the carbamoyl side chain (15%) by uridine diphosphate glycosyltransferase (UGT), presumably primarily by UGT2B7. These other pathways yield inactive metabolites.

Carbamazepine induces not only CYP3A3/4 and conjugation, but also presumably other cytochrome P450 isoforms (which remain to be characterized). Thus, carbamazepine decreases the serum levels of not only carbamazepine itself (autoinduction), but also many other medications (heteroinduction). Carbamazepine-induced decreases in serum levels of certain concurrent medications can render them ineffective. Moreover, if carbamazepine is discontinued, serum levels of these other medications can rise leading to toxic effects from these agents. Also, carbamazepine metabolism can be inhibited by CYP3A3/4 inhibitors yielding increased serum carbamazepine levels and intoxication (Figure 15.3).

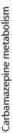
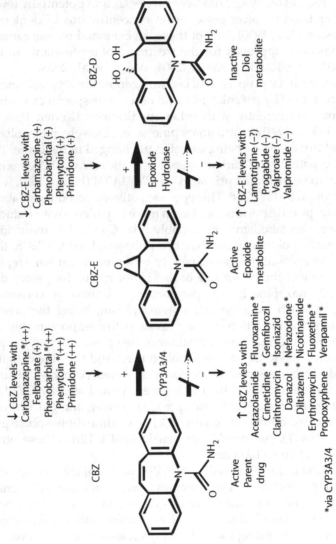

Figure 15.3 Metabolism of carbamazepine (CBZ) and drugs acting on its two major metabolic enzymes. CBZ-E=carbamazepine-10,11-epoxide. CBZ-D=carbamazepine-10,11-dihydro-dihydroxide. CYP3A3/4=cytochrome P450 3A3/4. + indicates enzyme induction; − indicates enzyme inhibition. (From Ketter, T. A., Post, R. M., & Worthington, K., *J. Clin. Psychopharmacol.*, 11, 198–203, 306–313, 1991.)

The active carbamazepine-epoxide metabolite can yield therapeutic and adverse effects similar to those of carbamazepine, but is not detected in conventional carbamazepine assays. The unwary clinician may misinterpret the significance of therapeutic or adverse effects associated with low or moderate serum carbamazepine levels. In addition, valproate displaces carbamazepine from plasma proteins, yielding an increase in free carbamazepine, which in combination with valproate-induced increases in carbamazepine-epoxide, can yield toxicity when utilizing carbamazepine plus valproate combination therapy.

Carbamazepine has a wide variety of drug-drug interactions (Tables 15.5 and 15.6), in excess of those seen with lithium or valproate, due to carbamazepine's constellation of pharmacokinetic properties (Table 15.7). Knowledge of carbamazepine drug-drug interactions and strategies for treating refractory symptoms is crucial in effective management. Carbamazepine drug–drug interactions are predominantly mediated by pharmacokinetic mechanisms. Recent advances in molecular pharmacology have characterized the specific cytochrome P450 isoforms responsible for metabolism of various medications (Ketter, Post, & Worthington, 1991a) (Table 15.8). This may allow clinicians to anticipate and avoid pharmacokinetic drug-drug interactions and thus provide more effective combination pharmacotherapies. The reader interested in detailed reviews of carbamazepine drug–drug interactions may find these in other articles (Ketter, Post, & Worthington, 1991a, 1991b).

Carbamazepine and lithium are frequently combined in treating bipolar disorder, and may provide additive or synergistic antimanic, antidepressant, and mood stabilizing effects. Although carbamazepine and lithium are not expected to have significant pharmacokinetic interactions with one another, systematic studies to confirm the absence of such interactions remain to be performed. A few case reports suggest that some individuals may experience neurotoxicity with the carbamazepine plus lithium combination despite having serum concentrations of both drugs within the therapeutic range, presumably related to a pharmacodynamic interaction. Nevertheless, the carbamazepine plus lithium combination is generally well tolerated, with merely additive neurotoxicity, which can be minimized by gradual dose escalation.

The carbamazepine plus valproate combination appears to be not only tolerated, but may show psychotropic synergy. Carbamazepine induces valproate metabolism, yielding decreased serum valproate concentrations. Carbamazepine appears to induce valproate metabolism by increasing clearance via both the conjugation and cytochrome P450 oxidation routes. Valproate inhibits epoxide hydrolase, increasing the serum carbamazepine-epoxide levels, at times without altering total serum carbamazepine levels. These interactions can potentially confound clinicians

Table 15.5 Selected Drugs with Increased Clearance
with Carbamazepine

Alprazolam (?)	Itraconazole
Amitriptyline	Lamotrigine
Aripiprazole	Levetiracetam (?)
Bupropion	Levothyroxine
Chlorpromazine (?)	Methadone
Citalopram	Midazolam
Clobazam	Mirtazapine
Clonazepam	Nortriptyline
Clozapine	Olanzapine
Cyclosporine (?)	Oxcarbazepine
Delavirdine	Oxiracetam (?)
Desipramine	Pancuronium
Dexamethasone	Phenytoin
Diazepam	Praziquantel
Dicumarol (?)	Prednisolone
Doxacurium	Primidone
Doxepin	Quetiapine
Doxycycline	Risperidone
Ethosuximide	Sertraline
Felbamate	Theophylline (?)
Felodipine	Thiothixene (?)
Fentanyl (?)	Tiagabine
Fluphenazine (?)	Topiramate
Glucocorticoids	Valproate
Haloperidol	Vecuronium
Hormonal contraceptives	Warfarin
Imipramine	Ziprasidone (?)
Indinavir	Zonisamide

as patients can have neurotoxicity due to elevated carbamazepine-epoxide or free carbamazepine concentrations in spite of therapeutic total carbamazepine levels. Thus, in view of increased carbamazepine-epoxide levels, carbamazepine levels as low as about one half of those seen without valproate may be required. Carbamazepine decreases serum valproate levels, and its discontinuation can yield increased serum valproate levels and toxicity. As a general rule, clinicians should carefully monitor patients on the carbamazepine plus valproate combination for side effects

Table 15.6 Selected Drugs That Decrease
Clearance of Carbamazepine

Acetazolamide
Cimetidine
Clarithromycin
Danazol
Diltiazem
d-Propoxyphene
Erythromycin
Fluoxetine
Flurithromycin
Fluvoxamine
Grapefruit juice
Isoniazid
Josamycin
Itraconazole
Ketoconazole
Nefazodone
Nelfinavir
Nicotinamide
Ponsinomycin
Propoxyphene
Quetiapine ($\uparrow$CBZ-E) (?)
Quinine
Ritonavir
Troleandomycin
Valproate ($\uparrow$CBZ-E)
Verapamil
Viloxazine

and consider decreasing the carbamazepine dose in advance (because of the expected displacement of carbamazepine from plasma proteins and increase in carbamazepine-epoxide) and ultimately increasing the valproate dose (because of expected carbamazepine-induced decrements in valproate).

Carbamazepine induces lamotrigine metabolism, so that as described below, lamotrigine therapy in the presence of carbamazepine requires higher doses of lamotrigine. Although lamotrigine does not yield clinically significant changes in serum carbamazepine concentrations, lamotrigine appears to enhance carbamazepine neurotoxicity, probably by a pharmacodynamic interaction.

Table 15.7 Mood Stabilizer Drug Interaction Potential

	Li	VPA	CBZ	LTG
Low therapeutic index	+	±	+	−
Long half-life	−	−	−	−
Nonlinear kinetics	−	±	±	−
Active metabolites	−	±	+	−
Enzyme inducer	−	−	++	−
Enzyme inhibitor	−	+	−	−
Single main elimination route	+	−	+	+
CYP substrate	−	±	3A3/4	−

++ indicates marked, + indicates moderate, ± indicates modest, − indicates none.

Carbamazepine increases metabolism of haloperidol and possibly other typical antipsychotics, such as chlorpromazine, fluphenazine and thiothixene, but not thioridazine. Some patients may have improvement or no deterioration in psychiatric status or fewer neuroleptic side effects during combination treatment, while others may have deterioration in psychiatric status. Haloperidol may increase carbamazepine levels, while loxapine and the amoxapine plus chlorpromazine combination may increase carbamazepine-epoxide levels, and thioridazine does not yield clinically significant changes in serum carbamazepine or carbamazepine-epoxide concentrations.

Carbamazepine induces clozapine metabolism, and this combination is not recommended in view of possible (but not proven) synergistic bone marrow suppression. Carbamazepine also increases metabolism of olanzapine, risperidone, quetiapine, aripiprazole, and ziprasidone. Although the clinical significance of carbamazepine-induced decreases in ziprasidone serum concentrations remains to be determined, carbamazepine interactions with other atypical antipsychotics can be clinically significant. For example, in a recent acute mania combination therapy study, carbamazepine decreased serum risperidone plus active metabolite concentrations by 40%, interfering with efficacy. In two patients, quetiapine appeared to increase carbamazepine-epoxide levels. The effects of clozapine, olanzapine, risperidone, ziprasidone, and aripiprazole on carbamazepine pharmacokinetics remain to be established.

Carbamazepine appears to induce metabolism of tricyclic antidepressants (TCAs), bupropion, citalopram, mirtazapine, mianserin, sertraline, and to some extent trazodone, but not viloxazine. Carbamazepine may increase rather than decrease serum levels of transdermal selegiline and its metabolites. Theoretical grounds have been stated for concern about

Table 15.8 Substrates, Inhibitors, and Inducers of Some Important Cytochrome P450 Isoforms

CYP	CYP1A2	CYP2C9/10	CYP2C19*	CYP2D6*	CYP2E1	CYP3A3/4
% of all CYP**	13	20 (for all 2C)		2	7	30 (for all 3A)
Substrates	Duloxetine Fuvoxamine 3° amine TCAs (N-demethy- lation) Clozapine (major) Olanzapine Caffeine Methadone Tacrine Acetaminophen Phenacetin Propranolol Theophylline	THC NSAIDs Phenytoin (major) Tolbutamide S-warfarin	Escitalopram (partly) Citalopram (partly) Moclobemide 3° amine TCAs (N-demethy- lation) Diazepam (N-demethy- lation) Hexobarbital Mephobarbital Lansoprazole Omeprazole (5-hydroxylation) Rabeprazole (demethylation)	Duloxetine Fluoxetine (partly) Mirtazepine (partly) Paroxetine Venlafaxine (O-demethy- lation) 2° & 3° amine TCAs (2,8,10- hyroxylation) Aripiprazole Chlorpromazine Clozapine (minor) Haloperidol (reduction)	Ethanol Acetamino- phen Chlorzoxa- zone Halothane Isoflurane Methoxy- flurane Sevoflurane	Carbamaze- pine Ethosuximide Tiagabine Zonisamide Alprazolam Diazepam (hydroxy- lation and N-demethy- lation) Midazolam Triazolam Zaleplon Zolpidem Zopiclone Buspirone Escitalopram (partly)	Amiodarone Disopyramide Lidocaine Propafenone Quinidine Erythromycin (Macrolides) Androgens Dexameth- asone Estrogens (Steroids) Astemizole Loratadine Terfenadine Lovastatin Simvastatin

(continued)

Table 15.8 Substrates, Inhibitors, and Inducers of Some Important Cytochrome P450 Isoforms (Continued)

CYP	CYP1A2	CYP2C9/10	CYP2C19*	CYP2D6*	CYP2E1	CYP3A3/4
% of all CYP**	13	20 (for all 2C)		2	7	30 (for all 3A)
			Phenytoin (minor)	Fluphenazine		Reboxetine
			S-mephenytoin	Perphenazine		Sertraline
			Nelfinavir	Risperidone		3° amine TCAs (N-demethylation)
				Sertindole		Trazodone
				Thioridazine		
						Aripiprazole
				Codeine (hydroxylation, O-demethylation)		Chlorpromazine
				Dextromethorphan (O-demethylation)		Sertindole
				Hydrocodone		Quetiapine
				Oxycodone		Ziprasidone
						Diltiazem
				Mexiletine		Felodipine
				Propafenone (1C antiarrhythmics)		Nimodipine
						Nifedipine
						Nisoldipine
				Beta blockers		Nitrendipine
				Donepezil (partly)		Verapamil
						Atorvastatin
						Cerivastatin (HMG-CoAR Inhib)
						Cyclophosphamide
						Tamoxifen
						Vincristine
						Vinblastine
						Ifosfamide
						Cyclosporine
						Tacrolimus
						Cisapride
						Donepezil (partly)
						Lovastatin
						Omeprazole/Rabeprazole (Sulfonation)
						Protease inhibitors

Inhibitors	Fluvoxamine Moclobemide Cimetidine Fluoroquinolines (ciprofloxacin, norfloxacin) Naringenin (grapefruit) Ticlopidine	Fluvoxamine Paroxetine Sertraline Disulfiram Cimetidine Amiodarone Azapropazone d-propoxyphene Fluconazole Fluvastatin Miconazole Phenylbutazone Stiripentol Sulphaphenazole Zafirlukast	Fluoxetine Fluvoxamine Imipramine Moclobemide Tranylcypromine Diazepam Felbamate Phenytoin Topiramate Cimetidine Omeprazole	Duloxetine Bupropion Fluoxetine Fluvoxamine (weak) iHydroxybupropion Paroxetine Sertraline (weak) Moclobemide Chlorpromazine Fluphenazine Haloperidol Perphenazine Thioridazine	d- and l-fenfluramine Diethyldithiocarbamate (disulfiram metabolite)	Acetaminophen Alfentanil Codeine (demethylation) Fentanyl Sufentanil Fluoxetine Fluvoxamine Nefazodone Sertraline (weak) Diltiazem Verapamil Dexamethasone Gestodene Ritonavir Indinavir Nelfinavir Saquinavir (protease inhibs)	Sildenafil Clarithromycin Erythromycin Troleandomycin (Macrolides) Fluconazole Itraconazole Ketoconazole (Azole antifungals) Amiodarone Cimetidine Mibefradil Naringenin (Grapefruit)

(continued)

Table 15.8 Substrates, Inhibitors, and Inducers of Some Important Cytochrome P450 Isoforms (*Continued*)

CYP	CYP1A2	CYP2C9/10	CYP2C19*	CYP2D6*	CYP2E1	CYP3A3/4
% of all CYP**	13	20 (for all 2C)		2	7	30 (for all 3A)
				Amiodarone Cimetidine Methadone Quinidine Ritonavir		
Inducers	Tobacco	Barbiturates Carbamazepine Phenytoin	Barbiturates Carbamazepine Phenytoin		Ethanol	Barbiturates Carbamazepine
	Omeprazole				Isoniazid	Monhydroxy-Rifampin derivative
	Charbroiled meats	Rifampin	Rifampin			Troglitazone
						Phenytoin
						Topiramate St. John's wort
						Dexamethasone Rifabutin

Source: Adapted from Ketter, T. A., Flockhart, D. A., Post, R. M., Denicoff, K., Pazzaglia, P. J., Marangell, L. B., et al., J. Clin. Psychopharmacol, 15(6), 387–398, 1995.

* Clinically significant human polymorphism reported.

** CYP percentages from Shimada et al., Activation of procarcinogens by human cytochrome P450 enzymes expressed in *Escherichia coli.* Simplified bacterial systems for genotoxicity assays. *Carcinogenesis.* 15(11), 2523–2529, 1994.

combining carbamazepine with monoamine oxidase inhibitors (MAOIs). However, preliminary data suggest that the addition of phenelzine or tranylcypromine to carbamazepine may be well tolerated, does not affect carbamazepine levels, and may provide relief of refractory depressive symptoms in some patients. The CYP3A3/4 inhibitors fluoxetine, fluvoxamine and nefazodone have been reported to inhibit carbamazepine metabolism, yielding increased carbamazepine levels and toxicity, while paroxetine, sertraline, and mirtazapine do not appear to yield clinically significant changes in carbamazepine levels. However, in one study in eight epilepsy patients, fluoxetine and fluvoxamine did not alter carbamazepine or carbamazepine-epoxide levels. Viloxazine and perhaps trazodone can also increase carbamazepine levels.

Carbamazepine is commonly administered along with benzodiazepines in patients with bipolar disorder, with merely additive central nervous system (e.g. sedation, ataxia) adverse effects. Indeed, contemporary controlled carbamazepine trials routinely permit some adjunctive benzodiazepine (e.g. lorazepam) administration. However, carbamazepine may decrease serum levels of clonazepam, alprazolam, clobazam, and midazolam, potentially decreasing the efficacy of these agents. The newer hypnotics eszopiclone and zolpidem may have drug interactions with carbamazepine, as these agents appear more susceptible than zaleplon to drugs that induce CYP3A4.

Carbamazepine induces the metabolism of multiple newer anticonvulsants, including topiramate, tiagabine, oxcarbazepine, zonisamide, and possibly levetiracetam, but not gabapentin or pregabalin. In contrast, none of these newer anticonvulsants yield clinically significant changes in carbamazepine pharmacokinetics. However, the anticonvulsants phenytoin, phenobarbital, primidone, felbamate, and methsuximide decrease serum carbamazepine levels. In addition, carbamazepine may have a pharmacodynamic interaction with levetiracetam.

The commonly used calcium channel blockers verapamil and diltiazem can increase carbamazepine levels and cause clinical toxicity, but this does not occur with the dihydropyridines nifedipine and nimodipine. Also, enzyme-inducing anticonvulsants like carbamazepine appear to decrease nimodipine and felodipine levels.

Carbamazepine decreases levothyroxine (T_4), free T_4 index, and less consistently liothyronine (T_3) concentrations. In contrast, thyroid binding globulin, reverse T_3, and basal plasma TSH concentrations, and basal metabolic rates are not substantially changed with carbamazepine therapy.

Drug–drug interactions between carbamazepine and other (nonpsychotropic) drugs are also of substantial clinical importance. Carbamazepine induces metabolism of diverse medications, raising the possibility of undermining the efficacy of steroids such as hormonal contraceptives (Crawford et al., 1990; Doose et al., 2003). In women taking carbamazepine, oral contraceptive preparations need to contain at least 50 ug of ethinylestradiol, levonorgestrel implants are contraindicated because of cases of contraceptive failure, and medroxyprogesterone injections need to be given every 10 rather than 12 weeks (Crawford, 2002). Carbamazepine also induces metabolism of prednisolone and methylprednisolone; the methylxanthines theophylline and aminophylline; the antibiotic doxycycline; the neuromuscular blockers pancuronium, vecuronium and doxacurium; and the anticoagulant warfarin, and possibly dicumarol. Coadministration of carbamazepine and delavirdine may lead to delavirdine inefficacy.

Similarly, a variety of medications can increase serum carbamazepine levels and potentially yield clinical toxicity, including nicotinamide, the antibiotics erythromycin, triacetyloleandomycin, clarithromycin, and isoniazid; the protease inhibitors ritonavir and nelfinavir; and the carbonic anhydrase inhibitor acetazolamide. In addition, other medications such as including cisplatin and doxorubicin may decrease serum carbamazepine levels, potentially yielding inefficacy.

Adverse events and their management

Carbamazepine therapy is associated with common (e.g. 1/10), benign, as well as rare (e.g. 1/100,000), serious, adverse events. The most common dose-related adverse effects with carbamazepine involve central nervous system (diplopia, blurred vision, fatigue, sedation, dizziness, and ataxia) or gastrointestinal system (nausea, vomiting) problems (Pellock, 1987). Carbamazepine central nervous system adverse effects tend to occur early in therapy before autoinduction and the development of some tolerance to carbamazepine's central adverse effects. Gradual initial dosing and careful attention to potential drug–drug interactions can help attenuate this problem. Carbamazepine-induced gastrointestinal disturbance can be approached in a fashion similar to that described for lithium.

The United States carbamazepine prescribing information includes a boxed warning regarding the risks of serious dermatological reactions and the HLA-B*1502 allele, as well as aplastic anemia (16 per million patient-years) and agranulocytosis (48 per million patient-years). Other warnings include the risks of teratogenicity, and serious rash. Thus, carbamazepine can yield hematologic (benign leukopenia, benign thrombocytopenia), dermatologic (benign rash), electrolyte (asymptomatic hyponatremia), and hepatic (benign transaminase elevations) problems. Much less commonly, carbamazepine can yield analogous serious problems. For example, mild leukopenia and benign rash occur in as many as 1/10 patients, with the slight possibility that these usually benign phenomena are heralding malignant aplastic anemia and Stevens-Johnson syndrome, seen in about 1/100,000 patients (Kramlinger, Phillips, & Post, 1994; Tohen et al., 1995). Hematologic monitoring needs to be intensified in patients with low or marginal leuko-cyte counts, and carbamazepine is generally discontinued if the leukocyte count falls below 3000/µL or the granulocyte count below 1000/µL. Recent evidence indicates that the risk of serious rash may be ten times as high in some Asian countries, and strongly linked to the HLA-B*1502 allele. Rash presenting with systemic illness, or involvement of the eyes, mouth, or blad-der (dysuria) constitutes a medical emergency and carbamazepine ought to be immediately discontinued and the patient assessed emergently. For more benign presentations, immediate dermatologic consultation is required to assess the risks of continuing therapy. In carefully selected cases, with the collaboration of dermatology, it may be safe to attempt desensitization by decreasing dose and adding antihistamine or prednisone. Carbamazepine, like valproate, can rarely cause clinically significant hepatic problems, and generally needs to be discontinued if hepatic indices rise above three times the upper limit of normal (Martinez et al., 1993).

Although carbamazepine can cause modest TSH increases, frank hypothyroidism is very uncommon. Like other agents with tricyclic struc-tures and sodium blocking properties, carbamazepine may affect cardiac conduction and should be used with caution in patients with cardiac dis-orders. A baseline electrocardiogram is worth consideration if there is any indication of cardiac problems.

Carbamazepine appears less likely than lithium or valproate to yield weight gain. For this reason, carbamazepine may provide an important alternative to other mood stabilizers for patients who struggle with this problem. Carbamazepine-induced hyponatremia is often tolerated in young physically well individuals, but can yield obtundation and other serious sequelae in frail elderly patients.

Carbamazepine, like the other mood stabilizers, is a teratogen (FDA pregnancy category D) (Gentile, 2006). Thus, carbamazepine can yield minor anomalies (craniofacial malformations and digital hypoplasia) in up to 20% (Jones et al., 1989), and spina bifida in about 1% (Rosa, 1991) of cases. For the latter, folate supplementation may attenuate the risk, and ultrasound may allow early detection. The issue of carbamazepine ther-apy in pregnancy can be approached in a fashion similar to that described above for lithium. Although carbamazepine concentrations in breast milk are variable, and there is very little evidence of adverse effects in new-borns exposed to carbamazepine via breast milk, the FDA recommends "a decision should be made whether to discontinue nursing or to discontinue the drug, taking into account the importance of the drug to the mother".

Dosing strategies

In acute settings, such as the inpatient treatment of mania, carbam-azepine therapy is commonly initiated at 200–400 mg/day, and increased as necessary and tolerated, by 200 mg/day every 2–4 days. In recent controlled studies, a beaded extended release capsule formulation was started at 200 mg twice per day and titrated by daily increments of 200 mg to final doses as high as 1600 mg/day (Weisler, Kalali, & Ketter, 2004; Weisler et al., 2005). In a recent report of open extension therapy after these controlled acute mania studies, beaded extended release capsule carbamazepine was started at 200 mg twice per day and titrated by increments of 200 mg every 3 days (vs every day in the acute studies) to final doses as high as 1600 mg/day (Ketter, Kalali, & Weisler, 2004). This approach decreased the incidence of central nervous system (dizziness, somnolence, ataxia), digestive (nausea, vomiting), and dermatologic (pruritus) adverse effects by about 50%. Euthymic or depressed patients tend to tolerate aggressive initiation less well than manic patients. Thus, in less acute situations, such as the initiation of prophylaxis or adjunctive use, carbamazepine is often started at 100–200 mg/day, and increased as necessary and tolerated, by 200 mg/day every 4–7 days. Even this gradual initiation may cause adverse effects. Thus, starting with 50 mg (half of a chewable 100 mg tablet) at bedtime and increasing by 50 mg every 4 days can yield a better tolerated initiation. Due to autoinduction, doses after 2–4 weeks of therapy may need to be twice as high as in the first week to yield comparable serum levels. Target doses are commonly between 600 and 1200 mg/day, yielding serum levels from 6 to 12 mcg/mL (20–60 μM/L), with the higher portion of the range used acutely, and lower doses used in prophylaxis or adjunctive therapy. In a carbamazepine versus lithium maintenance study, serum trough carbamazepine concentrations were maintained at 4–12 ug/mL, with a mean of 6.4 ug/mL (Greil et al., 1997). In another carbamazepine versus lithium maintenance study, serum trough carbamazepine concentrations were maintained at 4–12 ug/mL, with a mean of 7.7 ug/mL (Denicoff et al., 1997).

Clinical recommendations

Patients need to be advised of carbamazepine adverse effects and drug interactions. Clinical assessments with carbamazepine therapy include a baseline physical examination, and routinely querying patients regarding hepatic and hematologic disorders and adverse effects at baseline and during treatment. In the past, recommended laboratory monitoring during carbamazepine therapy has included baseline complete blood count, differential, platelets, hepatic indices, and serum sodium, with re-evaluation at 2, 4, 6, and 8 weeks, and then every 3 months, and as clinically indicated (American Psychiatric Association, 2002). Most of the dangerous hematologic reactions occur in the first 3 months of therapy (Tohen et al., 1995). In contemporary clinical practice, somewhat less focus is placed on scheduled monitoring, whereas clinically indicated (for example, when a patient becomes ill with a fever) monitoring is emphasized. Patients who have abnormal or marginal indices at any point merit careful scheduled and clinically indicated monitoring. The United States prescribing information for the beaded extended release capsule carbamazepine formulation that was recently approved for the treatment of acute mania includes monitoring baseline complete blood count, platelets, ±reticulocytes, ±serum iron, hepatic function tests, closely monitoring patients with low or decreased white blood cell count or platelets, and considering discontinuation of carbamazepine if there is evidence of bone marrow depression (Physicians' Desk Reference, 2007). Serum carbamazepine concentrations are typically assessed at steady state, and then as indicated by inefficacy or adverse effects. Titrating carbamazepine to the maximum dose that is well tolerated (commonly 6–12 mcg/mL in acute mania and 4–10 mcg/mL in bipolar depression and maintenance), and promptly addressing adverse effect concerns can help enhance adherence.

Lamotrigine

Lamotrigine (LTG) has a phenyltriazine structure and is a sodium channel and weak 5HT3 receptor blocker (this ionotropic receptor gates a cation channel), and decreases glutamate release (Ketter, Manji, & Post, 2003). Of interest, the latter property is also observed with the mood stabilizing anticonvulsants carbamazepine and oxcarbazepine. Although lamotrigine appears to modestly inhibit reuptake of serotonin, this effect does not appear to be clinically significant as sexual dysfunction is not a major concern. Although lamotrigine has anxiolytic activity in the Vögel (anticonflict) animal model, it does not appear to have robust clinical anxiolytic effects. In placebo controlled trials, lamotrigine appeared effective in bipolar prophylaxis (Bowden et al., 2003; Calabrese et al., 2003), and may have some utility in acute bipolar depression (Calabrese et al., 1999), rapid cycling bipolar disorder (Calabrese et al., 2000), and treatment refractory (primarily rapid cycling bipolar) mood disorder (Frye et al., 2000).

Lamotrigine has a bioavailability of about 98%. It is 55% bound to plasma proteins, and has a moderate volume of distribution of approximately 1 L/kg, and a linear dose to plasma concentration relationship (Mikati et al., 1989). In monotherapy its half-life is about 28 hours and clearance is about 40 mL/min. Lamotrigine is extensively metabolized, mostly by glucuronidation, primarily by UTG1A4 and UGT2B7 (Rowland et al., 2006), with only 10% excreted unchanged in the urine. Lamotrigine does not yield clinically significant induction or inhibition of CYP450 isoforms, and is thus more a target of than an instigator of drug interactions. Combined with the enzyme inducer carbamazepine, lamotrigine's half-life falls 50% to about 14 hours and clearance doubles to about 80 mL/min. Combined with the enzyme inhibitor valproate, lamotrigine's half-life doubles to about 56 hours, and clearance falls 50% to about 20 mL/min.

Thus, approximately 85% of lamotrigine is conjugated to yield inactive glucuronide metabolites, while about 10% is excreted unchanged in the urine (Cohen et al., 1987). As indicated by the above kinetic data, enzyme inducers such as carbamazepine decreases serum lamotrigine concentrations presumably mediated by induction of glucuronidation, while valproate increases lamotrigine levels, presumably mediated by inhibition of UGT2B7. In contrast, lamotrigine does not yield clinically significant changes in serum carbamazepine concentrations, and lamotrigine may only yield modest (25%) clinically insignificant decreases in valproate levels. However, lamotrigine appears to enhance carbamazepine neurotoxicity, probably by a pharmacodynamic interaction. Lamotrigine does not yield clinically significant changes in the pharmacokinetics of lithium. Although lithium is not expected to influence the pharmacokinetics of lamotrigine, the absence of such an interaction remains to be confirmed.

Lamotrigine does not generally yield clinically significant changes in serum clozapine, risperidone, or olanzapine concentrations. However, single cases of increased clozapine and risperidone with lamotrigine have been reported. Clozapine, risperidone, and olanzapine do not appear to alter lamotrigine pharmacokinetics. Systematic data are very limited or lacking regarding drug interactions between lamotrigine and typical antipsychotics as well as quetiapine, ziprasidone, and aripiprazole. Assessments from a therapeutic drug monitoring service suggested chlorpromazine, clozapine, haloperidol, perphenazine, and quetiapine may not generally alter lamotrigine serum concentration to dose ratios. In vitro experiments suggest that haloperidol minimally affects lamotrigine metabolism.

Although lamotrigine is commonly combined with antidepressants in patients with mood disorders with apparent good tolerability, there are only limited systematic data regarding drug interactions with such combinations. Bupropion does not appear to yield clinically significant changes in lamotrigine pharmacokinetics. In a controlled clinical trial, lamotrigine and paroxetine did not appear to have pharmacokinetic interactions—lamotrigine did not yield clinically significant changes in paroxetine concentrations, and serum lamotrigine concentrations were in the lower part of the epilepsy therapeutic range. In another controlled clinical trial, lamotrigine and fluoxetine did not appear yield adverse effects. Assessments of from a therapeutic drug monitoring service suggested citalopram, mirtazapine, nefazodone, venlafaxine, paroxetine, and sertraline may not generally alter lamotrigine serum concentration to dose ratios and the unexpected observation that fluoxetine may decrease lamotrigine serum concentration to dose ratios. In vitro experiments suggest that fluoxetine, phenelzine, trazodone do not affect lamotrigine metabolism and that amitriptyline and bupropion minimally affect lamotrigine metabolism. However, problems may occur with some individuals, as case reports suggest that sertraline may increase serum lamotrigine levels in some patients, that lamotrigine combined with escitalopram could yield myoclonus, and seizures, ventricular tachycardia, and rhabdomyolysis were observed after an overdose of venlafaxine and lamotrigine.

Lamotrigine is commonly administered along with benzodiazepines in patients with bipolar disorder, with merely additive central nervous system (e.g. sedation, ataxia) adverse effects. Indeed, contemporary controlled lithium trials routinely permit some adjunctive benzodiazepine (e.g. lorazepam) administration. Systematic data are very limited or lacking regarding drug interactions between lamotrigine and benzodiazepines. Assessments from a therapeutic drug monitoring service suggested clonazepam, diazepam, oxazepam, and zopiclone may not generally alter lamotrigine serum concentration to dose ratios. In vitro experiments suggest that clonzaepam and lorazepam minimally affect lamotrigine metabolism.

Lamotrigine does not appear to have clinically significant pharmacokinetic interactions with topiramate, levetiracetam, zonisamide, or pregabalin. Oxcarbazepine may decrease serum lamotrigine concentrations, but the clinical significance of this interaction remains to be established and could vary across patients, whereas lamotrigine does not appear to alter oxcarbazepine pharmacokinetics. A possible pharmacodynamic interaction has been reported with oxcarbazepine and lamotrigine. Although gabapentin and lamotrigine are not expected to influence one another's pharmacokinetics of lamotrigine, the absence of such interactions remains to be confirmed. Also, the presence or absence of pharmacokinetic interactions between lamotrigine and tiagabine remains to be assessed.

Lamotrigine has interactions with some non-psychotropic medications. Rifampin increases lamotrigine clearance, but cimetidine did not yield clinically significant changes in lamotrigine clearance. Although lamotrigine does not appear to yield clinically significant changes in the pharmacokinetics of hormonal contraceptives, hormonal contraceptives cause clinically significant decreases in serum lamotrigine concentrations (Christensen et al., 2007; Sabers et al., 2003; Sidhu et al., 2006).

Adverse events and their management

Lamotrigine is generally well tolerated, particularly in comparison to other treatment options for patients with bipolar disorder. The most common adverse events in bipolar disorder patients in clinical trials were headache, benign rash, dizziness, diarrhea, dream abnormality, and pruritus.

The United States lamotrigine prescribing information includes a boxed warning regarding the risk of serious rashes requiring hospitalization, which have included Stevens-Johnson syndrome, in 0.8% and 0.3% of pediatric and adult epilepsy patients receiving adjunctive therapy, respectively, and in 0.08% and 0.13% of adult mood disorder patients receiving monotherapy and adjunctive therapy, respectively. The risk of rash is higher in patients under age 16 years, and may be higher with coadministration with valproate, exceeding the recommended initial lamotrigine dose, and exceeding the recommended lamotrigine dose escalation. Benign rash may be seen in 10% of patients, but as any rash is potentially serious, rashes require discontinuation of lamotrigine, unless they are clearly not drug-related. Nearly all cases of life-threatening rashes have occurred within 2–8 weeks of starting lamotrigine. Other warnings in the prescribing information include the risks of hypersensitivity reactions (with fever and lymphadenopathy, but not necessarily rash), acute multiorgan failure (fatalities observed in about 1 in 400 pediatric and 1 in 1800 adult epilepsy patients, but not in bipolar disorder patients), blood dyscrasia, and possibly withdrawal seizures in bipolar disorder patients, so that unless safety concerns demand abrupt discontinuation, lamotrigine should be tapered over 2 weeks.

Lamotrigine can cause central nervous system (headache, somnolence, insomnia, dizziness, tremor) and gastrointestinal (nausea, diarrhea) (Bowden et al., 2003; Calabrese et al., 2003; Calabrese et al., 1999; Calabrese et al., 2000) adverse effects. In most instances these problems attenuate or resolve with time or lamotrigine dosage adjustment, but in occasional patients may require lamotrigine discontinuation. Unlike other mood stabilizers, lamotrigine has not been associated with weight gain. Also of clinical importance, lamotrigine may be less likely than SSRIs or other anticonvulsants to cause sexual dysfunction.

Lamotrigine, like the other mood stabilizers, is a teratogen (FDA pregnancy category C) (Gentile, 2006). Recent data suggest that overall rates of major congenital malformations with lamotrigine exposure could be comparable to rates with no anticonvulsant exposure and lower compared to rates with valproate exposure (Alsdorf et al., 2004; Cunnington, 2004; Vajda et al., 2004). Nevertheless, lamotrigine may increase the risk of subtypes of malformation, namely cleft lip and cleft palate. Lamotrigine concentrations in breast milk are variable, but in some instances may approach "therapeutic ranges". Despite the lack of evidence of adverse effects in newborns exposed to lamotrigine via breast milk, FDA has taken a conservative stance, considering lamotrigine administration "not recommended" during lactation.

Dosing strategies

Lamotrigine dosage is initially titrated *very slowly* in order to decrease the risk of rash. When given without valproate, the prescribing information recommends starting lamotrigine at 25 mg/day for 2 weeks, then increasing to 50 mg/day for the next 2 weeks, then increasing to 100 mg/day for 1 week, and then increasing to 200 mg/day in a single daily dose, with doses exceeding 200 mg/day not recommended unless concurrent hormonal contraceptives (which decrease serum lamotrigine concentrations) are administered (Physicians' Desk Reference, 2007). Nevertheless, even in the absence of hormonal contraceptive, selected patients may benefit from further gradual lamotrigine titration to final doses as high as 500 mg/day. Even more gradual titration, starting with 25 mg/day for 2 weeks, then increasing to 50 mg/day for the next 2 weeks, and then increasing as necessary and tolerated weekly by 25 mg/day may further decrease the risk of rash (Ketter et al., 2003).

When added to valproate, recommended doses are halved, so lamotrigine is started at 25 mg every other day (although 12.5 mg/day may be worth considering) for 2 weeks, then increasing to 25 mg/day for the next 2 weeks, then increasing to 50 mg/day for 1 week, and then increasing to 100 mg/day in a single daily dose, with doses exceeding 100 mg/day not recommended unless concurrent hormonal contraceptives (which decrease serum lamotrigine concentrations) are administered (Physicians' Desk Reference, 2007). Nevertheless, even in the absence of hormonal contraceptive, selected patients concurrently taking valproate may benefit from further gradual lamotrigine titration to final doses as high as 250 mg/day.

When given with carbamazepine, doses may be doubled, so that lamotrigine may be started at 50 mg/day for 2 weeks, then increasing to 100 mg/day for the next 2 weeks, then increasing to 300 mg/day for 1 week, and then increasing to 400 mg/day in divided doses, with doses exceeding 400 mg/day not recommended unless concurrent hormonal contraceptives (which decrease serum lamotrigine concentrations) are administered (Physicians' Desk Reference, 2007). Nevertheless, even in the absence of hormonal contraceptive, selected patients concurrently taking carbamazepine may benefit from further gradual lamotrigine titration to final doses as high as 800 mg/day.

Patients should be advised that if they fail to take lamotrigine for 5 half-lives (e.g. approximately 5 days in the absence of carbamazepine, or 3 days in the presence of carbamazepine), gradual reintroduction as described above is necessary, as rashes have been reported with rapid reintroduction.

Clinical recommendations

Patients need to be advised of lamotrigine adverse effects and drug interactions. Clinical assessments with lamotrigine therapy include a baseline physical examination, and routinely querying patients regarding rash at baseline and during treatment. Lamotrigine is generally well tolerated and serum concentrations have not been related to therapeutic effects in patients with bipolar disorder, so that therapeutic drug monitoring with lamotrigine is not generally performed. Nevertheless, in patients taking higher doses (e.g. 400 mg/day without valproate, 200 mg/day with valproate, or 800 mg/day with carbamazepine) with inadequate therapeutic response and good tolerability, assessing serum lamotrigine concentration may be worthwhile in order to provide an assessment of adherence and/or metabolic abnormalities. In epilepsy patients, serum lamotrigine concentrations range from approximately 3 to 15 mcg/mL (10–60 uM/L). Thus, in a patient with bipolar disorder is taking higher doses with inadequate therapeutic response a serum lamotrigine concentration of less than 3 mcg/mL or in excess of 15 mcg/mL may suggest adherence or nonresponse problems, respectively.

Antipsychotics

About 50% of patients with mania have psychotic symptoms, and bipolar depression may have psychotic features. Mood stabilizers may fail to provide adequate efficacy in such circumstances. Patients with acute mania with profound agitation may require parenteral medication, and patients with poor adherence may benefit from depot formulations. Unfortunately, mood stabilizers are not available in such formulations. Thus, due to both efficacy and formulation availability limitations of mood stabilizers, adjunctive antipsychotics are commonly used in the treatment of bipolar disorder patients.

Traditional antipsychotics

Traditional antipsychotics block dopamine D2 receptors, with the degree of blockade correlating with antipsychotic effects. These agents are effective in the acute and prophylactic treatment of mania, and are useful adjuncts in the management of psychotic depression. Chlorpromazine is approved by the FDA for the treatment of acute mania (Johnson et al., 1971; Okuma et al., 1979; Spring et al., 1970; Takahashi et al., 1975). In recent years, haloperidol, although not approved by the FDA for the treatment of acute mania, has demonstrated efficacy (as an active comparator in controlled trials of newer agents) in the treatment of acute mania as monotherapy (McIntyre et al., 2005; Tohen et al., 2003; Vieta et al., 2005) or as an adjunct to lithium or valproate (Sachs et al., 2002).

Severe acute agitation may be treated with parenteral combinations such as haloperidol 0.2 mg/kg i.m., plus lorazepam 2 mg i.m., plus diphenhydramine 50 mg i.m. Lorazepam and diphenhydramine provide additional sedation, with the latter also attenuating the risk of acute extra pyramidal symptoms (EPS). Injectible formulations of newer antipsychotics such as olanzapine, ziprasidone, and aripiprazole also appear useful in the treatment of acute agitation. Depot formulations of haloperidol, fluphenazine, and risperidone can prove useful in cases with poor medication compliance.

Traditional antipsychotics are generally well absorbed, with variable (20–80%) bioavailability, high (80–95%) protein binding, and variable volumes of distribution (10–40 L/kg), half-lives (12–24 hours), and clearances (70–600 mL/min) (Javaid, 1994). These agents have varying and in some cases complex metabolism, which is susceptible to induction by carbamazepine, phenobarbital, phenytoin, rifampin, and cigarettes. Several traditional antipsychotics (including haloperidol, perphenazine, and thioridazine) are CYP2D6 substrates, and hence susceptible to inhibition of metabolism. Thus, tricyclics, fluoxetine, beta blockers, and cimetidine can increase serum concentrations of some traditional antipsychotics. Some traditional antipsychotics (including perphenazine, thioridazine, chlorpromazine, haloperidol, and fluphenazine) are themselves CYP2D6 inhibitors, and may thus increase serum levels of tricyclic antidepressants and risperidone. Several traditional antipsychotics (including chlorpromazine, haloperidol, perphenazine, and thioridazine) are CYP3A4 substrates, and hence susceptible to inhibition of metabolism by nefazodone or induction of metabolism by carbamazepine. Oxcarbazepine compared to carbamazepine appears to have less of an effect upon serum levels of haloperidol and chlorpromazine. Tobacco smoking induces the metabolism of the traditional antipsychotics chlorpromazine and haloperidol, as well as the atypical antipsychotics clozapine and olanzapine.

Case reports have raised concerns regarding development of lithium toxicity and serious adverse events when combining lithium with typical antipsychotics. Systematic assessments and clinical trials suggest combining lithium with typical antipsychotics generally yields no more than merely additive adverse effects. Sporadic cases in which problems occur during such combination therapy may be due to pharmacodynamic interactions.

In view of recent controlled trials confirming the efficacy of haloperidol in acute mania (McIntyre et al., 2005; Sachs et al., 2002; Tohen et al., 2003; Vieta et al., 2005), potential drug interactions with this agent are considered in additional detail. Haloperidol is commonly administered with lithium and valproate with adequate tolerability (Sachs et al., 2002).

However, case reports have raised concerns that occasional patients treated with haloperidol combined with lithium may experience serious adverse effects, possibly due to a pharmacodynamic interaction. Haloperidol and valproate do not appear to have clinically significant pharmacokinetic interactions. In contrast, carbamazepine increases metabolism of haloperidol, and haloperidol may increase carbamazepine levels. Haloperidol may not generally alter lamotrigine serum concentration to dose ratios, and in vitro experiments suggest haloperidol minimally affects lamotrigine metabolism.

Fluoxetine may modestly increase serum concentrations for oral haloperidol, but could more than double serum concentrations for haloperidol decanoate. Fluvoxamine may modestly (23%) or more substantially (79%) increase serum haloperidol concentrations. In contrast, citalopram and sertraline do not appear to yield clinically significant changes in serum haloperidol concentrations. Similarly, in vitro, paroxetine did not markedly affect haloperidol metabolism. Venlafaxine may substantially increase (70%) serum haloperidol concentrations. Low dose haloperidol did not yield clinically significant changes in plasma trazodone concentrations. Nefazodone may modestly (36%) increase serum haloperidol concentrations.

Haloperidol is commonly administered along with benzodiazepines in patients with bipolar disorder, with merely additive central nervous system (e.g. sedation, ataxia) adverse effects. Indeed, contemporary controlled haloperidol acute mania trials routinely permit some adjunctive benzodiazepine (e.g. lorazepam) administration, and intramuscular haloperidol combined with lorazepam is commonly used to manage acute agitation. Alprazolam may modestly (23%) increase serum haloperidol concentrations, while lorazepam does not appear to yield clinically significant changes in haloperidol pharmacokinetics.

The role of traditional antipsychotics in the management of bipolar disorders is limited due to concerns over acute extrapyramidal symptoms (EPS) (Nasrallah et al., 1988), tardive dyskinesia (Kane & Smith, 1982), and induction of dysphoria (Ahlfors et al., 1981). Thus, attempts are often made to taper and discontinue these drugs after resolution of acute episodes. Nevertheless, a substantial number of bipolar disorder patients may be maintained on antipsychotics on a chronic basis (Sernyak et al., 1997), during which these neurological adverse effects, as well as sedation and weight gain are major concerns. High potency antipsychotics such as haloperidol may offer less sedation but more EPS, while molindone may cause less weight gain (Allison et al., 1999). Concerns have been raised around QTc prolongation with agents such as thioridazine and mesoridazine.

Atypical antipsychotics

Based on the novel efficacy profile, and lack of extrapyramidal symptoms and tardive dyskinesia seen with clozapine, a new generation of "atypical antipsychotics" has been developed. These agents block not only dopamine D_2 receptors (like the antimanic traditional antipsychotics) but also serotonin $5HT_2$ receptors (like the antidepressant nefazodone), and thus, perhaps depending on the relative size of these as well as other receptor blocking effects, could have antimanic, antidepressant, or even mood stabilizing properties. Clozapine appears effective in treatment-refractory bipolar disorder patients (Suppes et al., 1999). Between 2000 and 2004, five atypical antipsychotics (olanzapine, risperidone, quetiapine, ziprasidone and aripiprazole) received FDA monotherapy indications for acute mania (Ketter et al., 2005). In addition, in 2003 and 2004, three of these agents (olanzapine, risperidone, and quetiapine) also received FDA adjunctive (combined with lithium or valproate) therapy indications for acute mania. Moreover, two of these agents have received bipolar maintenance monotherapy indications (olanzapine in 2004 and aripiprazole in 2005), and olanzapine (combined with fluoxetine) in 2003 and quetiapine monotherapy in 2006 have received acute bipolar depression indications.

Clozapine

Clozapine (CLZ) is a dibenzodiazepine derivative that blocks serotonin $5HT_{2A}$, $5HT_{1C}$, and $5HT_3$, dopamine D_4, D_1, D_2, and D_3, muscarinic M_1, adrenergic alpha$_1$ and alpha$_2$, and histamine H_1 receptors (Bymaster et al., 1996). After its introduction in clinical studies in the United States in the early 1970s, clozapine was withdrawn in 1974 due to the risk of agranulocytosis, and was not approved for clinical use in the treatment of schizophrenia in United States until 1990. Although clozapine lacks an FDA indication for acute mania, this medication is of interest not only as it is the first atypical antipsychotic, but also as it is the only agent approved for treatment-resistant schizophrenia, and for decreasing suicidal behavior in patients with schizophrenia (Meltzer et al., 2003). Uncontrolled reports (for a review see Frye et al., 1998) and a controlled trial (Suppes et al., 1999) suggested that clozapine may be effective in treatment-refractory bipolar disorder patients.

Clozapine is well absorbed, with 70% bioavailability, 97% protein binding, a moderately large volume of distribution of 5 L/kg, a linear dose to serum concentration relationship, a half-life of 12 hours, and clearance of 750 mL/min (Ackenheil, 1989; Byerly & DeVane, 1996; Fitton & Heel, 1990; Jann et al., 1993). Clozapine is extensively metabolized with only trace amounts excreted unchanged in the urine. N-demethylation and N-oxidation are the predominant metabolic routes, yielding active N-desmethylclozapine (norclozapine) and inactive N-oxide metabolites. Clozapine is a CYP1A2 and to a lesser extent a CYP3A4 substrate. Clozapine does not appear to induce or inhibit most CYP450 isozymes, and thus is more of a target of than an instigator of drug interactions. Thus, other medications influencing clozapine pharmacokinetics account for the majority of pharmacokinetic drug interactions with clozapine.

Although clozapine and lithium are not expected to generally have clinically significant pharmacokinetic interactions, the absence of such interactions remains to be confirmed. Case reports suggest that sporadic individuals could develop serious adverse effects such as neuroleptic malignant syndrome when clozapine is combined with lithium. However, clinical data suggest this combination does not generally yield more than merely additive adverse effects. Valproate does not appear to generally yield clinically significant changes in serum clozapine concentrations, although limited data suggest valproate could decrease clozapine levels in some patients. Clozapine metabolism is increased with carbamazepine, and combination of clozapine with carbamazepine is not recommended in view of possible (but not proven) synergistic bone marrow suppression. The effects of clozapine upon valproate and carbamazepine pharmacokinetics remain to be established. Clozapine does not appear to generally have clinically significant pharmacokinetic interactions with lamotrigine, although a single case of increased serum clozapine with lamotrigine has been reported.

Studies suggest that risperidone does not generally alter serum clozapine concentrations, but case studies have reported risperidone-related increases in serum clozapine concentrations, and a case of a neurotoxic syndrome, characterized as mild NMS, after clozapine was added to risperidone, as well as clozapine-related increases in serum risperidone concentrations.

Clinically significant increases in serum clozapine concentrations occur with the CYP1A2 inhibitor fluvoxamine, and with fluoxetine. Although paroxetine may also yield increases in serum clozapine concentrations, the clinical significance of this interaction remains to be established. Pharmacokinetic studies suggest that sertraline does not generally yield clinically significant increases in serum clozapine concentrations, but case reports suggest this could occur in some individuals. Citalopram does not appear to generally yield clinically significant increases in serum clozapine concentrations, but a case report suggests this could occur in some individuals. Nefazodone may increase serum concentrations of clozapine, but the clinical significance of this interaction has been questioned. Mirtazapine does not appear to yield clinically significant increases in clozapine serum concentrations. Clozapine may modestly inhibit CYP2C9 and CYP2D6, and thus could increase serum nortriptyline concentrations.

Caution needs to be exercised when combining clozapine with benzodiazepines as some patients may develop respiratory depression or even arrest. Oxcarbazepine compared to carbamazepine appears to have less of an effect upon serum levels of clozapine. Topiramate does not generally yield clinically significant alterations in serum clozapine concentrations.

The CYP1A2 inducer omeprazole may modestly decrease serum clozapine concentrations in non-smokers, but this interaction could be clinically significant in some patients. The CYP3A4 inhibitor ketoconazole and erythromycin do not appear to generally yield clinically significant increases in serum clozapine concentrations, but case reports suggest some individuals may experience toxicity with the clozapine plus erythromycin combination. A single case report suggested that hormonal contraceptives could increase serum clozapine concentrations.

Tobacco smoking induces CYP1A2, apparently decreasing serum concentrations of clozapine in several but not all studies. In contrast, caffeine in excess of 400 mg/day modestly increases serum clozapine concentrations, presumably by inhibition of CYP1A2, but this could be clinically significant in some patients. The CYP3A4 inhibitor grapefruit juice does not appear to generally yield clinically significant increases in serum clozapine concentrations.

Clozapine generally has a challenging adverse effect profile compared to other treatment options (Baldessarini & Frankenburg, 1991; Marinkovic et al., 1994; Miller, 2000; Young, Bowers, & Mazure, 1998). Hence, this agent tends to be held in reserve for patients with treatment-resistant bipolar disorders (Suppes et al., 1999). The most common adverse effects associated with clozapine discontinuation include central nervous system (sedation, seizures, dizziness), cardiovascular (tachycardia, hypotension, syncope, electrocardiogram changes), gastrointestinal (nausea, vomiting), and hematologic (leucopenia, granulocytopenia, agranulocytosis) problems, and fever (Iqbal et al., 2003).

The United States clozapine prescribing information includes boxed warnings regarding the risks of: (1) agranulocytosis; (2) seizures; (3) myocarditis; (4) other adverse cardiovascular and respiratory effects; and (5) death (primarily cardiovascular or infectious) in elderly patients with dementia-related psychosis (an atypical antipsychotic class warning). The most serious adverse effect is agranulocytosis, which is seen in 1.3% of patients, and requires ongoing hematological monitoring (Grohmann et al., 1989). Seizures occur in 2% of patients on less than 300 mg/day, 4% on 300–600 mg/day, and 5% on 600–900 mg/day. Thus, combination with an anticonvulsant mood stabilizer could be desirable. Due to a pharmacokinetic interactions and concerns regarding potential synergy of marrow toxicity with carbamazepine, combination with other anticonvulsants such as valproate or lamotrigine are preferred. Myocarditis may occur at a rate of 0.3 cases per 100,000 patient-years. Other adverse cardiovascular and respiratory effects include orthostatic hypotension, syncope, respiratory/cardiac arrest (in 1/3,000 patients), tachycardia, and electrocardiogram repolarization changes.

Increasing concerns have been raised regarding the risks of hyperglycemia and diabetes mellitus with clozapine and newer antipsychotics. Indeed, the FDA has stipulated changes in the prescribing information for not only clozapine, but also for olanzapine, risperidone, quetiapine, ziprasidone, and aripiprazole, to include a warning of these risks, suggesting a class effect for such problems. Clozapine, olanzapine, risperidone, and quetiapine can also cause weight gain and cholesterol and triglyceride elevations. The report of a recent consensus development conference on antipsychotics and obesity, diabetes, and hyperlipidemia emphasized differences between atypical antipsychotics, with clozapine and olanzapine being the most, risperidone and quetiapine being less, and ziprasidone and aripiprazole being the least implicated (American Diabetes Association, 2004). Thus, clinical and (as indicated) laboratory monitoring for obesity, diabetes, and hyperlipidemia appears prudent for patients receiving clozapine. Clozapine-related weight gain can be approached in a fashion similar to that described above for lithium. Although in some instances clozapine-related weight gain and metabolic problems may be addressed by cautiously attempting to switch to another agent with fewer such adverse effects, this approach entails risk, as other agents may not be as effective or well tolerated as clozapine. In some instances, the efficacy/tolerability gap compared to other agents may be so great that, clinicians and patients with appropriate medical consultation, may decide to continue clozapine and treat the weight gain and metabolic disturbance symptomatically. Other warnings in the prescribing information include the risks of eosinophilia, neuroleptic malignant syndrome, and tardive dyskinesia.

Other clozapine adverse effects include cardiomyopathy (8.9 per 100,000 patient-years), fever, pulmonary embolism (fatal in 1 per 3450 patient-years), increased transaminases, hepatitis, anticholinergic symptoms (constipation, urinary retention), hypersalivation, and headache. To date, risperidone has not been associated with congenital malformations in humans (FDA Pregnancy Category B).

Dosing strategies Clozapine is commonly initiated at 25 mg/day and increased by 25–50 mg/day every 3–7 days, with 900 mg/day the maximum final dose in schizophrenia. In bipolar disorder patients, final doses of clozapine often range between 50 and 250 mg/day, given all or mostly at bedtime, and commonly in combination with other medications. Thus, in a controlled trial, mean doses of adjunctive clozapine in bipolar disorder and schizoaffective disorder patients were 234 and 623 mg/day, respectively (Suppes et al., 1999). In bipolar disorder patients, clozapine is often administered all or mostly at bedtime, and commonly in combination with other medications. Some data suggest that serum clozapine concentrations exceeding approximately 1.2 mM (400 ng/mL) are associated with better therapeutic effects in patients with treatment-resistant schizophrenia (Hasegawa et al., 1993; Kronig et al., 1995; Miller et al., 1994; Perry et al., 1991; Piscitelli et al., 1994; Potkin et al., 1994), while other data suggest that higher mean doses (mean 444 mg/day) used in the United States and lower mean doses (mean 284 mg/day) used in Europe yielded similar therapeutic effects (Fleischhacker et al., 1994). Serum clozapine concentrations exceeding 3.0 mM (1000 ng/mL) are associated with increased adverse effects (Freeman & Oyewumi, 1997).

Risperidone

Risperidone (RSP) is a benzisoxazole derivative that blocks serotonin 5HT2A and 5HT1A, dopamine D_1 and D_2, adrenergic alpha$_1$ and alpha$_2$, and histamine H_1 receptors (Bymaster et al., 1996). Risperidone is approved by the FDA for the treatment of acute mania as monotherapy (Hirschfeld et al., 2004; Khanna et al., 2003) and in combination with lithium or valproate (Sachs et al., 2002; Yatham et al., 2003). Risperidone is also available in a long-acting injectible formulation that is approved for the treatment of schizophrenia (Kane et al., 2003).

Risperidone is well absorbed, with 70% bioavailability, 90% protein binding, a moderate volume of distribution of 1 L/kg, a linear dose to serum concentration relationship, a clearance of 400 mL/min, and a half-life of 6 hours in extensive CYP2D6 metabolizers, and 24 hours in poor CYP2D6 metabolizers (He & Richardson, 1995; Mannens et al., 1993). Risperidone is substantially metabolized, with less than 30% excreted unchanged in the urine, whereas its main active 9-hydroxyrisperidone (paliperidone) metabolite is removed primarily by renal excretion. Risperidone is metabolized by CYP2D6 to (+)-9-hyrdroxyrisperidone, and to a lesser extent by CYP3A4 to (−)-9-hyrdroxyrisperidone. The 9-hydroxyrisperidone metabolite has activity similar to risperidone, and risperidone plus 9-hydroxyrisperidone are referred to collectively as the active moiety, which has a half-life of 20 hours, and protein binding of 90% for risperidone and 70% for 9-hydroxyrisperidone. Based upon pharmacokinetics related to the prominent renal excretion of the active moiety, risperidone dosage reduction and cautious dose titration may be necessary in the elderly and in patients with renal disease. Risperidone does not appear to induce or inhibit most CYP450 isozymes, and thus is more of a target of than an instigator of drug interactions.

Risperidone does not appear to generally yield clinically significant alterations in lithium pharmacokinetics, and one study found that changing patients from conventional antipsychotics plus lithium to risperidone plus lithium did not yield clinically significant alterations in lithium pharmacokinetics. Although lithium is not expected to influence the pharmacokinetics of risperidone, the absence of such an interaction remains to be confirmed. Case reports suggest that sporadic individuals could develop serious adverse effects such as neuroleptic malignant syndrome when lithium is combined with risperidone. However, controlled clinical trials suggest that this combination does not generally yield more than merely additive adverse effects. Carbamazepine yields clinically significant induction of risperidone metabolism, while the effects of risperidone on carbamazepine pharmacokinetics remain to be established. Risperidone does not appear to have clinically significant pharmacokinetic interactions with valproate, or lamotrigine. However, a single case of increased risperidone with lamotrigine has been reported.

Risperidone does not generally alter serum quetiapine or clozapine concentrations, but case studies suggest some individuals may experience risperidone-related increases in serum clozapine concentrations, and a case of a neurotoxic syndrome, characterized as mild NMS, after clozapine was added to risperidone, as well as clozapine-related increases in serum risperidone concentrations have been reported. The CYP2D6 inhibitor thioridazine increases risperidone serum concentrations.

CYP2D6 inhibitors such as paroxetine may decrease risperidone metabolism. Fluoxetine can yield clinically significant increases in serum risperidone concentrations. Fluvoxamine can yield modest increases in serum risperidone concentrations, but whether or not such an interaction explains a case report of neurotoxicity with adding fluvoxamine to risperidone remains to be determined. Sertraline does not appear to generally yield clinically significant increases in serum risperidone concentrations, although occasional patients may experience substantive increases. Venlafaxine and mirtazapine do not appear to yield clinically significant increases in serum risperidone concentrations. Although nefazodone does not appear to yield clinically significant increases in serum risperidone concentrations in general, occasional patients may experience substantive increases. Amitriptyline does not appear to generally yield clinically significant increases in serum risperidone concentrations.

Risperidone is commonly administered along with benzodiazepines in patients with bipolar disorder, with merely additive central nervous system (e.g. sedation, ataxia) adverse effects. Indeed, contemporary controlled risperidone trials routinely permit some adjunctive benzodiazepine (e.g. lorazepam) administration.

Oxcarbazepine does not yield clinically significant alterations in serum risperidone concentrations. Topiramate does not yield clinically significant alterations in serum risperidone or 9-hydroxyrisperidone concentrations.

Rifampin induces, while thioridazine and ketoconazole inhibit risperidone metabolism.

The most common adverse events associated with risperidone discontinuation in acute mania trails were somnolence, dizziness, and extrapyramidal disorders. Dose-related extrapyramidal symptoms are particularly evident above 6 mg/day.

The United States risperidone prescribing information includes a boxed warning regarding the increased risk of death (primarily cardiovascular or infectious) in elderly patients with dementia-related psychosis (an atypical antipsychotic class warning). The FDA has stipulated changes in the risperidone prescribing information to include a warning of the risks of hyperglycemia and diabetes mellitus. Risperidone can also yield weight gain and cholesterol and triglyceride elevations. The report of a recent consensus development conference suggests the risks of obesity, diabetes, and hyperlipidemia with this agent are intermediate, being less than with clozapine and olanzapine, but more than with ziprasidone and aripiprazole (2004). Thus, clinical and (as indicated) laboratory monitoring for obesity, diabetes, and hyperlipidemia appears prudent for patients receiving risperidone. Risperidone-related weight gain can be approached in a fashion similar to that described above for lithium. Although in some instances risperidone-related weight gain and metabolic problems may be addressed by cautiously attempting to switch to another agent with fewer such adverse effects, this approach entails risk, as other agents may not be as effective or well tolerated as risperidone. In some instances, the efficacy/tolerability gap compared to other agents may be so great that, clinicians and patients with appropriate medical consultation, may decide to continue risperidone and treat the weight gain and metabolic disturbance symptomatically.

Other warnings in the prescribing information include the risks of cerebrovascular adverse events, including stroke in elderly patients with dementia-related psychosis (a warning shared with olanzapine and aripiprazole), neuroleptic malignant syndrome, and tardive dyskinesia.

Other adverse effects include orthostatic hypotension, tachycardia, QT prolongation, seizures (in 0.3% of patients), hyperprolactinemia, amenorrhea, galactorrhea, decreased libido and sexual function, rhinitis, constipation, and dysphagia. There are case reports of mania induction or exacerbation in occasional patient with risperidone, but this phenomenon occurred no more often than with placebo in controlled adjunctive trials in acute mania. To date, risperidone has not been associated with congenital malformations in humans (FDA Pregnancy Category C).

Dosing strategies   Risperidone in acute mania is commonly initiated at 2–3 mg/day and increased by 1 mg/day on a daily basis as necessary and tolerated, with final doses ranging between 1 and 6 mg/day, and averaging approximately 4–6 mg/day in controlled trials (Hirschfeld et al., 2004; Khanna et al., 2003; Sachs et al., 2002; Yatham et al., 2003). In bipolar disorder patients, risperidone is often administered all or mostly at bedtime, and commonly in combination with other medications. Long-acting injectible risperidone in schizophrenia patients is initiated at 25 mg i.m. every 2 weeks, overlapping with oral risperidone or other oral antipsychotic, and increased monthly as necessary and tolerated to as high as 50 mg i.m. every 2 weeks.

Olanzapine

Olanzapine (OLZ) is a thienobenzodiazepine derivative that blocks serotonin $5HT_{2A}$, $5HT_{2C}$, $5HT_3$, and $5HT_6$, dopamine D_4, D_3, D_1, and D_2, muscarinic M_1-M_5, adrenergic alpha$_1$, and histamine H_1 receptors, and is a serotonin $5HT_{1A}$ agonist (Bymaster et al., 1996). Olanzapine is approved by the FDA for the treatment of acute mania as monotherapy (Tohen et al., 2000; Tohen et al., 1999) or added to lithium or valproate (Tohen et al., 2002), for acute bipolar I depression (combined with fluoxetine) (Tohen et al., 2003), and as monotherapy maintenance treatment for bipolar I disorder (Tohen et al., 2006). An intramuscular formulation is approved for the treatment of acute agitation in mania or schizophrenia (Meehan et al., 2001).

Olanzapine is well absorbed, with 80–100% bioavailability, 93% protein binding, a large volume of distribution of 15 L/kg, a half-life of 30 hours, linear pharmacokinetics at doses up to 20 mg, and clearance of 400 mL/min (Callaghan et al., 1999). Olanzapine is extensively (more than 80%) metabolized, primarily via glucuronidation by UGT1A4 to inactive 10-N-glucuronide olanzapine, as well as oxidation by CYP1A2 to inactive N-desmethyl olanzapine. Olanzapine does not induce or inhibit CYP450 isozymes, and is thus more a target of than an instigator of drug interactions.

Olanzapine does not generally have clinically significant pharmacokinetic interactions with lithium. Case reports suggest that sporadic individuals could develop serious adverse effects such as neuroleptic malignant syndrome when lithium is combined with olanzapine. However, controlled clinical data suggest that this combination does not generally yield more than merely additive adverse effects. In four patients, valproate appeared to lower serum olanzapine concentrations, but the clinical significance of this possible interaction remains to be established. Carbamazepine increases metabolism of olanzapine, presumably by induction of glucuronidation and possibly CYP1A2. The effects of olanzapine upon valproate and carbamazepine pharmacokinetics remain to be established. Olanzapine does not appear to have clinically significant pharmacokinetic interactions with lamotrigine.

The CYP1A2 inhibitor fluvoxamine yields clinically significant increases in serum olanzapine concentrations. Fluoxetine, sertraline, and mirtazapine do not yield clinically significant changes in serum olanzapine concentrations. Olanzapine lacks clinically significant pharmacokinetic interactions with imipramine.

Oxcarbazepine and topiramate do not generally yield clinically significant alterations in serum olanzapine concentrations.

Olanzapine is commonly administered along with benzodiazepines in patients with bipolar disorder, with merely additive central nervous system (e.g. sedation, ataxia) adverse effects. Indeed, contemporary controlled olanzapine trials routinely permit some adjunctive benzodiazepine (e.g. lorazepam) administration. Intramuscular lorazepam 1 hour after intramuscular aripiprazole did not yield clinically significant pharmacokinetic interactions, but was associated with additive sedation.

CYP1A2 inducers such as omeprazole might decrease serum olanzapine concentrations, but whether or not such putative interactions are clinically significant needs to be assessed. Ciprofloxacin may increase serum olanzapine concentrations. Tobacco smoking decreases serum olanzapine concentrations, presumably by induction of CYP1A2. Women compared to men may have slightly (approximately 25%) decreased olanzapine clearance, which in some individuals, especially if combined with other factors like tobacco smoking, could have clinical significance.

The most common adverse effects with oral olanzapine are somnolence, dry mouth, dizziness, asthenia, constipation, dyspepsia, increased appetite, and tremor. Olanzapine-related weight gain appears to be more of a problem than with lithium or valproate. Thus, in a 12-month maintenance trial, the incidence of weight gain was 30% with olanzapine and 10% with lithium (Tohen et al., 2005), and in a 47-week maintenance trial was 24% with olanzapine and 18% with valproate (Tohen et al., 2003). Olanzapine-related weight gain can be approached in a fashion similar to that described above for lithium. Somnolence is the most common adverse effect with intramuscular olanzapine. Maximal dosing of intramuscular olanzapine may yield substantial orthostatic hypotension, so that administration of additional doses to patients with clinically significant postural changes in systolic blood pressure is not recommended.

The United States olanzapine prescribing information includes a boxed warning regarding the increased risk of death (primarily cardiovascular or infectious) in elderly patients with dementia-related psychosis (an atypical antipsychotic class warning). The FDA has stipulated changes in the olanzapine prescribing information to include a warning of the risk of hyperglycemia and diabetes mellitus. Olanzapine can also yield weight gain and cholesterol and triglyceride elevations. The report of a recent consensus development conference suggested the risks of obesity, diabetes, and hyperlipidemia with this agent (and clozapine) are greater than with other newer antipsychotics (2004). Thus, clinical and (as indicated) laboratory monitoring for obesity, diabetes, and hyperlipidemia appears prudent for patients receiving olanzapine. Olanzapine-related weight gain can be approached in a fashion similar to that described above for lithium. Although in some instances olanzapinerelated weight gain and metabolic problems may be addressed by cautiously attempting to switch to another agent with fewer such adverse effects, this approach entails risk, as other agents may not be as effective or well tolerated as olanzapine. In some instances, the efficacy/tolerability gap compared to other agents may be so great that, clinicians and patients with appropriate medical consultation, may decide to continue olanzapine and treat the weight gain and metabolic disturbance symptomatically.

Other warnings in the prescribing information include the risks of cerebrovascular adverse events, including stroke, in elderly patients with dementia-related psychosis (a warning shared with risperidone and aripiprazole), neuroleptic malignant syndrome, and tardive dyskinesia.

Other adverse effects include orthostatic hypotension, syncope (in 0.6% of patients), seizures (in 0.9% of patients), hyperprolactinemia, and benign transaminase elevations (in 0.2% of patients) (Conley & Meltzer, 2000). Mania induction or exacerbation has been occasionally reported with olanzapine, but occurred no more often than with placebo in controlled trials. To date, olanzapine has not been associated with congenital malformations in humans (FDA Pregnancy Category C).

Dosing strategies   In acute mania monotherapy, olanzapine is commonly initiated at 10 mg/day and increased by 5 mg daily as necessary and tolerated, with final doses ranging between 5 and 20 mg/day, and averaging 15–16 mg/day in controlled trials (Tohen et al., 2000, 1999). In acute mania adjunctive therapy, olanzapine is commonly initiated at 10–15 mg/day and increased by 5 mg daily as necessary and tolerated, with final doses ranging between 5 and 20 mg/day, and averaging 10.4 mg/day in a controlled trial (Tohen et al., 2002). In acute agitation, intramuscular olanzapine is started with 10 mg i.m., with repeat doses of 10 mg i.m. as necessary and tolerated after 2 hours and 6 hours, with a maximum dose of 30 mg in a 24-hour period. Lower doses are recommended in elderly (5 mg i.m. once) or debilitated (2.5 mg i.m. once) patients. In acute bipolar I depression, olanzapine was dosed more conservatively, with a mean final dose of 7.4 mg/day (combined with a mean final dose of fluoxetine 39.3 mg/day) (Tohen et al., 2003). In monotherapy maintenance treatment for bipolar I disorder, the mean final olanzapine dose was 12.5 mg/day (Tohen et al., 2006). In bipolar disorder patients, olanzapine is often administered all or mostly at bedtime, and commonly in combination with other medications. Mean steady state serum olanzapine concentrations at endpoint in a 6-week schizophrenia trial at 5 and 15 mg/day were 10 ug/L and 31 ug/L, respectively, and were not related to clinical responses (Callaghan et al., 1999).

Quetiapine

Quetiapine (QTP) is a dibenzothiazepine derivative that blocks dopamine D_1 and D_2, serotonin $5HT_{2A}$ and $5HT_{1A}$, muscarinic M_1, adrenergic alpha$_1$ and alpha$_2$, histamine H_1, and sigma receptors (Bymaster et al., 1996). Quetiapine immediate release formulation and quetiapine extended release formulation (quetiapine XR) are approved by the FDA for the treatment of acute mania as monotherapy (Bowden et al., 2005; McIntyre et al., 2005; Yatham et al., 2004) or added to lithium or valproate (Sachs et al., 2004), and as monotherapy for acute bipolar I or II depression (Calabrese et al., 2005; Thase et al., 2006). In 2008, adjunctive (added to lithium or valproate) quetiapine and quetiapine XR were approved for maintenance treatment in bipolar disorder.

Quetiapine is well absorbed and 100% bioavailable, with 83% protein binding, a large volume of distribution of 10 L/kg, linear pharmacokinetics at doses between 200 and 750 mg/day, clearance of 1600 mL/min, and a short half-life of six hours (DeVane & Nemeroff, 2001). Quetiapine is extensively metabolized, primarily by CYP3A4 to inactive quetiapine sulfoxide (Hasselstrom & Linnet, 2006), with less than 1% excreted unchanged in the urine (DeVane & Nemeroff, 2001). Quetiapine does not have clinically significant effects on CYP isozymes, and is thus a target of rather than an instigator of drug interactions.

Quetiapine does not generally have clinically significant pharmacokinetic interactions with lithium. Controlled clinical trials suggest that combining lithium with quetiapine does not generally yield more than merely additive adverse effects. Valproate may or may not yield clinically significant increases in quetiapine serum concentrations, and the clinical significance of this potential interaction remains to be established, while quetiapine does not appear to yield clinically significant changes valproate pharmacokinetics. Quetiapine metabolism is increased with carbamazepine, and in two patients, quetiapine appeared to increase carbamazepine-epoxide levels. The effect of quetiapine upon carbamazepine pharmacokinetics, and the presence or absence of pharmacokinetic drug interactions between quetiapine and lamotrigine remain to be assessed.

Thioridazine (but not haloperidol or risperidone) can yield clinically significant decreases in serum quetiapine concentrations. There is a case report of blood dyscrasia with quetiapine and ziprasidone. Fluoxetine and imipramine do not appear to have clinically significant effects on quetiapine pharmacokinetics.

Quetiapine is commonly administered along with benzodiazepines in patients with bipolar disorder, with merely additive central nervous system (e.g. sedation, ataxia) adverse effects. Indeed, contemporary controlled quetiapine trials routinely permit some adjunctive benzodiazepine (e.g. lorazepam) administration. Quetiapine and lorazepam do not appear to have clinically significant pharmacokinetic interactions.

Quetiapine metabolism is increased with phenytoin. Topiramate does not generally yield clinically significant alterations in serum quetiapine concentrations. The CYP3A4 inhibitors ketoconazole and erythromycin yield clinically significant increases in serum quetiapine concentrations. In contrast to clozapine and olanzapine, tobacco smoking does not yield clinically significant decreases in serum quetiapine concentrations.

The most common adverse events with quetiapine are somnolence, dizziness (postural hypotension), dry mouth, constipation, increased serum glutamate pyruvate transaminase (SGPT), weight gain, and dyspepsia (Adler et al., 2007).

The United States quetiapine prescribing information includes boxed warnings regarding the increased risks of: (1) death (primarily cardiovascular or infectious) in elderly patients with dementia-related psychosis (an atypical antipsychotic class warning); and (2) suicidal thinking and behavior in children and adolescents (based on an antidepressant class warning). The FDA has stipulated changes in the quetiapine prescribing information to include a warning of the risks of hyperglycemia and diabetes mellitus. Quetiapine can also yield weight gain and cholesterol and triglyceride elevations. The report of a recent consensus development conference suggests the risks of obesity, diabetes, and hyperlipidemia with this agent are intermediate, being less than with clozapine and olanzapine, but more than with ziprasidone and aripiprazole (American Diabetes Association, American Psychiatric Association, American Association of Clinical Endocrinologists, & Obesity, 2004). Thus, clinical and (as indicated) laboratory monitoring for obesity, diabetes, and hyperlipidemia appears prudent for patients receiving quetiapine. Quetiapine-related weight gain can be approached in a fashion similar to that described above for lithium. Although in some instances quetiapine-related weight gain and metabolic problems may be addressed by cautiously attempting to switch to another agent with fewer such adverse effects, this approach entails risk, as other agents may not be as effective or well tolerated as quetiapine. In some instances, the efficacy/tolerability gap compared to other agents may be so great that, clinicians and patients with appropriate medical consultation, may decide to continue quetiapine and treat the weight gain and metabolic disturbance symptomatically.

Other warnings in the quetiapine prescribing information include the risks of neuroleptic malignant syndrome and tardive dyskinesia.

Other risks include syncope (in 1% of patients), seizures (in 0.5% of patients), hypothyroidism, and benign transaminse elevations (in 6% of patients). Concern regarding the development of cataracts in dogs has led to a recommendation of ophthalmologic examinations, but the risk in humans appears to be low (Nasrallah et al., 1999). To date, quetiapine has not been associated with congenital malformations in humans (FDA Pregnancy Category C).

Dosing strategies In acute mania, quetiapine immediate release formulation is commonly initiated at 100 mg/day in two divided doses, and increased daily by 100 mg as necessary and tolerated, with final doses ranging between 400 and 800 mg/day, and averaging approximately 500–600 mg/day in responders in controlled trials (Bowden et al., 2005; McIntyre et al., 2005; Sachs et al., 2004; Yatham et al., 2004). In acute mania, quetiapine extended release formulation (quetiapine XR) is started at 300 mg at bedtime, increased the next day to 600 mg at bedtime, and thereafter dosed between 400 mg and 800 mg at bedtime. In acute bipolar I or II depression, quetiapine and quetiapine XR are commonly initiated at 50 mg/day at bedtime, and increased by daily by 100 mg as necessary and tolerated, with final doses ranging between 300 and 600 mg/day in controlled trials (Calabrese et al., 2005; Thase et al., 2006). Mean steady state 12-hour trough serum quetiapine concentrations at 150 and 750 mg/day were 29 ug/L and 164 ug/L, respectively, and were not related to therapeutic effects in a 3-week trial in schizophrenia patients (DeVane & Nemeroff, 2001). The United States prescribing information for the longer-term adjunctive use of quetiapine and quetiapine XR notes that doses of 400 to 800 mg/day in divided doses were used in the registration studies, and that generally, in the maintenance phase, patients continued on the same dose on which they were stabilized in the stabilization phase. However, the information also states that patients should be treated with the lowest dose needed to maintain remission. The information does not provide recommendations for initiating quetiapine in euthymic patients. Given the risk of adverse effects, it is prudent to start quetiapine in euthymic patients in a gradual fashion similar to initiation in depressed patients, rather than the rapid initiation used in manic patients.

Ziprasidone

Ziprasidone (ZIP) is a benzisothiazole derivative that blocks serotonin $5-HT_{2A}$, $5-HT_{2C}$, and $5-HT_{1D}$, dopamine D_2 and D_3, adrenergic $alpha_1$, and histamine H_1 receptors (Stahl & Shayegan, 2003). It has a high ratio of $5HT2_A$ to D_2 receptor blockade, is an agonist at $5-HT_{1A}$ receptors, and is a serotonin and norepinephrine reuptake inhibitor. Ziprasidone is approved by the FDA for the treatment of acute mania as monotherapy (Keck et al., 2003b; Potkin et al., 2005). Intramuscular ziprasidone is approved for the treatment of acute agitation in schizophrenia patients (Brook, Lucey, & Gunn, 2000; Daniel et al., 2001; Lesem et al., 2001).

Concurrent ingestion of food doubles ziprasidone absorption (Hamelin et al., 1998), so that ziprasidone is 60% absorbed with food, and 30% unfed. Ziprasidone is 99% bound to plasma proteins, with a volume of distribution of 1.5 L/kg, a half-life of 6.6 hours, and clearance of 525 mL/min (Wilner et al., 2000). Ziprasidone is extensively metabolized, with less than 5% excreted unchanged in the urine (Prakash et al., 2000). Ziprasidone is metabolized 2/3 by aldehyde oxidase reduction to inactive S-methyldihydro ziprasidone, and 1/3 by CYP3A4 oxidation to inactive ziprasidone sulphoxide and other inactive metabolites. Ziprasidone does not have clinically significant effects on CYP isozymes, and is thus a target of rather than an instigator of drug interactions.

Ziprasidone does not generally affect serum concentrations of lithium. Although an interaction is not expected, the effect of lithium upon ziprasidone pharmacokinetics remains to be assessed. Case reports suggest that sporadic individuals could develop serious adverse effects such as neuroleptic malignant syndrome when lithium is combined with ziprasidone. However, clinical data suggest that this combination does not generally yield more than merely additive adverse effects. Carbamazepine decreases serum ziprasidone concentrations, but the clinical significance of this interaction remains to be determined. The effect of ziprasidone upon carbamazepine pharmacokinetics, and whether or not ziprasidone has pharmacokinetic interactions with valproate and lamotrigine remain to be assessed.

There are limited data regarding interactions between ziprasidone and other antipsychotics. Case reports describe blood dyscrasia with ziprasidone and quetiapine, and a possible serotonin syndrome with citalopram following cross-titration of clozapine to ziprasidone. Concerns have been raised regarding the ability of ziprasidone to yield QTc prolongation, and the possibility of exaggeration of this problem if combined with other agents such as chlorpromazine, thioridazine, pimozide, paliperidone, and quetiapine with this adverse effect. Systematic studies are lacking to assess the clinical significance of such putative pharmacodynamic interactions.

Ziprasidone is commonly administered along with benzodiazepines in patients with bipolar disorder, with merely additive central nervous system (e.g. sedation, ataxia) adverse effects. Indeed, contemporary controlled ziprasidone trials routinely permit some adjunctive benzodiazepine (e.g. lorazepam) administration.

Ketoconazole increases serum ziprasidone concentrations, but the clinical significance of this interaction remains to be determined. Ziprasidone does not effect serum concentrations of hormonal contraceptives.

The most common adverse events associated with discontinuation with ziprasidone in acute mania were akathisia, anxiety, depression, dizziness, dystonia, rash and vomiting (Goodnick, 2001). The most common adverse events with intramuscular ziprasidone for agitation in schizophrenia patients were headache, nausea, and somnolence.

Ziprasidone and aripiprazole, compared to risperidone, olanzapine and quetiapine, yield less sedation but more akathisia. In patients with acute mania, akathisia is commonly accompanied by and at times difficult to distinguish from agitation and anxiety. These overlapping symptoms may attenuate with adjunctive benzodiazepine therapy. Indeed, meta-analysis suggests that benzodiazepines (e.g. clonazepam 0.5–2.5 mg/day in two randomized, controlled, 1–2-week trials, with a total of 27 patients) can reduce symptoms of akathisia short term (Lima et al., 2002). There are more limited data regarding the utility of other agents for antipsychotic-related akathisia. Meta-analyses suggested that there is insufficient data to recommend beta-blockers (Lima et al., 2004), and that there is no reliable evidence to support or refute the utility of anticholinergics (Lima et al., 2004). In other controlled studies, mirtazapine 15 mg/day and propranolol 80 mg/day were superior to placebo in a 90-patient, 1-week trial (Poyurovsky et al., 2006), vitamin B_6 1200 mg/day tended to be superior to placebo in a 20 patient, 5-day trial (Lerner et al., 2004), and the 5-HT$_2$ antagonist mianserin 15 mg/day was superior to placebo in a 30-patient, 5-day trial (Poyurovsky et al., 1999).

The United States ziprasidone prescribing information includes a boxed warning regarding the increased risk of death (primarily cardiovascular or infectious) in elderly patients with dementia-related psychosis (an atypical antipsychotic class warning). The FDA has stipulated that the ziprasidone prescribing information include a warning of the risks of hyperglycemia and diabetes mellitus, but the report of a recent consensus development conference suggests the risks of obesity, diabetes, and hyperlipidemia with this agent are similar to those with aripiprazole, and are less than with other newer antipsychotics (American Diabetes Association, American Psychiatric Association, American Association of Clinical Endocrinologists, & Obesity, 2004). Nevertheless, clinical and (as indicated) laboratory monitoring for obesity, diabetes, and hyperlipidemia may be prudent for patients receiving ziprasidone. Although in some instances weight gain and metabolic problems associated with other agents may be addressed by cautiously attempting to switch to ziprasidone, this approach entails risk, as ziprasidone may not be as effective or well tolerated as the original agent.

Other warnings in the prescribing information include the risks of neuroleptic malignant syndrome, tardive dyskinesia, and QTc prolongation and risk of sudden death. Although premarketing studies suggested that ziprasidone yielded cardiac conduction delays, postmarketing experience to date has failed to indicate clinically significant problems with cardiac conduction (Daniel, 2003; Harvey & Bowie, 2005).

Other adverse effects include benign rash (in 5% of patients), orthostatic hypotension, syncope (in 0.6% of patients), and seizures (in 0.4% of patients). To date, ziprasidone has not been associated with congenital malformations in humans (FDA Pregnancy Category C).

Dosing strategies   In acute mania, ziprasidone is commonly initiated at 80 mg/day administered with food in two divided doses, and increased as necessary and tolerated on day 2 to 120–160 mg/day administered with food in two divided doses, with final doses ranging between 80 and 160 mg/day, and averaging approximately 125–130 mg/day in controlled trials (Keck et al., 2003b; Potkin et al., 2005). Intramuscular ziprasidone is administered as 10 mg i.m., repeating 10 mg i.m. as often as every 2 hours as necessary and tolerated with a maximum of 40 mg/day for 3 days.

Aripiprazole

Aripiprazole (ARI) is a quinolinone derivative that is a partial agonist at dopamine D_2 and serotonin 5-HT_{1A} receptors, and an antagonist at serotonin 5-HT_{2A} receptors (Lawler et al., 1999; Swainston, Harrison & Perry, 2004). As a D_2 partial agonist, aripiprazole may "stabilize" dopaminergic neurotransmission—decreasing dopamine neurotransmission in high dopamine states such as mania, and increasing dopamine neurotransmission in low dopamine states such as bipolar depression. Aripiprazole is approved by the FDA for the treatment of adults and adolescents with acute mania as monotherapy (Keck et al., 2003a; Sachs et al., 2006), as adjunctive (added to lithium or valproate) therapy (Vieta et al., 2008), and for monotherapy maintenance treatment for bipolar I disorder (Keck et al., 2006). Intramuscular aripiprazole is approved for the treatment of acute agitation associated with mania or schizophrenia (Andrezina et al., 2006; Tran-Johnson et al., 2007; Zimbroff et al., 2007).

Aripiprazole has a bioavailability of 87%, a volume of distribution of 4.9 L/kg, is 99% bound to plasma proteins, and has a long 72 hour half-life (Mallikaarjun, Salazar, & Bramer, 2004). Aripiprazole is metabolized to an active dehyro-aripiprazole metabolite that has a half-life of 94 hours. Aripiprazole is extensively metabolized, primarily oxidation by CYP2D6 and CYP3A4, with less than 1% excreted unchanged in the urine (Swainston, Harrison & Perry, 2004). Aripiprazole does not have clinically significant effects on CYP isozymes, and is thus a target of rather than an instigator of drug interactions. Although concerns have been raised regarding the possibility of inhibitors of CYP2D6 and CYP3A4 and inducers of CYP3A4 affecting aripiprazole pharmacokinetics, systematic data regarding such putative interactions are limited.

Lithium does not generally affect serum aripiprazole concentrations. Although an interaction is not expected, the effect of aripiprazole upon lithium pharmacokinetics remains to be assessed. Case reports suggest that sporadic individuals could develop serious adverse effects such as neuroleptic malignant syndrome when lithium is combined with aripiprazole. However, clinical data suggest that this combination does not generally yield more than merely additive adverse effects. Valproate does not generally affect serum aripiprazole concentrations, while the effect of aripiprazole upon valproate pharmacokinetics remains to be determined. Carbamazepine induces aripiprazole metabolism, while the effect of aripiprazole upon carbamazepine pharmacokinetics remains to be determined. Whether or not aripiprazole has pharmacokinetic interactions with lamotrigine remains to be assessed.

There are few data regarding interactions between aripiprazole and other antipsychotics. A case of a schizophrenia patient who experienced exacerbation of psychosis plus normalization of serum prolactin concentration when aripiprazole was added to haloperidol suggested a pharmacodynamic interaction wherein aripiprazole displaced haloperidol from dopamine D_2 receptors.

Case reports of problems with aripiprazole combined with antidepressants include a possible neuroleptic malignant syndrome with the aripiprazole plus fluoxetine combination, and urinary obstruction with the aripiprazole plus citalopram combination.

Aripiprazole is commonly administered along with benzodiazepines in patients with bipolar disorder, with merely additive central nervous system (e.g. sedation, ataxia) adverse effects. Indeed, contemporary controlled aripiprazole trials routinely permit some adjunctive benzodiazepine (e.g. lorazepam) administration. In healthy volunteers, intramuscular aripiprazole and intramuscular lorazepam did not have clinically significant pharmacokinetic interactions, but yielded additive sedation and orthostatic hypotension.

Quinidine and ketoconazole appear to increase serum aripiprazole concentrations. In contrast to clozapine and olanzapine, tobacco smoking does not yield clinically significant decreases in serum aripiprazole concentrations.

The most common adverse events with oral aripiprazole in acute mania trails were central nervous system (headache, agitation/anxiety/akathisia, insomnia, somnolence), and gastrointestinal (nausea, dyspepsia, vomiting, constipation) (Keck et al., 2003a; Marder et al., 2003; Sachs et al., 2006; Vieta et al., 2005). The most common adverse events with intramuscular aripiprazole in an acute agitation in mania trail were central nervous system (headache, dizziness, insomnia, somnolence), and gastrointestinal (nausea, vomiting) problems. Aripiprazole-related akathisia may respond to benzodiazepines, as described for ziprasidone. Decreasing dose may attenuate akathisia with aripiprazole, unlike with ziprasidone.

Gastrointestinal adverse effects such as nausea, dyspepsia, constipation, vomiting, and diarrhea, may be related to dopamine partial agonist effects and tend to diminish with ongoing exposure. Although in view of its long half-life, aripiprazole can be dosed once daily, during the first few days of treatment, the lower maximum concentrations associated with divided doses may offer enhanced tolerability. Thus, tolerability may be enhanced in patients with gastrointestinal or other adverse effects if aripiprazole is initiated at 15 mg per day (or lower if necessary) for a few days before increasing the dosage.

The United States aripiprazole prescribing information includes a boxed warning regarding the increased risk of death (primarily cardiovascular or infectious) in elderly patients with dementia-related psychosis (an atypical antipsychotic class warning). The FDA has stipulated that the aripiprazole prescribing information include a warning of the risks of hyperglycemia and diabetes mellitus. Although weight gain can occur with aripiprazole, this issue as well as metabolic disruption is generally less of a problem than with olanzapine (McQuade et al., 2004). Indeed, the report of a recent consensus development conference suggests the risks of obesity, diabetes, and hyperlipidemia with this agent are similar to those with ziprasidone, and less than with other newer antipsychotics (American Diabetes Association, American Psychiatric Association, American Association of Clinical Endocrinologists, & Obesity, 2004). Nevertheless, clinical and (as indicated) laboratory monitoring for obesity, diabetes, and hyperlipidemia may be prudent for patients receiving aripiprazole. Although in some instances weight gain and metabolic problems associated with other agents may be addressed by cautiously attempting to switch to aripiprazole, this approach entails risk, as aripiprazole may not be as effective or well tolerated as the original agent.

Other warnings in the prescribing information include the risks of cerebrovascular adverse events, including stroke, in elderly patients with dementia-related psychosis (a warning shared with risperidone and olanzapine), neuroleptic malignant syndrome and tardive dyskinesia.

Other adverse effects include orthostatic hypotension, syncope (in 0.5% of patients), seizures (in 0.1% of patients), and dysphagia. To date, aripiprazole has not been associated with congenital malformations in humans (FDA Pregnancy Category C).

Dosing strategies In acute manic and mixed episodes as monotherapy or as adjunctive (added to lithium or divalproex) treatment, oral aripiprazole is recommended in the United States prescribing information to be initiated in adults at 15 mg once per day, which is the recommended dose, and to be initiated in children and adolescents at 2 mg once per day, and titrated to the 10 mg/day recommended dose. The maximum dose is 30 mg/day for both adult and peditric patients with acute manic or mixed episodes. In early acute mania trials oral aripiprazole was initiated at 30 mg/day in a single daily dose, and decreased if necessary to 15 mg/day, with final doses ranging between 15 and 30 mg/day, and averaging approximately 28 mg/day in controlled trials (Keck et al., 2003a; Sachs et al., 2006; Vieta et al., 2005) and approximately 15% of patients had aripiprazole dosage decreased from 30 to 15 mg/day due to tolerability problems. Intramuscular aripiprazole is administered as 9.75 mg i.m. (or 5.25 mg i.m. if clinically indicated), repeating 9.75 mg i.m. as often as every 2 hours as necessary and tolerated, with a maximum of 30 mg/day. In monotherapy maintenance treatment for bipolar I disorder, the mean final aripiprazole dose was 24.3 mg/day (Keck et al., 2006). In two negative acute bipolar I nonpsychotic depression studies, aripiprazole monotherapy was initiated at 10 mg/day and flexibly dosed within a range of 5–30 mg/day, with a pooled mean dose of 16.5 mg/day (Thase et al., 2008). Citing high discontinuation rates, the authors speculated that this dosing may have been too aggressive for acute bipolar depression. Indeed, in adjunctive (added to antidepressants) treatment of unipolar major depressive disorder, oral aripiprazole is recommended in the United States prescribing information to be initiated in adults at 2–5 mg once per day, and titrated to a recommended dose of 5–10 mg/day (Berman et al., 2007; Marcus et al., 2008). It may be that the latter more conservative dosing would be better tolerated in depressed or euthymic bipolar disorder patients.

Adjunctive antidepressants

The mood stabilizers lithium, valproate and carbamazepine appear to offer more robust antimanic than antidepressant effects, and adjunctive antidepressant therapy is commonly used in treating bipolar disorder patients (Sharma et al., 1997). However there are limited systematic data to support the practice, and there is controversy regarding efficacy, with some evidence suggesting benefit (Gijsman et al., 2004; Tohen et al., 2003), and other data suggesting lack of benefit (Nemeroff et al., 2001; Sachs et al., 2007). Adjunctive antidepressants need to be administered with care, and in many cases for relatively brief periods, as these agents can induce mania, hypomania, mixed states, and cycle acceleration (Altshuler et al.,

1995). The United States FDA has stipulated that the prescribing information for antidepressants include a boxed warning regarding the risk of increased suicidal ideation and behavior in children and adolescents with antidepressants (4%) compared to placebo (2%) (Licinio & Wong, 2005), as well as warnings of similar problems in adults (Lenzer, 2005), and the need to screen depressed patients for bipolar disorder (Hirschfeld et al., 2000). However, in at least some (perhaps 15%) bipolar disorder patients, antidepressants combined with mood stabilizers or atypical antipsychotics administered longer-term may yield benefits (Altshuler et al., 2003). To date, the only antidepressant with FDA approval for bipolar depression is fluoxetine in combination with olanzapine (Tohen et al., 2003).

Selective serotonin reuptake inhibitors

Selective serotonin reuptake inhibitors (SSRIs) act primarily by blockade of synaptic serotonin uptake, but have a variety of secondary effects that confer these agents with some variability in therapeutic and adverse effects (Blier, de Montigny, & Chaput, 1990). These drugs have displaced tricyclic antidepressants as first line therapies for unipolar depression due to their superior adverse effect profiles, safety in overdose, and in some instances, broader range of therapeutic effects. SSRIs are commonly added to antimanic agents in the treatment of bipolar depression, although this has only been systematically studied to a limited extent (Cohn et al., 1989; Nemeroff et al., 2001; Post et al., 2006; Sachs et al., 2007; Simpson & DePaulo, 1991; Tohen et al., 2003; Vieta et al., 2002).

SSRIs are generally well absorbed with variable (fluvoxamine 53% to citalopram 80%) bioavailability, high (fluvoxamine 80% to sertraline 98%) protein binding, and variable volumes of distribution (citalopram 12 to fluoxetine up to 45 L/kg), half-lives (fluvoxamine 16 hours to fluoxetine 4 days), metabolite half-lives (norfluoxetine up to 7 days), and clearances (fluoxetine 300 to fluvoxamine 1600 mL/min) (Baumann, 1992).

Manufacturers have emphasized pharmacokinetic and drug interaction differences among these agents (Baker et al., 1998). SSRIs are metabolized by varying CYP450 isoforms, including CYP2D6 (fluoxetine, paroxetine), and CYP3A3/4 (sertraline, citalopram); and they can inhibit CYP2D6 (fluoxetine, paroxetine, and to a lesser extent sertraline), CYP3A3/4 (fluoxetine, fluvoxamine), CYP2C19 (fluvoxamine), and CYP1A2 (fluvoxamine) and CYP2C9 (fluoxetine, fluvoxamine) (Baumann, 1992). Fluvoxamine inhibits CYP1A2 to a greater extent than CYP2D6 and CYP3A4 (Olesen & Linnet, 2000). SSRIs can thus be instigators as well as targets of CYP450-mediated drug interactions. The most prominent clinical concerns have been raised with agents that inhibit CYP2D6 and CYP3A3/4, thus increasing serum levels of substrates of these isoforms. Administration of monoamine oxidase inhibitors (MAOIs) and SSRIs within 2 weeks of one another (in the case of fluoxetine a 5 week wait before starting MAOIs) is avoided due to potentially fatal pharmacodynamic interactions, possibly related to induction of hyperserotonergic states. The sections on mood stabilizers and antipsychotics above describe interactions between these agents and SSRIs.

Decreased libido and sexual function are common with SSRIs (Masand & Gupta, 2002; Vanderkooy, Kennedy, & Bagby, 2002), and various strategies used in treating (unipolar) major depressive disorder patients with these problems may be attempted (Hirschfeld, 1999; Keltner, McAfee, & Taylor, 2002). Other adverse effects vary across individual agents. For example, patients treated chronically with some of these medications can experience sedation, gastrointestinal disturbance, or weight gain. SSRI calming effects may be welcome in anxious patients but oversedating in anergic patients. SSRI initiation and titration varies across agents, as do the maximum recommended doses (across all indications): fluoxetine (up to 80 mg/day), sertraline (up to 200 mg/day), paroxetine (up to 60 mg/day), controlled release paroxetine (up to 75 mg/day), fluvoxamine (up to 300 mg/day), citalopram (up to 60 mg/day), and escitalopram (up to 20 mg/day). Mania induction can occur with SSRIs, but may be less of an issue than with tricyclic antidepressants (Peet, 1994; Stoll et al., 1994) or the serotonin-norepinephrine reuptake inhibitor venlafaxine (Post et al., 2006; Vieta et al., 2002).

Serotonin-norepinephrine reuptake inhibitors

Serotonin-norepinephrine reuptake inhibitors (SNRIs) act primarily by dual blockade of synaptic serotonin and norepinephrine uptake (Horst & Preskorn, 1998; Kasamo, Blier, & De Montigny, 1996). In view of the serotonin uptake blockade, SNRI therapeutic (e.g. antidepressant, anxiolytic) and adverse (e.g. sexual dysfunction) effects overlap those of SSRIs. As with SSRIs, administration within 2 weeks of MAOIs should be avoided. The added norepinephrine uptake blockade may confer upon SNRIs additional therapeutic (e.g. analgesic) and adverse (e.g. hypertension, increased switching into mania) effects compared to SSRIs.

Venlafaxine is an SNRI that may be effective in bipolar depression (Amsterdam, 1998; Post et al., 2006; Vieta et al., 2002). Venlafaxine is only 27% protein bound, and has a volume of distribution of 8 L/kg, a half-life of 5 hours, and a clearance of 1400 mL/min (Taft et al., 1997). The extended release formulation is preferred in view of the brief half-life of immediate release venlafaxine which can result in withdrawal symptoms (Fava et al., 1997). Venlafaxine is metabolized by CYP2D6, and has minimal effects on CYP450 isoforms, decreasing the risk of drug interactions. Adverse effects include abnormal ejaculation, gastrointestinal complaints (nausea, dry mouth, and anorexia), central nervous system complaints (dizziness, somnolence, and abnormal dreams), and sweating. Venlafaxine is commonly started at 37.5–75 mg/day to avoid early nausea, and increased as necessary and tolerated every 4–7 days by 75 mg/day, with recommended final doses ranging between 375 mg/day for immediate-release and 225 mg/day for extended-release formulations, although clinicians occasionally utilize doses as high as 450 mg/day of either formulation. In the higher part of the dosage range, venlafaxine can increase blood pressure. Experience with this agent in bipolar depression suggests that mania induction can occur, perhaps at a rate higher than that seen with SSRIs (such as sertraline and paroxetine) and bupropion (Post et al., 2006; Vieta et al., 2002).

Duloxetine is a newer SNRI with antidepressant and analgesic effects. Duloxetine is 90% protein bound, and has a volume of distribution of 23 L/kg, and a half-life of 12 hours (Lantz et al., 2003). Duloxetine is metabolized by CYP1A2 and CYP2D6, and in view of the former, smoking may reduce and fluvoxamine may increase serum duloxetine concentrations. Duloxetine has minimal effects on CYP450 isoforms, decreasing the risk of hepatically mediated drug interactions. Adverse effects include sexual dysfunction, nausea, dry mouth, constipation, decreased appetite, fatigue, somnolence, and increased sweating. Duloxetine is commonly started at 30 mg/day to avoid early nausea, and increased as necessary and tolerated every 4–7 days by 30 mg/day, with final doses range between 60 mg/day for depression and 120 mg/day for diabetic neuropathy. In the higher part of the dosage range, duloxetine can increase blood pressure. As duloxetine is a newer drug, there are few data regarding the effects of this agent in patients with bipolar disorder. To date, there is insufficient data to assess the risk of mood elevation with duloxetine compared to other agents such as SSRIs.

Bupropion and atypical antidepressants

A variety of other antidepressants with diverse mechanisms of action have been introduced. In general, these agents have favorable adverse effect profiles compared to tricyclic antidepressants, and some do not cause the sexual difficulties encountered with SSRIs.

Bupropion has nonserotonergic, presumably dopaminergic/noradrenergic, mechanism(s) (Horst & Preskorn, 1998). Bupropion is well absorbed, 85% protein bound, and has a large volume of distribution of 20 L/kg, a half-life of 21 hours, and a clearance of 2300 mL/min (Goodnick, 1991). Immediate-release, sustained-release, and extended-release formulations are available. Bupropion is metabolized by CYP2B6, and can inhibit CYP2D6, suggesting potential drug interactions mediated by these isoforms. Carbamazepine (but not valproate) dramatically decreases bupropion and increases (active) metabolite levels. Administration of bupropion within 2 weeks of MAOIs should be avoided. Bupropion is generally well tolerated, lacks the sexual, weight gain, and sedation problems seen with at least some SSRIs, and has energizing effects that may be welcome in anergic patients, but overstimulating in anxious patients, and can cause seizures. Abdominal pain, agitation, anxiety, dizziness, dry mouth, insomnia, myalgia, nausea, palpitation, pharyngitis, sweating, tinnitus, and urinary frequency can also occur. The sustained-release and extended-release formulations of bupropion are preferred, as they lower peak serum levels, attenuating the risk of seizures. For example, sustained-release bupropion given in divided doses of up to 300 mg/day, decreases the risk of seizures to 0.1%. Adjunctive bupropion commonly used in treating bipolar depression (Post et al., 2006; Sachs et al., 1994, 2007), and has the advantage of helping with smoking cessation (Tonnesen et al., 2003). Bupropion appears less likely than tricyclic antidepressants (Sachs et al., 1994) and venlafaxine (Post et al., 2006) to cause switches into mania.

Trazodone blocks $5HT_1$, $5HT_2$, and $alpha_2$ receptors (Marek et al., 1992), and has more prominent sedative than antidepressant properties, and thus is commonly used as an adjunctive hypnotic agent in (unipolar) major depressive disorder and in bipolar disorder, despite concerns regarding the limited systematic data to support this practice (Mendelson, 2005). Trazodone is well absorbed, and has 80% bioavailability, 90% protein binding, a moderate volume of distribution of 1 L/kg, a half-life of 4 hours, and a clearance of 120–200 mL/min (Nilsen, Dale, & Husebo, 1993). Trazodone has relatively few metabolic drug-drug interactions. It is typically given in doses of 50–200 mg at bedtime, but some patients may tolerate doses as high as 600 mg/day. The main adverse effects are sedation, dizziness, and psychomotor impairment. Priapism can occur but is rare. Trazodone has been reported to induce mania, but limited experience precludes assessment of this risk relative to other agents. However, perhaps due to its rather modest antidepressant effects, the practice of low dose adjunctive trazodone does not appear clinically to yield much risk of inducing manic switches, but this issue has not been systematically explored.

Nefazodone blocks $5HT_1$, $5HT_2$, and $alpha_2$ receptors and serotonin uptake (Horst & Preskorn, 1998). It is well absorbed, but has only 20% bioavailability, and 99% protein binding, a low volume of distribution of 0.5 L/kg, a short half-life of three hours, and a clearance of 500–2000 mL/min (Greene & Barbhaiya, 1997). Nefazodone is a CYP3A3/4 substrate and inhibitor, and thus can increase serum levels of CYP3A3/4 substrates such as alprazolam, triazolam, and carbamazepine. Nefazodone may increase serum concentrations of clozapine, but the clinical significance of this interaction has been questioned.

Nefazodone labeling includes contraindications to combination with terfenadine, astemizole, cisapride, and pimozide out of concern that elevated levels of these CYP3A3/4 substrates will yield potentially fatal cardiac adverse events. It is recommended not to administer nefazodone within 2 weeks of MAOIs. Nefazodone is typically given in doses of 300–600 mg, with the bulk of the dose at bedtime. Nefazodone does not cause sexual problems, and initially its most prominent adverse effects were considered to be sedation, dry mouth, and gastrointestinal disturbance. However, serious hepatotoxicity has markedly decreased the utilization of this agent (Stewart, 2002). There are few data regarding nefazodone use in bipolar disorders. Mania induction has been reported with nefazodone, but limited experience precludes assessment of this risk relative to other agents.

Mirtazapine blocks $alpha_2$, $5HT_2$, $5HT_3$, and H_1 receptors (Gillman, 2006). It has only 50% bioavailability, and is 85% protein bound, with a volume of distribution of 4 L/kg, a half-life of 30 hours, and a clearance of 500 mL/min (Timmer, Sitsen, & Delbressine, 2000). Mirtazapine is a CYP2D6, more than CYP1A2 or CYP3A4, substrate and is not a clinically significant enzyme inhibitor. Carbamazepine induces the metabolism of mirtazapine, and tricyclic antidepressants and mirtazapine inhibit metabolism of one another, but lithium and mirtazapine do not alter the pharmacokinetics of one another. Administration within 2 weeks of MAOIs should be avoided. Adverse effects include sedation, dizziness, weight gain, cholesterol increases, agranulocytosis (in 0.1% of patients), and transaminase elevation above three times the upper limit of normal (in 2% of patients). There are few data regarding mirtazapine in bipolar disorders. Mania induction with mirtazapine has been reported, but limited experience precludes assessment of this risk relative to other agents.

Monoamine oxidase inhibitors

Monoamine oxidase inhibitors (MAOIs) block the metabolism of serotonin, norepinephrine, and dopamine (Goodman & Charney, 1985). Older agents such as phenelzine, tranylcypromine, and isocarboxazid inhibit both MAO-A and MAO-B irreversibly and are thus called irreversible MAOIs, while some newer agents such as moclobemide are reversible inhibitors of monoamine oxidase-A (RIMAs).

Irreversible MAOIs are potent antidepressants, effective in treating refractory depression and bipolar depression (Thase et al., 1992). They have brief half-lives that are not directly related to their clinical effects, presumably due to the irreversible nature of their MAO inhibition, which provides a MAO deficit until a sufficient amount of new enzyme is produced (in about 2 weeks) (Mallinger & Smith, 1991). Thus, foods and drugs incompatible with MAOIs must not be ingested within 2 weeks of discontinuing MAOIs. In addition, MAOIs should not be initiated within about five (parent or metabolite, which ever is greater) half-lives after discontinuing incompatible medications. For most drugs, this means waiting about 2 weeks. However, after discontinuing drugs with long half-lives, or metabolite half-lives, such as fluoxetine, up to 5 weeks should elapse prior to starting MAOIs. Irreversible MAOIs have complex and incompletely characterized metabolism, which has a "suicide" inhibition component, whereby they are inactivated by covalently bonding to monoamine oxidase. Older irreversible MAOIs have serious and potentially fatal interactions with a variety of high tyramine foods such as aged meats, cheese, Chianti wine, and fava beans (Gardner et al., 1996); and drugs such as SSRIs, clomipramine, venlafaxine, stimulants, decongestants, and opiates (Livingston & Livingston, 1996). They appear compatible with lithium, valproate, antipsychotics, trazodone, and anxiolytics. Although concerns have been raised around combining these agents with carbamazepine, limited evidence suggests this may be tolerated and confers benefit in some treatment-refractory bipolar disorder patients (Ketter et al., 1995). Irreversible MAOIs can cause sedation, sleep fragmentation, orthostasis, gastrointestinal disturbance, urinary retention, and decreased libido and sexual function (Blackwell, 1981; Pollack & Rosenbaum, 1987; Rabkin et al., 1984). Irreversible MAOIs, compared to tricyclic antidepressants, may be more effective in bipolar depression and less likely to trigger severe manic switches (Himmelhoch et al., 1991; Thase et al., 1992).

RIMAs, such as moclobemide, may have more modest antidepressant effects than reversible MAOIs, but may have utility in bipolar depression (Angst & Stabl, 1992; Silverstone, 2001). Moclobemide is a benzamide derivative, which inhibits MAO-A for about 24 hours (Cesura et al., 1992). It is well absorbed with 90% bioavailability, and has low 50% protein binding, a moderate volume of distribution of 1 L/kg, and a short half-life of 2 hours, which increases with escalating doses (Mayersohn & Guentert, 1995). Moclobemide is a CYP2C19 substrate and inhibits CYP1A2, CYP2C19, and CYP2D6. Unlike irreversible MAOIs, moclobemide lacks serious interactions with high tyramine foods. However, caution is still necessary with respect to some of the drug–drug interactions described for irreversible MAOIs. Coadministration with SSRIs, SNRIs or other MAOIs should be avoided. Moclobemide can cause dry mouth, headache, sedation, gastrointestinal disturbance, and sleep fragmentation, but not sexual problems or orthostasis. Mania induction has been reported, and may be less frequent than with tricyclic antidepressants, but limited experience precludes assessment of this risk relative to other agents.

Recently, a transdermal formulation of the irreversible MAOI selegiline has been approved for the treatment of (unipolar) major depressive disorder in the United States. This formulation has a bioavailability of 30%, so that a 20 mg/20 cm² patch yields the equivalent of 6 mg of selegiline per 24 hours. Absorption is independent of dose, which ranges from 6 to 12 mg/24 hours (Rohatagi et al., 1997). Selegiline is 90% bound to plasma proteins, and has a half-life of 24 hours, and a clearance of 1400 mL/min. The transdermal formulation has no first-pass effect, and is metabolized by N-dealkylation to N-desmethylselegiline, and by N-deproparglyation to R(-) methamphetamine. This formulation avoids the high gastrointestinal exposure seen with oral MAOIs, so that dietary tyramine ingestion is *not* restricted for the lowest dose of 6 mg/24 hours. There are insufficient data to ascertain the need for dietary restrictions with doses of 9 or 12 mg/24 hours. Like oral MAOIs, multiple concurrent medications (such as antidepressants, carbamazepine, oxcarbazepine, opiates, and sympatomimetics) are contraindicated within 2 weeks, due to the potential for pharmacodynamic interactions. Carbamazepine may increase rather than decrease serum levels of transdermal selegiline and its metabolites (Physicians' Desk Reference, 2007). As transdermal selegiline is a relatively new treatment, there are limited data regarding its use in patients with bipolar disorder.

Tricyclic antidepressants

Tricyclic antidepressants (TCAs) block reuptake of serotonin and norepinephrine to varying degrees (Goodman & Charney, 1985), and in the past were first line agents in the treatment of (unipolar) major depressive disorder. TCAs are generally well absorbed, and have variable (20–70%) bioavailability, high (90%) protein binding, half-lives around 24 hours, and variable volumes of distribution (10–30 L/kg), and clearances (300–1700 mL/min) (Gram, 1980). Hydroxylation by CYP2D6 is the rate-limiting metabolic step, and thus serum TCA levels rise with CYP2D6 inhibitors such as fluoxetine, sertraline, paroxetine, haloperidol, methadone, propafenone, and quinidine. TCA serum levels can also rise with methylphenidate, disulfiram, acute ethanol, hormonal contraceptives, cimetidine, chloramphenicol, and possibly valproate and azole antifungals, although the mechanism(s) of these phenomena are less clear. TCA levels fall with carbamazepine, phenobarbital, phenytoin, chronic ethanol, tobacco smoking, and possibly rifampin. Administration within 2 weeks of MAOIs is generally avoided.

TCAs can yield tremor, sedation, orthostasis, and anticholinergic (dry mouth, tachycardia, blurred vision) adverse effects (Beaumont, 1988; Kusturica et al., 2002; Pollack & Rosenbaum, 1987; Rabkin et al., 1984). Although TCAs may be well-tolerated by some individuals, safety and tolerability problems with these agents have led them to be generally replaced by newer antidepressants (Blackwell, 1981; Kusturica et al., 2002). Thus, TCA therapy is generally considered a low priority strategy in treating bipolar depression due to adverse effects, danger in overdose, and TCAs being the antidepressants most implicated in causing manic switches (Altshuler et al., 1995; Peet, 1994; Sachs et al., 1994; Silverstone, 2001; Stoll et al., 1994).

Benzodiazepines and mechanistically related drugs

Benzodiazepines (BZs) and mechanistically related compounds (such as zaleplon, zolpidem, and eszopiclone) modulate $GABA_A$ receptor function and produce anxiolytic and hypnotic effects. Patients with bipolar disorders commonly have comorbid anxiety disorders, and may need more anxiolytic and sedative effects than those obtained with mood stabilizers. Thus, adjunctive benzodiazepines and mechanistically related drugs are commonly used in the management of bipolar disorders. Indeed, benzodiazepines are commonly administered along with mood stabilizers and antipsychotics in patients with bipolar disorder, with merely additive central nervous system (e.g. sedation, ataxia) adverse effects.

Benzodiazepines and mechanistically related compounds are generally well absorbed, and tend to be extensively (95%) protein bound, have moderate volumes of distribution around 1 L/kg, and have half-lives which are short (less than 6 hours with triazolam, clorazepate, flurazepam, zaleplon, zolpidem, and eszopiclone), intermediate (6–20 hours with alprazolam, lorazepam, oxazepam, and temazepam), and long (more than 20 hours with diazepam and clonazepam).

The 2-keto-benzodiazepines, clorazepate, diazepam, and flurazepam, are metabolized by CYP2C19 and CYP3A3/4. Serum levels of these agents are decreased by tobacco smoking, barbiturates, and rifampin; and increased by fluoxetine, fluvoxamine, disulfiram, hormonal contraceptives, ketoconazole, cimetidine, isoniazid, omeprazole, and propranolol. The triazolo-benzodiazepines alprazolam and triazolam have substantial CYP3A3/4 metabolic components. Serum levels of these agents are to varying degrees decreased by carbamazepine, and increased by fluoxetine, fluvoxamine, nefazodone, diltiazem, hormonal contraceptives, ketoconazole, cimetidine, erythromycin, and propoxyphene. In addition, eszopiclone and zolpidem appear susceptible agents that induce CYP3A4, more so than zaleplon. Also, eszopiclone appears susceptible agents that inhibit CYP3A4, more so than zaleplon and zolpidem. The 7-nitro-benzodiazepines, clonazepam and nitrazepam, and the 3-hydroxy-benzodiazepines lorazepam, oxazepam, and temazepam are metabolized by robust N-reduction and conjugation reactions, respectively.

Benzodiazepines and mechanistically related drugs are commonly administered along with mood stabilizers, antipsychotics, and antidepressants in patients with bipolar disorder, in most cases with merely additive central nervous system (e.g. sedation, ataxia) adverse effects. Indeed, contemporary controlled acute mania trials of mood stabilizers and antipsychotics routinely permit some adjunctive benzodiazepine (e.g. lorazepam) administration. However, limited data suggest that for at least some patients, caution is indicated with such combinations. Interactions between benzodiazepines and individual mood stabilizers and antipsychotics are described in the above sections on these agents.

Although benzodiazepines and mechanistically related drugs are generally safe and well-tolerated in acute treatment, with sedation, memory problems, incoordination, and occasional disinhibition being the main adverse effects, with chronic use concerns around abuse, tolerance, and withdrawal arise (Vgontzas, Kales, & Bixler, 1995). Thus, efforts are made to make benzodiazepines and mechanistically related drug exposure brief and to find alternative agents such as trazodone for insomnia, or gabapentin for anxiety. In some patients, very low dose olanzapine (0.625–2.5 mg) or quetiapine (6.25–25 mg) may allow tapering or discontinuation of benzodiazepines and mechanistically related drugs. Nevertheless, some patients with comorbid anxiety disorders and persistent insomnia may need, tolerate, and responsibly use adjunctive benzodiazepines and mechanistically related drugs on a chronic basis. Benzodiazepines and mechanistically related drugs do not commonly trigger manic switches, although concern has been raised around alprazolam at the level of case reports, in view of its putative modest antidepressant effects.

Newer anticonvulsants

A series of newer anticonvulsants have been marketed over the last decade (LaRoche & Helmers, 2004), and more are in development (Bialer, 2006). Compared to older anticonvulsants, several of the new medications have enhanced tolerability, simpler kinetics, and fewer drug-drug interactions. These drugs have a variety of mechanisms, including enhancing neural inhibition by increasing GABAergic function, and/or decreasing neural excitation by decreasing glutamatergic function (Macdonald & Kelly, 1995). Such agents could yield psychotropic effects as these amino acid neurotransmitters have been implicated in psychiatric disorders. The psychotropic profiles of these new anticonvulsants have not yet been fully characterized, but important kinetic differences between them have already emerged. In

2008, the FDA released an alert regarding increased risk of suicidality (suicidal behavior or ideation) in patients with epilepsy as well as psychiatric disorders for eleven anticonvulsants (carbamazepine, felbamate gabapentin, lamotrigine, levetiracetam, oxcarbazepine, pregabalin, tiagabine, topiramate, valproate, and zonisamide). In the FDA's analysis, anticonvulsants compared to placebo yielded approximately twice the risk of suicidality (0.43% vs 0.22%). The relative risk for suicidality was higher in the patients with epilepsy compared to psychiatric disorders. As of mid-2008, a class warning regarding this risk had not yet been added to the United States prescribing information for anticonvulsants, but it is anticipated that this may occur.

Felbamate

The use of felbamate (FBM) is restricted to patients with refractory epilepsy due to its associations with aplastic anemia and fatal hepatitis, perhaps related to toxic metabolite formation. However, felbamate is of considerable theoretical interest in view of its novel mechanisms, pharmacokinetics, and psychiatric effects. Felbamate has a dicarbamate structure similar to meprobamate, and several mechanisms which include sodium channel blockade, modest GABAergic, and more robust antiglutamatergic actions (Palmer & McTavish, 1993). Felbamate appears to possess a novel stimulant-like psychotropic profile in epilepsy patients (Ketter et al., 1996).

Gabapentin

Gabapentin (GBP) and the related anticonvulsant pregabalin have structures similar to gamma-aminobutyric acid (GABA), but do not appear to be direct functional analogs of GABA. These agents have selective inhibitory effects on voltage-gated calcium channels containing the alpha-2 delta subunit (Gee et al., 1996; Taylor, Angelotti, & Fauman, 2007; Taylor et al., 1993), reducing depolarization-induced calcium influx at nerve terminals (Fink et al., 2002), resulting in decreased release of excitatory neurotransmitters such as glutamate (Dooley, Mieske, & Borosky, 2000) and noradrenaline (Dooley et al., 2002; Dooley, Donovan, & Pugsley, 2000). In rat forebrain, these drugs acutely decreased cellular glutamate, but did not alter GABA or glutamine concentrations (Errante & Petroff, 2003). These agents are inactive at $GABA_A$, $GABA_B$, and benzodiazepine receptors, and are not metabolized to GABA or GABA agonists. However, gabapentin increases nonsynaptic GABA release from glia, and is also a substrate and a competitive inhibitor of the large (L) neutral amino acid carrier system, and may modulate (but does not directly block) sodium channels.

Gabapentin has an anxiolytic preclinical profile. Emerging data suggested that open gabapentin augmentation was well tolerated and could help some patients with mood disorders. Controlled data suggest efficacy in social phobia (Pande et al., 1999) and panic disorder (Pande et al., 2000b), neuropathic pain (Serpell, 2002), chronic daily headache (Spira & Beran, 2003), and post-herpetic neuralgia (Rowbotham et al., 1998), but were less encouraging in acute mania (Pande et al., 2000a) and treatment-refractory (primarily rapid cycling bipolar) mood disorder patients (Frye et al., 2000).

Although gabapentin has generally favorable pharmacokinetic properties, it has saturable (sublinear) absorption (Stewart et al., 1993) and a bioavailability of 60%, which declines further if individual doses are greater than 900 mg (McLean, 1994). Thus, many patients may need to take divided doses of gabapentin. Also, aluminum/magnesium hydroxide antacids modestly decrease gabapentin bioavailability. Like lithium, gabapentin is not bound to plasma proteins, has moderate volume of distribution of about 1 L/kg, is not metabolized, and is >95% excreted unchanged in the urine. gabapentin has a half-life of about six hours and a clearance similar to that of creatinine (120 mL/min, similar to the glomerular filtration rate), so that in a fashion similar to lithium, decreased renal function decreases gabapentin clearance (so that dosage may need to be decreased in patients with decreased renal function), and physical activity may increase gabapentin clearance. gabapentin levels could thus fall with the increase in activity seen in hypomania or mania.

As gabapentin is excreted unchanged in the urine and lacks effects on hepatic metabolism, it appears to lack hepatically mediated drug-drug interactions (Richens, 1993). Thus, gabapentin lacks pharmacokinetic drug interactions with carbamazepine and valproate and with pregabalin in patients with epilepsy. Also, gabapentin also fails to alter lithium kinetics in mood disorder patients with normal renal function (Frye et al., 1998). The effect of lithium upon gabapentin pharmacokinetics remains to be established. Although pharmacokinetic interactions between gabapentin and lamotrigine are not expected, the absence of such interactions remains to be confirmed. Gabapentin does not yield clinically significant changes in the kinetics of hormonal contraceptives.

Gabapentin is generally well tolerated, but can cause sedation, dizziness, ataxia, fatigue, and weight gain (Goa & Sorkin, 1993). Some evidence suggests that gabapentin can cause behavioral deterioration in some pediatric epilepsy patients who also suffer from cognitive or behavioral disorders (Lee et al., 1996). Gabapentin can be rapidly initiated in epilepsy patients with 300 mg, 600 mg, and 900 mg on the first, second and third days. Final gabapentin doses usually range between 900 mg/day and an approved maximum of 3600 mg/day in three or four divided doses

(Physicians' Desk Reference, 2007), which yields serum concentrations of approximately 12–20 ug/mL (70–120 uM/L) (Johannessen et al., 2003). In controlled trials, final gabapentin doses ranged between 600 and 3600 mg/day in an adjunctive acute mania study (Pande et al., 2000a), and the mean final gabapentin dose was approximately 4000 mg/day as monotherapy in treatment-resistant (primarily rapid cycling bipolar) mood disorder patients (Frye et al., 2000). Lower doses have been reported to benefit some patients with bipolar disorders (Schaffer & Schaffer, 1997). In other controlled trials, final gabapentin doses ranged between 900 and 3600 mg/day in social phobia (Pande et al., 1999), 600 and 3600 mg/day in panic disorder (Pande et al., 2000), 900 and 2400 mg/day in neuropathic pain (Serpell, 2002), 1200 and 3600 mg/day in post-herpetic neuralgia (Rowbotham et al., 1998), and had a mean of 2400 mg/day in chronic daily headache (Spira & Beran, 2003).

Topiramate

Topiramate (TPM) is a fructopyranose sulfamate which blocks sodium channels (Zona, Ciotti, & Avoli, 1997) and AMPA/kainate gated ion channels (Poulsen et al., 2004). Topiramate also positively modulates GABA-A receptors (Gordey, DeLorey, & Olsen, 2000; White et al., 2000), and inhibits carbonic anhydrase (Shank et al., 1994). Although early open reports of topiramate in bipolar disorders were encouraging, later multicenter, randomized, double-blind, placebo-controlled studies were discouraging. Thus, in several trials topiramate proved no better or worse than placebo in adults with acute mania (Kushner et al., 2006). However, topiramate appeared effective in several comorbid conditions seen in patients with bipolar disorders, with randomized, double-blind, placebo-controlled trails demonstrating efficacy in eating disorders such as bulimia (Hoopes et al., 2003), binge eating disorder with obesity (McElroy et al., 2003), and obesity (Bray et al., 2003), as well as in alcohol dependence (Johnson et al., 2003) and the prevention of migraine headaches (Brandes et al., 2004). Weight loss has been consistently observed in controlled trials with topiramate, not only in patients with eating disorders as noted above, but also in manic (Kushner et al., 2006) and depressed (McIntyre et al., 2002) patients with bipolar disorders.

Topiramate has a bioavailability of 80%, absorption independent of food, low (15%) binding to plasma proteins, saturable binding to erythrocytes (which contain carbonic anhydrase) which correlates with hematocrit (Gidal & Lensmeyer, 1999), and a moderate volume of distribution of about 0.8 L/kg (Bourgeois, 1999). topiramate has a half-life of about 24 hours, a clearance of about 25 mL/min, and linear elimination kinetic between doses of 100 and 800 mg/day. During monotherapy, topiramate is 70% excreted unchanged in the urine, however, when combined with enzyme inducers, this figure falls to about 50%.

The large renal component of topiramate disposition yields it resistant to effects of enzyme inhibitors, yet the limited monotherapy hepatic metabolism component makes it susceptible to enzyme inducers. For example, in epilepsy patients, carbamazepine yields clinically significant decreases in topiramate serum concentrations, but topiramate does not yield clinically significant changes in carbamazepine serum concentrations. The enzyme(s) responsible for the metabolic component of topiramate elimination, and the mechanism of carbamazepine induction of topiramate metabolism, remain to be definitively characterized, but stimulation of oxidative pathways yielding 2,3-diol-topiramate and 10-OH-topiramate has been implicated. In contrast, valproate and lamotrigine do not appear to have clinically significant pharmacokinetic interactions with topiramate in patients with epilepsy. In an unpublished study, topiramate yielded clinically insignificant decreases in serum lithium concentrations in healthy volunteers, but case reports have raised the possibility that topiramate cause clinically significant increases in serum lithium concentrations in some individuals. The effects of lithium on topiramate pharmacokinetics remain to be established.

Although levetiracetam does not alter topiramate concentrations, the combination may yield adverse effects through a pharmacodynamic interaction. In addition, combination of topiramate with other carbonic anhydrase inhibitors such as acetazolamide and zonisamide, is not recommended due to concerns about increasing the risk of nephrolithiasis or heat-related problems (oligohydrosis and hyperthermia). Topiramate is a mild enzyme inducer, and can decrease blood concentrations of hormonal contraceptives, potentially compromising their efficacy (Rosenfeld et al., 1997). This effect may be less problematic at doses of 200 mg/day or less (Doose et al., 2003).

Topiramate does not generally yield clinically significant alterations in serum haloperidol, clozapine, risperidone, olanzapine, or quetiapine concentrations. Administration of topiramate with amitriptyline did not yield clinically significant changes in plasma amitriptyline or nortriptyline concentrations, but could modestly decrease topiramate clearance or increase topiramate bioavailability. Oxcarbazepine may modestly decrease serum concentrations of topiramate.

Topiramate can cause impaired concentration, weight loss, dizziness, speech problems, somnolence, ataxia, and paresthesias (Froscher et al., 2005). Topiramate appears associated with renal calculi in 1–2% of epilepsy patients, presumably due to carbonic anhydrase inhibition (Shorvon, 1996). Topiramate has been associated with dose-related hyperchloremic, non-anion gap metabolic acidosis, oligohydrosis and hyperthermia, and rarely with acute myopia with secondary angle closure glaucoma. Affective disturbance, psychosis, aggression, and irritability have been occasionally seen in epilepsy patients treated with topiramate (Mula et al., 2003).

In epilepsy patients, topiramate is started at 50 mg/day and increased by 50 mg/day each week with a recommended maximum dose of 400 mg/day in two divided doses (Physicians' Desk Reference, 2007), which yields serum concentrations of approximately 5–20 ug/mL (15–60 uM/L) (Johannessen et al., 2003). In epilepsy studies, doses up to 1000 mg/day did not improve responses compared to those seen with doses of 400 mg/day. In migraine patients, initiation, titration, and final doses are about half the amounts used in epilepsy. In controlled trials, final topiramate doses ranged between 200 and 600 mg/day in acute mania (Kushner et al., 2006), between 50 and 200 mg/day in migraine (Brandes et al., 2004), between 64 and 384 mg/day in obesity (Bray et al., 2003), and were approximately 200 mg/day for obesity with binge eating (McElroy et al., 2003), and alcohol dependence (Johnson et al., 2003), and 100 mg/day for bulimia (Hoopes et al., 2003).

Tiagabine

Tiagabine (TGB) is a nipecotic acid derivative, which inhibits GABA reuptake in neurons and glial cells (Suzdak & Jansen, 1995). There are no controlled studies of tiagabine in bipolar disorders. Although some experience with open low dose tiagabine in bipolar disorders was encouraging (Schaffer, Schaffer, & Howe, 2002), other open reports suggested problems with both efficacy and tolerability. For example, rapid loading of open primarily adjunctive tiagabine, starting at 20 mg/day (five times the recommended starting dose) in eight acute mania inpatients not only was ineffective, but also yielded unacceptable adverse effects, with one patient having a seizure (Grunze et al., 1999). This suggests not only inefficacy in mania, but also that loading or rapid dosage escalation should be avoided, and caution exercised in using tiagabine, particularly in the initial titration phase. However, even more gradual initiation may be problematic. Thus, open primarily adjunctive tiagabine initiated at 4 mg/day and increased weekly as tolerated by 4 mg/day (mean dose 8.7 mg/day, mean duration 38 days) in outpatients with treatment-refractory bipolar disorder had limited efficacy, and raised tolerability concerns, as 2/13 (15%) patients had seizures attributed as likely due to the medication (Suppes et al., 2002). Thus, open studies have raised both efficacy and tolerability concerns regarding tiagabine in bipolar disorders. In contrast, small controlled trials have reported that low dose (≤16 mg/day) tiagabine was generally well tolerated and yielded benefit in generalized anxiety disorder (Rosenthal, 2003) and primary insomnia (Roth & Walsh, 2004).

Tiagabine is well absorbed with a bioavailability of about 90%, and is extensively (96%) bound to plasma proteins, and has linear kinetics at doses between 2 and 24 mg/day (Brodie, 1995; Gustavson & Mengel, 1995). In monotherapy, tiagabine has a half-life of about eight hours and clearance of about 110 mL/min, and with enzyme inducers the half-life falls to about four hours and clearance doubles to about 220 mL/min. Tiagabine is a CYP3A substrate, and is extensively transformed into inactive 5-oxo-tiagabine and glucuronide metabolites, with only 2% being excreted unchanged in the urine. The remainder is excreted as metabolites in feces (65%) and urine (25%).

Tiagabine neither induces nor inhibits hepatic enzymes, and hence is a target rather than an instigator of pharmacokinetic drug interactions. Thus, enzyme inducers such as carbamazepine can yield clinically significant decreases in serum tiagabine concentrations, possibly by induction of CYP3A, while tiagabine does not yield clinically significant changes in the pharmacokinetics of carbamazepine or phenytoin, or valproate. Valproate does not yield clinically significant changes in serum total tiagabine concentrations, but appears to displace tiagabine from protein binding sites yielding an increase in free tiagabine. The presence or absence of pharmacokinetic interactions between tiagabine and lamotrigine and tiagabine and lithium remains to be established. Tiagabine does not yield clinically significant changes in the kinetics of hormonal contraceptives.

Tiagabine can cause dizziness, fatigue, sedation, tremor, weakness and gastrointestinal disturbance (Leppik, 1995). In epilepsy patients also taking enzyme inducers, tiagabine is typically initiated at four mg/day and increased weekly by 4–8 mg/day as tolerated with an approved maximum dose of 56 mg/day in two to four divided doses (Physicians' Desk Reference, 2007), which yields serum concentrations of approximately 20–100 ng/mL (50–250 nM/L) (Johannessen et al., 2003). A 50% decrease in these doses may be required in patients not taking concurrent enzyme inducers. As noted above, rapid loading of open primarily adjunctive tiagabine in patients with acute mania, starting at 20 mg/day yielded unacceptable adverse effects, with one patient having a seizure (Grunze et al., 1999), and even more gradual initiation in outpatients with bipolar disorder at 4 mg/day and increased weekly as tolerated by 4 mg/day (mean final dose 8.7 mg/day) raised tolerability concerns, with 2/13 patients having seizures (Suppes et al., 2002).

Oxcarbazepine

Oxcarbazepine (OXC), the 10-keto analog of carbamazepine, has both structural and mechanistic similarities to carbamazepine (Ambrosio et al., 2002; McLean et al., 1994). Oxcarbazepine's structural similarity to carbamazepine suggests the possibility that oxcarbazepine could have psychotropic effects that overlap those of carbamazepine, and as noted below, compared to carbamazepine it has more favorable adverse effect and drug interactions profiles. Unfortunately, there is very little controlled evidence of efficacy for oxcarbazepine in bipolar disorders, far less than for carbamazepine. Specifically, to date, there are no large double-blind, placebo-controlled trials demonstrating oxcarbazepine efficacy in bipolar disorder. Although small, multicenter, active-comparator studies failed to find difference between oxcarbazepine and haloperidol and oxcarbazepine and lithium in adults with acute mania, insufficient statistical power precludes making conclusions regarding the efficacy of oxcarbazepine in acute mania (Emrich, 1990). A more recent somewhat larger study in pediatric acute mania failed to demonstrate an overall advantage of oxcarbazepine compared placebo, but in post hoc analyses found an advantage in children but not in adolescents (Wagner et al., 2006).

Oxcarbazepine has >95% absorption with no clinically significant effect of food upon absorption, and may be considered a prodrug that is rapidly and extensively metabolized by cytosol arylketone reductase to its active 10-monohydroxyderivative (MHD), which is appears to be the primary component responsible for clinical effects (May, Korn-Merker, & Rambeck, 2003). Oxcarbazepine and MHD have half-lives of 2 and 9 hours, protein binding of 60% and 40%, respectively, linear elimination kinetics, and no autoinduction of metabolism. MHD has a volume of distribution of 0.5 L/kg, with clearance of 20 mL/min, which is primarily by renal excretion, so that oxcarbazepine dosage may need to be decreased in patients with renal impairment (Rouan et al., 1994).

In contrast to carbamazepine, oxcarbazepine has no autoinduction and less heteroinduction, yielding fewer drug interactions. Thus, oxcarbazepine does not yield clinically significant alterations in serum concentrations of carbamazepine or valproate, and compared to carbamazepine, oxcarbazepine yields less robust decreases in serum lamotrigine concentrations. Although oxcarbazepine may decrease serum lamotrigine concentrations, the clinical significance of this interaction remains to be established and could vary across patients. Lamotrigine does not appear to alter oxcarbazepine pharmacokinetics. A possible pharmacodynamic interaction has been reported with oxcarbazepine and lamotrigine. Valproate and lamotrigine do not yield clinically significant changes in serum oxcarbazepine concentrations. In contrast, carbamazepine induces oxcarbazepine metabolism, yielding decreased serum MHD concentrations. The presence or absence of pharmacokinetic interactions between oxcarbazepine and lithium remains to be established.

Oxcarbazepine does not yield clinically significant alterations in serum olanzapine or risperidone concentrations. Replacing carbamazepine with oxcarbazepine may increase serum concentrations of citalopram, and haloperidol, chlorpromazine, and clozapine. Oxcarbazepine may modestly decrease serum concentrations of topiramate and levetiracetam.

Like carbamazepine, oxcarbazepine yields clinically significant (about 50%) decreases in serum concentrations of ethinylestradiol and levonorgestrel derived from hormonal contraceptives, presumably related to CYP3A4 induction (Fattore et al., 1999; Klosterskov et al., 1992). Oxcarbazepine also yields decreases in serum concentrations of the dihydropyridine calcium channel blocker felodipine (which is also a CYP3A4 substrate). In contrast to carbamazepine, the CYP3A4 inhibitor erythromycin, and the antidepressant viloxazine do not yield clinically significant increases in serum oxcarbazepine concentrations.

Oxcarbazepine adverse effects most frequently involve the central nervous system, including dizziness, sedation, and fatigue (Friis et al., 1993). Oxcarbazepine appears to yield less neurotoxicity and rash than carbamazepine, and unlike carbamazepine, has not been associated with blood dyscrasias (Dam et al., 1989; Reinikainen et al., 1987). Cross-allergy between oxcarbazepine and carbamazepine occurs in about 25% of patients (Van Parys & Meinardi, 1994). Hyponatremia occurs with oxcarbazepine (Friis et al., 1993), and may be the main adverse effect that occurs more commonly than with carbamazepine. Adverse effects with oxcarbazepine therapy appear related to serum MHD concentrations, which if over 30 ug/mL indicate increased risk (Striano et al., 2006).

Dosing strategies

In epilepsy patients, oxcarbazepine is commonly started at 600 mg/day and increased weekly by 600 mg/day, with final doses commonly ranging between 900 and 2400 mg/day in two divided doses (Physicians' Desk Reference, 2007), which yield serum concentrations of approximately 13–35 ug/mL (50–140 uM/L) (Johannessen et al., 2003). In an early, small, double-blind, on-off-on acute mania trial, the mean oxcarbazepine dose was 1886 mg/day (range 1800–2100) (Emrich et al., 1983). In small, multicenter, active-comparator acute mania studies, mean oxcarbazepine doses were 2400 mg/day and 1400 mg/day, when compared to haloperidol and lithium, respectively (Emrich, 1990). In a recent pediatric acute mania study oxcarbazepine was increased every 2 days by 300 mg/day to a maximum of 900–2400 mg/day, with mean doses of 1200 mg/day and 2040 mg/day in children and adolescents, respectively (Wagner et al., 2006).

Levetiracetam

Levetiracetam (LEV) is the *S*-enantimor of the ethyl analog of the nootropic agent piracetam (Shorvon, 2001), and has GABAergic (Loscher,

Honack, & Bloms-Funke, 1996) and antikindling (Loscher, Honack, & Rundfeldt, 1998) effects, reduces voltage-dependent potassium currents (Madeja et al., 2003), and binds to the synaptic vesicle protein SV2A (Lynch et al., 2004), and thus could have effects on release of neurotransmitters from synaptic vesicles. Open studies suggest that levetiracetam may have efficacy in patients with bipolar disorder (Bersani, 2004; Braunig & Kruger, 2003; Goldberg & Burdick, 2002; Grunze et al., 2003; Kaufman, 2004; Kyomen, 2006; Post et al., 2005), although there also are reports of levetiracetam-related depression (Wier et al., 2006) and aggressive behavior (Mula, Trimble, & Sander, 2004). In a controlled pilot studies, levetiracetam was no better than placebo in patients with social anxiety disorder (Zhang, Connor, & Davidson, 2005), autism (Wasserman et al., 2006), and essential tremor (Handforth & Martin, 2004). Levetiracetam was effective in an animal model of mania (Lamberty, Margineanu, & Klitgaard, 2001), and a series of uncontrolled case reports (Braunig & Kruger, 2003; Goldberg & Burdick, 2002; Kaufman, 2004) and case series (Bersani, 2004; Grunze et al., 2003; Kyomen, 2006; Post et al., 2005) have been encouraging. Controlled studies are needed to assess the effects of levetiracetam in patients with bipolar disorder.

Levetiracetam has a favorable pharmacokinetic profile, with absorption that is not related to food, bioavailability of >95%, less than 10% binding to plasma proteins, a moderate volume of distribution of about 0.6 L/kg, linear elimination pharmacokinetics at clinically relevant doses (between 500 and 5000 mg/day), a half-life of 8 hours, and clearance of 40 mL/min (Patsalos, 2000). Levetiracetam is 66% excreted unchanged in the urine, and is 24% hydrolyzed (in blood rather than in liver) to an inactive metabolite (Coupez, Nicolas, & Browne, 2003). In view of the substantive renal clearance, levetiracetam dosage may need to be decreased in patients with impaired renal function. As the minor metabolic component of levetiracetam disposition involves hydrolysis rather than oxidation or glucuronidation, and levetiracetam does not yield clinically significant changes in hepatic oxidation or glucuronidation, these properties yield a low potential for pharmacokinetic drug interactions.

Hence, levetiracetam does not appear to have clinically significant pharmacokinetic interactions with valproate or lamotrigine in epilepsy patients. Carbamazepine appears to decrease serum levetiracetam concentrations, but there are variable assessments of the potential clinical significance of this interaction. Although levetiracetam does not yield clinically significant alterations in serum concentrations of carbamazepine or carbamazepine-epoxide in epilepsy patients, levetiracetam plus carbamazepine may yield adverse effects through a pharmacodynamic interaction. The presence or absence of pharmacokinetic interactions between levetiracetam and lithium remains to be established.

Levetiracetam does not appear to have clinically significant pharmacokinetic interactions with gabapentin or topiramate in epilepsy patients, although the levetiracetam plus topiramate combination may yield adverse effects through a pharmacodynamic interaction. Levetiracetam does not yield clinically significant alterations in serum concentrations of phenytoin, phenobarbital, or primidone in epilepsy patients. Oxcarbazepine may modestly decrease serum concentrations of levetiracetam. Levetiracetam does not yield clinically significant changes in the metabolism of hormonal contraceptives.

Levetiracetam is generally well tolerated, but can cause somnolence, asthenia, dizziness, coordination problems, and mood/anxiety/behavioral problems (Harden, 2001; Mula, Trimble, & Sander, 2004; Mula et al., 2003). In epilepsy patients, the latter occur in 13.3% of adults (vs. 6.2% with placebo), and in 37.6% of children (vs. 18.6% with placebo) (Physicians' Desk Reference, 2007). Levetiracetam-related behavioral problems appeared more common in patients with epilepsy than in patients with cognitive or anxiety disorders (Cramer et al., 2003).

In epilepsy patients, levetiracetam is commonly started at 500–1000 mg/day, and increased as necessary and tolerated every 2 weeks by 1000 mg/day up to 3000 mg/day in two divided doses (Physicians' Desk Reference, 2007), yielding serum concentrations of approximately 6–20 ug/mL (35–120 uM/L) (Johannessen et al., 2003).

Zonisamide

Zonisamide (ZNS) is a sulfonamide that blocks sodium channels (Schauf, 1987), reduces T-type calcium currents (Kito, Maehara, & Watanabe, 1996), facilitates dopaminergic and serotonergic neurotransmission (Kaneko et al., 1993), and is a weak carbonic anhydrase inhibitor (Masuda & Karasawa, 1993). Although zonisamide binds to the GABA/benzodiazepine receptor complex, it does not alter chloride currents, and does not appear to have major GABAergic activity. Open studies suggest that zonisamide may have efficacy in patients with bipolar disorder (Anand et al., 2005; Baldassano et al., 2004; Ghaemi et al., 2006; Kanba et al., 1994; McElroy et al., 2005; Wilson & Findling, 2007), although there also are reports of zonisamide-related affective disturbance (Charles, Stoesz, & Tollefson, 1990; Ozawa et al., 2004; Sullivan, Ward, & Zesiewicz, 2006). Controlled studies are needed to assess the effects of zonisamide in patients with bipolar disorder.

Zonisamide has generally favorable pharmacokinetic properties, with good (close to 100%) bioavailability, only 40–60% binding to plasma proteins (but extensive binding to erythrocytes), a clearance of 20 mL/min, and a moderate volume of distribution of 1.5 L/kg (Leppik, 2004;

Sills & Brodie, 2007). Zonisamide has linear pharmacokinetics between 200 and 400 mg/day, but has disproportionate serum concentrations at 800 mg, presumably related to saturable binding to carbonic anhydrase in erythrocytes. As monotherapy, zonisamide has a half-life of 60 hours, which falls to 30 hours if administered with enzyme inducers. Zonisamide is reduced to 2-sulfamoylacetylphenol (SMAP), primarily by CYP3A4, and is only 30% excreted unchanged in the urine. Zonisamide does not inhibit CYP450 isoenzymes, does not induce its own metabolism, and is a target rather than an instigator of drug interactions.

Thus, carbamazepine decreases serum zonisamide concentrations, while zonisamide does not appear to yield clinically significant changes in carbamazepine pharmacokinetics. Zonisamide and valproate and zonisamide and lamotrigine do have clinically significant pharmacokinetic interactions in patients with epilepsy. The presence or absence of pharmacokinetic interactions between zonisamide and lithium remains to be established.

Phenytoin, and phenobarbital decrease serum zonisamide concentrations. Combination of zonisamide with other carbonic anhydrase inhibitors such as acetazolamide and topiramate is not recommended due to concerns about increasing the risk of nephrolithiasis or heat-related problems (oligohydrosis and hyperthermia). Zonisamide does not alter hormonal contraceptive pharmacokinetics.

Zonisamide is generally well tolerated, but can cause somnolence, anorexia, dizziness, headache, nausea, and agitation/irritability (Faught, 2004; Peters & Sorkin, 1993). Zonisamide has been associated with nephrolithiasis in approximately 4% of patients (but only symptomatic in approximately 1% of patients) (Physicians' Desk Reference, 2007), presumably due to carbonic anhydrase inhibition. In patients with epilepsy, zonisamide is started at 100 mg/day, and increased every 2 weeks as necessary and tolerated by 100 mg/day, with final doses commonly ranging between 300 and 600 mg/day in two divided doses (Physicians' Desk Reference, 2007), yielding serum concentrations of approximately 10–38 ug/mL (45–180 uM/L) (Johannessen et al., 2003). In a controlled study in obesity, the mean final zonisamide dose was 427 mg/day.

Pregabalin

Pregabalin (PGB), or S-(+)-3-isobutylGABA, has a structure and mechanisms that overlap those of gabapentin (Ben-Menachem, 2004; Sills, 2006; Taylor et al., 2007). Both of these agents are structural but not direct functional analogs of GABA, that have selective inhibitory effects on voltage-gated calcium channels containing the alpha-2 delta subunit (Gee et al., 1996; Taylor et al., 2007, 1993), reducing depolarization-induced calcium influx at nerve terminals (Fink et al., 2002), resulting in decreased release of excitatory neurotransmitters such as glutamate (Dooley, Mieske, & Borosky, 2000) and noradrenaline (Dooley et al., 2002; Dooley, Donovan, & Pugsley, 2000). In rat forebrain, these drugs acutely decreased cellular glutamate, but did not alter GABA or glutamine concentrations (Errante & Petroff, 2003). These agents are inactive at $GABA_A$, $GABA_B$, and benzodiazepine receptors, and are not metabolized to GABA or GABA agonists.

In controlled trials, pregabalin appeared effective for generalized anxiety disorder (Feltner et al., 2003; Montgomery et al., 2006; Pande et al., 2003; Pohl et al., 2005; Rickels et al., 2005), social anxiety disorder (Pande et al., 2004), neuropathic pain associated with postherpetic neuralgia (Dworkin et al., 2003; Freynhagen et al., 2005; Sabatowski et al., 2004), diabetic peripheral neuropathy (Freynhagen et al., 2005; Richter et al., 2005; Rosenstock et al., 2004), and spinal cord injury (Siddall et al., 2006), as well as for relief of pain, disturbed sleep, and fatigue in fibromyalgia syndrome (Crofford et al., 2005). As pregabalin is a newer medicine, its effects in patients with bipolar disorder remain to be assessed.

PBG appears to have generally favorable pharmacokinetic properties (Ben-Menachem, 2004). Similar to gabapentin, pregabalin is not bound to plasma proteins, has a moderate volume of distribution of 0.5 L/kg, a half-life of 6 hours (requiring t.i.d. dosing), is not metabolized, >95% excreted unchanged in urine, has clearance of 80 mL/min that varies with creatinine clearance. Thus, decreased renal function decreases gabapentin clearance, and dosage reduction may be necessary in patients with decreased renal function (Randinitis et al., 2003). Pregabalin lacks hepatic metabolism, does not induce or inhibit hepatic metabolism, and lacks metabolic drug interactions. Unlike gabapentin, pregabalin has higher (>90%) bioavailability, and absorption that is proportional to dose. Food has no clinically relevant effect on pregabalin absorption.

Like gabapentin, in view of the absence of hepatic metabolism, pregabalin lacks metabolic drug interactions. Thus, in patients with epilepsy, pregabalin lacks clinically significant pharmacokinetic drug interactions with carbamazepine, valproate, and lamotrigine. The presence or absence of pregabalin pharmacokinetic interactions with lithium remains to be established.

In patients with epilepsy, pregabalin lacks clinically significant pharmacokinetic drug interactions with gabapentin and topiramate. Although tiagabine does not affect pregabalin pharmacokinetics, the presence or absence of a pregabalin effect on tiagabine pharmacokinetics remains to be established. The presence or absence of pregabalin pharmacokinetic interactions with oxcarbazepine, levetiracetam , and zonisamide remains to be established.

Pregabalin does not yield clinically significant changes in the kinetics of hormonal contraceptives.

Pregabalin is generally well tolerated, but can cause dizziness, somnolence, dry mouth, edema, blurred vision, weight gain, and problems with concentration/attention (Montgomery, 2006). In pain syndromes pregabalin is started at 150 mg/day and increased to 300 mg/day over 1 week, with a maximum recommended dose of 600 mg in three divided doses. In controlled trials, doses have ranged from 150 to 600 mg/day in generalized anxiety disorder (Feltner et al., 2003; Montgomery et al., 2006; Pande et al., 2003; Pohl et al., 2005; Rickels et al., 2005) and social anxiety disorder (Pande et al., 2004).

Conclusion

Effective pharmacotherapy of bipolar disorder patients requires not only familiarity with mood stabilizer pharmacodynamics, dosing, pharmacokinetics, drug interactions, adverse effects, and their management, but also similar knowledge of antipsychotics, antidepressants, benzodiazepines, and increasingly the newer anticonvulsants. In the past, clinicians have relied on observational drug interaction information, but recent characterization of substrates, inhibitors and inducers of drug metabolism now allows not only the development of mechanistic models, but also enhanced anticipation and avoidance of clinical drug–drug interactions (Table 15.8). These developments promise to yield safer and more effective therapeutics when psychotropics are combined with one another in treatment of patients with bipolar disorders.

References

Ackenheil, M. (1989). Clozapine—pharmacokinetic investigations and biochemical effects in man. *Psychopharmacology (Berl)*, *99*(Suppl), S32–S37.

Adler, C. M., Fleck, D. E., Brecher, M., & Strakowski, S. M. (2007). Safety and tolerability of quetiapine in the treatment of acute mania in bipolar disorder. *J. Affect. Disord.*, *100*(Suppl 1), S15–S22.

Ahlfors, U. G., Baastrup, P. C., Dencker, S. J., Elgen, K., Lingjaerde, O., Pedersen, V., et al. (1981). Flupenthixol decanoate in recurrent manic-depressive illness. A comparison with lithium. *Acta Psychiatr. Scand.*, *64*(3), 226–237.

Aldenkamp, A. P., Alpherts, W. C., Moerland, M. C., Ottevanger, N., & Van Parys, J. A. (1987). Controlled release carbamazepine: cognitive side effects in patients with epilepsy. *Epilepsia*, *28*(5), 507–514.

Allen, M. H., Hirschfeld, R. M., Wozniak, P. J., Baker, J. D., & Bowden, C. L. (2006). Linear relationship of valproate serum concentration to response and optimal serum levels for acute mania. *Am. J. Psychiatry*, *163*(2), 272–275.

Allison, D. B., Mentore, J. L., Heo, M., Chandler, L. P., Cappelleri, J. C., Infante, M. C., et al. (1999). Antipsychotic-induced weight gain: a comprehensive research synthesis. *Am J Psychiatry, 156*(11), 1686–1696.

Alsdorf, R. M., Wyszynski, D. F., Holmes, L. B., & Nambisan, M. (2004). Evidence of increased birth defects in the offspring of women exposed to valproate during pregnancy: findings from the AED pregnancy registry. *Birth Defects Res: Clin. Mol. Ter., 70*, 245.

Altshuler, L., Suppes, T., Black, D., Nolen, W. A., Keck, P. E., Jr., Frye, M. A., et al. (2003). Impact of antidepressant discontinuation after acute bipolar depression remission on rates of depressive relapse at 1-year follow-up. *Am. J. Psychiatry, 160*(7), 1252–1262.

Altshuler, L. L., Post, R. M., Leverich, G. S., Mikalauskas, K., Rosoff, A., & Ackerman, L. (1995). Antidepressant-induced mania and cycle acceleration: a controversy revisited. *Am. J. Psychiatry, 152*(8), 1130–1138.

Aly, M. I., & Abdel-Latif, A. A. (1980). Studies on distribution and metabolism of valproate in rat brain, liver, and kidney. *Neurochem. Res., 5*(12), 1231–1242.

Ambrosio, A. F., Soares-Da-Silva, P., Carvalho, C. M., & Carvalho, A. P. (2002). Mechanisms of action of carbamazepine and its derivatives, oxcarbazepine, BIA 2-093, and BIA 2-024. *Neurochem. Res., 27*(1–2), 121–130.

Amdisen, A. (1982). Lithium and drug interactions. *Drugs, 24*(2), 133–139.

Amdisen, A., & Andersen, C. J. (1982). Lithium treatment and thyroid function. A survey of 237 patients in long-term lithium treatment. *Pharmacopsychiatria, 15*(5), 149–155.

American Diabetes Association, American Psychiatric Association, American Association of Clinical Endocrinologists, & Obesity, N. A. A. f. t. S. o. (2004). Consensus development conference on antipsychotic drugs and obesity and diabetes. *Diabetes Care, 27*(2), 596–601.

American Psychiatric Association. (2002). Practice guideline for the treatment of patients with bipolar disorder (revision). *Am. J. Psychiatry, 159*(4 Suppl), 1–50.

Amsterdam, J. (1998). Efficacy and safety of venlafaxine in the treatment of bipolar II major depressive episode. *J. Clin. Psychopharmacol., 18*(5), 414–417.

Anand, A., Bukhari, L., Jennings, S. A., Lee, C., Kamat, M., Shekhar, A., et al. (2005). A preliminary open-label study of zonisamide treatment for bipolar depression in 10 patients. *J. Clin. Psychiatry, 66*(2), 195–198.

Anderson, G. D. (1998). A mechanistic approach to antiepileptic drug interactions. *Ann. Pharmacother., 32*(5), 554–563.

Andrezina, R., Josiassen, R. C., Marcus, R. N., Oren, D. A., Manos, G., Stock, E., et al. (2006). Intramuscular aripiprazole for the treatment of acute agitation in patients with schizophrenia or schizoaffective disorder: a double-blind, placebo-controlled comparison with intramuscular haloperidol. *Psychopharmacology (Berl), 188*(3), 281–292.

Angst, J., & Stabl, M. (1992). Efficacy of moclobemide in different patient groups: a meta-analysis of studies. *Psychopharmacology (Berl), 106*(Suppl), S109–S113.

Baillie, T. A. (1992). Metabolism of valproate to hepatotoxic intermediates. *Pharm. Weekbl. Sci., 14*(3A), 122–125.

Baker, G. B., Fang, J., Sinha, S., & Coutts, R. T. (1998). Metabolic drug interactions with selective serotonin reuptake inhibitor (SSRI) antidepressants. *Neurosci. Biobehav. Rev., 22*(2), 325–333.

Baldassano, C. F., Ghaemi, S. N., Chang, A., Lyman, A., & Lipari, M. (2004). Acute treatment of bipolar depression with adjunctive zonisamide: a retrospective chart review. *Bipolar Disord., 6*(5), 432–434.

Baldessarini, R. J., & Frankenburg, F. R. (1991). Clozapine. A novel antipsychotic agent. *N. Engl. J. Med., 324*(11), 746–754.

Baldessarini, R. J., Tondo, L., Davis, P., Pompili, M., Goodwin, F. K., & Hennen, J. (2006). Decreased risk of suicides and attempts during long-term lithium treatment: a meta-analytic review. *Bipolar Disord., 8*(5 Pt 2), 625–639.

Baldessarini, R. J., Tondo, L., Faedda, G. L., Suppes, T. R., Floris, G., & Rudas, N. (1996). Effects of the rate of discontinuing lithium maintenance treatment in bipolar disorders. *J. Clin. Psychiatry, 57*(10), 441–448.

Baptista, T., Teneud, L., Contreras, Q., Alastre, T., Burguera, J. L., de Burguera, M., et al. (1995). Lithium and body weight gain. *Pharmacopsychiatry, 28*(2), 35–44.

Baumann, P. (1992). Clinical pharmacokinetics of citalopram and other selective serotonergic reuptake inhibitors (SSRI). *Int. Clin. Psychopharmacol., 6*(Suppl 5), 13–20.

Beaumont, G. (1988). Adverse effects of tricyclic and non-tricyclic antidepressants. *Int. Clin. Psychopharmacol., 3*(Suppl 2), 55–61.

Bell, A. J., Cole, A., Eccleston, D., & Ferrier, I. N. (1993). Lithium neurotoxicity at normal therapeutic levels. *Br. J. Psychiatry, 162*, 689–692.

Ben-Menachem, E. (2004). Pregabalin pharmacology and its relevance to clinical practice. *Epilepsia, 45*(Suppl 6), 13–18.

Bersani, G. (2004). Levetiracetam in bipolar spectrum disorders: first evidence of efficacy in an open, add- on study. *Hum. Psychopharmacol., 19*(5), 355–356.

Bertilsson, L. (1978). Clinical pharmacokinetics of carbamazepine. *Clin. Pharmacokinet., 3*(2), 128–143.

Bertilsson, L., & Tomson, T. (1986). Clinical pharmacokinetics and pharmacological effects of carbamazepine and carbamazepine-10,11-epoxide. An update. *Clin. Pharmacokinet., 11*(3), 177–198.

Bialer, M. (2006). New antiepileptic drugs that are second generation to existing antiepileptic drugs. *Expert Opin. Investig Drugs, 15*(6), 637–647.

Blackwell, B. (1981). Adverse effects of antidepressant drugs. Part 1: monoamine oxidase inhibitors and tricyclics. *Drugs, 21*(3), 201–219.

Blier, P., de Montigny, C., & Chaput, Y. (1990). A role for the serotonin system in the mechanism of action of antidepressant treatments: preclinical evidence. *J. Clin. Psychiatry, 51*(Suppl), 14–20; discussion 21.

Bocchetta, A., Mossa, P., Velluzzi, F., Mariotti, S., Zompo, M. D., & Loviselli, A. (2001). Ten-year follow-up of thyroid function in lithium patients. *J. Clin. Psychopharmacol., 21*(6), 594–598.

Bourgeois, B. F. (1988). Pharmacologic interactions between valproate and other drugs. *Am. J. Med., 84*(1A), 29–33.

Bourgeois, B. F. (1999). Pharmacokinetics and metabolism of topiramate. *Drugs Today (Barc), 35*(1), 43–48.

Bowden, C. L., Brugger, A. M., Swann, A. C., Calabrese, J. R., Janicak, P. G., Petty, F., et al. (1994). Efficacy of divalproex vs lithium and placebo in the treatment of mania. The Depakote Mania Study Group. *JAMA, 271*(12), 918–924.

Bowden, C. L., Calabrese, J. R., Ketter, T. A., Sachs, G. S., White, R. L., & Thompson, T. R. (2006). Impact of lamotrigine and lithium on weight in obese and nonobese patients with bipolar I disorder. *Am. J. Psychiatry, 163*(7), 1199–1201.

Bowden, C. L., Calabrese, J. R., McElroy, S. L., Gyulai, L., Wassef, A., Petty, F., et al. (2000). A randomized, placebo-controlled 12-month trial of divalproex and lithium in treatment of outpatients with bipolar I disorder. Divalproex Maintenance Study Group. *Arch. Gen. Psychiatry, 57*(5), 481–489.

Bowden, C. L., Calabrese, J. R., Sachs, G., Yatham, L. N., Asghar, S. A., Hompland, M., et al. (2003). A placebo-controlled 18-month trial of lamotrigine and lithium maintenance treatment in recently manic or hypomanic patients with bipolar I disorder. *Arch. Gen. Psychiatry, 60*(4), 392–400.

Bowden, C. L., Grunze, H., Mullen, J., Brecher, M., Paulsson, B., Jones, M., et al. (2005). A randomized, double-blind, placebo-controlled efficacy and safety study of quetiapine or lithium as monotherapy for mania in bipolar disorder. *J. Clin. Psychiatry, 66*(1), 111–121.

Bowden, C. L., Janicak, P. G., Orsulak, P., Swann, A. C., Davis, J. M., Calabrese, J. R., et al. (1996). Relation of serum valproate concentration to response in mania. *Am. J. Psychiatry, 153*(6), 765–770.

Bowden, C. L., Swann, A. C., Calabrese, J. R., Rubenfaer, L. M., Wozniak, P. J., Collins, M. A., et al. (2006). A randomized, placebo-controlled, multicenter study of divalproex sodium extended release in the treatment of acute mania. *J. Clin. Psychiatry, 67*(10), 1501–1510.

Brandes, J. L., Saper, J. R., Diamond, M., Couch, J. R., Lewis, D. W., Schmitt, J., et al. (2004). Topiramate for migraine prevention: a randomized controlled trial. *JAMA, 291*(8), 965–973.

Braunig, P., & Kruger, S. (2003). Levetiracetam in the treatment of rapid cycling bipolar disorder. *J. Psychopharmacol., 17*(2), 239–241.

Bray, G. A., Hollander, P., Klein, S., Kushner, R., Levy, B., Fitchet, M., et al. (2003). A 6-month randomized, placebo-controlled, dose-ranging trial of topiramate for weight loss in obesity. *Obes. Res., 11*(6), 722–733.

Brodie, M. J. (1995). Tiagabine pharmacology in profile. *Epilepsia, 36*(Suppl 6), S7–9.

Brook, S., Lucey, J. V., & Gunn, K. P. (2000). Intramuscular ziprasidone compared with intramuscular haloperidol in the treatment of acute psychosis. Ziprasidone I.M. Study Group. *J. Clin. Psychiatry, 61*(12), 933–941.

Bryant, A. E., 3rd., & Dreifuss, F. E. (1996). Valproic acid hepatic fatalities. III. U.S. experience since 1986. *Neurology, 46*(2), 465–469.

Byerly, M. J., & DeVane, C. L. (1996). Pharmacokinetics of clozapine and risperidone: a review of recent literature. *J. Clin. Psychopharmacol., 16*(2), 177–187.

Bymaster, F. P., Calligaro, D. O., Falcone, J. F., Marsh, R. D., Moore, N. A., Tye, N. C., et al. (1996). Radioreceptor binding profile of the atypical antipsychotic olanzapine. *Neuropsychopharmacology, 14*(2), 87–96.

Calabrese, J. R., Bowden, C. L., Sachs, G., Yatham, L. N., Behnke, K., Mehtonen, O. P., et al. (2003). A placebo-controlled 18-month trial of lamotrigine and lithium maintenance treatment in recently depressed patients with bipolar I disorder. *J. Clin. Psychiatry, 64*(9), 1013–1024.

Calabrese, J. R., Bowden, C. L., Sachs, G. S., Ascher, J. A., Monaghan, E., & Rudd, G. D. (1999). Lamictal 602 Study Group. A double-blind placebo-controlled study of lamotrigine monotherapy in outpatients with bipolar I depression. *J. Clin. Psychiatry, 60*(2), 79–88.

Calabrese, J. R., Keck, P. E., Jr., Macfadden, W., Minkwitz, M., Ketter, T. A., Weisler, R. H., et al. (2005). A randomized, double-blind, placebo-controlled trial of quetiapine in the treatment of bipolar I or II depression. *Am. J. Psychiatry, 162*(7), 1351–1360.

Calabrese, J. R., Suppes, T., Bowden, C. L., Sachs, G. S., Swann, A. C., McElroy, S. L., et al. (2000). Lamictal 614 Study Group. A double-blind, placebo-controlled, prophylaxis study of lamotrigine in rapid-cycling bipolar disorder. *J. Clin. Psychiatry, 61*(11), 841–850.

Callaghan, J. T., Bergstrom, R. F., Ptak, L. R., & Beasley, C. M. (1999). Olanzapine. Pharmacokinetic and pharmacodynamic profile. *Clin. Pharmacokinet., 37*(3), 177–193.

Castrogiovanni, P. (2002). A novel slow-release formulation of lithium carbonate (Carbolithium Once-A-Day) vs. standard Carbolithium: a comparative pharmacokinetic study. *Clin. Ter., 153*(2), 107–115.

Cesura, A. M., Kettler, R., Imhof, R., & Da Prada, M. (1992). Mode of action and characteristics of monoamine oxidase-A inhibition by moclobemide. *Psychopharmacology (Berl), 106*(Suppl), S15–16.

Chapman, A., Keane, P. E., Meldrum, B. S., Simiand, J., & Vernieres, J. C. (1982). Mechanism of anticonvulsant action of valproate. *Prog. Neurobiol., 19*(4), 315–359.

Charles, C. L., Stoesz, L., & Tollefson, G. (1990). Zonisamide-induced mania. *Psychosomatics, 31*(2), 214–217.

Chen, C., Veronese, L., & Yin, Y. (2000). The effects of lamotrigine on the pharmacokinetics of lithium. *Br. J. Clin. Pharmacol., 50*(3), 193–195.

Chen, G., Manji, H. K., Hawver, D. B., Wright, C. B., & Potter, W. Z. (1994). Chronic sodium valproate selectively decreases protein kinase C alpha and epsilon in vitro. *J. Neurochem., 63*(6), 2361–2364.

Christensen, J., Petrenaite, V., Atterman, J., Sidenius, P., Ohman, I., Tomson, T., et al. (2007). Oral contraceptives induce lamotrigine metabolism: Evidence from a double-blind, placebo-controlled trial. *Epilepsia, 48*(3), 484–489.

Cohen, A. F., Land, G. S., Breimer, D. D., Yuen, W. C., Winton, C., & Peck, A. W. (1987). Lamotrigine, a new anticonvulsant: pharmacokinetics in normal humans. *Clin. Pharmacol. Ther., 42*(5), 535–541.

Cohen, L. S., Friedman, J. M., Jefferson, J. W., Johnson, E. M., & Weiner, M. L. (1994). A reevaluation of risk of in utero exposure to lithium. *JAMA, 271*(2), 146–150.

Cohen, L. S., Sichel, D. A., Robertson, L. M., Heckscher, E., & Rosenbaum, J. F. (1995). Postpartum prophylaxis for women with bipolar disorder. *Am. J. Psychiatry, 152*(11), 1641–1645.

Cohn, J. B., Collins, G., Ashbrook, E., & Wernicke, J. F. (1989). A comparison of fluoxetine imipramine and placebo in patients with bipolar depressive disorder. *Int. Clin. Psychopharmacol., 4*(4), 313–322.

Conley, R. R., & Meltzer, H. Y. (2000). Adverse events related to olanzapine. *J. Clin. Psychiatry, 61*(Suppl 8), 26–29; discussion 30.

Coupez, R., Nicolas, J. M., & Browne, T. R. (2003). Levetiracetam, a new antiepileptic agent: lack of in vitro and in vivo pharmacokinetic interaction with valproic acid. *Epilepsia, 44*(2), 171–178.

Cramer, J. A., De Rue, K., Devinsky, O., Edrich, P., & Trimble, M. R. (2003). A systematic review of the behavioral effects of levetiracetam in adults with epilepsy, cognitive disorders, or an anxiety disorder during clinical trials. *Epilepsy Behav., 4*(2), 124–132.

Crawford, P. (2002). Interactions between antiepileptic drugs and hormonal contraception. *CNS Drugs, 16*(4), 263–272.

Crawford, P., Chadwick, D. J., Martin, C., Tjia, J., Back, D. J., & Orme, M. (1990). The interaction of phenytoin and carbamazepine with combined oral contraceptive steroids. *Br. J. Clin. Pharmacol., 30*(6), 892–896.

Crofford, L. J., Rowbotham, M. C., Mease, P. J., Russell, I. J., Dworkin, R. H., Corbin, A. E., et al. (2005). Pregabalin for the treatment of fibromyalgia syndrome: results of a randomized, double-blind, placebo-controlled trial. *Arthritis Rheum., 52*(4), 1264–1273.

Cunnington, M. C. (2004). The International Lamotrigine pregnancy registry update for the epilepsy foundation. *Epilepsia, 45*(11), 1468.

Dam, M., Ekberg, R., Loyning, Y., Waltimo, O., & Jakobsen, K. (1989). A double-blind study comparing oxcarbazepine and carbamazepine in patients with newly diagnosed, previously untreated epilepsy. *Epilepsy Res., 3*(1), 70–76.

Daniel, D. G. (2003). Tolerability of ziprasidone: an expanding perspective. *J. Clin. Psychiatry, 64*(Suppl 19), 40–49.

Daniel, D. G., Potkin, S. G., Reeves, K. R., Swift, R. H., & Harrigan, E. P. (2001). Intramuscular (IM) ziprasidone 20 mg is effective in reducing acute agitation associated with psychosis: a double-blind, randomized, trial. *Psychopharmacology (Berl), 155*(2), 128–134.

De Leon, J. (2003). Glucuronidation enzymes, genes and psychiatry. *Int. J. Neuropsychopharmacol., 6*(1), 57–72.

Delva, N. J., & Hawken, E. R. (2001). Preventing lithium intoxication. Guide for physicians. *Can. Fam. Physician, 47*, 1595–1600.

Denicoff, K. D., Smith-Jackson, E. E., Disney, E. R., Ali, S. O., Leverich, G. S., & Post, R. M. (1997). Comparative prophylactic efficacy of lithium, carbamazepine, and the combination in bipolar disorder. *J. Clin. Psychiatry, 58*(11), 470–478.

DeVane, C. L. (2003). Pharmacokinetics, drug interactions, and tolerability of valproate. *Psychopharmacol. Bull., 37*(Suppl 2), 25–42.

DeVane, C. L., & Nemeroff, C. B. (2001). Clinical pharmacokinetics of quetiapine: an atypical antipsychotic. *Clin. Pharmacokinet., 40*(7), 509–522.

Dinan, T. G. (2002). Lithium in bipolar mood disorder. *BMJ, 324*(7344), 989–990.

Dooley, D. J., Donovan, C. M., Meder, W. P., & Whetzel, S. Z. (2002). Preferential action of gabapentin and pregabalin at P/Q-type voltage-sensitive calcium channels: inhibition of K+-evoked [3H]-norepinephrine release from rat neocortical slices. *Synapse, 45*(3), 171–190.

Dooley, D. J., Donovan, C. M., & Pugsley, T. A. (2000). Stimulus-dependent modulation of [(3)H]norepinephrine release from rat neocortical slices by gabapentin and pregabalin. *J. Pharmacol. Exp. Ther., 295*(3), 1086–1093.

Dooley, D. J., Mieske, C. A., & Borosky, S. A. (2000). Inhibition of K(+)-evoked glutamate release from rat neocortical and hippocampal slices by gabapentin. *Neurosci. Lett., 280*(2), 107–110.

Doose, D. R., Wang, S. S., Padmanabhan, M., Schwabe, S., Jacobs, D., & Bialer, M. (2003). Effect of topiramate or carbamazepine on the pharmacokinetics of an oral contraceptive containing norethindrone and ethinyl estradiol in healthy obese and nonobese female subjects. *Epilepsia, 44*(4), 540–549.

Dreifuss, F. E., & Langer, D. H. (1988). Side effects of valproate. *Am. J. Med., 84*(1A), 34–41.

Dworkin, R. H., Corbin, A. E., Young, J. P., Jr., Sharma, U., LaMoreaux, L., Bockbrader, H., et al. (2003). Pregabalin for the treatment of postherpetic neuralgia: a randomized, placebo-controlled trial. *Neurology, 60*(8), 1274–1283.

Emrich, H. M. (1990). Studies with (Trileptal) oxcarbazepine in acute mania. *Int. Clin. Psychopharmacol., 5*(Suppl 1), 83–88.

Emrich, H. M., Altmann, H., Dose, M., & von Zerssen, D. (1983). Therapeutic effects of GABA-ergic drugs in affective disorders. A preliminary report. *Pharmacol. Biochem. Behav., 19*(2), 369–372.

Errante, L. D., & Petroff, O. A. (2003). Acute effects of gabapentin and pregabalin on rat forebrain cellular GABA, glutamate, and glutamine concentrations. *Seizure, 12*(5), 300–306.

Ethell, B. T., Anderson, G. D., & Burchell, B. (2003). The effect of valproic acid on drug and steroid glucuronidation by expressed human UDP-glucuronosyltransferases. *Biochem. Pharmacol., 65*(9), 1441–1449.

Fattore, C., Cipolla, G., Gatti, G., Limido, G. L., Sturm, Y., Bernasconi, C., et al. (1999). Induction of ethinylestradiol and levonorgestrel metabolism by oxcarbazepine in healthy women. *Epilepsia, 40*(6), 783–787.

Faught, E. (2004). Review of United States and European clinical trials of zonisamide in the treatment of refractory partial-onset seizures. *Seizure, 13*(Suppl 1), S59–S65; discussion S71–S52.

Fava, M., Mulroy, R., Alpert, J., Nierenberg, A. A., & Rosenbaum, J. F. (1997). Emergence of adverse events following discontinuation of treatment with extended-release venlafaxine. *Am. J. Psychiatry, 154*(12), 1760–1762.

Feltner, D. E., Crockatt, J. G., Dubovsky, S. J., Cohn, C. K., Shrivastava, R. K., Targum, S. D., et al. (2003). A randomized, double-blind, placebo-controlled, fixed-dose, multicenter study of pregabalin in patients with generalized anxiety disorder. *J. Clin. Psychopharmacol., 23*(3), 240–249.

Fink, K., Dooley, D. J., Meder, W. P., Suman-Chauhan, N., Duffy, S., Clusmann, H., et al. (2002). Inhibition of neuronal Ca(2+) influx by gabapentin and pregabalin in the human neocortex. *Neuropharmacology, 42*(2), 229–236.

Finley, P. R., Warner, M. D., & Peabody, C. A. (1995). Clinical relevance of drug interactions with lithium. *Clin. Pharmacokinet., 29*(3), 172–191.

Fitton, A., & Heel, R. C. (1990). Clozapine. A review of its pharmacological properties, and therapeutic use in schizophrenia. *Drugs, 40*(5), 722–747.

Fleischhacker, W. W., Hummer, M., Kurz, M., Kurzthaler, I., Lieberman, J. A., Pollack, S., et al. (1994). Clozapine dose in the United States and Europe: implications for therapeutic and adverse effects. *J. Clin. Psychiatry, 55*(Suppl B), 78–81.

Freeman, D. J., & Oyewumi, L. K. (1997). Will routine therapeutic drug monitoring have a place in clozapine therapy? *Clin. Pharmacokinet., 32*(2), 93–100.

Freynhagen, R., Strojek, K., Griesing, T., Whalen, E., & Balkenohl, M. (2005). Efficacy of pregabalin in neuropathic pain evaluated in a 12-week, randomised, double-blind, multicentre, placebo-controlled trial of flexible- and fixed-dose regimens. *Pain, 115*(3), 254–263.

Friis, M. L., Kristensen, O., Boas, J., Dalby, M., Deth, S. H., Gram, L., et al. (1993). Therapeutic experiences with 947 epileptic out-patients in oxcarbazepine treatment. *Acta Neurol. Scand., 87*(3), 224–227.

Froscher, W., Schier, K. R., Hoffmann, M., Meyer, A., May, T. W., Rambeck, B., et al. (2005). Topiramate: a prospective study on the relationship between concentration, dosage and adverse events in epileptic patients on combination therapy. *Epileptic Disord., 7*(3), 237–248.

Frye, M. A., Ketter, T. A., Altshuler, L. L., Denicoff, K., Dunn, R. T., Kimbrell, T. A., et al. (1998). Clozapine in bipolar disorder: treatment implications for other atypical antipsychotics. *J. Affect. Disord., 48*(2–3), 91–104.

Frye, M. A., Ketter, T. A., Kimbrell, T. A., Dunn, R. T., Speer, A. M., Osuch, E. A., et al. (2000). A placebo-controlled study of lamotrigine and gabapentin monotherapy in refractory mood disorders. *J. Clin. Psychopharmacol., 20*(6), 607–614.

Frye, M. A., Kimbrell, T. A., Dunn, R. T., Piscitelli, S., Grothe, D., Vanderham, E., et al. (1998). Gabapentin does not alter single-dose lithium pharmacokinetics. *J. Clin. Psychopharmacol., 18*(6), 461–464.

Gardner, D. M., Shulman, K. I., Walker, S. E., & Tailor, S. A. (1996). The making of a user friendly MAOI diet. *J. Clin. Psychiatry, 57*(3), 99–104.

Garnett, W. R., Levy, B., McLean, A. M., Zhang, Y., Couch, R. A., Rudnic, E. M., et al. (1998). Pharmacokinetic evaluation of twice-daily extended-release carbamazepine (CBZ) and four-times-daily immediate-release CBZ in patients with epilepsy. *Epilepsia, 39*(3), 274–279.

Gee, N. S., Brown, J. P., Dissanayake, V. U., Offord, J., Thurlow, R., & Woodruff, G. N. (1996). The novel anticonvulsant drug, gabapentin (Neurontin), binds to the alpha2delta subunit of a calcium channel. *J. Biol. Chem., 271*(10), 5768–5776.

Gelenberg, A. J. (1988). Lithium efficacy and adverse effects. *J. Clin. Psychiatry, 49* (Suppl), 8–11.

Gelenberg, A. J., Kane, J. M., Keller, M. B., Lavori, P., Rosenbaum, J. F., Cole, K., et al. (1989). Comparison of standard and low serum levels of lithium for maintenance treatment of bipolar disorder. *N. Engl. J. Med., 321*(22), 1489–1493.

Gentile, S. (2006). Prophylactic treatment of bipolar disorder in pregnancy and breastfeeding: focus on emerging mood stabilizers. *Bipolar Disord., 8*(3), 207–220.

Ghaemi, S. N., Zablotsky, B., Filkowski, M. M., Dunn, R. T., Pardo, T. B., Isenstein, E., et al. (2006). An open prospective study of zonisamide in acute bipolar depression. *J. Clin. Psychopharmacol., 26*(4), 385–388.

Gidal, B. E., Anderson, G. D., Spencer, N. W., Maly, M., Murty, J., Pitterle, M., et al. (1994). Valproic acid (VPA) associated weight gain in monotherapy patients with epilepsy. Paper presented at the Annual Meeting of the American Epilepsy Society, New Orleans, LA, December 2–8.

Gidal, B. E., & Lensmeyer, G. L. (1999). Therapeutic monitoring of topiramate: evaluation of the saturable distribution between erythrocytes and plasma of whole blood using an optimized high-pressure liquid chromatography method. *Ther. Drug Monit., 21*(5), 567–576.

Gijsman, H. J., Geddes, J. R., Rendell, J. M., Nolen, W. A., & Goodwin, G. M. (2004). Antidepressants for bipolar depression: a systematic review of randomized, controlled trials. *Am. J. Psychiatry, 161*(9), 1537–1547.

Gillman, P. K. (2006). A systematic review of the serotonergic effects of mirtazap-ine in humans: implications for its dual action status. *Hum. Psychopharmacol.,* 21(2), 117–125.

Gitlin, M. J., Cochran, S. D., & Jamison, K. R. (1989). Maintenance lithium treat-ment: side effects and compliance. *J. Clin. Psychiatry,* 50(4), 127–131.

Goa, K. L., & Sorkin, E. M. (1993). Gabapentin. A review of its pharmacological properties and clinical potential in epilepsy. *Drugs,* 46(3), 409–427.

Goldberg, J. F., & Burdick, K. E. (2002). Levetiracetam for acute mania. *Am. J. Psychiatry,* 159(1), 148.

Goodman, W. K., & Charney, D. S. (1985). Therapeutic applications and mecha-nisms of action of monoamine oxidase inhibitor and heterocyclic antidepres-sant drugs. *J. Clin. Psychiatry,* 46(10 Pt 2), 6–24.

Goodnick, P. J. (1991). Pharmacokinetics of second generation antidepressants: bupropion. *Psychopharmacol. Bull.,* 27(4), 513–519.

Goodnick, P. J. (2001). Ziprasidone: profile on safety. *Expert Opin. Pharmacother.,* 2(10), 1655–1662.

Gordey, M., DeLorey, T. M., & Olsen, R. W. (2000). Differential sensitivity of recom-binant GABA(A) receptors expressed in Xenopus oocytes to modulation by topiramate. *Epilepsia,* 41(Suppl 1), S25–29.

Gram, L. F. (1980). Pharmacokinetics and clinical response to tricyclic antidepres-sants. *Acta Psychiatr. Scand. Suppl.,* 280, 169–180.

Granneman, G. R., Schneck, D. W., Cavanaugh, J. H., & Witt, G. F. (1996). Pharmacoki-netic interactions and side effects resulting from concomitant administration of lithium and divalproex sodium. *J. Clin. Psychiatry,* 57(5), 204–206.

Graves, N. M. (1995). Neuropharmacology and drug interactions in clinical prac-tice. *Epilepsia,* 36(Suppl 2), S27–33.

Graves, N. M., Brundage, R. C., Wen, Y., Cascino, G., So, E., Ahman, P., et al. (1998). Population pharmacokinetics of carbamazepine in adults with epilepsy. *Pharmacotherapy,* 18(2), 273–281.

Greene, D. S., & Barbhaiya, R. H. (1997). Clinical pharmacokinetics of nefazodone. *Clin. Pharmacokinet.,* 33(4), 260–275.

Greil, W., Ludwig-Mayerhofer, W., Erazo, N., Schochlin, C., Schmidt, S., Engel, R. R., et al. (1997). Lithium versus carbamazepine in the maintenance treatment of bipolar disorders--a randomised study. *J. Affect. Disord.,* 43(2), 151–161.

Grohmann, R., Ruther, E., Sassim, N., & Schmidt, L. G. (1989). Adverse effects of clozapine. *Psychopharmacology (Berl),* 99(Suppl), S101–104.

Grunze, H., Erfurth, A., Marcuse, A., Amann, B., Normann, C., & Walden, J. (1999). Tiagabine appears not to be efficacious in the treatment of acute mania. *J. Clin. Psychiatry,* 60(11), 759–762.

Grunze, H., Langosch, J., Born, C., Schaub, G., & Walden, J. (2003). Levetiracetam in the treatment of acute mania: an open add-on study with an on-off-on design. *J. Clin. Psychiatry,* 64(7), 781–784.

Gustavson, L. E., & Mengel, H. B. (1995). Pharmacokinetics of tiagabine, a gamma-aminobutyric acid-uptake inhibitor, in healthy subjects after single and mul-tiple doses. *Epilepsia,* 36(6), 605–611.

Hamelin, B. A., Allard, S., Laplante, L., Miceli, J., Wilner, K. D., Tremblay, J., et al. (1998). The effect of timing of a standard meal on the pharmacokinetics and pharmacodynamics of the novel atypical antipsychotic agent ziprasidone. *Pharmacotherapy,* 18(1), 9–15.

Handforth, A., & Martin, F. C. (2004). Pilot efficacy and tolerability: a randomized, placebo-controlled trial of levetiracetam for essential tremor. *Mov. Disord.*, *19*(10), 1215–1221.

Hansen, H. E., & Amdisen, A. (1978). Lithium intoxication. (Report of 23 cases and review of 100 cases from the literature). *Q. J. Med.*, *47*(186), 123–144.

Harden, C. (2001). Safety profile of levetiracetam. *Epilepsia*, *42*(Suppl 4), 36–39.

Harvey, N. S., & Merriman, S. (1994). Review of clinically important drug interactions with lithium. *Drug Saf.*, *10*(6), 455–463.

Harvey, P. D., & Bowie, C. R. (2005). Ziprasidone: efficacy, tolerability, and emerging data on wide-ranging effectiveness. *Expert Opin. Pharmacother.*, *6*(2), 337–346.

Hasegawa, M., Gutierrez-Esteinou, R., Way, L., & Meltzer, H. Y. (1993). Relationship between clinical efficacy and clozapine concentrations in plasma in schizophrenia: effect of smoking. *J. Clin. Psychopharmacol.*, *13*(6), 383–390.

Hasselstrom, J., & Linnet, K. (2006). In vitro studies on quetiapine metabolism using the substrate depletion approach with focus on drug-drug interactions. *Drug Metabol. Drug Interact.*, *21*(3–4), 187–211.

He, H., & Richardson, J. S. (1995). A pharmacological, pharmacokinetic and clinical overview of risperidone, a new antipsychotic that blocks serotonin 5-HT2 and dopamine D2 receptors. *Int. Clin. Psychopharmacol.*, *10*(1), 19–30.

Henry, C. (2002). Lithium side-effects and predictors of hypothyroidism in patients with bipolar disorder: sex differences. *J. Psychiatry Neurosci.*, *27*(2), 104–107.

Himmelhoch, J. M., Thase, M. E., Mallinger, A. G., & Houck, P. (1991). Tranylcypromine versus imipramine in anergic bipolar depression. *Am. J. Psychiatry*, *148*(7), 910–916.

Hirschfeld, R. M. (1999). Management of sexual side effects of antidepressant therapy. *J. Clin. Psychiatry*, *60*(Suppl 14), 27–30; discussion 31–25.

Hirschfeld, R. M., Keck, P. E., Jr., Kramer, M., Karcher, K., Canuso, C., Eerdekens, M., et al. (2004). Rapid antimanic effect of risperidone monotherapy: a 3-week multicenter, double-blind, placebo-controlled trial. *Am. J. Psychiatry*, *161*(6), 1057–1065.

Hirschfeld, R. M., Williams, J. B., Spitzer, R. L., Calabrese, J. R., Flynn, L., Keck, P. E., Jr., et al. (2000). Development and validation of a screening instrument for bipolar spectrum disorder: the Mood Disorder Questionnaire. *Am. J. Psychiatry*, *157*(11), 1873–1875.

Hoopes, S. P., Reimherr, F. W., Hedges, D. W., Rosenthal, N. R., Kamin, M., Karim, R., et al. (2003). Treatment of bulimia nervosa with topiramate in a randomized, double-blind, placebo-controlled trial, part 1: improvement in binge and purge measures. *J. Clin. Psychiatry*, *64*(11), 1335–1341.

Horst, W. D., & Preskorn, S. H. (1998). Mechanisms of action and clinical characteristics of three atypical antidepressants: venlafaxine, nefazodone, bupropion. *J. Affect. Disord.*, *51*(3), 237–254.

Iqbal, M. M., Rahman, A., Husain, Z., Mahmud, S. Z., Ryan, W. G., & Feldman, J. M. (2003). Clozapine: a clinical review of adverse effects and management. *Ann. Clin. Psychiatry*, *15*(1), 33–48.

Isojarvi, J. I., Laatikainen, T. J., Pakarinen, A. J., Juntunen, K. T., & Myllyla, V. V. (1993). Polycystic ovaries and hyperandrogenism in women taking valproate for epilepsy. *N. Engl. J. Med.*, *329*(19), 1383–1388.

Jann, M. W., Grimsley, S. R., Gray, E. C., & Chang, W. H. (1993). Pharmacokinetics and pharmacodynamics of clozapine. *Clin. Pharmacokinet., 24*(2), 161–176.

Javaid, J. I. (1994). Clinical pharmacokinetics of antipsychotics. *J. Clin. Pharmacol., 34*(4), 286–295.

Jefferson, J. W., Greist, J. H., Ackerman, D. L., & Carroll, J. A. (1987). *Lithium Encyclopedia for Clinical Practice* (2nd Edition). Washington, DC: American Psychiatric Press, Inc.

Jefferson, J. W., Greist, J. H., & Baudhuin, M. (1981). Lithium: interactions with other drugs. *J. Clin. Psychopharmacol., 1*(3), 124–134.

Joffe, H., Cohen, L. S., Suppes, T., McLaughlin, W. L., Lavori, P., Adams, J. M., et al. (2006). Valproate is associated with new-onset oligoamenorrhea with hyperandrogenism in women with bipolar disorder. *Biol. Psychiatry, 59*(11), 1078–1086.

Johannessen, S. I., Battino, D., Berry, D. J., Bialer, M., Kramer, G., Tomson, T., et al. (2003). Therapeutic drug monitoring of the newer antiepileptic drugs. *Ther. Drug Monit., 25*(3), 347–363.

Johnson, B. A., Ait-Daoud, N., Bowden, C. L., DiClemente, C. C., Roache, J. D., Lawson, K., et al. (2003). Oral topiramate for treatment of alcohol dependence: a randomised controlled trial. *Lancet, 361*(9370), 1677–1685.

Johnson, G., Gershon, S., Burdock, E. I., Floyd, A., & Hekimian, L. (1971). Comparative effects of lithium and chlorpromazine in the treatment of acute manic states. *Br. J. Psychiatry, 119*(550), 267–276.

Jones, K. L., Lacro, R. V., Johnson, K. A., & Adams, J. (1989). Pattern of malformations in the children of women treated with carbamazepine during pregnancy. *N. Engl. J. Med., 320*(25), 1661–1666.

Jope, R. S. (1999). Anti-bipolar therapy: mechanism of action of lithium. *Mol. Psychiatry, 4*(2), 117–128.

Kanba, S., Yagi, G., Kamijima, K., Suzuki, T., Tajima, O., Otaki, J., et al. (1994). The first open study of zonisamide, a novel anticonvulsant, shows efficacy in mania. *Prog. Neuropsychopharmacol. Biol. Psychiatry, 18*(4), 707–715.

Kane, J. M., Eerdekens, M., Lindenmayer, J. P., Keith, S. J., Lesem, M., & Karcher, K. (2003). Long-acting injectable risperidone: efficacy and safety of the first long-acting atypical antipsychotic. *Am. J. Psychiatry, 160*(6), 1125–1132.

Kane, J. M., & Smith, J. M. (1982). Tardive dyskinesia: prevalence and risk factors, 1959 to 1979. *Arch. Gen. Psychiatry, 39*(4), 473–481.

Kaneko, S., Okada, M., Hirano, T., Kondo, T., Otani, K., & Fukushima, Y. (1993). Carbamazepine and zonisamide increase extracellular dopamine and serotonin levels in vivo, and carbamazepine does not antagonize adenosine effect in vitro: mechanisms of blockade of seizure spread. *Jpn. J. Psychiatry Neurol., 47*(2), 371–373.

Kasamo, K., Blier, P., & De Montigny, C. (1996). Blockade of the serotonin and norepinephrine uptake processes by duloxetine: in vitro and in vivo studies in the rat brain. *J. Pharmacol. Exp. Ther., 277*(1), 278–286.

Kaufman, K. R. (2004). Monotherapy treatment of bipolar disorder with levetiracetam. *Epilepsy Behav., 5*(6), 1017–1020.

Keck, P. E., Calabrese, J. R., McQuade, R. D., Carson, W. H., Carlson, B. X., Rollin, L. M., et al. (2006). A randomized, double-blind, placebo-controlled 26-week trial of aripiprazole in recently manic patients with bipolar I disorder. *J. Clin. Psychiatry, 67*(4), 626–637.

Keck, P. E., Jr., Marcus, R., Tourkodimitris, S., Ali, M., Liebeskind, A., Saha, A., et al. (2003a). A placebo-controlled, double-blind study of the efficacy and safety of aripiprazole in patients with acute bipolar mania. *Am. J. Psychiatry, 160*(9), 1651–1658.

Keck, P. E., Jr., Versiani, M., Potkin, S., West, S. A., Giller, E., & Ice, K. (2003b). Ziprasidone in the treatment of acute bipolar mania: a three-week, placebo-controlled, double-blind, randomized trial. *Am. J. Psychiatry, 160*(4), 741–748.

Keltner, N. L., McAfee, K. M., & Taylor, C. L. (2002). Mechanisms and treatments of SSRI-induced sexual dysfunction. *Perspect. Psychiatr. Care, 38*(3), 111–116.

Ketter, T. A., Flockhart, D. A., Post, R. M., Denicoff, K., Pazzaglia, P. J., Marangell, L. B., et al. (1995). The emerging role of cytochrome P450 3A in psychopharmacology. *J. Clin. Psychopharmacol., 15*(6), 387–398.

Ketter, T. A., Kalali, A. H., & Weisler, R. H. (2004). A 6-month, multicenter, open-label evaluation of beaded, extended-release carbamazepine capsule monotherapy in bipolar disorder patients with manic or mixed episodes. *J. Clin. Psychiatry, 65*(5), 668–673.

Ketter, T. A., Malow, B. A., Flamini, R., Ko, D., White, S. R., Post, R. M., et al. (1996). Felbamate monotherapy has stimulant-like effects in patients with epilepsy. *Epilepsy Res., 23*(2), 129–137.

Ketter, T. A., Manji, H. K., & Post, R. M. (2003). Potential mechanisms of action of lamotrigine in the treatment of bipolar disorders. *J. Clin. Psychopharmacol., 23*(5), 484–495.

Ketter, T. A., Post, R. M., Parekh, P. I., & Worthington, K. (1995). Addition of monoamine oxidase inhibitors to carbamazepine: preliminary evidence of safety and antidepressant efficacy in treatment-resistant depression. *J. Clin. Psychiatry, 56*(10), 471–475.

Ketter, T. A., Post, R. M., & Worthington, K. (1991a). Principles of clinically important drug interactions with carbamazepine. Part I. *J. Clin. Psychopharmacol., 11*(3), 198–203.

Ketter, T. A., Post, R. M., & Worthington, K. (1991b). Principles of clinically important drug interactions with carbamazepine. Part II. *J. Clin. Psychopharmacol., 11*(5), 306–313.

Ketter, T. A., Wang, P. W., Chandler, R. A., Alarcon, A. M., Becker, O. V., Nowakowska, C., et al. (2005). Dermatology precautions and slower titration yield low incidence of lamotrigine treatment-emergent rash. *J. Clin. Psychiatry, 66*(5), 642–645.

Ketter, T. A., Wang, P. W., Nowakowska, C., Marsh, W. K., & Bonner, J. C. (2005). Treatment of acute mania in bipolar disorder. In T. A. Ketter (Ed.), *Advances in the Treatment of Bipolar Disorder* (pp. 11–55). Washington, DC: American Psychiatric Publishing, Inc.

Khanna, S., Hirschfeld, R. M. A., Karcher, K., Grossman, F., & Kramer, M. L. (2003). Risperidone monotherapy in acute bipolar mania. Paper presented at the 156th Annual Meeting of the American Psychiatric Association, San Francisco, CA, May 17–22.

Kiang, T. K., Ho, P. C., Anari, M. R., Tong, V., Abbott, F. S., & Chang, T. K. (2006). Contribution of CYP2C9, CYP2A6, and CYP2B6 to valproic acid metabolism in hepatic microsomes from individuals with the CYP2C9*1/*1 genotype. *Toxicol. Sci., 94*(2), 261–271.

Kito, M., Maehara, M., & Watanabe, K. (1996). Mechanisms of T-type calcium channel blockade by zonisamide. *Seizure, 5*(2), 115–119.

Kleiner, J., Altshuler, L., Hendrick, V., & Hershman, J. M. (1999). Lithium-induced subclinical hypothyroidism: review of the literature and guidelines for treatment. *J. Clin. Psychiatry, 60*(4), 249–255.

Klosterskov Jensen, P., Saano, V., Haring, P., Svenstrup, B., & Menge, G. P. (1992). Possible interaction between oxcarbazepine and an oral contraceptive. *Epilepsia, 33*(6), 1149–1152.

Kramlinger, K. G., Phillips, K. A., & Post, R. M. (1994). Rash complicating carbamazepine treatment. *J. Clin. Psychopharmacol., 14*(6), 408–413.

Kronig, M. H., Munne, R. A., Szymanski, S., Safferman, A. Z., Pollack, S., Cooper, T., et al. (1995). Plasma clozapine levels and clinical response for treatment-refractory schizophrenic patients. *Am. J. Psychiatry, 152*(2), 179–182.

Kushner, S. F., Khan, A., Lane, R., & Olson, W. H. (2006). Topiramate monotherapy in the management of acute mania: results of four double-blind placebo-controlled trials. *Bipolar Disord., 8*(1), 15–27.

Kusturica, J., Zulic, I., Loga-Zec, S., Mulabegovic, N., Loga, S., & Kapic, E. (2002). Frequency and characteristics of side effects associated with antidepressant drugs. *Bosn. J. Basic Med. Sci., 2*(1–2), 5–11.

Kyomen, H. H. (2006). The use of levetiracetam to decrease mania in elderly bipolar patients. *Am. J. Geriatr. Psychiatry, 14*(11), 985.

Lamberty, Y., Margineanu, D. G., & Klitgaard, H. (2001). Effect of the new antiepileptic drug levetiracetam in an animal model of mania. *Epilepsy Behav., 2*(5), 454–459.

Lantz, R. J., Gillespie, T. A., Rash, T. J., Kuo, F., Skinner, M., Kuan, H. Y., et al. (2003). Metabolism, excretion, and pharmacokinetics of duloxetine in healthy human subjects. *Drug Metab. Dispos., 31*(9), 1142–1150.

LaRoche, S. M., & Helmers, S. L. (2004). The new antiepileptic drugs: scientific review. *JAMA, 291*(5), 605–614.

Lawler, C. P., Prioleau, C., Lewis, M. M., Mak, C., Jiang, D., Schetz, J. A., et al. (1999). Interactions of the novel antipsychotic aripiprazole (OPC-14597) with dopamine and serotonin receptor subtypes. *Neuropsychopharmacology, 20*(6), 612–627.

Lee, D. O., Steingard, R. J., Cesena, M., Helmers, S. L., Riviello, J. J., & Mikati, M. A. (1996). Behavioral side effects of gabapentin in children. *Epilepsia, 37*(1), 87–90.

Lenox, R. H., & Hahn, C. G. (2000). Overview of the mechanism of action of lithium in the brain: fifty-year update. *J. Clin. Psychiatry, 61*(Suppl 9), 5–15.

Lenzer, J. (2005). FDA warns that antidepressants may increase suicidality in adults. *BMJ, 331*(7508), 70.

Leppik, I. E. (1995). Tiagabine: the safety landscape. *Epilepsia, 36* (Suppl 6), S10–S13.

Leppik, I. E. (2004). Zonisamide: chemistry, mechanism of action, and pharmacokinetics. *Seizure, 13*(Suppl 1), S5–9; discussion S10.

Lerner, V., Bergman, J., Statsenko, N., & Miodownik, C. (2004). Vitamin B6 treatment in acute neuroleptic-induced akathisia: a randomized, double-blind, placebo-controlled study. *J. Clin. Psychiatry, 65*(11), 1550–1554.

Lesem, M. D., Zajecka, J. M., Swift, R. H., Reeves, K. R., & Harrigan, E. P. (2001). Intramuscular ziprasidone, 2 mg versus 10 mg, in the short-term management of agitated psychotic patients. *J. Clin. Psychiatry, 62*(1), 12–18.

Li, X., Ketter, T. A., & Frye, M. A. (2002). Synaptic, intracellular, and neuroprotective mechanisms of anticonvulsants: are they relevant for the treatment and course of bipolar disorders? *J. Affect. Disord., 69*(1–3), 1–14.

Licinio, J., & Wong, M. L. (2005). Depression, antidepressants and suicidality: a critical appraisal. *Nat. Rev. Drug Discov., 4*(2), 165–171.

Lima, A. R., Bacalcthuk, J., Barnes, T. R., & Soares-Weiser, K. (2004). Central action beta-blockers versus placebo for neuroleptic-induced acute akathisia. *Cochrane Database Syst. Rev.* (4), CD001946.

Lima, A. R., Soares-Weiser, K., Bacaltchuk, J., & Barnes, T. R. (2002). Benzodiazepines for neuroleptic-induced acute akathisia. *Cochrane Database Syst. Rev.* (1), CD001950.

Lima, A. R., Weiser, K. V., Bacaltchuk, J., & Barnes, T. R. (2004). Anticholinergics for neuroleptic-induced acute akathisia. *Cochrane Database Syst. Rev.* (1), CD003727.

Lima, W. J., Dopheide, J. A., Kramer, B. A., Earhart, C. A., & Wincor, M. Z. (1999). A naturalistic comparison of adverse effects between slow titration and loading of divalproex sodium in psychiatric inpatients. *J. Affect. Disord., 52*(1–3), 261–267.

Lin, J. H., & Lu, A. Y. (1998). Inhibition and induction of cytochrome P450 and the clinical implications. *Clin. Pharmacokinet., 35*(5), 361–390.

Livingston, M. G., & Livingston, H. M. (1996). Monoamine oxidase inhibitors. An update on drug interactions. *Drug Saf., 14*(4), 219–227.

Livingstone, C., & Rampes, H. (2006). Lithium: a review of its metabolic adverse effects. *J. Psychopharmacol., 20*(3), 347–355.

Loscher, W., Honack, D., & Bloms-Funke, P. (1996). The novel antiepileptic drug levetiracetam (ucb L059) induces alterations in GABA metabolism and turnover in discrete areas of rat brain and reduces neuronal activity in substantia nigra pars reticulata. *Brain Res., 735*(2), 208–216.

Loscher, W., Honack, D., & Rundfeldt, C. (1998). Antiepileptogenic effects of the novel anticonvulsant levetiracetam (ucb L059) in the kindling model of temporal lobe epilepsy. *J. Pharmacol. Exp. Ther., 284*(2), 474–479.

Lynch, B. A., Lambeng, N., Nocka, K., Kensel-Hammes, P., Bajjalieh, S. M., Matagne, A., et al. (2004). The synaptic vesicle protein SV2A is the binding site for the antiepileptic drug levetiracetam. *Proc. Natl. Acad. Sci. USA, 101*(26), 9861–9866.

Macdonald, R. L., & Kelly, K. M. (1995). Antiepileptic drug mechanisms of action. *Epilepsia, 36*(Suppl 2), S2–12.

Mackenzie, P. I., Owens, I. S., Burchell, B., Bock, K. W., Bairoch, A., Belanger, A., et al. (1997). The UDP glycosyltransferase gene superfamily: recommended nomenclature update based on evolutionary divergence. *Pharmacogenetics, 7*(4), 255–269.

Madeja, M., Margineanu, D. G., Gorji, A., Siep, E., Boerrigter, P., Klitgaard, H., et al. (2003). Reduction of voltage-operated potassium currents by levetiracetam: a novel antiepileptic mechanism of action? *Neuropharmacology, 45*(5), 661–671.

Mallikaarjun, S., Salazar, D. E., & Bramer, S. L. (2004). Pharmacokinetics, tolerability, and safety of aripiprazole following multiple oral dosing in normal healthy volunteers. *J. Clin. Pharmacol., 44*(2), 179–187.

Mallinger, A. G., & Smith, E. (1991). Pharmacokinetics of monoamine oxidase inhibitors. *Psychopharmacol. Bull., 27*(4), 493–502.

Mannens, G., Huang, M. L., Meuldermans, W., Hendrickx, J., Woestenborghs, R., & Heykants, J. (1993). Absorption, metabolism, and excretion of risperidone in humans. *Drug Metab. Dispos., 21*(6), 1134–1141.

Marcus, W. L. (1994). Lithium: a review of its pharmacokinetics, health effects, and toxicology. *J. Environ. Pathol. Toxicol. Oncol., 13*(2), 73–79.

Marder, S. R., McQuade, R. D., Stock, E., Kaplita, S., Marcus, R., Safferman, A. Z., et al. (2003). Aripiprazole in the treatment of schizophrenia: safety and tolerability in short-term, placebo-controlled trials. *Schizophr. Res., 61*(2–3), 123–136.

Marek, G. J., McDougle, C. J., Price, L. H., & Seiden, L. S. (1992). A comparison of trazodone and fluoxetine: implications for a serotonergic mechanism of anti-depressant action. *Psychopharmacology (Berl), 109*(1–2), 2–11.

Marinkovic, D., Timotijevic, I., Babinski, T., Totic, S., & Paunovic, V. R. (1994). The side-effects of clozapine: a four year follow-up study. *Prog. Neuropsychopharmacol. Biol. Psychiatry, 18*(3), 537–544.

Martinez, P., Gonzalez de Etxabarri, S., Ereno, C., Lopez, G., Hinojal, C., & Teira, R. (1993). [Acute severe hepatic insufficiency caused by carbamazepine]. *Rev. Esp. Enferm Dig., 84*(2), 124–126.

Masand, P. S., & Gupta, S. (2002). Long-term side effects of newer-generation anti-depressants: SSRIS, venlafaxine, nefazodone, bupropion, and mirtazapine. *Ann. Clin. Psychiatry, 14*(3), 175–182.

Masuda, Y., & Karasawa, T. (1993). Inhibitory effect of zonisamide on human carbonic anhydrase in vitro. *Arzneimittelforschung, 43*(4), 416–418.

May, T. W., Korn-Merker, E., & Rambeck, B. (2003). Clinical pharmacokinetics of oxcarbazepine. *Clin. Pharmacokinet., 42*(12), 1023–1042.

Mayersohn, M., & Guentert, T. W. (1995). Clinical pharmacokinetics of the monoamine oxidase-A inhibitor moclobemide. *Clin. Pharmacokinet., 29*(5), 292–332.

McElroy, S. L., Arnold, L. M., Shapira, N. A., Keck, P. E., Jr., Rosenthal, N. R., Karim, M. R., et al. (2003). Topiramate in the treatment of binge eating disorder associated with obesity: a randomized, placebo-controlled trial. *Am. J. Psychiatry, 160*(2), 255–261.

McElroy, S. L., Keck, P. E., Stanton, S. P., Tugrul, K. C., Bennett, J. A., & Strakowski, S. M. (1996). A randomized comparison of divalproex oral loading versus haloperidol in the initial treatment of acute psychotic mania. *J. Clin. Psychiatry, 57*(4), 142–146.

McElroy, S. L., Suppes, T., Keck, P. E., Jr., Black, D., Frye, M. A., Altshuler, L. L., et al. (2005). Open-label adjunctive zonisamide in the treatment of bipolar disorders: a prospective trial. *J. Clin. Psychiatry, 66*(5), 617–624.

McIntyre, R. S., Brecher, M., Paulsson, B., Huizar, K., & Mullen, J. (2005). Quetiapine or haloperidol as monotherapy for bipolar mania-a 12-week, double-blind, randomised, parallel-group, placebo-controlled trial. *Eur. Neuropsychopharmacol., 15*(5), 573–585.

McIntyre, R. S., Mancini, D. A., McCann, S., Srinivasan, J., Sagman, D., & Kennedy, S. H. (2002). Topiramate versus bupropion SR when added to mood stabilizer therapy for the depressive phase of bipolar disorder: a preliminary single-blind study. *Bipolar Disord., 4*(3), 207–213.

McLean, M. J. (1994). Clinical pharmacokinetics of gabapentin. *Neurology, 44*(6 Suppl 5), S17–22; discussion S31–12.

McLean, M. J., Schmutz, M., Wamil, A. W., Olpe, H. R., Portet, C., & Feldmann, K. F. (1994). Oxcarbazepine: mechanisms of action. *Epilepsia, 35*(Suppl 3), S5–9.

McQuade, R. D., Stock, E., Marcus, R., Jody, D., Gharbia, N. A., Vanveggel, S., et al. (2004). A comparison of weight change during treatment with olanzapine or aripiprazole: results from a randomized, double-blind study. *J. Clin. Psychiatry, 65*(Suppl) *18*, 47–56.

Meehan, K., Zhang, F., David, S., Tohen, M., Janicak, P., Small, J., et al. (2001). A double-blind, randomized comparison of the efficacy and safety of intramuscular injections of olanzapine, lorazepam, or placebo in treating acutely agitated patients diagnosed with bipolar mania. *J. Clin. Psychopharmacol., 21*(4), 389–397.

Meltzer, H. Y., Alphs, L., Green, A. I., Altamura, A. C., Anand, R., Bertoldi, A., et al. (2003). Clozapine treatment for suicidality in schizophrenia: International Suicide Prevention Trial (InterSePT). *Arch. Gen. Psychiatry, 60*(1), 82–91.

Mendelson, W. B. (2005). A review of the evidence for the efficacy and safety of trazodone in insomnia. *J. Clin. Psychiatry, 66*(4), 469–476.

Meyer, U. A. (1994). The molecular basis of genetic polymorphisms of drug metabolism. *J. Pharm. Pharmacol., 46*(Suppl 1), 409–415.

Mikati, M. A., Schachter, S. C., Schomer, D. L., Keally, M., Osborne-Shafer, P., Seaman, C. A., et al. (1989). Long-term tolerability, pharmacokinetic and preliminary efficacy study of lamotrigine in patients with resistant partial seizures. *Clin. Neuropharmacol., 12*(4), 312–321.

Miller, D. D. (2000). Review and management of clozapine side effects. *J. Clin. Psychiatry, 61*(Suppl 8), 14–17; discussion 18–19.

Miller, D. D., Fleming, F., Holman, T. L., & Perry, P. J. (1994). Plasma clozapine concentrations as a predictor of clinical response: a follow-up study. *J. Clin. Psychiatry, 55*(Suppl B), 117–121.

Minov, C. (2004). [Risk of QTc prolongation due to combination of ziprasidone and quetiapine]. *Psychiatr. Prax, 31*(Suppl 1), S142–S144.

Molden, E., Garcia, B. H., Braathen, P., & Eggen, A. E. (2005). Co-prescription of cytochrome P450 2D6/3A4 inhibitor-substrate pairs in clinical practice. A retrospective analysis of data from Norwegian primary pharmacies. *Eur. J. Clin. Pharmacol., 61*(2), 119–125.

Montgomery, S. A. (2006). Pregabalin for the treatment of generalised anxiety disorder. *Expert Opin. Pharmacother., 7*(15), 2139–2154.

Montgomery, S. A., Tobias, K., Zornberg, G. L., Kasper, S., & Pande, A. C. (2006). Efficacy and safety of pregabalin in the treatment of generalized anxiety disorder: a 6-week, multicenter, randomized, double-blind, placebo-controlled comparison of pregabalin and venlafaxine. *J. Clin. Psychiatry, 67*(5), 771–782.

Mula, M., Trimble, M. R., Lhatoo, S. D., & Sander, J. W. (2003). Topiramate and psychiatric adverse events in patients with epilepsy. *Epilepsia, 44*(5), 659–663.

Mula, M., Trimble, M. R., & Sander, J. W. (2004). Psychiatric adverse events in patients with epilepsy and learning disabilities taking levetiracetam. *Seizure, 13*(1), 55–57.

Mula, M., Trimble, M. R., Yuen, A., Liu, R. S., & Sander, J. W. (2003). Psychiatric adverse events during levetiracetam therapy. *Neurology, 61*(5), 704–706.

Murray, M. (2006). Role of CYP pharmacogenetics and drug-drug interactions in the efficacy and safety of atypical and other antipsychotic agents. *J. Pharm. Pharmacol., 58*(7), 871–885.

Nasrallah, H. A., Churchill, C. M., & Hamdan-Allan, G. A. (1988). Higher frequency of neuroleptic-induced dystonia in mania than in schizophrenia. *Am. J. Psychiatry*, 145(11), 1455–1456.

Nasrallah, H. A., Dev, V., Rak, I., & Raniwalla, J. (1999). Safety update on quetiapine and lenticular examinations: experience with 300,000 patients. Paper presented at the 38th Annual Meeting of the American College of Neuropsychopharmacology, Acapulco, Mexico, December 13–17.

Nelson, D. R., Koymans, L., Kamataki, T., Stegeman, J. J., Feyereisen, R., Waxman, D. J., et al. (1996). P450 superfamily: update on new sequences, gene mapping, accession numbers and nomenclature. *Pharmacogenetics*, 6(1), 1–42.

Nemeroff, C. B., Evans, D. L., Gyulai, L., Sachs, G. S., Bowden, C. L., Gergel, I. P., et al. (2001). Double-blind, placebo-controlled comparison of imipramine and paroxetine in the treatment of bipolar depression. *Am. J. Psychiatry*, 158(6), 906–912.

Nilsen, O. G., Dale, O., & Husebo, B. (1993). Pharmacokinetics of trazodone during multiple dosing to psychiatric patients. *Pharmacol. Toxicol.*, 72(4–5), 286–289.

Obach, R., Borja, J., Prunonosa, J., Valles, J. M., Torrent, J., Izquierdo, I., et al. (1988). Lack of correlation between lithium pharmacokinetic parameters obtained from plasma and saliva. *Ther. Drug Monit.*, 10(3), 265–268.

Okuma, T., Inanaga, K., Otsuki, S., Sarai, K., Takahashi, R., Hazama, H., et al. (1979). Comparison of the antimanic efficacy of carbamazepine and chlorpromazine: a double-blind controlled study. *Psychopharmacology*, 66(3), 211–217.

Olesen, O. V., & Linnet, K. (2000). Fluvoxamine-Clozapine drug interaction: inhibition in vitro of five cytochrome P450 isoforms involved in clozapine metabolism. *J. Clin. Psychopharmacol.*, 20(1), 35–42.

Ozawa, K., Kobayashi, K., Noda, S., & Iyo, M. (2004). Zonisamide-induced depression and mania in patients with epilepsy. *J. Clin. Psychopharmacol.*, 24(1), 110–111.

Palmer, K. J., & McTavish, D. (1993). Felbamate. A review of its pharmacodynamic and pharmacokinetic properties, and therapeutic efficacy in epilepsy. *Drugs*, 45(6), 1041–1065.

Pande, A. C., Crockatt, J., Janney, C. A., Werth, J. L., & Tsaroucha, G. (2000). Gabapentin Bipolar Disorder Study Group. Gabapentin in bipolar disorder: a placebo-controlled trial of adjunctive therapy. *Bipolar Disord.*, 2(3 pt 2), 249–255.

Pande, A. C., Crockatt, J. G., Feltner, D. E., Janney, C. A., Smith, W. T., Weisler, R., et al. (2003). Pregabalin in generalized anxiety disorder: a placebo-controlled trial. *Am. J. Psychiatry*, 160(3), 533–540.

Pande, A. C., Davidson, J. R., Jefferson, J. W., Janney, C. A., Katzelnick, D. J., Weisler, R. H., et al. (1999). Treatment of social phobia with gabapentin: a placebo-controlled study. *J. Clin. Psychopharmacol.*, 19(4), 341–348.

Pande, A. C., Feltner, D. E., Jefferson, J. W., Davidson, J. R., Pollack, M., Stein, M. B., et al. (2004). Efficacy of the novel anxiolytic pregabalin in social anxiety disorder: a placebo-controlled, multicenter study. *J. Clin. Psychopharmacol.*, 24(2), 141–149.

Pande, A. C., Pollack, M. H., Crockatt, J., Greiner, M., Chouinard, G., Lydiard, R. B., et al. (2000). Placebo-controlled study of gabapentin treatment of panic disorder. *J. Clin. Psychopharmacol.*, 20(4), 467–471.

Patsalos, P. N. (2000). Pharmacokinetic profile of levetiracetam: toward ideal characteristics. *Pharmacol. Ther.*, 85(2), 77–85.

Peet, M. (1994). Induction of mania with selective serotonin re-uptake inhibitors and tricyclic antidepressants. *Br. J. Psychiatry, 164*(4), 549–550.

Pellock, J. M. (1987). Carbamazepine side effects in children and adults. *Epilepsia, 28*(Suppl 3), S64–70.

Perry, P. J., Miller, D. D., Arndt, S. V., & Cadoret, R. J. (1991). Clozapine and norclozapine plasma concentrations and clinical response of treatment-refractory schizophrenic patients. *Am. J. Psychiatry, 148*(2), 231–235.

Persson, L. I., Ben-Menachem, E., Bengtsson, E., & Heinonen, E. (1990). Differences in side effects between a conventional carbamazepine preparation and a slow-release preparation of carbamazepine. *Epilepsy Res., 6*(2), 134–140.

Peselow, E. D., Dunner, D. L., Fieve, R. R., & Lautin, A. (1980). Lithium carbonate and weight gain. *J. Affect. Disord., 2*(4), 303–310.

Peters, D. H., & Sorkin, E. M. (1993). Zonisamide. A review of its pharmacodynamic and pharmacokinetic properties, and therapeutic potential in epilepsy. *Drugs, 45*(5), 760–787.

Physicians' Desk Reference (61st edition). (2007). Montvale, NJ: Thomson PDR.

Piscitelli, S. C., Frazier, J. A., McKenna, K., Albus, K. E., Grothe, D. R., Gordon, C. T., et al. (1994). Plasma clozapine and haloperidol concentrations in adolescents with childhood-onset schizophrenia: association with response. *J. Clin. Psychiatry, 55*(Suppl B), 94–97.

Pohl, R. B., Feltner, D. E., Fieve, R. R., & Pande, A. C. (2005). Efficacy of pregabalin in the treatment of generalized anxiety disorder: double-blind, placebo-controlled comparison of BID versus TID dosing. *J. Clin. Psychopharmacol., 25*(2), 151–158.

Pollack, M. H., & Rosenbaum, J. F. (1987). Management of antidepressant-induced side effects: a practical guide for the clinician. *J. Clin. Psychiatry, 48*(1), 3–8.

Pope, H. G., Jr., McElroy, S. L., Keck, P. E., Jr., & Hudson, J. I. (1991). Valproate in the treatment of acute mania. A placebo-controlled study. *Arch. Gen. Psychiatry, 48*(1), 62–68.

Post, R. M., Altshuler, L. L., Frye, M. A., Suppes, T., McElroy, S. L., Keck, P. E., Jr., et al. (2005). Preliminary observations on the effectiveness of levetiracetam in the open adjunctive treatment of refractory bipolar disorder. *J. Clin. Psychiatry, 66*(3), 370–374.

Post, R. M., Altshuler, L. L., Leverich, G. S., Frye, M. A., Nolen, W. A., Kupka, R. W., et al. (2006). Mood switch in bipolar depression: comparison of adjunctive venlafaxine, bupropion and sertraline. *Br. J. Psychiatry, 189*, 124–131.

Post, R. M., Weiss, S. R. B., Chuang, D. M., & Ketter, T. A. (1994). Mechanisms of action of carbamazepine in seizure and affective disorders. In R. T. Joffe & J. R. Calabrese (Eds.), *Anticonvulsants in Psychiatry* (pp. 43–92). New York, NY: Marcel Dekker, Inc.

Potkin, S. G., Bera, R., Gulasekaram, B., Costa, J., Hayes, S., Jin, Y., et al. (1994). Plasma clozapine concentrations predict clinical response in treatment-resistant schizophrenia. *J. Clin. Psychiatry, 55*(Suppl B), 133–136.

Potkin, S. G., Keck, P. E., Jr., Segal, S., Ice, K., & English, P. (2005). Ziprasidone in acute bipolar mania: a 21-day randomized, double-blind, placebo-controlled replication trial. *J. Clin. Psychopharmacol., 25*(4), 301–310.

Potter, W. Z., & Ketter T. A. (1993). Pharmacological issues in the treatment of bipolar disorder: focus on mood-stabilizing compounds. *Can. J. Psychiatry, 38*, S51–S56.

Poulsen, C. F., Simeone, T. A., Maar, T. E., Smith-Swintosky, V., White, H. S., & Schousboe, A. (2004). Modulation by topiramate of AMPA and kainate mediated calcium influx in cultured cerebral cortical, hippocampal and cerebellar neurons. *Neurochem. Res., 29*(1), 275–282.

Poyurovsky, M., Pashinian, A., Weizman, R., Fuchs, C., & Weizman, A. (2006). Low-dose mirtazapine: a new option in the treatment of antipsychotic-induced akathisia. A randomized, double-blind, placebo- and propranolol-controlled trial. *Biol. Psychiatry, 59*(11), 1071–1077.

Poyurovsky, M., Shardorodsky, M., Fuchs, C., Schneidman, M., & Weizman, A. (1999). Treatment of neuroleptic-induced akathisia with the 5-HT2 antagonist mianserin. Double-blind, placebo-controlled study. *Br. J. Psychiatry, 174,* 238–242.

Prakash, C., Kamel, A., Cui, D., Whalen, R. D., Miceli, J. J., & Tweedie, D. (2000). Identification of the major human liver cytochrome P450 isoform(s) responsible for the formation of the primary metabolites of ziprasidone and prediction of possible drug interactions. *Br. J. Clin. Pharmacol., 49*(Suppl 1), 35S–42S.

Quiroz, J. A., Gould, T. D., & Manji, H. K. (2004). Molecular effects of lithium. *Mol. Interv., 4*(5), 259–272.

Rabkin, J., Quitkin, F., Harrison, W., Tricamo, E., & McGrath, P. (1984). Adverse reactions to monoamine oxidase inhibitors. Part I. A comparative study. *J. Clin. Psychopharmacol., 4*(5), 270–278.

Randinitis, E. J., Posvar, E. L., Alvey, C. W., Sedman, A. J., Cook, J. A., & Bockbrader, H. N. (2003). Pharmacokinetics of pregabalin in subjects with various degrees of renal function. *J. Clin. Pharmacol., 43*(3), 277–283.

Rasgon, N. (2004). The relationship between polycystic ovary syndrome and antiepileptic drugs: a review of the evidence. *J. Clin. Psychopharmacol., 24*(3), 322–334.

Rasgon, N. L., Altshuler, L. L., Fairbanks, L., Elman, S., Bitran, J., Labarca, R., et al. (2005). Reproductive function and risk for PCOS in women treated for bipolar disorder. *Bipolar Disord., 7*(3), 246–259.

Reinikainen, K. J., Keranen, T., Halonen, T., Komulainen, H., & Riekkinen, P. J. (1987). Comparison of oxcarbazepine and carbamazepine: a double-blind study. *Epilepsy Res., 1*(5), 284–289.

Rendic, S., & Di Carlo, F. J. (1997). Human cytochrome P450 enzymes: a status report summarizing their reactions, substrates, inducers, and inhibitors. *Drug Metab. Rev., 29*(1–2), 413–580.

Richens, A. (1993). Clinical pharmacokinetics of gabapentin. In D. Chadwick (Ed.), *New Trends in Epilepsy Management: the Role of Gabapentin* (pp. 41–46). London: Royal Society of Medicine Services.

Richter, R. W., Portenoy, R., Sharma, U., Lamoreaux, L., Bockbrader, H., & Knapp, L. E. (2005). Relief of painful diabetic peripheral neuropathy with pregabalin: a randomized, placebo–controlled trial. *J. Pain, 6*(4), 253–260.

Rickels, K., Pollack, M. H., Feltner, D. E., Lydiard, R. B., Zimbroff, D. L., Bielski, R. J., et al. (2005). Pregabalin for treatment of generalized anxiety disorder: a 4-week, multicenter, double-blind, placebo-controlled trial of pregabalin and alprazolam. *Arch. Gen. Psychiatry, 62*(9), 1022–1030.

Rohatagi, S., Barrett, J. S., DeWitt, K. E., & Morales, R. J. (1997). Integrated pharmacokinetic and metabolic modeling of selegiline and metabolites after transdermal administration. *Biopharm. Drug Dispos., 18*(7), 567–584.

Rosa, F. W. (1991). Spina bifida in infants of women treated with carbamazepine during pregnancy. *N. Engl. J. Med., 324*(10), 674–677.

Rosenfeld, W. E., Doose, D. R., Walker, S. A., & Nayak, R. K. (1997). Effect of topiramate on the pharmacokinetics of an oral contraceptive containing norethindrone and ethinyl estradiol in patients with epilepsy. *Epilepsia, 38*(3), 317–323.

Rosenstock, J., Tuchman, M., LaMoreaux, L., & Sharma, U. (2004). Pregabalin for the treatment of painful diabetic peripheral neuropathy: a double-blind, placebo-controlled trial. *Pain, 110*(3), 628–638.

Rosenthal, M. (2003). Tiagabine for the treatment of generalized anxiety disorder: a randomized, open-label, clinical trial with paroxetine as a positive control. *J. Clin. Psychiatry, 64*(10), 1245–1249.

Roth, T., & Walsh, J. K. (2004). Sleep-consolidating effects of tiagabine in patients with primary insomnia. Paper presented at the 157th Annual Meeting of the American Psychiatric Association, New York, NY, May 1–6.

Rouan, M. C., Lecaillon, J. B., Godbillon, J., Menard, F., Darragon, T., Meyer, P., et al. (1994). The effect of renal impairment on the pharmacokinetics of oxcarbazepine and its metabolites. *Eur. J. Clin. Pharmacol., 47*(2), 161–167.

Rowbotham, M., Harden, N., Stacey, B., Bernstein, P., & Magnus-Miller, L. (1998). Gabapentin for the treatment of postherpetic neuralgia: a randomized controlled trial. *JAMA, 280*(21), 1837–1842.

Rowland, A., Elliot, D. J., Williams, J. A., Mackenzie, P. I., Dickinson, R. G., & Miners, J. O. (2006). In vitro characterization of lamotrigine N2-glucuronidation and the lamotrigine-valproic acid interaction. *Drug Metab. Dispos., 34*(6), 1055–1062.

Sabatowski, R., Galvez, R., Cherry, D. A., Jacquot, F., Vincent, E., Maisonobe, P., et al. (2004). Pregabalin reduces pain and improves sleep and mood disturbances in patients with post-herpetic neuralgia: results of a randomised, placebo-controlled clinical trial. *Pain, 109*(1–2), 26–35.

Sabers, A., Ohman, I., Christensen, J., & Tomson, T. (2003). Oral contraceptives reduce lamotrigine plasma levels. *Neurology, 61*(4), 570–571.

Sachs, G., Bowden, C., Calabrese, J. R., Ketter, T., Thompson, T., White, R., et al. (2006). Effects of lamotrigine and lithium on body weight during maintenance treatment of bipolar I disorder. *Bipolar Disord., 8*(2), 175–181.

Sachs, G., Chengappa, K. N., Suppes, T., Mullen, J. A., Brecher, M., Devine, N. A., et al. (2004). Quetiapine with lithium or divalproex for the treatment of bipolar mania: a randomized, double-blind, placebo-controlled study. *Bipolar Disord., 6*(3), 213–223.

Sachs, G., Sanchez, R., Marcus, R., Stock, E., McQuade, R., Carson, W., et al. (2006). Aripiprazole in the treatment of acute manic or mixed episodes in patients with bipolar I disorder: a 3-week placebo-controlled study. *J. Psychopharmacol., 20*(4), 536–546.

Sachs, G. S., Grossman, F., Ghaemi, S. N., Okamoto, A., & Bowden, C. L. (2002). Combination of a mood stabilizer with risperidone or haloperidol for treatment of acute mania: a double-blind, placebo-controlled comparison of efficacy and safety. *Am. J. Psychiatry, 159*(7), 1146–1154.

Sachs, G. S., Lafer, B., Stoll, A. L., Banov, M., Thibault, A. B., Tohen, M., et al. (1994). A double-blind trial of bupropion versus desipramine for bipolar depression. *J. Clin. Psychiatry, 55*(9), 391–393.

Sachs, G. S., Nierenberg, A. A., Calabrese, J. R., Marangell, L. B., Wisniewski, S. R., Gyulai, L., et al. (2007). Effectiveness of adjunctive antidepressant treatment for bipolar depression. *N. Engl. J. Med., 356*(17), 1711–1722.

Schaffer, C. B., & Schaffer, L. C. (1997). Gabapentin in the treatment of bipolar disorder. *Am. J. Psychiatry, 154*(2), 291–292.

Schaffer, L., Schaffer, C., & Howe, J. (2002). An open case series on the utility of tiagabine as an augmentation in refractory bipolar outpatients. *J. Affect. Disord., 71*(1–3), 259.

Schauf, C. L. (1987). Zonisamide enhances slow sodium inactivation in Myxicola. *Brain Res., 413*(1), 185–188.

Schmidt, D. (1984). Adverse effects of valproate. *Epilepsia, 25*(Suppl 1), S44–49.

Sernyak, M. J., Godleski, L. S., Griffin, R. A., Mazure, C. M., & Woods, S. W. (1997). Chronic neuroleptic exposure in bipolar outpatients. *J. Clin. Psychiatry, 58*(5), 193–195.

Serpell, M. G. (2002). Gabapentin in neuropathic pain syndromes: a randomised, double-blind, placebo-controlled trial. *Pain, 99*(3), 557–566.

Shank, R. P., Gardocki, J. F., Vaught, J. L., Davis, C. B., Schupsky, J. J., Raffa, R. B., et al. (1994). Topiramate: preclinical evaluation of structurally novel anticonvulsant. *Epilepsia, 35*(2), 450–460.

Sharma, V., Mazmanian, D. S., Persad, E., & Kueneman, K. M. (1997). Treatment of bipolar depression: a survey of Canadian psychiatrists. *Can. J. Psychiatry, 42*(3), 298–302.

Shen, W. W. (1997). The metabolism of psychoactive drugs: a review of enzymatic biotransformation and inhibition. *Biol. Psychiatry, 41*(7), 814–826.

Shorvon, S. (2001). Pyrrolidone derivatives. *Lancet, 358*(9296), 1885–1892.

Shorvon, S. D. (1996). Safety of topiramate: adverse events and relationships to dosing. *Epilepsia, 37* (Suppl 2), S18–S22.

Siddall, P. J., Cousins, M. J., Otte, A., Griesing, T., Chambers, R., & Murphy, T. K. (2006). Pregabalin in central neuropathic pain associated with spinal cord injury: a placebo-controlled trial. *Neurology, 67*(10), 1792–1800.

Sidhu, J., Job, S., Singh, S., & Philipson, R. (2006). The pharmacokinetic and pharmacodynamic consequences of the co-administration of lamotrigine and a combined oral contraceptive in healthy female subjects. *Br. J. Clin. Pharmacol., 61*(2), 191–199.

Sills, G. J. (2006). The mechanisms of action of gabapentin and pregabalin. *Curr. Opin. Pharmacol., 6*(1), 108–113.

Sills, G. J., & Brodie, M. J. (2007). Pharmacokinetics and drug Interactions with zonisamide. *Epilepsia., 48*(3), 435–41.

Silverstone, T. (2001). Moclobemide vs. imipramine in bipolar depression: a multicentre double-blind clinical trial. *Acta Psychiatr. Scand., 104*(2), 104–109.

Simpson, S. G., & DePaulo, J. R. (1991). Fluoxetine treatment of bipolar II depression. *J. Clin. Psychopharmacol., 11*(1), 52–54.

Sindrup, S. H., Brosen, K., & Gram, L. F. (1992). Pharmacokinetics of the selective serotonin reuptake inhibitor paroxetine: nonlinearity and relation to the sparteine oxidation polymorphism. *Clin. Pharmacol. Ther., 51*(3), 288–295.

Smith, M. C., Centorrino, F., Welge, J. A., & Collins, M. A. (2004). Clinical comparison of extended-release divalproex versus delayed-release divalproex: pooled data analyses from nine trials. *Epilepsy Behav., 5*(5), 746–751.

Spira, P. J., & Beran, R. G. (2003). Gabapentin in the prophylaxis of chronic daily headache: a randomized, placebo-controlled study. *Neurology, 61*(12), 1753–1759.

Spring, G., Schweid, D., Gray, C., Steinberg, J., & Horwitz, M. (1970). A double-blind comparison of lithium and chlorpromazine in the treatment of manic states. *Am. J. Psychiatry, 126*(9), 1306–1310.

Sproule, B. (2002). Lithium in bipolar disorder: can drug concentrations predict therapeutic effect? *Clin. Pharmacokinet., 41*(9), 639–660.

Stahl, S. M., & Shayegan, D. K. (2003). The psychopharmacology of ziprasidone: receptor-binding properties and real-world psychiatric practice. *J. Clin. Psychiatry, 64*(Suppl 19), 6–12.

Stewart, B. H., Kugler, A. R., Thompson, P. R., & Bockbrader, H. N. (1993). A saturable transport mechanism in the intestinal absorption of gabapentin is the underlying cause of the lack of proportionality between increasing dose and drug levels in plasma. *Pharm. Res., 10*(2), 276–281.

Stewart, D. E. (2002). Hepatic adverse reactions associated with nefazodone. *Can. J. Psychiatry, 47*(4), 375–377.

Stoll, A. L., Mayer, P. V., Kolbrener, M., Goldstein, E., Suplit, B., Lucier, J., et al. (1994). Antidepressant-associated mania: a controlled comparison with spontaneous mania. *Am. J. Psychiatry, 151*(11), 1642–1645.

Striano, S., Striano, P., Di Nocera, P., Italiano, D., Fasiello, C., Ruosi, P., et al. (2006). Relationship between serum mono-hydroxy-carbazepine concentrations and adverse effects in patients with epilepsy on high-dose oxcarbazepine therapy. *Epilepsy Res., 69*(2), 170–176.

Sullivan, K. L., Ward, C. L., & Zesiewicz, T. A. (2006). Zonisamide-induced mania in an essential tremor patient. *J. Clin. Psychopharmacol., 26*(4), 439–440.

Suppes, T., Chisholm, K. A., Dhavale, D., Frye, M. A., Altshuler, L. L., McElroy, S. L., et al. (2002). Tiagabine in treatment refractory bipolar disorder: a clinical case series. *Bipolar Disord., 4*(5), 283–289.

Suppes, T., Dennehy, E. B., Hirschfeld, R. M., Altshuler, L. L., Bowden, C. L., Calabrese, J. R., et al. (2005). The Texas Implementation of Medication Algorithms: update to the algorithms for treatment of bipolar I disorder. *J. Clin. Psychiatry, 66*(7), 870–886.

Suppes, T., Webb, A., Paul, B., Carmody, T., Kraemer, H., & Rush, A. J. (1999). Clinical outcome in a randomized 1-year trial of clozapine versus treatment as usual for patients with treatment-resistant illness and a history of mania. *Am. J. Psychiatry, 156*(8), 1164–1169.

Suzdak, P. D., & Jansen, J. A. (1995). A review of the preclinical pharmacology of tiagabine: a potent and selective anticonvulsant GABA uptake inhibitor. *Epilepsia, 36*(6), 612–626.

Svinarov, D. A., & Pippenger, C. E. (1995). Valproic acid-carbamazepine interaction: is valproic acid a selective inhibitor of epoxide hydrolase? *Ther. Drug Monit., 17*(3), 217–220.

Swainston Harrison, T., & Perry, C. M. (2004). Aripiprazole: a review of its use in schizophrenia and schizoaffective disorder. *Drugs, 64*(15), 1715–1736.

Taft, D. R., Iyer, G. R., Behar, L., & DiGregorio, R. V. (1997). Application of a first-pass effect model to characterize the pharmacokinetic disposition of venlafaxine after oral administration to human subjects. *Drug Metab. Dispos., 25*(10), 1215–1218.

Takahashi, R., Sakuma, A., Itoh, K., Itoh, H., & Kurihara, M. (1975). Comparison of efficacy of lithium carbonate and chlorpromazine in mania. Report of collaborative study group on treatment of mania in Japan. *Arch. Gen. Psychiatry, 32*(10), 1310–1318.

Taylor, C. P., Angelotti, T., & Fauman, E. (2007). Pharmacology and mechanism of action of pregabalin: the calcium channel alpha(2)-delta (alpha(2)-delta) subunit as a target for antiepileptic drug discovery. *Epilepsy Res., 73*(2), 137–150.

Taylor, C. P., Vartanian, M. G., Yuen, P. W., Bigge, C., Suman-Chauhan, N., & Hill, D. R. (1993). Potent and stereospecific anticonvulsant activity of 3-isobutyl GABA relates to in vitro binding at a novel site labeled by tritiated gabapentin. *Epilepsy Res., 14*(1), 11–15.

Thakker, K. M., Mangat, S., Garnett, W. R., Levy, R. H., & Kochak, G. M. (1992). Comparative bioavailability and steady state fluctuations of Tegretol commercial and carbamazepine OROS tablets in adult and pediatric epileptic patients. *Biopharm. Drug Dispos., 13*(8), 559–569.

Thase, M. E., Macfadden, W., Weisler, R. H., Chang, W., Paulsson, B., Khan, A., et al. (2006). Efficacy of quetiapine monotherapy in bipolar I and II depression: a double-blind, placebo-controlled study (the BOLDER II study). *J. Clin. Psychopharmacol., 26*(6), 600–609.

Thase, M. E., Mallinger, A. G., McKnight, D., & Himmelhoch, J. M. (1992). Treatment of imipramine-resistant recurrent depression, IV: A double-blind crossover study of tranylcypromine for anergic bipolar depression. *Am. J. Psychiatry, 149*(2), 195–198.

Timmer, C. J., Sitsen, J. M., & Delbressine, L. P. (2000). Clinical pharmacokinetics of mirtazapine. *Clin. Pharmacokinet., 38*(6), 461–474.

Timmer, R. T., & Sands, J. M. (1999). Lithium intoxication. *J. Am. Soc. Nephrol., 10*(3), 666–674.

Tohen, M., Calabrese, J. R., Sachs, G. S., Banov, M. D., Detke, H. C., Risser, R., et al. (2006). Randomized, placebo-controlled trial of olanzapine as maintenance therapy in patients with bipolar I disorder responding to acute treatment with olanzapine. *Am. J. Psychiatry, 163*(2), 247–256.

Tohen, M., Castillo, J., Baldessarini, R. J., Zarate, C., Jr., & Kando, J. C. (1995). Blood dyscrasias with carbamazepine and valproate: a pharmacoepidemiological study of 2,228 patients at risk. *Am. J. Psychiatry, 152*(3), 413–418.

Tohen, M., Chengappa, K. N., Suppes, T., Zarate, C. A., Jr., Calabrese, J. R., Bowden, C. L., et al. (2002). Efficacy of olanzapine in combination with valproate or lithium in the treatment of mania in patients partially nonresponsive to valproate or lithium monotherapy. *Arch. Gen. Psychiatry, 59*(1), 62–69.

Tohen, M., Goldberg, J. F., Gonzalez-Pinto Arrillaga, A. M., Azorin, J. M., Vieta, E., Hardy-Bayle, M. C., et al. (2003). A 12-week, double-blind comparison of olanzapine vs haloperidol in the treatment of acute mania. *Arch. Gen. Psychiatry, 60*(12), 1218–1226.

Tohen, M., Greil, W., Calabrese, J. R., Sachs, G. S., Yatham, L. N., Oerlinghausen, B. M., et al. (2005). Olanzapine versus lithium in the maintenance treatment of bipolar disorder: a 12-month, randomized, double-blind, controlled clinical trial. *Am. J. Psychiatry, 162*(7), 1281–1290.

Tohen, M., Jacobs, T. G., Grundy, S. L., McElroy, S. L., Banov, M. C., Janicak, P. G., et al. (2000). Efficacy of olanzapine in acute bipolar mania: a double-blind, placebo-controlled study. The Olanzapine HGGW Study Group. *Arch. Gen. Psychiatry, 57*(9), 841–849.

Tohen, M., Ketter, T. A., Zarate, C. A., Suppes, T., Frye, M., Altshuler, L., et al. (2003). Olanzapine versus divalproex sodium for the treatment of acute mania and maintenance of remission: a 47-week study. *Am. J. Psychiatry, 160*(7), 1263–1271.

Tohen, M., Sanger, T. M., McElroy, S. L., Tollefson, G. D., Chengappa, K. N., Daniel, D. G., et al. (1999). Olanzapine versus placebo in the treatment of acute mania. Olanzapine HGEH Study Group. *Am. J. Psychiatry, 156*(5), 702–709.

Tohen, M., Vieta, E., Calabrese, J., Ketter, T. A., Sachs, G., Bowden, C., et al. (2003). Efficacy of olanzapine and olanzapine-fluoxetine combination in the treatment of bipolar I depression. *Arch. Gen. Psychiatry, 60*(11), 1079–1088.

Tonnesen, P., Tonstad, S., Hjalmarson, A., Lebargy, F., Van Spiegel, P. I., Hider, A., et al. (2003). A multicentre, randomized, double-blind, placebo-controlled, 1-year study of bupropion SR for smoking cessation. *J. Intern. Med., 254*(2), 184–192.

Tran-Johnson, T. K., Sack, D. A., Marcus, R. N., Auby, P., McQuade, R. D., & Oren, D. A. (2007). Efficacy and safety of intramuscular aripiprazole in patients with acute agitation: a randomized, double-blind, placebo-controlled trial. *J. Clin. Psychiatry, 68*(1), 111–119.

Vajda, F., Lander, C., O'Brien, T., Hitchcock, A., Graham, J., Solinas, C., et al. (2004). Australian pregnancy registry of women taking antiepileptic drugs. *Epilepsia, 45*(11), 1466.

Van Parys, J. A., & Meinardi, H. (1994). Survey of 260 epileptic patients treated with oxcarbazepine (Trileptal) on a named-patient basis. *Epilepsy Res., 19*(1), 79–85.

Vanderkooy, J. D., Kennedy, S. H., & Bagby, R. M. (2002). Antidepressant side effects in depression patients treated in a naturalistic setting: a study of bupropion, moclobemide, paroxetine, sertraline, and venlafaxine. *Can. J. Psychiatry, 47*(2), 174–180.

Vayer, P., Cash, C. D., & Maitre, M. (1988). Is the anticonvulsant mechanism of valproate linked to its interaction with the cerebral gamma-hydroxybutyrate system? *Trends Pharmacol. Sci., 9*(4), 127–129.

Vendsborg, P. B., Bech, P., & Rafaelsen, O. J. (1976). Lithium treatment and weight gain. *Acta Psychiatr. Scand., 53*(2), 139–147.

Vestergaard, P., & Amdisen, A. (1981). Lithium treatment and kidney function. A follow-up study of 237 patients in long-term treatment. *Acta Psychiatr. Scand., 63*(4), 333–345.

Vestergaard, P., Amdisen, A., Hansen, H. E., & Schou, M. (1979). Lithium treatment and kidney function. A survey of 237 patients in long-term treatment. *Acta Psychiatr. Scand., 60*(5), 504–520.

Vestergaard, P., Amdisen, A., & Schou, M. (1980). Clinically significant side effects of lithium treatment. A survey of 237 patients in long-term treatment. *Acta Psychiatr. Scand., 62*(3), 193–200.

Vgontzas, A. N., Kales, A., & Bixler, E. O. (1995). Benzodiazepine side effects: role of pharmacokinetics and pharmacodynamics. *Pharmacology, 51*(4), 205–223.

Vieta, E., Bourin, M., Sanchez, R., Marcus, R., Stock, E., McQuade, R., et al. (2005). Effectiveness of aripiprazole v. haloperidol in acute bipolar mania: double-blind, randomised, comparative 12-week trial. *Br. J. Psychiatry, 187*, 235–242.

Vieta, E., Martinez-Aran, A., Goikolea, J. M., Torrent, C., Colom, F., Benabarre, A., et al. (2002). A randomized trial comparing paroxetine and venlafaxine in the treatment of bipolar depressed patients taking mood stabilizers. *J. Clin. Psychiatry, 63*(6), 508–512.

Vieta E, T'Joen C, McQuade RD, Carson WH, Jr., Marcus RN, Sanchez R, et al. (2008). Efficacy of adjunctive aripiprazole to either valproate or lithium in bipolar mania patients partially nonresponsive to valproate/lithium monotherapy: a placebo-controlled study. *Am. J. Psychiatry, 165*, 1316–1325.

Viguera, A. C., Newport, D. J., Ritchie, J., Stowe, Z., Whitfield, T., Mogielnicki, J., et al. (2007). Lithium in breast milk and nursing infants: clinical implications. *Am. J. Psychiatry, 164*(2), 342–345.

Wagner, K. D., Kowatch, R. A., Emslie, G. J., Findling, R. L., Wilens, T. E., McCague, K., et al. (2006). A double-blind, randomized, placebo-controlled trial of oxcarbazepine in the treatment of bipolar disorder in children and adolescents. *Am. J. Psychiatry, 163*(7), 1179–1186.

Ward, M. E., Musa, M. N., & Bailey, L. (1994). Clinical pharmacokinetics of lithium. *J. Clin. Pharmacol., 34*(4), 280–285.

Wasserman, S., Iyengar, R., Chaplin, W. F., Watner, D., Waldoks, S. E., Anagnostou, E., et al. (2006). Levetiracetam versus placebo in childhood and adolescent autism: a double-blind placebo-controlled study. *Int. Clin. Psychopharmacol., 21*(6), 363–367.

Weisler, R. H., Kalali, A. H., & Ketter, T. A. (2004). A multicenter, randomized, double-blind, placebo-controlled trial of extended-release carbamazepine capsules as monotherapy for bipolar disorder patients with manic or mixed episodes. *J. Clin. Psychiatry, 65*(4), 478–484.

Weisler, R. H., Keck, P. E., Jr., Swann, A. C., Cutler, A. J., Ketter, T. A., & Kalali, A. H. (2005). Extended-release carbamazepine capsules as monotherapy for acute mania in bipolar disorder: a multicenter, randomized, double-blind, placebo-controlled trial. *J. Clin. Psychiatry, 66*(3), 323–330.

Wen, X., Wang, J. S., Kivisto, K. T., Neuvonen, P. J., & Backman, J. T. (2001). In vitro evaluation of valproic acid as an inhibitor of human cytochrome P450 isoforms: preferential inhibition of cytochrome P450 2C9 (CYP2C9). *Br. J. Clin. Pharmacol., 52*(5), 547–553.

White, H. S., Brown, S. D., Woodhead, J. H., Skeen, G. A., & Wolf, H. H. (2000). Topiramate modulates GABA-evoked currents in murine cortical neurons by a nonbenzodiazepine mechanism. *Epilepsia, 41*(Suppl 1), S17–20.

Wier, L. M., Tavares, S. B., Tyrka, A. R., Price, L. H., & Carpenter, L. L. (2006). Levetiracetam-induced depression in a healthy adult. *J. Clin. Psychiatry, 67*(7), 1159–1160.

Wilkinson, G. R. (2005). Drug metabolism and variability among patients in drug response. *N. Engl. J. Med., 352*(21), 2211–2221.

Wilner, K. D., Tensfeldt, T. G., Baris, B., Smolarek, T. A., Turncliff, R. Z., Colburn, W. A., et al. (2000). Single- and multiple-dose pharmacokinetics of ziprasidone in healthy young and elderly volunteers. *Br. J. Clin. Pharmacol., 49*(Suppl 1), 15S–20S.

Wilson, M. S., & Findling, R. L. (2007). Zonisamide for bipolar depression. *Expert Opin. Pharmacother., 8*(1), 111–113.

Winsberg, M. E., DeGolia, S. G., Strong, C. M., & Ketter, T. A. (2001). Divalproex therapy in medication-naive and mood-stabilizer-naive bipolar II depression. *J. Affect. Disord., 67*(1–3), 207–212.

Yatham, L. N., Grossman, F., Augustyns, I., Vieta, E., & Ravindran, A. (2003). Mood stabilisers plus risperidone or placebo in the treatment of acute mania. International, double-blind, randomised controlled trial. *Br. J. Psychiatry, 182*, 141–147.

Yatham, L. N., Kennedy, S. H., O'Donovan, C., Parikh, S., Macqueen, G., McIntyre, R., et al. (2005). Canadian Network for Mood and Anxiety Treatments (CANMAT) guidelines for the management of patients with bipolar disorder: consensus and controversies. *Bipolar Disord., 7*(Suppl 3), 5–69.

Yatham, L. N., Paulsson, B., Mullen, J., & Vagero, A. M. (2004). Quetiapine versus placebo in combination with lithium or divalproex for the treatment of bipolar mania. *J. Clin. Psychopharmacol., 24*(6), 599–606.

Young, C. R., Bowers, M. B., Jr., & Mazure, C. M. (1998). Management of the adverse effects of clozapine. *Schizophr. Bull., 24*(3), 381–390.

Zarate, C. A., Jr., Tohen, M., Narendran, R., Tomassini, E. C., McDonald, J., Sederer, M., et al. (1999). The adverse effect profile and efficacy of divalproex sodium compared with valproic acid: a pharmacoepidemiology study. *J. Clin. Psychiatry, 60*(4), 232–236.

Zhang, W., Connor, K. M., & Davidson, J. R. (2005). Levetiracetam in social phobia: a placebo controlled pilot study. *J. Psychopharmacol., 19*(5), 551–553.

Zimbroff, D. L., Marcus, R. N., Manos, G., Stock, E., McQuade, R. D., Auby, P., et al. (2007). Management of acute agitation in patients with bipolar disorder: efficacy and safety of intramuscular aripiprazole. *J. Clin. Psychopharmacol., 27*(2), 171–176.

Zona, C., Ciotti, M. T., & Avoli, M. (1997). Topiramate attenuates voltage-gated sodium currents in rat cerebellar granule cells. *Neurosci Lett., 231*(3), 123–126.

chapter sixteen

Practical issues in psychological approaches to individuals with bipolar disorders

Jan Scott
University of Newcastle upon Tyne

Francesc Colom
IDIBAPS Hospital Clínic

Contents

Introduction 551
The start of the process 552
The keys to engagement 554
Understanding the client's "illness" model 554
Integrating the client's and clinician's goals 558
Enhancing medication adherence 561
Insight, awareness, adjustment, and guilt 567
Regularity without misery 569
Controlling what you can control: Psychiatrist agreement 570
Being alert 571
Don't do this at home: Who to refer 572
References 572

Introduction

This chapter focuses on practicalities of providing psychological input to individuals with bipolar disorders (BP) in day-to-day clinical practice. The first and most obvious thing to state is that it is impossible for clinicians *not* to be psychologically important to clients with BP. There are however, three key models of psychological input-general clinical management, supportive therapy, and specific therapies (now commonly referred to as empirically supported psychotherapies). The latter are usually delivered in a course of about 20–25 sessions by trained therapists and these therapies have been the focus of a number of recent randomized controlled treatment trials (RCTs)—details of the outcomes and implications of the findings of these RCTs are discussed in Chapter 17. As such, this chapter will not review these therapies any further, but will discuss simple, basic interventions that can and should form part of a clinical management package for the many individuals with BP who are not receiving a formal course of individual, family or group psychotherapy. The approaches we describe are usually integrated within the care and treatment program in general clinical settings and are most likely to be delivered clinically by general psychiatrists or professionals working in a mental health team. The interventions are derived from the core elements of the systematic therapies. However, these brief, selected techniques are not currently the subject of formal direct empirical evaluations specifically in BP (although there is indirect evidence to support the use of these approaches), but are selected from the perspective that they represent an appropriate set of skills for all clinicians working in the field.

This chapter will outline some approaches that could be incorporated into clinical interviews with no or minimum additional training. The key themes explored in the chapter are: collaborative approaches to service engagement and treatment adherence; enhancing life style regularity; and encouraging the self-directed use of relapse prevention skills by individuals with BP (Scott, 2002). The chapter will also identify which clients may benefit from a referral for a formal course of one of the specific therapies now developed for BP.

The start of the process

The effective delivery of treatment relies upon the client's (and frequently the carer's) ability and willingness to accept the services offered, and to adhere to an agreed treatment plan. For many individuals, the aftermath of the first acute episode of mania and/or being given a diagnosis of BP for the first time can be a confusing and distressing time (Scott, 1995). To ensure the individual and their family have an opportunity to benefit from the care and treatments available, it is first necessary to engage them in the "disease management" process. The development of a therapeutic alliance is the vehicle through which engagement proceeds. This is such an intuitive part of clinical practice that many readers will be surprised to see this discussed. However, developing a "working alliance" and engagement are essential for the success of any interventions in BP and what is intuitive to one clinician may need to be practiced by another. As such, we provide a brief overview if only to provide an *aide memoir* when training or supervising less experienced clinicians or when trying to uncover the reasons why any client on their own current caseload is not fully "signed up" to the treatment package.

The importance of the therapeutic alliance and its impact upon outcome in formal psychotherapy settings is frequently highlighted in the literature (e.g. Scott & Colom, 2008). A recent review of studies measuring the therapeutic alliance in the treatment of severe mental disorders showed it is also a reliable predictor of client outcome in general adult psychiatry services (McCabe & Priebe, 2004). Various models have been proposed for conceptualizing a healthy alliance; essential components appear to be having an equal partnership between clinician and client, negotiation, and collaborative decision-making (see Tacchi & Scott, 2009). An overview of the factors that promote a positive doctor–client interaction (based on DiMatteo, 1979) is provided in Box 16.1.

A positive working alliance will aid engagement. But engagement in the treatment process incorporates a spectrum of behaviors and the degree of engagement a person exhibits may change over time, so it is important to view it in a multi-dimensional way, rather than as an "all or nothing" concept. In order to monitor the degree of engagement, we suggest briefly reviewing this aspect of the treatment process at regular intervals. Hall et al. (2001) suggest engagement can be assessed on six dimensions: appointment keeping, client-therapist interactions, communication, openness, collaboration with treatment and medication adherence. Priebe et al. (2005) reported that individuals with severe mental disorders identified that two of the most important factors in promoting their engagement were the employment of a "partnership model" in the therapeutic relationship, and clinical interactions that did not exclusively focus on medication. In contrast, their most important reasons for disengagement from the treatment services were: a desire to be independent, a negative therapeutic alliance, and a feeling they were not in control (which they attributed to the prescribed medications or sometimes to involuntary hospitalizations).

BOX 16.1   DEVELOPING A POSITIVE THERAPEUTIC ALLIANCE

- Affective qualities: Warmth, positive regard, lack of tension, nonverbal expressiveness
- Communication style: Ask not tell, listen
- Client participation: Answer client concerns, allow discussion
- Collaboration: Mutual understanding and goal setting
- Psychotherapeutic Qualities: Empathy and respect
- Time: Don't rush

The keys to engagement

The themes that emerge from the above and other studies suggest that in order to promote a healthy alliance and begin the process of engagement, the clinician particularly needs to pay attention to:

1. Listening to the client and taking the time to find out about their perspective, (rather than the clinician simply assuming they know what the client believes or jumping to conclusions on the basis of their answers to a limited range of questions).
2. Fostering a collaborative approach.
3. Negotiating shared goals for treatment sessions.

A common barrier to exploring the details of the client's perspective—rather than completing a diagnostic interview or a mental state assessment at a follow-up appointment—is a perceived shortage of time. There is no simple solution to this, but it is essential that sessions do not appear hurried, and time is clearly needed with new clients to start to build a rapport and understand their current thinking on what is happening to them (so the clinician is aware of any misconceptions and their expectations from the outset). The only comfort we can offer busy clinicians is that the periods spent establishing a collaborative relationship where both clinician and client understand each other's viewpoints and goals is never wasted and indeed may save several hours of more challenging work at a later date (e.g. when trying to repair the therapeutic alliance with a disenchanted client who has disengaged from treatment). An important aspect of the interaction is to create an atmosphere of open, honest communication so a client can reveal any difficulties. It is particularly important that a client at risk of treatment non-adherence is able to talk about this without feeling that their behavior will be disapproved. Any sense of this is likely to lead to reluctance on the part of the client to voice his or her concerns about treatment or adhering with medications. The critical skill for the clinician is to focus more on asking questions and listening, and gradually "shaping" and guiding the client's discovery rather than telling the client your views. Providing information is necessary but on its own it is not sufficient to change views and behaviors.

Understanding the client's "illness" model

Most clinicians would rightly state that they listen to the client's views, but few will explore the client's own theory about their disorder in a structured way. The use of a health beliefs model (which is commonly employed in the psychological management of persistent physical disorders), allows a clinician to explore and understand the client's perspective by providing crucial insights into the client's beliefs about BP and their attitudes towards and expectations about treatment. Scott and Tacchi (2002) advocate the use of a modified version of the cognitive representation of illness model (Leventhal, Diefenbach, & Levanthal, 1992) in the assessment of individuals with a probable diagnosis of BP. The model describes how an individual constructs an internal representation of what is happening to them when they experience physical or mental symptoms and how they react to this scenario. It is an example of a self-regulatory model and so it is particularly useful approach when trying to encourage the client's active participation in the treatment process as a self-regulation theory assumes an individual tries to be an active problem-solver and that their behaviors represent their personal effort to resolve the problem caused by a health "threat". The cognitive representation of illness model has three core elements:

1. A cognitive representation, which reflects the meaning of the health threat to the individual. This can be activated by internal (symptoms) or external (information in the media) cues.
2. An action plan, which is the coping strategy developed and instigated by the individual to deal with the threat.
3. The individual's appraisal of the outcome of the coping strategy.

It is suggested that, no matter what the nature of the symptoms, most individuals organize their thinking about any health threat around five key themes (Scott & Tacchi, 2002). These are: What is it (identity)? Why has it happened (cause)? How long will it last, will it recur (timeline)? What effects will it have (consequences)? What can I do to make it go away (cure/control)? Thus the structure of the representation is a stable aspect of the model but the content of the cognitive representations may be idiosyncratic and can be influenced by culture, past experiences or the views of significant others.

The second component of the model suggests that if symptoms occur, individuals will make some attempt to cope with them. Crucially their choice of a particular coping strategy to cure or control the problem (e.g. taking medication or not) will be influenced by whether that seems to be a logical step given their ideas about the perceived identity, cause, timeline, controllability and consequences of the symptoms they have experienced. Taking medication or indeed seeking professional help may be one of a number of coping behaviors employed by the individual. The individual will next appraise their coping strategy and come to a decision about how effective it has been. They will then continue to use or modify this coping strategy accordingly. If the many alternative coping strategies are all ineffective the individual may re-appraise their cognitive representation, and then institute a further sequence of actions based on the new view they adopt.

Finally, the model suggests that individuals who perceive coherence between their concrete experiences of the symptoms, the meaning they have attached to them, and the explanation offered to them by a significant other (this may be a health professional) are more likely to engage with health services or adhere with the interventions that are suggested. This is predictable as the coherence in between the clients' view and the external feedback mean that any suggested course of action (such as a program of treatment) appears logical.

Despite some criticisms of this theory, a core strength of the model is that it sees the individual's cognitive representation and coping strategies as a dynamic process evolving over time. Furthermore, it identifies the individual's pattern of behavior as being "logical" in that it makes sense to them as the problem solving strategies employed are a direct result of the attributions and evaluation of the problems BP is posing to them. For this reason, the model is sometimes referred to as a "common sense" model and failure to engage or accept treatment may be viewed as "intelligent non-adherence" because this behavior is entirely consistent with the client's perceptions about the identity and causes of the problem and what would be an effective strategy to control the threat. For example, if the individual believes their mood swings are a function of their personality rather than BP, they may be reluctant to take medication, but may initially prefer to try to resolve the problem on their own, trying relaxation or "self-improvement" classes.

The most direct way of using the model in clinical practice is to systematically elicit the client's ideas and views about the five key areas of the model, namely: identify, cause, time line, consequences, control; examples of questions are given in Box 16.2. It cannot be stressed enough that this information is needed *before* the clinician offers their own professional opinions on the formulation or the exposition of the problems. By asking questions and eliciting the clients' views of their experiences it is possible to be aware of any gaps in their knowledge or any misunderstandings they have about the nature or cause of their difficulties. This means the clinician is aware of any likely areas of immediate discordance and can also start to predict when and how other problems might arise in the treatment process. As such, they can proactively attend to engagement and concordance issues, rather than being in the situation of having to react after the event (e.g. trying to offer education to an individual who stopped treatment when feeling) better because the client did not understand the likelihood of relapse in BP nor the difference between medications that get them well and those that help them stay well).

> ## BOX 16.2 QUESTIONS TO ESTABLISH THE CLIENT'S VIEWS OF THEIR PROBLEMS
>
> - *What is it?* What brought you here today? Can you describe what is happening to you? What concerns do you have?
> - *What caused it?* What do you think is happening to you? What do you think has lead to this? What explanation have you considered? Has anyone else offered an explanation to you?
> - *Timeline?* How long do you think this will last? What can you or anyone else do to affect this? Was there something that happened before that you can recognise?
> - *How has it affected you?* What have been the consequences so far? What have been the costs to you and to others? In future how could we avoid the negative consequences?
> - *Can it be controlled?* What have you done to try to control this problem? What can you or anyone else do to affect it/control it? Are there any problem-solving techniques or coping strategies that you have tried?

Exploring the clients' views of whether the problem can be cured or controlled also allows the clinician to establish the individuals coping style: Did they show evidence of avoidance (ignoring their symptoms in the hope they would go away), did they try to actively problem solve, did they use maladaptive strategies (e.g. using drugs or alcohol to try to reduce depression or dampen their overactivity)? Certain behaviors that may have seemed eccentric can be viewed as having some logic when understood from the perspective of the client's idiosyncratic model. In addition, as discussed next, effective strategies can be encouraged and built upon increasing the client's perception that they have some control on their problems, and also increasing collaboration.

The coping strategies that the client has used to-date can be seen in the context of the clients' beliefs about themselves and about BP. If strategies have been effective with regard to symptom management or their quality of life these can be incorporated into the treatment plan (e.g. advocating regular sleep–wake cycles to reduce instability in daily routines). If the client's strategies have been ineffective this information can be used to help the client reappraise whether this is an approach that should be revised, (e.g. the benefit of trying to "self-medicate" mood changes with drugs or alcohol), or can be replaced with an alternative coping strategy. A client may have tried a number of strategies; indeed the decision to seek help may be a problem-solving strategy that they only try after they have

BOX 16.3 EXPLORING COPING STRATEGIES

- What was the first thing you did to try and cope with this problem?
- What happened as a result?
- How effective did you think that approach was?
- What (symptoms) changed as a result?
- Did you try anything else?
- How effective was that approach?
- What would you do differently next time?

made other unsuccessful attempts to cope with their symptoms. Box 16.3 outlines some simple questions to help explore these issues.

Integrating the client's and clinician's goals

When there is coherence between the client's concrete experience of symptoms, the meaning that they have attached to these and the explanation given to them by the clinician (and others), there is much greater likelihood of engagement with and adherence with treatment. The task for the clinician is to use the client's model as a starting point reinforcing accurate information and perceptions, and adaptive coping strategies, using questions to guide discovery of other important facts and providing information as necessary in a targeted manner (e.g. about the risk of recurrence). In this way, the clinician uses the client's initial model as the starting point for their discussion but then builds on this to develop an accurate shared understanding of BP. Having incorporated the client's model into the clinician's model and produced a jointly agreed formulation of the clients problems, it is then possible to put forward a logical set of treatment goals that incorporates the adaptive or appropriate elements of the client's current coping strategies and the treatment components the clinician also sees as critical. Introduced in this way, the treatment package then makes sense to the client, which increases the acceptability of the regime to the client and, therefore, makes it more likely it will be followed. However, the goals of treatment also have to be individualized to facilitate engagement and adherence. It is rarely that the primary goal of an individual given the diagnosis of BP would be "to take medication daily for the rest of my life". The primary goals of clients are usually to return to work or to enjoy their previous level of functioning. A clinician's primary goal is usually to initially achieve a stable mental state and to use this as a platform from which improvements in the client's quality of daily life can be achieved. These goals are overlapping but need to be reframed to be fully coherent.

However, a simple set of questions will allow the clinician and client to quickly achieve concordance. For example, the clinician might ask:

'Your main wish is to be able to do ...X.... In order for us to achieve this, can we list the things you need to be able to do?'

If the client's desire is to return to work, the list of steps to allow them to achieve this goal might include, being able to get a restful night of sleep and get up at a regular time, to be able to concentrate for extended periods, to be able to complete a full day of activities and being able to plan such a day. The clinician and client can then discuss how to achieve each of these steps and the use of medication to improve sleep, concentration and reduce symptoms is now a logical part of the process, whilst planning daily activities and keeping a diary of what the client did compared with what they planned also an essential part of working towards an agreed goal. This shared decision making is a constructive way of educating clients about the process of change whilst retaining their sense of autonomy and/or control over treatment decisions that affect their well-being (Tacchi & Scott, 2005).

Later in the treatment process, clinicians need to retain the clients' commitment to treatment. Horne (1997) stated that an individual needs a prompt (a reminder of the threat of illness or the action that must be taken against it) to continue to engage in health-related behaviors. These "cues" to action can be internal such as the clients' recognition of prodromal symptoms of a BP relapse or external such as spontaneous statements made by others, information in the media etc. The skill of the clinician is how to ensure that their interventions have a positive effect on behavior, rather than leading the client to give up hope for the future. In general this is best achieved by reinforcing the benefits of treatment (e.g. effective problem-solving behaviors undertaken by the client, likelihood that of adherence will increase their chances of achieving their personal goals) rather than emphasizing the negative outcomes of not taking medications (e.g. non-adherence may lead to negative family interactions). One way is to assist the client in drawing up a checklist of the positive and negatives about treatment such as shown in Box 16.4.

Any treatment regime must be acceptable, understandable and manageable for that particular individual. So before a client leave an interview, the clinician needs to ask questions about these issues. If any of these three criteria are not met, the clinician needs to ask himself or herself why they are letting the client leave the consultation as there is less than a 30% likelihood that the client will not adhere with that treatment package (Scott, 2000).

It is often helpful for individuals to write the details of the agreed treatment plan for themselves. We usually encourage that they have five subheadings for this plan (Tacchi & Scott, 2005):

BOX 16.4   EXPLORING THE BENEFITS AND BARRIERS FOR ADHERENCE

Benefits of Treatment

- Being symptom free
- Enjoying hobbies, socializsing, studies
- Return to usual daily activities, being able to work
- Increased concentration
- No hassle from others about taking treatment

Barriers to Treatment

- Treatment regime not fitting in with lifestyle
- Beliefs, e.g. I should be able to cope without tablets/the help of professionals
- Views of significant others e.g. my father took lithium and didn't like it
- Stigma of illness e.g. taking tablets reminds me I have a chronic illness
- Forgetting tablets/concerns about side effects

- Overall treatment plan
  - Who is seen (doctor, psychologist, nurse, etc.) and how regularly
  - Contact with other services (attendance at work training courses, etc.)
- Medications
  - Name of medication, what dose is taken and how often
- Benefits of treatment
  - Three or four key points (such as shown in Box 16.4)
- Barriers to treatment
  - The key barriers as described by the clients
- Ways to overcome these barriers
  - For each barrier, the client is encouraged to note a coping strategy

Some individuals with BP like to keep a full page copy of such a plan in a prominent place at home and/or a credit card sized copy in their wallet so they can remind themselves of what the plan is and why it is beneficial to them (Scott, 2002). Despite such approaches, medication non-adherence is a significant problem in BP, so the next section particularly looks at this issue.

Enhancing medication adherence

The process of engagement and the development of a shared set of treatment goals will usually involve, at the very least, a trial of medication, and in most clients this is accompanied by an expectation of long-term prophylaxis. Before offering any medication it is useful to establish if the client has heard of the medication, do they know anyone else who has taken it or a similar medication, what do they know about it, do they have any concerns about it, etc. This approach, followed by fielding any specific questions and filling in gaps in knowledge or correcting misconceptions, allows the clinician to be aware of any general issues about medications (clients reluctant to take any tablets for anything, even a headache) or specific issues (e.g. a client who had a family member who had a bad reaction to lithium, or has read about controversies about certain medications may be unlikely to take those particular medications). This approach is usually far more effective in engaging the client with the treatment and promoting adherence than the clinician giving a brief didactic presentation on the medication in question and a synopsis of the side effects accompanied by a prescription (5% of which are never taken to the pharmacy for dispensing).

The most important approach to minimizing the risk of non-adherence is for clinicians to recognize that it is likely to be a problem for all clients receiving long-term treatment at some point. Bearing this in mind it is possible to identify some simple interventions that can be used to try to ensure adherence with newly prescribed treatments. In the first instance it is helpful to:

- Emphasize that medication is only one part of the treatment program Link adherence with medication to the clients' personal goals, e.g. "if we can stabilize your mood state with medication this will give us a window of opportunity to work on how you handle your relationship with XXX, that you tell me is causing you concern..."
- Reinforce that you are keen to develop a regime that is acceptable, understandable and manageable for the individual.
- Use the minimum possible number of medications and of doses.
- Regularly review benefits of and barriers to adherence.
- Expect non-adherence.

It is useful to remember that adherence is unlikely to be an all or nothing phenomena. Some clients take their medication regularly, others miss some doses, and others show cycles of adherence where they take treatment regularly when they feel unwell but become less committed to taking medication when they feel better. It is important to repeat the question about adherence on a regular basis, but the clinician should try to do so in a non-judgmental way so that the client feels able to give accurate answers to the questions posed. Box 16.5 offers suggestions of different questions that can be used depending on the client and the different situations in which the interviews will take place.

If there appears to be evidence of non-adherence or the client is perceived to be at high risk of becoming non-adherent, it is helpful to establish the actual pattern of adherence, in order to intervene effectively and appropriately. Diary keeping or enlisting significant others to provide information may be helpful in some cases. It is good clinical practice to establish patterns of adherence right at the beginning of prescribing any medication and to encourage clients to continue to monitor this throughout treatment for example by the use of a calendar. This will prevent an accusatory feel from discussions at a later date, as both the clinician and client can examine the evidence from a diary if non-adherence is a risk.

It is worth considering the nature or possible drivers of medication non-adherence when trying to determine the techniques to overcome this problem. Scott (1999) distinguishes between non-intentional and intentional non-adherence, which require different approaches. Unintentional non-adherence usually occurs when clients forget medications or find it difficult to establish regular patterns of adherence. A review of records of taking medication may, however, expose a different type of problem, namely that certain situations increase the individuals risk for non-adherence or that the primary problem relates to negative attitudes towards medication rather than difficulty in establishing a pattern of behavior. Intentional non-adherence is usually an indication of cognitive barriers to engaging with medication such as beliefs that trying harder would allow the individual to deal with the symptoms without recourse to the health services.

BOX 16.5 QUESTIONS TO ESTABLISH OR MONITOR ADHERENCE

- Many individuals find it hard to stick with a course of tablets—Do you ever have any trouble taking all of your medication as prescribed?
- Are there times when it is more difficult to remember to take your medication?
- Does your medication regime fit in with your lifestyle or activities?
- Do you ever try and cope without your tablets?

Unintentional non-adherence is likely to respond to a behavioral approach but in practice all forms of non-adherence will initially be tackled with behavioral approaches. Highly complex treatment regimens can increase the risk of non-adherence so a simple schedule should be negotiated wherever possible (Goodwin & Jamison, 1990). Use of once-a-day medication or longer-acting medications should be considered if preferred by the client. Use of a medi-pack or dosette that allows the daily medication regime to be organized in advance and self-monitoring of adherence is also helpful. Matching the prescription to the client's lifestyle or activities and concordance with the client's preferences with regard to dosing regimes should also be considered. Lastly, discussing client preferences for the type of drug or mode of administration (oral, depot) usually increase the likelihood of adherence.

Use of medication can be improved by writing the essential details on a small card that can be carried in a pocket or wallet. This may include information about the regime, situations or symptoms that may prompt changes in medication dose and recommended action if a dose or doses of medication are missed, plus what action to take or who to contact in a crisis.

Other behavioral interventions include prompts or cues to action and the use of reinforcements or pairing medication routines with other regular activities (see Box 16.6). For example, notes stuck in a prominent place that is visited daily such as the bathroom mirror may act as a reminder to take morning doses of medication. Pairing tablet taking with a routine daily activity for example brushing teeth may also aid adherence.

BOX 16.6 BEHAVIORAL TECHNIQUES FOR INCREASING MEDICATION ADHERENCE

- Give written instructions
- Use prompts, e.g. notes stuck in prominent places, text message alerts
- Pair tablet taking with routine activities e.g. brushing teeth
- Rehearse each step of adherence with the regime, particularly
- when anticipating exposure to high risk situations where non-adherence is likely
- Engage families, significant others or support workers in the process
- Keep a diary
- Simplify the regime
- Match the prescription to the client's lifestyle

Reminders provided in real time such as pre-arranged telephone calls, text messaging or using the alarm clock functions on mobile phones or other electronic equipment can help. Rehearsal, where the client visualizes each step in their medication routine and rehearsing additional coping strategies for novel situations is also beneficial. Family members or significant others can be engaged to offer reinforcement however this should only be considered when relationships are stable and the client feels this would be constructive rather than undermining their independence. The benefits of each strategy can be monitored through keeping a simple medication diary that can be reviewed with the clinician to monitor progress and the effectiveness of the intervention. For some of these interventions it may be possible to recruit the help of the clinical pharmacist or another team member to reinforce these strategies when prescriptions are collected.

Cognitive techniques are less likely to be used in general day-to-day practice, as they can require more clinical time or training. However, basic cognitive approaches can be useful particularly when non-adherence is intentional (see Box 16.7). In intentional non-adherence the client should be provided with a realistic appraisal of BP and his or her prognosis. This can take the form of an educational discussion supplemented by reading or video material. A worthwhile approach is to ask the client to take the first step and seek information about BP as a "homework assignment" either by obtaining leaflets from appropriate organizations, audiovisual aids or the internet etc. Obviously this strategy can only be implemented if the clinician judges this approach would be a positive experience and within the capability of a particular individual. However, the benefit is that the client finds out about the nature and course of BP in general and can compare

---

BOX 16.7　COGNITIVE TECHNIQUES

- Explore understanding
- Realistic appraisal of progress—in clinic education or homework assignment undertaken by the client
- Explore pattern of non-adherence e.g. specific thoughts that prevent adherence
- Identify negative thoughts associated with disorder or its treatment
- Test out ideas through simple experiments
- Facilitate client in identifying alternative explanations to modify these views
- Help client reframe general views e.g. attitudes and expectations of treatment

their findings with their current attitudes, beliefs or expectations of treatment. The next task is to explore the individual pattern of non-adherence. This information is mainly used to identify specific situations where there is a high risk of omitting prescribed medication. Again the emphasis is on guiding the client to examine his or her own cognitions and behaviors, for example a business man who omitted lithium prior to important contract meetings because he thought it would make him "dopey". Any alternative explanations about the reasons for omitting doses and ratings of the degree of belief and thoughts need to be generated by the client and not the doctor. Experiments are devised to test out the negative thoughts and can also provide further data on which to base discussions to generate alternative views e.g. carefully monitoring how he felt if he did take lithium before one contract meeting and then a meeting when he did not take it.

The approach taken will vary with the point in the clients history at which non-adherence occurs. The client who has relapsed as a result of stopping medication may be easier to engage in a discussion about the costs and benefits of treatment, as difficulties are fresh and tangible. However, reasons for stopping medication need to be explored as these may establish possible barriers to treatment in the future.

For clients experiencing their first BP episode, it is likely that this is also the first occasion they have contact with mental health services. There is no past pattern with regard to medication adherence to review and some of the discussion will be hypothetical, trying to establish general attitudes towards medication and likely behaviors and potential periods of increased risk of non-adherence. In trying to encourage adherence, it is important to strike a balance between instilling hope about future prospects for remission and/or a good quality of life despite being diagnosed as having a BP against warnings about the adverse effects of non-adherence on prognosis, which may be regarded by the client as "scare mongering" or may demoralize the individual because it emphasizes the negative impact of the disorder on the individual's adult life.

A different scenario is a client on maintenance treatment who is currently well. It is common in this instance for a client to start to doubt the benefits of or necessity of treatment. In this case a constructive way forward is to discuss the costs and benefits of medication and to undertake a careful assessment of knowledge about the difference between the treatment of acute symptoms as compared with treatments that prevent symptom return or keep people well. This may also require a review of the initial presentation and rationale for treatment. This can sometimes be difficult as memories of a past relapse have faded or are being avoided. Reality testing perhaps by involving significant others or gaining information from other sources, for example the internet, may be useful.

Consideration should be given to the client who refuses medication, but is prepared to remain in contact with the clinic. There are many reasons why a client decides not to engage in treatment, some of which include a poor doctor–client relationship, a decision made whilst being unwell, side effects of medication, media reports of negative effects such as suggestions of dependency, the views of significant others or a reduction in insight. If it is possible to identify a specific reason this can be amenable to intervention using the behavioral and cognitive strategies identified. However, in some instances, particularly if the client has the mental capacity to make this decision, it may be necessary as a clinician to agree with the client to a period of no treatment as an experiment. Whilst unlikely to be the clinicians preferred course of action, it is better to help manage this process rather than seeing the client vote with their feet and leave the service entirely and risk sudden medication withdrawal and early symptomatic relapse. Maintaining regular, indeed ideally, increased contact with the client has the advantage of keeping the dialogue open with the prospect of a return to medication without this decision being seen as a failure on anyone's part.

The client who is refusing treatment should also be encouraged to review his or her decision by listing advantages and disadvantages of the choice and considering if there is anything else that might change his or her mind and lead to continued acceptance of medication. Clients should be encouraged to talk to others to check out their views and to read about what interventions might protect them from relapse. If a client is to stop medication, it is crucial they are given advice to do this slowly and to avoid using non-prescription drugs in their place.

In some instances, clinicians may have to accept the client is NOT going to take medication. However, the first thing to establish is whether this is a "NO MEDICATION" or a "NO TREATMENT" option. If the client chooses to stop medication (and assuming compulsory treatment is not being considered nor justified at that moment) then it is vital that both parties plan the medication withdrawal program. Rather than giving up on the client at this point, the clinician needs to enter a dialogue about the need for gradual withdrawal to avoid relapse, the need for the client to feel able to inform the clinician if they stop the medication more quickly than they plan, the length of time this medication-free experiment will last and the frequency of future clinical reviews. Most importantly, the clinician and client need to agree clear criteria in advance about how they will identify the end point of an unsuccessful experiment, that is under what circumstances would the client accept medication again. Clients should be encouraged to look at enhancing all other coping strategies, to regularize their day-to-day activities and utilize any other strategies that may control symptoms. A record should then be kept of symptoms and agreed outcomes to make an accurate assessment of progress and the client is also encouraged to be honest in consultations with regard to their well-being and behavior. Ideally the client should also identify someone outside the clinical setting whom they trust who will also help monitor their progress and can advocate on their behalf, particularly if they experience symptoms of a recurrence. At this point, the clinician will hopefully have a further opportunity to negotiate a further treatment trial using a regime that the client now believes is acceptable, understandable and manageable. By viewing BP and its treatment from a long-term perspective, the clinician can hopefully maintain a therapeutic alliance with the client and work through these potentially difficult periods and help the client gradually adjust to BP and achieve better clinical outcomes and quality of life in the future.

Insight, awareness, adjustment, and guilt

Lack of illness insight is a major problem for a good number of individuals suffering from BD. Unfortunately, because of this issue, many of them will never show up at the psychiatrist's office. Hence, complete lack of insight in mental disorders is a major health problem we will have to deal with from the perspective of health politics. But what really matters for us in our clinical practice is the partial awareness that some bipolar patients may show. Many bipolar patients visit their psychiatrist just looking for help in their depressive phase and mostly ignoring the problems related with their "ups" that may be interpreted simply as a period of happiness or as a restitution of normality after depression. Some patients may even excuse their hyperactivity as a need of recovering from all the "wasted time" when they have been depressed.

Improving illness awareness is very often a difficult task as the therapist has to directly confront many of the issues and beliefs that may reinforce patients' reluctance to accept the diagnosis. These may relate to stigma, misattributions regarding the etiology of bipolar disorder (basically linking ups and downs to personality) or their family's negative view of mental illnesses. Trying to "convince" the patient makes little sense especially before a strong therapeutic alliance has been developed. Some exercises may enhance patient awareness and enhance his readiness to accept help. One very simple exercise that has proven to be very useful in group psychoeducation programs and that can be easily translated into routine individual practice is the retrospective illness chart (Colom & Vieta, 2006; Scott, 2002). This consists of helping the patient to draw a two-axis diagram representing the last 5–10 years of their bipolar swings, writing down possible triggering factors, potential consequences of each episodes, treatments prescribed and their response and degree of adherence. The patient can usually learn to do this graphic in no more than 30 minutes, whilst drawing it at home (possibly with the help of a friend, partner or relative) may not take more than 2 hours. This provides extremely useful material to work with during the next few sessions. We invite the patient to draw a retrospective and not a prospective chart, as many patients may become anxious or obsessive about checking their mood day by day, something that may even complicate the therapy. Some especially sensitive patients may feel uncomfortable at being reminded of negative events when drawing the illness chart. If this is the case, we could offer these patients to compose a fictitious illness chart "just to acquire the skills". This will usually reduce anxiety and allow them to then compose their own illness chart.

Another useful and user-friendly technique for changing patient's attitude toward the disorder is teaching them on how to talk about the illness. Patients often make several mistakes when talking about their illness that reflect their own underlying beliefs. The most common one is, perhaps, using the expression "I am bipolar" instead of "I have bipolar disorder". This description shows up the inner attitudes of some patients who regard bipolar disorder as the sole determinant of their identity and not a diagnosis. This may have several consequences including difficulty in differentiating the self from the disorder, which may even lead to non-adherence, as most individuals would rarely accept a medication to change their personality. Hence, although such self-descriptions may seem just as a minor detail, they are not, and it is important to "model" statements for the patient to help talk about the disorder and to start the process of subtly changing their attitude toward the disorder. Some advice can also be given to help our patients talk about bipolar disorder with other people. We basically focus on three issues:

1. Focus on the biological etiology in order to talk about the underlying processes in bipolar disorder.
2. Focus on behavioral and physical symptoms (such as the lack of energy, hypersomnia or fatigue) more than in "mental" symptoms. It may help to avoid stigma as it is generally easier for people to understand the former as "real" symptoms of "a real illness".
3. Consciously avoid comments on suicide attempts, psychotic symptoms or hypersexuality as these may attract some sort of curiosity or attention that would not lead to understanding but fear.

Following this very simple advice, patients can practice or role play talking about bipolar disorder in a less stigmatized manner, and feel more confident of explaining the problems in a understandable way to significant others.

Regarding guilt and related issues, some of these ideas are partly relieved by inviting the patient to compare bipolar disorders with other non-psychiatric conditions such as diabetes, as both share certain characteristics such as chronicity, the need for both pharmacological and behavioral care and the benefiting from self-monitoring. However, therapists should be careful of the risks that some patients may view such explanations as absolving them of responsibility for their actions and abandon the general non-pharmacological care of his illness by stressing the biological condition. Thus, the patient should be reminded that in the same way that anyone is not guilty of having a myocardial infarction but can reduce future risk by taking responsibility for healthy habits (i.e. stop smoking, regulate stress, practice moderate physical exercise, follow a low-cholesterol diet and so on), the patient with bipolar disorder is not guilty of suffering from such a condition but should be encouraged to take responsibility for taking the medications prescribed and also of instituting regular sleeping habits, learning to deal with stress, monitoring early warning signs, avoiding the use of street drugs and alcohol and so forth.

Regularity without misery

Therapists need to be very careful when dealing with the issue of lifestyle regularity. Often the patient may feel that, by establishing certain rules about how they organize their personal agenda, what we are *really* trying to do is to change the way they are. This will, of course, raise resistance. Thus, when suggesting a "healthier" lifestyle we should first acknowledge the experience of loss of the former self, especially if that person had many habits and behaviors that may seriously interfere with bipolar disorder maintenance. In a way, for some patients, redesigning their lifestyle can be seen as an attempt by others to control their future or, even as a sort of an aggression. It is, then, crucial to let the patients learn the difference between who they are and what they do. For some patients the clinician needs to deal with grief feelings regarding (a) the healthy self or (b) the "wild" self. Not acknowledging and coping with this situation will reinforce denial and hinder the therapeutic relationship.

A very important issue related to lifestyle is whether the patient should or should not do physical exercise. Physical exercise is known to have benefits for many physical and psychiatric conditions, including unipolar depression. As it is known also to be a sort of "natural" stimulant, it will require some monitoring as a potential elation-inductor. Very simple advice for our patients would be to do moderate physical exercise when euthymic but stop it in case they suspect a (hypo)manic episode is starting. On the other hand, patients should be discouraged from practicing sports in the late evening, as it may disrupt sleep patterns.

Dealing with the issue of night-life and sleep pattern regulation will be more difficult in young patients. Patients usually argue that they do not want to "become a bore" and that, by not going out at night increases their sense of being different from their peers and actually makes relapse into depression much more likely. We should not discourage young patients from their usual social networking but we should balance this need with that of a regular sleep pattern. It may be acceptable to negotiate initially with the patient how many nights-out per month they treat themselves. Later, the patient should be able to self-regulate them with limited guidance from others.

Controlling what you can control: Psychiatrist agreement

In an ideal world a clinician would wish to help a patient with BD to design a desirable healthy life-style, but in the real world, the first goal is to collaborate in achieving a possible (and less health damaging) life-style. Unfortunately, some clinicians still attempt to push the patients towards the "ideal" life-style that not even they or their grandmothers can achieve. The clinician needs first and foremost to remember the patient is a human being and, like most of us, has a number of habits and attitudes that at times appear harmful rather than helpful to their existence. However, as clinicians, we should try to ascertain which habits destabilize the patient and worsen their BD and which ones do not, which attitudes towards the disorder need to be modified and which ones are still acceptable. Next, the clinician needs to identify which changes need to be addressed at a later time and which changes may be possible at an early stage.

Let us consider the case of an imaginary patient called "Howl". Howl goes out four nights a week and his entire world revolves around night-life; Howl's hair-dress gives him free entrance to most of the trendy pubs in town and it is fantastic for being a rock-band drummer, but would be barely acceptable for an engineer school student—which he tries to be every morning, sometimes unsuccessfully. The same applies to Howl's behavior and clothing. Howl smokes cigarettes (30 a day), cannabis (2–4 joints a day) and, occasionally, takes cocaine or NDMA when going out at night. He maintains parallel relationships with two different women. He regularly drinks alcohol to excess. He is 23 and he has been suffering from bipolar II disorder since he was 18. Interestingly he has no problem acknowledging his mental disorder and he is adherent with medication.

Clearly, the prognosis for Howl is quite poor unless many changes can be achieved (reduced or, better, fully stop street-drugs and alcohol intake, control sleep disruption, and improve life-style regulation). The problem is that if the clinician tries, even in general terms, to suggest all these possible changes to Howl, he will probably feel personally attacked or even refuse therapy. In order to maintain a working alliance with Howl—and achieve long-term changes—the first issue is not "which changes need to be made in order to enhance euthymia?" but "which changes are acceptable for this person right here and right now?"

The clinician decided that the most urgent issue that needed to be addressed was street-drugs intake, especially cocaine and NDMA. Thus, they focused their therapeutic efforts on this single issue to begin with. For Howl, it might be acceptable to limit his cocaine consumption only to "special times" (i.e. nights when he has a gig with his rock band). Of course for a clinician it is not acceptable to negotiate with a patient "how many cocaine lines you may have per month", but better "which cocaine dosing would be easiest for you to omit?" Whilst not an ideal clinical situation, the clinician has to balance this approach against loosing Howl altogether from follow-up. The therapist should always consider the gap between what is needed and what is possible/acceptable for the patient at this stage in the treatment process. To begin with, we would not ask Howl to focus on his day routines or to give up his night-life, as Howl would surely see this proposal as unrealistic and unacceptable. It is vital to maintain a dialogue with Howl and the clinician needs to show patience and maintain a long-term view of the treatment goals.

Being alert

A common component of all psychological interventions that have proved to be efficacious for bipolar patients is the improvement in the detection of early warning signs of relapse. Group psychoeducation provides an ideal setting for enhancing prodromes detection, thanks to its format that allows patients to learn by observation of others. However, in day by day clinical practice, it is not always possible to put together a group of euthymic patients with BD or to have a specialized group therapist to undertake the program. Hence, clinicians need to give patients the tools for identifying new episodes during regular individual appointments.

We suggest a very simple method that can be used no matter what setting the clinician is working in: Helping the patient to write down a short and practical list of early warning signs. These warning signs, ideally, should be single behaviors that are easy to identify, are memorable to the patient and are known to be indicative of relapse at the time they occur (not retrospectively). The patient should be encouraged to write down a short list (approximately ten items for (hypo)mania and ten for depression). Sometimes, patients need someone else's help with the list (partner, friends or family members) to confirm the suggested items or generate new ones, or even the clinician help (if the patient is well known to them). It is recommended that the patient choose the most well-known early warning signs for them and their family. However, it is very important not to choose symptoms, mistaking them for warning signs. A warning sign must, by definition, be very subtle and sensitive more than a specific. Most commonly mentioned warning signs for mania include sleeping problems, irritability or mood lability (not elation) and excessive spending. However, we should ask the patient to accurately define each item in order to be useful. For instance, we may ask the patient to specify what does he mean by sleeping problems and try to be highly specific: an acceptable warning sign definition would be, for instance, "sleeping less than 7 hours" or "waking up before the alarm rings". This way, the clinician and the patient avoid conflict when a relapse seems to be starting. In the case of irritability, it is much better to define it according to the number of discussions or fights that the patient had had during the day more than according to the perception of irritability itself.

Don't do this at home: Who to refer

In this chapter, we have tried to address some relevant issues that might be easily covered in routine treatment sessions. However, we should be aware that some therapeutic issues should be addressed by the specialist. It is very important for clinicians to know the limits of what they can and what they can not do in routine settings and to know when to refer. This would of course include some patients with personality disorder, some with refractory bipolar depressions, patients with an added anxiety disorder, substance abuse, and so on. In the same way that a patient may become medication refractory, another patient may become so to speak resistant to psychotherapy, due to a very bad experience. This is why we advise not to perform psychotherapy, if it is not highly likely to work.

References

Colom F., & Vieta E. (2006). *Psychoeducation Manual for Bipolar Disorder.* England: Cambridge University Press.

DiMatteo M. (1979). A social-psychological analysis of physician patient rapport: Toward a science of the art of medicine. *Journal of Social Issues, 35,* 12–33.

Goodwin F. K., & Jamison K. R. (1990). *Manic-Depressive Illness.* New York: Oxford University Press.

Hall M., Meaden A., & Smith J. et al. (2001). Brief report: The development and psychometric properties of an observer-rated measure of engagement with mental health services. *Journal of Mental Health, 10*(4), 457–465.

Horne R. (1997). Representations of medication and treatment: advances in theory and measurement. In: K. J. Petrie, & J. Weinman (Eds), *Perceptions of Health and Illness: Current Research and Applications.* London: Harwood Academic Publishers.

Levanthal H., Diefenbach M., & Levanthal E. (1992). Illness cognition: using common sense to understand treatment adherence and affect cognition interactions. *Cognitive Therapy and Research, 6,* 143–163.

McCabe R., & Priebe S. (2004). The therapeutic relationship in the treatment of severe mental illness. *International Journal of Social Psychiatry, 50*(2), 115–128.

Priebe S., Watts J., & Chase M. et al. (2005). Processes of disengagement and engagement in assertive outreach patients: qualitative study. *British Journal of Psychiatry, 187,* 438–443.

Scott J. (1995). Psychotherapy for bipolar disorder. *British Journal of Psychiatry, 167*: 581–588.

Scott J. (1999). Cognitive and behavioural approaches to medication adherence. *Advances in Psychiatric Treatment, 5,* 338–347.

Scott J. (2000). Predicting medication non-adherence in severe affective disorders. *Acta Neurolopsychiatrica, 12,* 128–130.

Scott J. (2002). *Overcoming Mood Swings.* England: Constable Robinson.

Scott J., & Colom F. (2008). Gaps and limitations of psychological interventions for bipolar disorders. *Psychotherapy & Psychosomatics, 77,* 4–11.

Scott J., & Tacchi M.J. (2002). A pilot study of concordance therapy for individuals with bipolar disorder who are non-adherent with lithium prophylaxis. *Bipolar Disorders, 4,* 286–293.

Tacchi M.J., & Scott J. (2005). *Improving Adherence in Schizophrenia and Bipolar Disorders.* England: J Wiley & Sons Ltd.

Tacchi M.J., & Scott J. (2009). Strategies for promoting engagement and adherence with treatment in severe mental disorders. In: S. Waters, & G. Thornicroft (Eds), *Community Psychiatry.* England: J Wiley & Sons, in press.

chapter seventeen

Psychosocial interventions for bipolar disorder: A critical review of evidence for efficacy

David J. Miklowitz
University of Colorado
Oxford University

Contents

Introduction 575
    Historical roots of current psychosocial approaches 576
    The biopsychosocial approach to treatment 577
Testing psychosocial interventions: Design considerations.................... 578
Cognitive-behavior therapy 579
    Conclusion 580
Individual and group psychoeducation 580
    Conclusion 582
Family-focused therapy 582
    Conclusion 584
Interpersonal and social rhythm therapy 584
    Conclusion 585
Comparing different forms of psychosocial intervention:
    The STEP-BD trial 585
Conclusions and future directions.. 586
    Moderators and mediators 586
    Cost-effectiveness.. 587
    Psychosocial treatment as preventative intervention.................... 587
References.. 588

Introduction

Bipolar disorder is one of biological psychiatry's greatest success stories. Pharmacotherapy is the first-line offense against episodes of mania and depression, as well as in maintaining long-term stability. Nonetheless, clinicians and researchers are increasingly recognizing the value of psychosocial interventions as adjunctive to pharmacotherapy. The past decade has seen a substantial increase in the number of randomized clinical trials of psychotherapy and pharmacotherapy, most of which find strong evidence for the efficacy of combined approaches. What kinds of psychosocial interventions are effective for bipolar disorder, for what domains of outcome, at what point in the patient's illness, and over what period of time? This chapter reviews the literature on psychosocial interventions (with an emphasis on randomized clinical trials), draws conclusions about the area as a whole, and points to directions for future research.

Historical roots of current psychosocial approaches

In the 1950s and 1960s, before the advent of lithium treatment, psychoanalytic approaches prevailed (e.g. Cohen et al., 1954). Bipolar disorder was widely seen as having a strong biological and genetic basis, but psychoanalysis was seen as a means of addressing historical traumas and neurotic or interpersonal conflicts associated with emerging symptom states. No empirical data on these approaches were produced, although studies of psychoanalytic couple treatments emerged in the 1970s as a means of supplementing and augmenting medication strategies (e.g. Fitzgerald, 1972; Davenport et al., 1977).

In the mid- to late 1980s, investigators took a different approach: how could psychosocial treatments help patients adjust to the community after an illness episode, and could it help them stay on their medications? Clarkin et al. (1990; Glick et al., 1991) enrolled 186 psychotic and bipolar or unipolar depressed patients in a trial involving nine sessions of inpatient family intervention. The model focused on enhancing post-hospital adjustment and family functioning. Those patients who were randomly assigned to family intervention had better symptomatic and global functioning than patients who were assigned to standard care alone in the 6–18 months after hospital discharge, although the treatment effects were specific to the female patients.

Cochran (1984) constructed a six-session cognitive behavioral therapy (CBT) for stable bipolar patients in an outpatient affective disorders clinic. The purpose of treatment was to keep patients compliant with their lithium regimens through challenging distorted thoughts or assumptions about the role of medication in their lives. Relative to pharmacotherapy alone, the intervention was successful at 6-month follow-up in promoting lithium compliance and reducing the number of hospitalizations attributable to noncompliance.

These early studies contributed to two assumptions that we now largely take for granted: psychosocial treatment of bipolar illness can be systematically studied through randomized controlled trials, and treatments are likely to be most successful if they are oriented toward illness management and coping. These assumptions mirrored trends in schizophrenia research in the late 1970s and 1980s. Family psychoeducational treatments for schizophrenia were found to be quite effective as adjunctive to neuroleptics in delaying psychotic relapse and enhancing functioning (Pitschel-Walz et al., 2001). The consistency of the psychoeducational treatment findings in schizophrenia were striking, and contributed to emerging biopsychosocial approaches to bipolar and unipolar affective disorder, as well as more traditional medical illnesses (Dixon et al., 2001).

The biopsychosocial approach to treatment

On the face of it, biopsychosocial approaches to the treatment of bipolar disorder are straightforward: integrated treatments consisting of pharmacotherapy, active collaboration with the patient in choosing medications and managing side effects, and adjunctive psychotherapy to enhance medication adherence, illness adaptations, interpersonal relationships, and job functioning. Implicit in biopsychosocial approaches, however, is a recognition of the role of stress in the course and outcome of the disease, and that psychosocial interventions can positively influence these processes. What findings within the bipolar/stress literature have been influential in the design of models of psychotherapy?

Family psychoeducational approaches to bipolar disorder and schizophrenia have been influenced by the research on *expressed emotion* (EE), which has consistently shown that patients who return following a hospitalization (or following outpatient treatment for an acute episode) to families in which relatives express high levels of criticism, hostility, or emotional overinvolvement are two- to three-times more likely to relapse in the next 9–12 months than patients who return to "low EE" families (for reviews, see Butzlaff & Hooley, 1998; Miklowitz, 2004). These longitudinal observations suggested that altering the emotional atmosphere of the family during the post-episode period might be central to providing protection against early recurrences of psychotic or affective disorder.

The interpersonal and cognitive approaches to bipolar disorder (reviewed below) draw more heavily on evidence that stress from life events contributes to bipolar recurrences. Several investigators have shown that negative life events such as loss experiences can slow down recovery from bipolar depressive episodes (e.g. Johnson & Miller 1997), whereas stress that causes significant changes in sleep/wake rhythms (Malkoff-Schwartz et al., 1998, 2000), or that accelerates goal attainment (Johnson et al., 2000) can precipitate manic episodes. Psychosocial interventions targeting a person's emotional, cognitive, or behavioral reactions to events could therefore be useful adjuncts to pharmacotherapy.

In conclusion, most models of psychosocial intervention draw from the assumption that certain stressors—and the psychological processes associated with them—interact to produce episodes of bipolar disorder. These stressors and associated processes operate against the background of biological and genetic vulnerabilities. The nature and relative strength of these interactive processes will change at different phases of development (Miklowitz & Cicchetti, 2006). Let us now turn our attention to specific models of psychosocial intervention and their empirical support.

Testing psychosocial interventions: Design considerations

In evaluating the literature on psychosocial interventions, it is useful to keep several design distinctions in mind. First, the most convincing data usually come from randomized controlled trials rather than open trials. Open trials are usually reserved for the early phases of development of a treatment, and can be useful in demonstrating that a treatment is worth testing in a randomized trial. The primary outcome from an open trial is usually a pre/post effect size, which measures the amount of change in a single group over time. Within-group effect sizes are often confused with between-group effect sizes, which measure the degree to which two groups differ in change of an outcome variable over time. Typically, within-group effect sizes are much larger than between-group effect sizes.

Second, most psychosocial intervention studies—with some notable exceptions below—are oriented toward prevention of recurrence over 1–2 year periods rather than acute efficacy following an episode. Most, although not all pharmaceutical trials are aimed at acute stabilization rather than maintenance treatment, and use a strict time window, usually the 8–12 weeks after onset of an acute episode. Moreover, the primary outcome variable in drug trials is often time until a change in pharmacological intervention, whereas psychosocial studies generally focus on recurrence or reduction in residual symptoms. Thus, the effect sizes observed within drug and psychosocial studies are rarely directly comparable.

Third, psychosocial studies vary as to whether the targeted population is acutely depressed, acutely manic, or remitted. Studies of cognitive-behavioral therapy (CBT) and group psychoeducation typically begin when patients have been recovered for at least 6 months. Studies of family-focused therapy (FFT) and interpersonal and social rhythm therapy (IPSRT) have typically begun immediately after an acute episode, often for which the patient was hospitalized.

Finally, in evaluating the trials, it is important to note differences in comparison groups, which can make all the difference in whether a novel treatment is deemed effective or not. The easiest contrasts are between an active treatment and treatment as usual, especially if usual treatment means pharmacotherapy alone. This is analogous to a drug/placebo comparison. Tougher contrasts are between active psychotherapies and briefer (e.g. two to three sessions) psychosocial treatments. The most conservative contrasts are between active psychotherapies which are the same length and intensity (analogous to comparing two drugs whose relative dosages or dosing frequencies are equated). The latter studies provide an "attention control" over the opportunity that clinical personnel have to observe and intervene with new illness episodes.

Cognitive-behavior therapy

There have been two major trials of CBT as adjunctive to medications for bipolar disorder, both conducted in the United Kingdom. The first (Lam et al., 2003) randomly assigned 103 patients to pharmacotherapy alone or pharmacotherapy with CBT (12–18 sessions over 6 months). Patients had been in remission for at least 6 months but had had ≥3 episodes in the last 5 years. Over 1 year, patients in adjunctive CBT were healthier on a number of measures: they were less likely to relapse, relapsed later in the follow-up, spent fewer days in episode, coped better with prodromal symptoms, and had better social functioning than patients in usual care. The results, however, were less striking at 12–30 month follow-up, as the differences between the groups in relapse were no longer significant. Nonetheless, patients in CBT continued to report better mood states and fewer days in episode over the 30 months than those in usual care.

The multicenter randomized effectiveness trial of Scott et al. (2006), conducted in the United Kingdom across five sites and with a substantial sample size (N=253), had mixed results. Patients received 22 sessions of CBT plus pharmacotherapy or pharmacotherapy alone (treatment as usual, or TAU). Unlike the study by Lam and colleagues, the patients had been in various clinical states before entry into the trial. Also, the CBT was structured somewhat differently than the version of Lam and colleagues, in that therapists and patients began treatment with cognitive restructuring (challenging of dysfunctional thoughts and attitudes) before moving onto behavioral strategies such as pleasurable life events scheduling or relapse prevention planning.

A majority (60%) of the patients had recurrences during the 18-month follow-up, but patients in CBT and TAU did not differ in time to recurrence over the 18-month study. Post-hoc exploratory analyses revealed that patients with fewer than 12 prior episodes had recurrences later in treatment if they received CBT than if they received TAU. In contrast, patients with more than 12 episodes had later recurrences in TAU than CBT.

How do we make sense of these conflicting results? The study by Scott et al. suggests that CBT may be most suited to patients in the early stages of their disorder (or those with a less cyclic course). It is unclear, however, why patients with more than 12 episodes would have a worse outcome in CBT than TAU. Possibly, an intensive treatment that focuses on intrapsychic processes such as distorted beliefs or assumptions is unsettling to the highly relapse-prone patient. These patients might have responded better to a more traditional behavioral strategy such as pleasant events scheduling (behavioral activation). The two studies also differed in clinical status at study entry: whereas patients in the Lam sample were in recovery, patients in the Scott study could be in any clinical state. Finally, the Scott study was conducted across multiple sites. Although this is clearly a strength of the study, therapists at the sites may have differed in their experience in treating people with bipolar disorder.

Conclusion

Although the results of the Scott trial cast doubt on the effectiveness of CBT for bipolar disorder, other trials have found benefits (Lam et al., 2005; Cochran, 1984). Moreover, the recently completed Systematic Treatment Enhancement Program for Bipolar Disorder (STEP-BD) found benefits for CBT and other forms of psychotherapy in stabilizing depressive episodes (reviewed below). Clearly, more research on the optimal format of CBT, and what course of illness features are associated with the greatest benefits, will be essential in the next phase of research on this modality.

Individual and group psychoeducation

Guidelines for the treatment of bipolar disorder (Yatham et al., 2005) often point to the importance of educating the individual patient about the nature, course, and treatment/self-management of bipolar disorder. Surprisingly, however, individual psychoeducation has received the least empirical investigation. Only one trial (Perry et al., 1999) has examined the benefits of a specific form of individual psychoeducation – how to identify early warning signs of recurrence and obtain emergency treatment. This form of psychoeducation was given in seven to 12 individual sessions and compared with routine care, both given with standard medication treatment. They randomly assigned 69 patients who had had a relapse within the prior 12 months. Over 18 months, there was a 30% reduction in manic relapses, greater intervals of stability prior to manic recurrences, and better social and employment functioning in the psychoeducation condition than in the routine care condition. The intervention had no impact on the frequency or timing of depressive recurrences. This form of individual psychoeducation may be a cost-effective way of reducing manic symptoms and enhancing functioning when given alongside of pharmacotherapy.

Other studies have examined psychoeducation within a group setting. Colom and associates (2003) randomly assigned patients to a 21-session structured, didactic psychoeducation group or an unstructured support group, both in combination with standard pharmacotherapy. Like the study by Lam et al., the 120 patients had been in remission for at least 6 months. At the end of 2 years, fewer of the group psychoeducation patients (67%) than the control patients (92%) had relapsed, and fewer had been hospitalized. Broad effects of group psychoeducation could be observed for manic, mixed, and depressive symptoms. Patients in the structured groups were more likely to maintain higher and more stable lithium levels, and were less likely to require hospitalization. One study limitation is that rates of attrition were somewhat higher (27%) in the structured than in the unstructured groups. Nonetheless, this trial is a breakthrough in the study of group psychoeducation as an adjunct to medication in preventative maintenance.

The largest randomized trial of individual and group psychoeducation to date (Simon et al., 2006) evaluated a 2-year multicomponent care-management intervention against continued treatment-as-usual among 441 patients receiving health care within the same managed care network. The care-management intervention consisted of pharmacotherapy, monthly telephone monitoring of moods and medication adherence, facilitating the patient's access to community services, crisis intervention (as needed), interdisciplinary care planning, and a structured group psychoeducational treatment following the life skills model of Bauer & McBride (1996). Over 2 years, patients in the multicomponent program had significantly lower mania scores and spent less time in manic or hypomanic episodes than those in a treatment-as-usual comparison group, but there were no effects on depressive symptoms. Importantly, the patients who benefited were those who had clinically significant symptoms at baseline. The treatment was delivered with only marginal increases in the costs of services (approximately US $1300/patient), suggesting that it was cost-effective given its powerful effects on preventing manic symptoms.

One study examined the relative efficacy of two group psychoeducational treatments for bipolar adults who had comorbid substance dependence (Weiss et al., 2007). A total of 62 patients with substance dependence were randomly assigned to 20 weeks of integrated group therapy or group drug counseling. The integrated group used a cognitive behavioral relapse prevention model focused on the relationships between the two disorders (i.e. similarities in cognitions and behaviors during the recovery and relapse processes). The group counseling did not address mood issues, and instead focused on encouraging abstinence and teaching ways to cope with substance craving.

Over 8 months, the integrated, dual-focus groups were better in maintaining abstinence: patients in these groups had half as many days of substance use as those receiving only drug counseling. The results were only significant for days of alcohol use, not drug use. The groups did not differ in the number of episodes of bipolar disorder, and patients in the integrated groups had higher subsyndromal depression and mania scores during treatment and follow-up than patients in drug counseling. The significance of this higher level of subsyndromal symptoms is unclear; it is possible that the dual diagnosis focus of the groups increased the likelihood that patients would recognize and report such symptoms. Integrated group treatment deserves further study in randomized trials involving substance dependent patients.

Conclusion

Psychoeducation, notably as delivered in groups, has been shown to be an effective intervention for manic episodes and comorbid substance dependence. Its effects on depression are less consistent. The absence in these models of traditional psychological methods for treating depression— such as cognitive restructuring, behavioral activation, interpersonal problem solving, and increasing family or marital support and communication effectiveness—may limit their effectiveness in stabilizing depression. However, teaching patients strategies for recognizing and preventing the escalation of prodromal symptoms, coping with craving for alcohol or substances, and the importance of medication adherence may be core ingredients in preventing manic episodes. We will return to the theme of common ingredients shortly.

Family-focused therapy

Several research groups have examined the utility of FFT as adjunctive to pharmacotherapy for bipolar patients. FFT targets patients who are stabilizing from an acute manic or depressive episode and is typically initiated during the immediate post-hospital phase. In the first published randomized trial (Miklowitz et al., 2003a), 101 acutely ill patients, 80% of whom were initially assessed while in the hospital, were randomly assigned at discharge to FFT and pharmacotherapy or a brief psychosocial control called crisis management (CM) and pharmacotherapy. FFT was given in 21 sessions over 9 months and consisted of psychoeducation (didactic strategies for managing illness episodes as a family, including relapse prevention planning), communication skills training, and problem-solving skills training. Patients in CM received two sessions of psychoeducation and crisis intervention sessions as needed over 9 months.

Over a 2-year follow-up, patients in FFT were three times more likely to finish the study without relapsing (52% vs 17%) and had longer periods of stability without relapse (73.5 weeks vs 53.2 weeks). FFT was also associated with lower depression and mania severity scores over 2 years. Post-hoc analyses revealed two mechanisms by which FFT achieves its effects: via improving the emotional tone of family interactions, which in turn predicts improvements in depressive symptoms (Simoneau et al., 1999) and enhancing the consistency of medication adherence, which predicts stabilization of mania symptoms (Miklowitz et al., 2003a).

A second trial examined the effects of FFT and pharmacotherapy when compared to an equally intensive (21 session) individual therapy and medications (Rea et al., 2003). Patients in the individual treatment received 21 sessions of psychoeducation, relapse prevention planning, medication adherence monitoring, and support against the social stigma of the illness. All patients began in a hospitalized manic episode and were randomly assigned to treatments just after hospital discharge. Patients did not differ in relapse or rehospitalization rates in the first year of treatment, during which the psychosocial treatments were given. However, in a 1–2 year post-treatment follow-up, patients in FFT had lower rates of relapse (28%) and even lower rates of rehospitalization (12%) than patients in individual therapy (60% and 60%, respectively). Moreover, when patients in FFT did have relapses, they were less likely to require rehospitalization (55%) than patients in individual treatment (88%). Medication regimens and compliance with those regimens were comparable across conditions (Rea et al., 2003).

FFT has also been investigated in an open trial of adolescent patients (Miklowitz, Biuckians, & Richards, 2006). A total of 20 patients (mean age 15) received 21 sessions of FFT in combination with pharmacotherapy and were followed over 2 years. Adolescents showed improvements in depression (withing-group Cohen's $d=0.87$), mania ($d=1.19$), and total mood symptom scores ($d=1.05$) over time. The improvements were not linear: patients tended to improve month by month until 9 months, and then showed a partial return of symptoms after regular sessions were withdrawn. Then, they improved again in the second year of post-treatment follow-up. The fluctuating trajectory of symptoms over time emphasizes the importance of considering non-linear patterns of change among bipolar patients.

In the absence of a control group, one cannot conclude that the FFT caused these changes among adolescent patients. A three-site randomized trial of FFT for bipolar adolescents is nearing completion.

Conclusion

FFT has been found to be consistently effective in randomized trials. However, not all patients have family members who are either accessible or wish to be involved in treatment. The STEP program estimated that 54% of patients who were eligible for psychosocial intervention were eligible for family treatment. The rate of family accessibility is higher among patients in childhood, adolescence or young adulthood than among patients who are middle-aged and highly recurrent. FFT should be considered whenever patients have access to family members and especially when family or marital conflict is one unintended side effect of the bipolar disorder.

Interpersonal and social rhythm therapy

Ehlers and colleagues (1988, 1993) have proposed a model in which bipolar symptoms are viewed as the final common pathway of disruptions in daily routines and sleep/wake cycles, which is turn disrupt circadian rhythms. The interpersonal and social-rhythm therapy (IPSRT; Frank, 2005), which derives from the interpersonal therapy for depression (Weissman, Markowitz, & Klerman, 2000) has two objectives: to stabilize social rhythms (i.e. when patients arise, go to sleep, exercise, socialize, etc.) and resolve interpersonal problems that co-occurred with the most recent episode of bipolar disorder. Following an acute episode, patients learn to to track their daily routines and sleep/wake cycles and identify events (e.g. changes in job hours; upcoming vacations) that may provoke further changes in these routines.

In the Pittsburgh Maintenance Therapies study (Frank et al., 2005), 175 acutely ill bipolar patients were assigned randomly during a stabilization phase to IPSRT or active clinical management in conjunction with pharmacological treatment. Once stabilized, patients were again assigned randomly to IPSRT or clinical management for a 2-year maintenance treatment period. Patients who received IPSRT in the acute phase had longer intervals prior to recurrences in the maintenance phase than patients assigned to clinical management in the acute phase. Acute phase IPSRT was most effective in delaying recurrences in the maintenance phase when patients succeeded in stabilizing their social rhythms (daily routines and sleep/wake cycles) during the acute phase. IPSRT during the maintenance phase, however, did not differently influence recurrence rates during the maintenance phase when compared to clinical management.

IPSRT was also examined in a treatment development study. Miklowitz and colleagues (2003b) hypothesized that patients—especially those with high levels of family conflict and social stress—would be more likely to stabilize social rhythms if their family members were involved in treatment. They examined a model of integrated family and individual therapy (IFIT) in which patients received individual IPSRT sessions during one week and family or marital FFT sessions the next. In an open trial, 30 patients received pharmacotherapy and an average of 29 individual or family sessions for the year following an illness episode. The outcomes of patients in the combined treatment were then compared to the outcomes of 70 historical control patients who received pharmacotherapy, two sessions of family education, and CM over one year. Patients in the integrated family and individual treatment had longer intervals prior to relapse and had less severe depressive symptoms during the study year than patients in CM, even after the effects of medication regimens and compliance were statistically controlled. The integrated treatment did not affect manic symptoms.

Conclusion

The large scale randomized trial of Frank and colleagues finds that IPSRT given acutely offers long-term maintenance protection. The mechanisms of action probably include the stabilization of social rhythms, although unmeasured variables—such as whether patients resolved the initial problem that brought them into treatment—may have also played a mediational role. Questions remain about who benefits from IPSRT and whether it has equal impact on depressive and manic symptoms.

Comparing different forms of psychosocial intervention: The STEP-BD trial

All of the aforementioned trials compared an active treatment arm to a control intervention. None compared two or more empirically supported treatments. To use a pharmacotherapy analogy, most of the trials had placebo controls, but none compared one active agent to another.

The Systematic Treatment Enhancement Program (STEP-BD) examined the effectiveness of pharmacologic and psychosocial interventions in a practical clinical trial in 15 centers across the US (Sachs et al., 2003). One innovative aspect of the program was a study in which acutely depressed bipolar patients ($N = 293$) were assigned randomly to medication and one of four psychosocial treatments: 30 sessions of FFT, IPSRT, or CBT, or a three-session psychoeducational control treatment called collaborative care (CC). Over 1 year, being in any intensive psychotherapy was associated with a higher recovery rate from depression (105/163, or 64.4%) than being in CC (67/130, or 51.5%; hazard ratio=1.47) (Miklowitz et al., 2007). Patients in intensive treatment were also more likely to remain well during any given month of the 1-year study than patients in the CC group.

Rates of recovery for the specific modalities were as follows: FFT, 77% (20/26) recovered, IPSRT, 65% (40/62) recovered, and CBT, 60% (45/75) recovered. In the CC condition, 51.5% recovered. The study was under-powered to detect statistically significant differences between the intensive modalities.

The results of the STEP-BD program suggest that bipolar patients with acute depression require a more intensive psychotherapy than is typically offered in community mental health centers. Possibly, the common ingredients of intensive treatments—such as teaching coping strategies to manage mood, intervening early with prodromal symptoms, enhancing patients' consistency with mood stabilizing medications, and working toward resolution of key interpersonal or family problems—contributed to more rapid recoveries. Further analyses of the STEP-BD dataset will consider functional outcomes (i.e. work, social relationships, satisfaction with life) and moderators of treatment outcome (patient subgroups who show greater or lesser benefit from intensive psychotherapy).

Conclusions and future directions

This review of the literature on adjunctive psychotherapy for bipolar disorder finds supportive evidence for group psychoeducation (with and without individual care management), family-focused therapy, interpersonal and social rhythm therapy, and cognitive-behavioral therapy. One study has provided evidence for individual psychoeducation (Perry et al., 1999). The forthcoming generation of psychotherapy research should address several key issues, as reviewed in this section.

Moderators and mediators

There are few clues as to who will benefit most from the various forms of psychotherapy (moderators). Moderators refer to variables measured before treatment begins and which specify the circumstances under which the treatments will be more and less effective (Kraemer et al., 2002). For example, Frank and colleagues (2005) found that patients who had medical comorbidities did better with active clinical management than IPSRT. Subsequent analyses revealed that medical comorbidity was a proxy for other poor prognosis illness attributes, such as longer duration of lifetime depression and slower recovery from depression (Thompson et al., 2006). In contrast, Simon et al. (2006) found that their multicomponent care management was only effective among patients with clinically significant symptoms at baseline. Analyzing data from two trials of FFT, Kim and Miklowitz (2004) found that the association between EE-criticism in relatives and poor outcomes of mania among patients was stronger in

CM treatment than in FFT, suggesting that FFT may have "blunted" the impact of EE on subsequent patient outcomes. Finally, Scott et al. (2006) found that CBT was more effective in preventing recurrences among patients with fewer than 12 illness episodes, whereas treatment-as-usual was more effective among patients with more than 12 episodes.

This kind of pragmatic clinical data may prove more useful in practice than simple univariate comparisons of the effectiveness of various treatments. Nonetheless, studies of moderators have to be powered with adequate sample sizes to reliably identify treatment by moderator interactions.

Mediators refer to variables that explain *how* treatments work (Kraemer et al., 2002). They typically refer to "change variables" measured before, during, and after treatment. To be a mediator of symptomatic change, the mediator must change before the symptom indicator, and must predict the level of change in the symptom indicator. Moreover, the association between treatment type and symptomatic outcomes must become non-significant once the mediator is covaried. Studies of FFT have identified several possible mediators of effects, including improvements in medication adherence (Miklowitz et al., 2003a), improvements in patient/relative interaction patterns (Simoneau et al., 1999), and the ability of patients and family members to identify and intervene early with prodromal symptoms (Rea et al., 2003). The Pittsburgh Maintenance Therapies trial has identified stabilization of sleep/wake rhythms as a possible mediator (Frank et al., 2005). It is not yet clear what variables mediate the clinical effects of group psychoeducation or CBT (for example, whether changes in dysfunctional attitudes or core dysfunctional beliefs are necessary to observe clinical change).

Cost-effectiveness

With the notable exception of the Simon et al. (2006) study, few studies have examined what treatments cost relative to their effects. Treatment costs can be very hard to calculate, because costs for patients can include transportation, child care, or lost days from work. Ideally, when comparing two or more treatments, investigators should calculate the effect size for the difference in treatment costs and compare it to the effect sizes for treatment-related changes in mood symptoms, functioning, and quality of life.

Psychosocial treatment as preventative intervention

We are entering an era in which the initial presentations of bipolar disorder in childhood or early adolescence can be reliably measured, along with risk factors for subsequent syndromal onset (i.e. presence of a first degree relative with bipolar I disorder). In the environmental domain, early adversity (i.e. sexual or physical abuse in childhood or adolescence) is associated with an earlier age at illness onset, a poorer prognosis course of illness, more suicidality, more comorbidity, and a lack of response to treatment (Post et al., 2001). These findings argue for the development of age-appropriate psychosocial interventions to be given earlier rather than later, as a means of addressing early adversity in genetically high-risk children and staving off the fully syndromal onset of the disorder (or at least decreasing its severity once manifest). Children who have not yet developed the full syndrome of bipolar disorder may be amenable to psychosocial interventions to learn stress management skills, and families may benefit from learning strategies for coping with the onset of symptoms that do occur. Thus, the protective benefits of family relationships could be maximized, which could alter the developmental trajectory of the disorder when other risk factors (i.e. genetic vulnerability, early adversity) are present. These questions should be addressed in the next generation of studies on psychosocial interventions for bipolar disorder.

References

Bauer, M. S., & McBride, L. (1996). *Structured Group Psychotherapy for Bipolar Disorder: The Life Goals Program.* New York, NY: Springer.

Butzlaff, R. L., & Hooley, J. M. (1998). Expressed emotion and psychiatric relapse: A meta-analysis. *Archives of General Psychiatry, 55,* 547–552.

Clarkin, J. F., Glick, I. D., Haas, G. L., et al. (1990) A randomized clinical trial of inpatient family intervention: V. Results for affective disorders. *Journal of Affective Disorders, 18,* 17–28.

Cochran, S. D. (1984). Preventing medical noncompliance in the outpatient treatment of bipolar affective disorders. *Journal of Consulting and Clinical Psychology, 52,* 873–878.

Cohen, M., Baker, G., Cohen, R. A., Fromm-Reichmann, F., & Weigert, V. (1954). An intensive study of 12 cases of manic-depressive psychosis. *Psychiatry, 17,* 103–137.

Colom, F., Vieta, E., Martinez-Aran, A., et al. (2003). A randomized trial on the efficacy of group psychoeducation in the prophylaxis of recurrences in bipolar patients whose disease is in remission. *Archives of General Psychiatry, 60,* 402–407.

Davenport, Y. B., Ebert, M. H., Adland, M. L., & Goodwin, F. K. (1977). Couples group therapy as adjunct to lithium maintenance of the manic patient. *American Journal of Orthopsychiatry, 47,* 495–502.

Dixon, L., McFarlane, W. R., Lefley, H., et al. (2001). Evidence-based practices for services to families of people with psychiatric disabilities. *Psychiatric Services, 52,* 903–910.

Ehlers, C. L., Frank, E., & Kupfer, D. J. (1988). Social zeitgebers and biological rhythms: a unified approach to understanding the etiology of depression. *Archives of General Psychiatry, 45,* 948–952.

Ehlers, C. L., Kupfer, D. J., Frank, E., & Monk, T. H. (1993): Biological rhythms and depression: the role of zeitgebers and zeitstorers. *Depression, 1,* 285–293.

Fitzgerald, R. G. (1972). Mania as a message: treatment with family therapy and lithium carbonate. *American Journal of Psychotherapy, 26,* 547–555.

Frank, E., (2005). *Treating Bipolar Disorder: A Clinician's Guide to Interpersonal and Social Rhythm Therapy*. New York, NY: Guilford Publications.

Frank, E. Kupfer, D. J., Thase, M. E., et al. (2005). Two-year outcomes for interpersonal and social rhythm therapy in individuals with bipolar I disorder. *Archives of General Psychiatry, 62,* 996–1004.

Glick, I. D., Clarkin, J. F., Haas, G. L., Spencer, J. H., & Chen, C. L. (1991). A randomized clinical trial of inpatient family intervention: VI. Mediating variables and outcome. *Family Process, 30,* 5–99.

Johnson, S. L., & Miller, I. (1997). Negative life events and time to recovery from episodes of bipolar disorder. *Journal of Abnormal Psychology, 106,* 449–457.

Johnson, S. L., Sandrow, D., & Meyer, B., et al. (2000). Increases in manic symptoms following life events involving goal-attainment. *Journal of Abnormal Psychology, 109,* 721–727.

Kim, E. Y., & Miklowitz, D. J. (2004). Expressed emotion as a predictor of outcome among bipolar patients undergoing family therapy. *Journal of Affective Disorders, 82,* 343–352.

Kraemer, H. C., Wilson, T., Fairburn, C. G., & Agras, W. S. (2002). Mediators and moderators of treatment effects in randomized clinical trials. *Archives of General Psychiatry, 59,* 877–883.

Lam, D. H., Hayward, P., Watkins, E. R., Wright, K., & Sham. P. (2005). Relapse prevention in patients with bipolar disorder: cognitive therapy outcome after 2 years. *American Journal of Psychiatry, 162,* 324–329.

Lam, D. H., Watkins, E. R., Hayward, P., et al. (2003). A randomized controlled study of cognitive therapy of relapse prevention for bipolar affective disorder: outcome of the first year. *Archives of General Psychiatry, 60,* 145–152.

Malkoff-Schwartz, S., Frank, E., Anderson, B., et al. (1998). Stressful life events and social rhythm disruption in the onset of manic and depressive bipolar episodes: A preliminary investigation. *Archives of General Psychiatry, 55,* 702–707.

Malkoff-Schwartz, S., Frank, E., Anderson, B. P., et al. (2000). Social rhythm disruption and stressful life events in the onset of bipolar and unipolar episodes. *Psychological Medicine, 30,* 1005–1016.

Miklowitz, D. J. (2004). The role of family systems in severe and recurrent psychiatric disorders: a developmental psychopathology view. *Development and Psychopathology, 16,* 667–688.

Miklowitz, D. J., Biuckians, A., & Richards, J. A. (2006). Early-onset bipolar disorder: a family treatment perspective. *Development and Psychopathology, 18,* 1247–1265.

Miklowitz, D. J., & Cicchetti, D. (2006). Toward a lifespan developmental psychopathology perspective on bipolar disorder. *Development and Psychopathology, 18,* 935–938.

Miklowitz, D. J., George, E. L., Richards, J. A., Simoneau, T. L., & Suddath, R. L. (2003a). A randomized study of family-focused psychoeducation and pharmacotherapy in the outpatient management of bipolar disorder. *Archives of General Psychiatry, 60,* 904–912.

Miklowitz, D. J., Otto, M. W., Frank, E., Reilly-Harrington, N. A., Wisniewski, S. R., Kogan, J. N., Nierenberg, A. A., Calabrese, J. R., Marangell, L. B., Gyulai, L., Araga, M., Gonzalez, J. M., Shirley, E. R., Thase, M. E., & Sachs, G. S. (2007). Psychosocial treatments for bipolar depression: a 1-year randomized trial from the Systematic Treatment Enhancement Program. *Archives of General Psychiatry, 64,* 419–427.

Miklowitz, D. J., Richards, J. A., George, E. L., et al. (2003b). Integrated family and individual therapy for bipolar disorder: results of a treatment development study. *Journal of Clinical Psychiatry, 64*, 182–191.

Perry, A., Tarrier, N., Morriss, R., McCarthy, E., & Limb, K. (1999). Randomised controlled trial of efficacy of teaching patients with bipolar disorder to identify early symptoms of relapse and obtain treatment. *British Medical Journal, 16*, 149–153.

Pitschel-Walz, G., Leucht, S., Bäuml, J., Kissling, W., & Engel, R. R. (2001). The effect of family interventions on relapse and rehospitalization in schizophrenia: A meta-analysis. *Schizophrenia Bulletin, 27*, 73–92.

Post, R. M., Leverich, G. S., Xing, G., & Weiss, R. B. (2001). Developmental vulnerabilities to the onset and course of bipolar disorder. *Development and Psychopathology, 13*, 581–598.

Rea, M. M., Tompson, M., Miklowitz, D. J., Goldstein, M. J., Hwang, S., & Mintz, J. (2003). Family focused treatment vs. individual treatment for bipolar disorder: results of a randomized clinical trial. *Journal of Consulting and Clinical Psychology, 71*, 482–492.

Sachs, G. S., Thase, M. E., Otto, M. W., et al. (2003). Rationale, design, and methods of the systematic treatment enhancement program for bipolar disorder (STEP-BD). *Biological Psychiatry, 53*, 1028–1042.

Scott, J., Paykel, E., Morriss, R., et al. (2006). Cognitive behaviour therapy for severe and recurrent bipolar disorders: a randomised controlled trial. *British Journal of Psychiatry, 188*, 313–320.

Simon, G. E., Ludman, E. J., Bauer, M. S., Unutzer, J., Operskalski, B. (2006). Long-term effectiveness and cost of a systematic care program for bipolar disorder. *Archives of General Psychiatry, 63*, 500–508.

Simoneau, T. L., Miklowitz, D. J., Richards, J. A., Saleem, R., & George, E. L. (1999). Bipolar disorder and family communication: Effects of a psychoeducational treatment program. *Journal of Abnormal Psychology, 108*, 588–597.

Thompson, W. K., Kupfer, D. J., Fagiolini, A., Scott, J. A., & Frank, E. (2006). Prevalence and clinical correlates of medical comorbidities in patients with bipolar I disorder: analysis of acute-phase data from a randomized controlled trial. *Journal of Clinical Psychiatry, 67*, 783–788.

Weiss, R. D., Griffin, M. L., Kolodziej, M. E., et al. (2007). A randomized trial of integrated group therapy versus group drug counseling for patients with bipolar disorder and substance dependence. *American Journal of Psychiatry, 164*, 100–107.

Weissman, M. M., Markowitz, J., & Klerman, G. L. (2000). *Comprehensive Guide to Interpersonal Psychotherapy*. New York, NY: Basic Books.

Yatham, L. N., Kennedy, S. H., O'Donovan, C., et al. (2005). Canadian Network for Mood and Anxiety Treatments (CANMAT) guidelines for the management of patients with bipolar disorder: consensus and controversies. *Bipolar Disorders, 7*, 5–69.

chapter eighteen

Novel treatments in bipolar disorder: Future directions

Jorge A. Quiroz
Johnson & Johnson Pharmaceutical Research and Development

Robert M. Post
George Washington University

Contents

Introduction 592
Neurotrophic cascades 593
    Potential role for brain derived neurotrophic factor (BDNF) 593
        Phosphodiesterase Inhibitors 594
        BCL-2 596
Intracellular signaling cascades 597
    PKC: The legacy of one of lithium's putative mechanisms of
        action 597
    Glycogen synthase kinase-3 beta: A similar approach 598
    Increased intercellular calcium 598
    Other second messenger targets 599
Neuropeptides, stress and the HPA axis 600
    Glucocorticoids 600
    CRF1 receptor antagonists 601
    Glucocorticoid receptor antagonists 602
    Thyrotropin-releasing hormone (TRH) 603
    Cytokines and inflammation 603
    Glutamatergic system of neurotransmission 603
        Glutamatergic release inhibition: Riluzole 604
        NMDA receptor antagonism: Ketamine 604
        AMPA and Kainate Receptors 605
        Metabotropic glutamate receptors (mGluR) 606
Other strategies 606
    Heavy metals 606

Neurostimulation for regional effects 607
Conclusions 607
References 609

Introduction

Bipolar disorder is a common, severe, recurring and, often, chronic disease marked by episodes of hypomania, mania and or depression. Although the course can be episodic with intervening periods of euthymia, chronic subthreshold mood symptoms can commonly result in dysfunction in a variety of domains in patients' lives. It is also associated with high rates of mortality, both because of suicide and increased risk of medical illnesses like cardiovascular disease. The data are substantial that if the illness is not treated or if it is inadequately treated, there is a tendency for accelerated cycling and shorter intervals of wellness between episodes (reviewed in Post, 2007b). Consequently, the outcome is associated with high rates of relapse, chronicity, residual symptoms, comorbidities, cognitive and functional impairment, and psychosocial disability. Few current treatments have bimodal efficacy and most have undesirable side effects. The need for discovering new therapeutic agents that are both efficacious and have fewer side effects is, therefore, compelling.

The search for new therapeutic strategies can be guided by (a) the understanding of the pathophysiology of bipolar disorder, to control core symptomatology and attenuate or prevent the systemic effects of the illness (reviewed in Quiroz et al., 2004) or by (b) the understanding of the precise biochemical targets of antimanic and or mood stabilizer agents currently in use (reviewed in Gould et al., 2004a). A comprehensive approach should include the extensive new genetic knowledge currently being generated combined with the knowledge obtained in the fields of epidemiology, neuroimaging, and neuropathology, that altogether will allow for a more precise understanding of the disease process(s) involved.

Taking into consideration these approaches, the phenomena of episode-sensitization and stress-sensitization—the sensitization/kindling model—that has been generally validated in the literature, may offer a window of opportunity to understand the underlying pathophysiology of the disorder. In fact, as observed by Kraepelin (1921) almost a century ago, untreated or inadequately treated successive affective episodes, on average, not only recur with increasing frequency, but with greater autonomy and independence from exogenous stressors (Post, 2007b). As paralleled in the amygdala-kindled seizure model, there is also substantial evidence that with multiple recurrences, both unipolar and bipolar mood episodes that were initially triggered by notable stressors can also begin to emerge spontaneously (Post, 1992). As such, the clinical data on faster and more autonomous occurrences in their own right speak to the importance of early, consistent, long-term prophylactic treatment of the mood disorders.

In this chapter, we review new approaches for the development of novel therapeutics for the treatment of bipolar disorder, based on the strategies mentioned above, that could lead to improved quality of life of patients and of their families.

Neurotrophic cascades

Recent structural neuroimaging studies in bipolar disorder have demonstrated regional volumetric reductions that include reduced grey matter volumes in areas of the orbital and medial prefrontal cortex (PFC), temporal lobe, and enlargement of third ventricle (Manji et al., 2003). Post-mortem neuropathological studies are complementary, showing reductions in cortical volume, and region- and layer-specific reductions in number, density, and/or size of neurons and glial cells in the subgenual PFC, orbital cortex, dorsal anterolateral PFC, amygdala, basal ganglia, and dorsal raphe nuclei in individuals with bipolar disorder and other severe mood disorders compared to controls (Manji et al., 2003). Thus, in addition to its neurochemical basis, bipolar disorder is associated with structurally-related abnormalities, as well. With the capacity of neuronal and glial cells to resist or adapt to environmental stressors (cellular resilience), this is translated into the ability to undergo re-modeling of synaptic connections (synaptic plasticity), cell regeneration (neurogenesis), phenomena known as cellular plasticity, in general. (sentence is difficult to read, suggest rewording to: "Bipolar disorder is associated with impairments in cellular plasticity, with reduced capacity of neuronal and glial cells to resist or adapt to environmental stressors (cellular resilience), remodeling of synaptic connections (synaptic plasticity), and cell regeneration (neurogenesis)")

Potential role for brain derived neurotrophic factor (BDNF)

BDNF, and other neurotrophic factors are necessary for the survival and function of neurons, implying that a sustained reduction of them could affect neuronal viability, synaptic plasticity, and modulation of synaptic transmission (including glutamate, GABA, dopamine and serotonin neurotransmitter release (Du, Gould, & Manji, 2003). In particular, the defeat-stress animal model of depression (which has an inherent component of stress sensitization), provides a clear link to the necessary and specific role for BDNF decreases in the hippocampus and increased in the ventral striatum in the depression-like behaviors (Berton et al., 2006; Tsankova et al., 2006). BDNF appears to play an important role in multiple aspects of genetic and environmentally mediated vulnerability to bipolar illness (Figure 18.1) (Post, 2007b,c). Moreover, increasing amount of evidence demonstrating that pharmacotherapeutic interventions for recurrent unipolar illness (antidepressants and ECT as reviewed in Duman & Monteggia, 2006), and for bipolar illness (lithium, valproate, carbamazepine, and the atypical antipsychotics quetiapine and ziprasidone as reviewed in Chuang et al., 2002; Einat & Manji, 2006; Post, 2007a) all has a substantial impact on BDNF expression (Post, 2007c). Therefore additional strategies that directly or indirectly target this factor's expression may result in areas of new therapeutic developments for the disease.

One attempt to directly increase BDNF brain availability, used recombinant methionyl human brain derived neurotrophic factor (mBDNF) infused intrathecally in patients with amyotrophic lateral sclerosis (Ochs et al., 2000). A myriad of side effects (including sensory symptoms, paresthesias or a sense of warmth, sleep disturbance, dry mouth, agitation and other behavioral effects) were described, and further studies are required to assess the potential effects of intrathecal BDNF. Some other potential strategies are described below.

Phosphodiesterase Inhibitors

BDNF expression may be increased by activation of several intracellular pathways. The cyclic adenosine monophosphate (cAMP)-mediated signaling cascade may well be a pathway to increase BDNF expression. The effects of cAMP appear to be mediated by activation of protein kinase A (PKA), an enzyme that phosphorylates and regulates many proteins including ion channels, cytoskeletal elements, and transcription factors. Among them, PKA activation produces phosporylation and activation of cyclic AMP response element binding protein (CREB), which in turn promotes the transcription of several genes, including those for BDNF and Bcl-2. Thus, it is understandable that the inhibition of phosphodiesterase (PDE) (Wachtel & Schneider, 1986), the enzymes responsible for the breakdown of cAMP, leads to an activation of the entire cascade, including increases in the transcription of BDNF (see Duman, 2002 for review). In fact, chronic antidepressant administration increases the expression of cAMP-specific phosphodiesterase (PDE) 4A and 4B isoforms (Takahashi et al., 1999) as a compensatory response (Nibuya, Nestler, & Duman, 1996).

In a confirmatory manner, PDE inhibitors have been demonstrated to produce antidepressant-like effects in animal behavioral models (Griebel et al., 1991; O'Donnell, 1993; Wachtel & Schneider, 1986) and more importantly, in open (Zeller et al., 1984) and controlled clinical trials (Bertolino et al., 1988; Bobon et al., 1988; Fleischhacker et al., 1992;

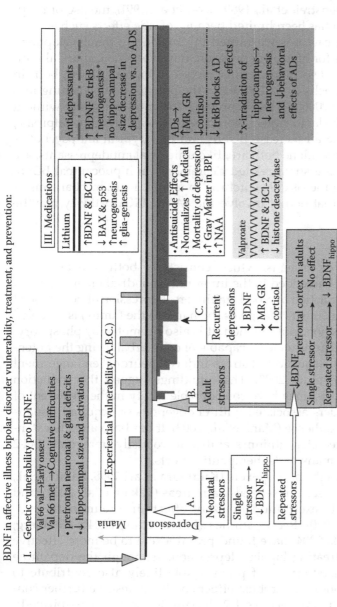

Figure 18.1 Summary of the effects of BDNF on affective illness vulnerability, treatment, and revention. The interaction of BDNF with the life course of a patient and his or her treatment are schematized on the backdrop of a life chart; increasing mania is represented above the midline, and increasing depression is represented below the midline. The three general areas are i) genetic vulnerability, ii) experiential vulnerability, and iii) medications (treatment) are shown, as well as the specific implications of the interactions of each with BDNF. BDNF, brain-derived neurotrophic factor; MRs, mineralocorticoid receptors; MRI, magnetic resonance imaging; MRS, magnetic resonance spectroscopy; GRs, glucocorticoid receptors; AD, antidepressant; hippo, hippocampus; NAA, N-acetyl aspartate; hippo, hippocampus; pfc, prefrontal cortex. (Reprinted from Post RM, Kindling and sensitization as models for affective episode recurrence, cyclicity, and tolerance phenomena, *Neurosci. and Biobehav. Rev.*, 31(16), 858–873, 2007b. With permission from Elsevier.)

Hebenstreit et al., 1989). These studies showed that rolipram, a specific inhibitor of the high-affinity cAMP PDE4, may have antidepressant efficacy in depressed patients. In addition to contradictory evidence about the response (Hebenstreit et al., 1989; Scott et al., 1991), the use of rolipram for depression has been limited because of side effects such as nausea and emesis. A caveat is warranted in considering the development of PDE4 inhibitors for bipolar depression, however. The unimodal antidepressants have a less than sterling record in bipolar illness, both in terms of efficacy (Sachs et al., 2007) and the potential for switching into mania (Post et al., 2006b). Thus searching for antidepressants without switch liability (like lamotrigine) would be the ideal. Lithium, valproate, and carbamazepine all increase BDNF, and the atypical antipsychotics quetiapine and ziprasidone both are, like unimodal antidepressants, are capable of preventing stress-related decrements in hippocampal BDNF without increasing the risk of switching to mania. Thus, mechanisms of increasing BDNF that do not involve the cAMP. PKA pathway may be more promising.

BCL-2

The bcl-2 family of proteins, which consists of both pro- and anti-apoptotic proteins embedded in the inner mitochondrial membrane, is a major target for the action of mood stabilizers. Expression of bcl-2 (one of the antiapoptotic members that gives the name to the family) is involved in regulating mitochondrial function. It is also promoted by phosphorylation of CREB and appears to be capable of counterbalancing the potentially damaging consequences of stress-induced neuronal endangerment (reviewed in Manji et al., 2003). These findings suggest that induction (upregulation) of bcl-2 may have considerable utility in the treatment of a variety of disorders associated with endogenous or acquired impairments of cellular resilience (Manji et al., 2003). It has been already extensively demonstrated that lithium's ability to robustly upregulate bcl-2 may play a role in many of its therapeutic effects.

Most interestingly, pramipexole (Kitamura et al., 1998; Zarate et al., 2004b) upregulates bcl-2 in several brain areas (Takata et al., 2000), and has been shown to exert antidepressant effects in preliminary studies (Sporn et al., 2000). Recent studies (Zarate et al., 2004b; Goldberg, Burdick, & Endick, 2004) have found pramipexole to be more effective than placebo in treating bipolar depression. Although the dopamine D2 and D3 agonistic effects of pramipexole likely also contribute to the observed response, the robust effects on bcl-2 deserve further consideration. Other more selective D2 dopaminergic agonists (piribedil and bromocriptine) induce antidepressant responses in some subjects (Post et al., 1978), and whether they also increases bcl-2 has not been studied.

In a randomized double-blind, placebo-controlled study, 21 patients with DSM-IV bipolar II disorder, depressive phase on therapeutic levels of lithium or valproate were studied for 6 weeks. A therapeutic response occurred in 60% of patients taking pramipexole and 9% taking placebo, while hypo-manic switches were equally observed in both groups (Zarate et al., 2004b). A second trial involved 22 depressed nonpsychotic bipolar subjects in a similar design. Eight (67%) of 12 patients taking pramipexole and two (20%) of ten taking placebo had an improvement of at least 50% in their Hamilton depression scale scores (Goldberg, Burdick, & Endick, 2004). In both these trials subjects were treated with a mood stabilizer, which was augmented with pramipexole, resulting in antidepressant response and prevention of switches of mood states in this limited duration. The dual neurotrophic and dopaminergic roles of pramipexole open a window to further investigate the roles of these targets in the pathophysiology and treatment of bipolar disorder.

Intracellular signaling cascades

PKC: The legacy of one of lithium's putative mechanisms of action

PKC is a family of enzymes of intracellular mediators of signals, highly enriched in the brain where it plays a major role in regulating pre- and postsynaptic neurotransmission. PKC plays a crucial role in the regulation of neuronal excitability, neurotransmitter release, synaptic plasticity, and various forms of learning and memory. Several neurotransmitters acting on cell surface receptors induce PKC activity that in turn produces the hydrolysis of various membrane phospholipids.

The potential involvement of PKC and its substrates in bipolar disorder have been extensively studied, particularly the changes in PKC signaling pathways after treatment with lithium (and valproate) (Chen et al., 1994; Friedman et al., 1993; Hahn & Friedman, 1999; Manji et al., 1993; Manji & Lenox, 1999; Young et al., 1999). Lithium treatment results in significant decreases in membrane-associated PKC, particularly isozymes alpha and epsilon in discrete brain areas. Interestingly, valproate (which is structurally highly dissimilar to lithium) was also found to cause the same isozyme-specific decrease in PKC (Chen et al., 1994; Manji & Lenox, 1999). Of clinical relevance is that, currently, there is only one other patent PKC inhibitor that crosses the blood-brain barrier available for human use, namely tamoxifen. Based on the hypothesis that inhibition of PKC may be relevant to treat bipolar disorder during manic episodes, a single-blind study was conducted in patients (Bebchuk et al., 2000). This study found that tamoxifen significantly decreased manic symptoms within a short period of time of 3–7 days.

More recently, a randomized, placebo-controlled, double-blind study was conducted at the National Institute of Mental Health. In it, 16 subjects with bipolar disorder, in an acute or mixed manic episode, with or without psychotic features, were given oral tamoxifen or placebo for 3 weeks. The authors confirmed that tamoxifen was associated with significant antimanic effects in individuals with bipolar disorder, as early as day 5 with sustained efficacy throughout the 3 week trial. The response rates were 63% for tamoxifen and 13% for placebo (Zarate et al., 2007). A similar study, still unpublished, replicated these findings (Yildiz et al., 2008). In addition, a pilot study of hormone modulation as a new treatment for mania in women with bipolar affective disorder utilizing this medication was also recently conducted (Kulkarni et al., 2006). All the evidence suggests that inhibition of PKC may be a relevant target in the development of new treatment for bipolar mania. This approach has not yet been studied in bipolar depression, however.

Glycogen synthase kinase-3 beta: A similar approach

Targeting glycogen synthase kinase-3 (GSK-3) for the treatment of bipolar disorders has also been based on the findings of lithium's putative mechanism of action. Lithium produces direct inhibition of the enzyme GSK-3 (probably by competing with magnesium). It is also probable that beta-catenin—a transcription factor downstream target of GSK-3—might be mediating the changes associated with the action of lithium (and other mood stabilizers, as well), as reviewed in Gould et al. (2006). However the targets of GSK-3 are multiple, including other transcription factors (CREB, c-Jun), proteins bound to microtubules (Tau, microtubule-associated protein [MAP]-1B, kinesin light chain), cell cycle mediators (cyclin D, human ninein), and regulators of metabolism (glycogen synthase, pyruvate dehydrogenase) (Frame & Cohen, 2001; Gould et al., 2004b). Although many of these functions are likely to be critically important to both cellular and organism functioning, GSK-3 is currently receiving increased attention as a regulator of apoptosis and cellular resilience. Generally, increased activity of GSK-3 is pro-apoptotic, whereas inhibiting GSK-3 attenuates or prevents apoptosis (Gould & Manji, 2002; Jope & Bijur, 2002). Taken together the current evidence suggests that inhibition of GSK-3 may represent a target for novel medication development to treat mood disorders (Gould et al., 2006).

Increased intercellular calcium

Another highly replicated finding in both unipolar and bipolar disorder is evidence of increased intracellular calcium as measured in platelets and blood elements. This evidence led Dubovski and colleagues to consider L-type calcium channel blockers, such as the phenylalkylamin verapamil in clinical approaches to mania (Dubovsky et al., 1986). A series of small double-blind studies in acute mania were generally positive, although one randomized study found verapamil no more effective than treatment as usual in bipolar depression. These only partially positive data led Pazzaglia and collaborators to explore another class of L-type calcium channel blockers with the hope that they might have a broader spectrum of effects in mania and depression, in this case the dihydropyridine L-type calcium channel blocker nimodipine (Pazzaglia et al., 1998).

Nimodipine has a variety of properties that differ from verapamil including: blocking dopamine overflow induced by cocaine, blocking cocaine-induced hyperactivity, and being positive in animal models of depression. In a small series of subjects, nimodipine proved to be effective in some highly treatment-resistant individuals with ultradian cycling bipolar disorder or in recurrent brief unipolar depression (Pazzaglia et al., 1998, 1993). These studies were done in a double-blind off-on-off-on fashion in order to confirm responsivity within individual subjects. These data, which did confirm cross-responsivity among nimodipine and other dihydropyridine compounds, but not to verapamil, suggest the potential utility of exploring other dihydropyridine-L-type calcium channel blockers. However, a recent report showed that a promising dihydro-pyridine showed no efficacy in a small double-blind, placebo-controlled trial in acute mania (Murray et al., 2007). Thus, nimodipine and its close congeners remain candidates for further development, but uncertainty remains about the generalizability of responsiveness to this whole class of compounds.

Other second messenger targets

The comparison of lithium and valproate actions during chronic administration raises the issue of PKC inhibition as potentially important to antimanic efficacy, as discussed previously. However, inhibition of other second messenger systems also appears a promising target of therapeutics, because both lithium and carbamazepine inhibit stimulated-induced adenylate cyclase. Based on this hypothesis, Belmaker and associates who found that an antibiotic which selectively inhibits cyclase also appears to posses antimanic properties (Belmaker, Roitman, & Birchet, 1988).

Lithium also has marked effects in inhibiting phosphoinositol (PI) turnover, and this has theoretically been linked to its mechanism of action. However, in this case, its actions are not shared by carbamazepine or valproate, but all three compounds do inhibit inositol uptake. The findings of lithium inhibiting a variety of second messenger systems, including adenylate cyclase, G proteins at multiple levels, intercellular calcium and PI turnover suggest the possibility that modulating or muting excessive neurotransmitter activity in a variety of systems by diverse actions in inhibiting second messenger amplification of signal transduction may be important to its antimanic or antidepressant effects.

This would particularly be the case if one conceptualized both mania and depression as excessive over-swings in either excitatory or inhibitory neurotransmitter systems that needed to be dampened in order to prevent such over reactivity. This may be one way of conceptualizing how common effects in modulating one or more second messengers may be capable of exerting bimodal mood stabilizing effects. This would appear to be a key concept in developing novel treatments for bipolar illness, wherein one would want to avoid the potential adverse effect of switching patients into mania (which is prominent with the older tricyclic antidepressants and the second generation antidepressant venlafaxine—with its dual effects on reuptake blockade of both serotonin and norepinephrine). Initiating unidirectional enhancement of norepinephrine or serotonergic systems via reuptake blockade, changes in turnover, or by release mechanisms, may not be optimal for stabilizing the bi-directional mood swings in bipolar illness. Thus, second and third messenger signal transduction systems involved in multiple excitatory and inhibitory neurotransmitter systems may be particularly appealing targets of therapeutics in bipolar disorder.

The lack of good animal models for cyclic alterations in behavior characteristic of bipolar illness also has limited new drug development in bipolar disorder. One potential exception to this paucity is the cocaine-related hyperactivity model developed by Antelman and colleagues (1995), which appears to show notable oscillations and marked motor hyper- and hyporesponsivity. They found, additionally, that inositol showed promise in inhibiting some of the associated biochemical and behavioral oscillations observed. Given the highly preliminary data suggesting the potential clinical utility of inositol in humans with mood and anxiety disorders, this target appears to be worthy of further exploration.

Neuropeptides, stress and the HPA axis

Glucocorticoids

Preclinical data indicate that early life stressors have long-term effects on behavior and underlying neural function (Duman & Monteggia, 2006; Meaney et al., 1988; Roceri et al., 2004). These preclinical data are paralleled by those in the clinic whereby early childhood psychosocial adversity is associated with a more turbulent course of bipolar illness (Brown et al., 2005; Garno et al., 2005; Leverich et al., 2002) and with adult onset unipolar depression (Heim et al., 2001) as a function of gene–environment interactions (Caspi et al., 2003). In addition, stress sensitization and cocaine sensitization and their cross-sensitization to each other can occur in adult animals (Kalivas, 2004; Kalivas & Stewart, 1991), suggesting differential potential stress vulnerabilities throughout one's developmental life span and an explanation of the high incidence of co-morbid substance abuse in the affective disorder (Post, 2007b; Post et al., 2006a).

The activation of the hypothalamus-pituitary-adrenal (HPA) axis associated with stress response is then a natural candidate to be investigated in mood disorders; in fact, stress and glucocorticoid abnormalities have been associated with abnormalities in neural plasticity (particularly mediating stress-induced cellular atrophy (McEwen, 1999; Sapolsky, 1996; Sapolsky, Romero, & Munck, 2000). One of the most consistent effects of stress on cellular morphology in preclinical models is atrophy of hippocampal neurons (for reviews see McEwen, 1999 and Sapolsky, 2000). Interestingly, the overactivity of the HPA axis in depression (either unipolar or bipolar) is among the most consistently replicated biological findings in psychiatry (including the lack of dexamethasone suppression of plasma cortisol levels, increased ACTH response to CRH, and altered responses to the combined dexamethasone/corticotropin release hormone (DEX/CRF) challenge test) (Ising et al., 2007; Plotsky, Owens, & Nemeroff, 1998).

It is natural that targeting the HPA axis has become a relevant strategy for the development of novel therapeutics for severe mood disorders. Published double-blind, placebo-controlled clinical studies to modulate the HPA axis have employed inhibitors of glucocorticoid synthesis (Malison et al., 1999; Wolkowitz et al., 1999a) to downregulate the axis. Antagonists of the GR (Belanoff et al., 2001; Young, 2004), hydrocortisone, to downregulate the HPA axis (DeBattista et al., 2000), utilization of dehydroepiandrosterone (Bloch et al., 1999; Wolkowitz et al., 1999b), and CRF 1R antagonists (Zobel et al., 2000) are some of the approaches reviewed in Quiroz et al. (2004). We describe here some compelling evidence on two of these strategies:

CRF1 receptor antagonists

Several classes of CRF 1R inhibitors have been identified (astressin, α-helCRF, CP-154526, antalarmin, DMP-695, DMP-696, CRA-1000, R-121919, SSR-125543, NBI 35965, NBI 27914, among others) (see Holmes et al., 2003; Saunders & Williams, 2003 for review), and abundant pre-clinical data has been generally supported the potential role of this target in the development of new antidepressant strategies. In fact, antalarmin, besides exploratory findings in rodents (Ducottet, Griebel, & Belzung, 2003), significantly diminishes the CRF-stimulated ACTH release in non-human primates, and decreases the pituitary-adrenal, sympathetic, and adrenal medullary responses to stress, additionally reverting stress-induced inhibition of exploratory and sexual behaviors (Webster et al., 1996; Habib et al., 2000).

Of most relevance, R-121919 was showed to reduce anxiety and depressive symptoms in patients with major depression in an open label clinical trial (Zobel et al., 2000). The clinical development of the compound was discontinued due to two cases of healthy volunteers who developed elevated liver enzymes while receiving a high dose of R-121919 (Kunzel et al., 2003). Recently, however, in an extended data report of the clinical study in major depression patients, no serious side effected were noted in the hypothalamic-pituitary-gonadal system, the hypothalamic-pituitary-thyroid axis, the renin-angiotensin system, and prolactin or vasopressin secretion, encouraging the development of CRF 1R antagonists as potential antidepressant medications (Kunzel et al., 2003). However, it is important to note that contrary to this premise, a recent controlled study reported negative results ultilizing this strategy.

Glucocorticoid receptor antagonists

Clinical studies that have pursued the alteration of the HPA axis through pharmacological antagonism of glucocorticoids in depression and bipolar disorder have been published. Mifepristone (RU-486) is a non-selective antagonist of the GR receptor with activity in psychotic depression (Belanoff et al., 2001; Belanoff et al., 2002; Murphy, Filipini, & Ghadirian, 1993; DeBattista et al., 2006; Flores et al., 2006; Simpson et al., 2005). Recently, peripheral BDNF levels were measured in patients with bipolar disorder, schizophrenia, and healthy controls after 7 days of adjunctive mifepristone, in a double-blind, placebo-controlled crossover design study (Mackin et al., 2007). The authors found that cortisol levels were significantly increased and BDNF levels decreased in both schizophrenia and bipolar disorder, although correlation between both levels differed depending on the diagnosis (Mackin et al., 2007). In addition, a role for mifepristone in bipolar patients was further evaluated after a double-blind crossover, 1 week, placebo controlled trial. Interestingly, improvement in neurocognitive functioning—including spatial working memory performance, verbal fluency, and spatial recognition memory—was observed with mifepristone treatment when compared with placebo. HAM-D and MADRS scores were also significantly reduced when compared to baseline. The authors concluded that, although still requiring replication, the data showed preliminary evidence that glucocorticoid receptor antagonists may have useful cognitive-enhancing and possibly antidepressant properties in bipolar disorder (Young et al., 2004).

Thyrotropin-releasing hormone (TRH)

The strategy to target peptide systems involved in the final common pathway of antidepressant or mood stabilizing action of treatments, has opened the door to the enhancement of the thyrotropin-releasing hormone (TRH). TRH is a particularly interesting neuropeptide, co-secreted with both serotonin and dopamine, and appears to have bi-modal effects in animal models of interest for bipolar illness. In animals that are hyperactive, it appears to inhibit this behavior, and in those that are inactive or even hibernating, TRH appears to be activating.

There are also clinical data suggesting both potential antimanic and antidepressant effects of parenterally administered TRH, but questions remain about its brain penetrability and duration of action, as well as the rapid development of tolerance or tachyphylaxis. One study, attempting to circumvent the problem of penetration into the brain, delivered TRH directly into spinal fluid of those with treatment-refractory affective disorders and found notable antidepressant, antianxiety, and anti-suicide effects of TRH compared with a sham lumbar puncture control condition (Callahan et al., 1997; Frye et al. 1999). Winokur and colleagues have been exploring the possible use of longer acting TRH analogs, and this approach has a neurobiological basis to recommend it (Gary et al., 2003; Szuba et al., 2005).

Cytokines and inflammation

A small, but rapidly growing literature suggests that there are alterations in cytokines in bipolar disorder, potentially mediating a diverse array of CNS effects on neurotransmitter systems as well as altering inflammatory and oxidative stress effects. Several promising studies have found that TNF-alpha antagonists appear to have antidepressant effects, and this as well as exploration of other cytokines found to be hyper-secreted in bipolar illness would be useful.

A direct attempt to approach the issue of oxidative stress has been tested recently by administering N-acetyl cysteine to patients with inadequately treatment responsive subjects with bipolar disorder (Berk, 2008). The authors reported that this glutathione precurson, after several months, yielded significant improvements on a variety of indices compared with placebo. These data suggest the potential importance of trying to decrease oxidative stress, which has been directly associated with episodes of mania and depression.

Glutamatergic system of neurotransmission

Increasing amounts of evidence suggest that abnormal activity of the glutamatergic system are partly regulated via glucocorticoids and stress mechanisms, and consequently, might be involved in the pathogenesis of impairments in cellular neuroplasticity observed in subjects with bipolar disorder (Zarate, 2002). Glutamate is the major excitatory synaptic neurotransmitter in the brain that regulates numerous physiological functions in the mammalian central nervous system (CNS) such as synaptic plasticity, learning, and memory (Bannerman et al., 1995; Collingridge, 1994; Collingridge & Bliss, 1995; Watkins & Collingridge, 1994). Glutamatergic neurotransmission involves a complex system of receptors that include ionotropic receptors (ion channels that, after activation, allow the interchange of ions, mainly entrance of calcium to the neuronal cytoplasm) and metabotropic receptors (G protein-coupled receptors that induce direct activation of intracellular signaling pathways). The ionotropic receptors are categorized according to its pharmacological ability of binding to N-methyl-D-aspartate (NMDA), AMPA, or kainate. Metabotropic receptors are classified instead by their ability to activate inhibitory or excitatory G protein subunits. We review here some ongoing strategies to target this system.

Glutamatergic release inhibition: Riluzole

Riluzole (2-amino-6-trifluoromethoxybenzothiazole), an inhibitor of glutamate release, is an FDA approved medication for the treatment of ALS (Bensimon, Lacomblez, & Meininger, 1994). After a positive finding in subjects with major depression treated with riluzole for 6 weeks (Zarate et al., 2004a), the concept was tested, interestingly, in subjects with bipolar depression (Zarate et al., 2005). In this 8-week study of riluzole in combination with lithium, a significant treatment effect was observed suggesting that riluzole may indeed have antidepressant efficacy in this population (Zarate et al., 2005). A confirmatory double blind, placebo controlled study is currently underway.

NMDA receptor antagonism: Ketamine

A strategy aimed to target the post-synaptic glutamatergic receptor is to directly block the N-methyl-D-aspartate (NMDA) ionotropic receptor. Ketamine, primarily used for the induction and maintenance of general anesthesia, was initially utilized to determine the feasibility of this approach in depressed subjects (Berman et al., 2000). Recently, a randomized, double blind, placebo controlled study was conducted to investigate if a rapid antidepressant effect could be achieved by means of ketamine i.v. infusion in subjects with major depression (Zarate et al., 2006). Very interestingly, the patients receiving ketamine showed significant improvement in depression compared with placebo within 2 hours, an effect that lasted three to five days, and without the dissociative symptoms usually induced by this medication (Zarate et al., 2006). Due to the psychomimetic properties of ketamine at higher doses the potential utilization of this strategy in subjects with bipolar disorder is suspect. However, the findings confirm that blockade of the NMDA channel might well be a pathway that deserves further exploration to obtain an improvement of depressive symptoms in a rapid manner, and further in finding ways to sustain this acute improvement.

Consistent with this observation, a selective glutamate NR2B sub-unit antagonist has also shown rapid onset of antidepressant effects (Preskorn et al., 2007). These and the ketamine data—in addition to the, sometimes dramatic, overnight antidepressant effect of one night's sleep deprivation—indicate that attaining rapid onset attain rapid antidepressant affects is possible and deserves further clinical therapeutic investigation. Glutamatergic neurotransmission is linked to the pathophysiology of mood disorders, and may provide targets for novel drug development.

AMPA and Kainate Receptors
AMPA receptors mediate the fast component of excitatory neurotransmission physiologically involved in processes of learning and memory. A series of compounds that slow the rate of the AMPA receptor desensitization and/or deactivation in the presence of an agonist (e.g., glutamate and AMPA) but do not activate the receptor themselves, are thought to have a role in the treatment of schizophrenia (Goff et al., 2001), as well as in depression. These compounds, called AMPA receptor positive modulators/potentiators (Bleakman & Lodge, 1998; Borges & Dingledine, 1998) or AMPAkines, allosterically modify the post-synaptic receptor. They have been shown to posses antidepressant properties in animal models of depression These include paradigms of inescapable stressors, e.g. forced-swim test, tail-suspension-induced immobility tests, learned-helplessness, and animals exposed to chronic mild stress procedure (Li et al., 2001). Some of these treatments mediated through AMPA show a faster onset of activity when compared with SSRIs (Knapp et al., 2002). Their action has been related to increased levels of BDNF mRNA and protein (Lauterborn et al., 2000) and to phenomena of neurogenesis in the hippocampus (Bai, Bergeron, & Nelson, 2003). Although the impact of this target remains to be proved in patients with depressive symptomatology, this strategy may represent an exciting new avenue for the development of novel compounds.

Conversely, AMPA receptors mediate the sustained maintenance phase of long-term potentiation (LTP), which is strongly implicated in the etiopathogenesis of PTSD and recurrent mood disorders. The blockade of AMPA (or, better yet, its modulation by partial agonists) may be valuable in some syndromes involving overlearned, unwanted behaviors, such as in PTSD or even in stress-triggered recurrent mood disorders. In this regard, topiramate, an antagonist of AMPA/kainate receptors, has shown promising results in PTSD and many other common comorbidities of bipolar illness, including alcohol and cocaine abuse, and eating disorders. Kainate receptor modulation remains virtually unexplored, but is a very intriguing target for therapy given the high concentrations of these receptors in the amygdala and their potential role in neurotoxicity.

Metabotropic glutamate receptors (mGluR)

Metabotropic glutamate receptors (mGluR) function is to regulate glutamate neuronal transmission by altering the release of neurotransmitter or modulating the post-synaptic responses to glutamate. They have been demonstrated to be involved in the early phase of memory formation and the mechanism of long-term depression (Riedel, Platt, & Micheau, 2003; Salinska & Stafiej, 2003; Tan, Hori, & Carpenter, 2003). In addition to a potential role in several CNS related disorders, including schizophrenia and anxiety (see Zarate, 2002 for review), accumulating evidence from biochemical and behavioral studies support the idea that the regulation of glutamatergic neurotransmission via mGlu receptors is altered in mood disorders and that these receptors may serve as targets for antidepressant drug development, as well (Witkin et al., 2007). In fact compounds that antagonize mGlu2, mGlu3 and/or mGlu5 receptors (which are different subtypes of mGlu receptors associated with different intracellular activity) have been shown to have antidepressant effects in animal models. To date no mGlu receptor agonist or antagonist has been proven to posses antidepressant effects in humans, but again, this target may represent an opportunity for the development of novel treatments.

The idea of indirect modulation of glutamatergic transmission has much appeal in light of the potential difficulties of direct glutamatergic receptor antagonism (PCP psychosis) or agonism (seizures and neurotoxicity). Modulation of the NMDA receptor indirectly with agents such as d-cycloserine has some evidence for altering the negative symptoms of schizophrenia and deserves further exploration in bipolar disorder.

Other strategies

Heavy metals

Lithium is a metal ion and the potential effects of other heavy metals remain to be explored more systematically. There is a promising preliminary literature surrounding that of zinc, which is a co-transmitter with glutamate in dentate granule cells, and exerts a variety of post-synaptic effects on both NMDA and GABA receptors. Recently, homocysteine had been linked to deficits in cognition and inability of patients with bipolar disorder to re-acquire the euthymic state between episodes. Directly targeting this pathway with folate, B12 and other substances to reduce homocysteine levels may also have merit. In this regard, it is noteworthy that a complex combination of multiple heavy metals, folate, and nutritional supplements has shown promise in very preliminary clinical trials in adults and young people with bipolar illness, (Kaplan et al., 2001) and this micro-nutrient strategy deserves further attention.

Neurostimulation for regional effects

A variety of neurostimulatory techniques are now available or in different phases of clinical testing, including repeated transcranial magnetic stimulation (rTMS) and vagal nerve stimulation (VNS), reviewed in (Herrmann & Ebmeier, 2006; Loo & Mitchell, 2005; Nahas et al., 2006; Nemeroff et al., 2006). These have the advantage of not requiring anesthesia or seizures, which carries the potential for memory loss with ECT treatment. The mechanism of action of TMS and VNS are not yet well delineated, but these neurostimulatory treatments offer the possibility of being used in conjunction with pharmacological approaches. This might enhance or inhibit neurotransmitter systems in a fashion that could have regional specificity, synergistic effects, or effects mirroring those induced with experience dependent neuroplasaticity (Post & Speer, 2007).

Conclusions

New progress in understanding the mechanisms of action of mood stabilizing agents and pathophysiological processes in the illness itself has yielded panoply of new targets for future treatments for bipolar disorder. However, a sobering thought should be borne in mind: a substance like lithium has a myriad of mechanisms of action, and we know little about which of these in particular are crucial to its effects in bipolar disorder, despite studies over a half century. While this must give us pause on the one hand, it also suggests the possibility that it is lithium's diverse effects on multiple neurotransmitter, second messenger systems in the signal transduction cascade, including effects at the gene transcriptional level, that may combine to make it such a powerful therapeutic agent.

Thus, single targeting of novel systems may ultimately turn out to be not so productive as utilizing multiple targets of action in combination. Interestingly, clinical therapeutics has driven us in this direction with the findings that many treatment-resistant patients, in fact, have substantial response or remission when highly complex combination treatments are utilized. Therefore, the search for a novel "clean" drug with a specific target of action may ultimately prove not to be as clinically efficacious as a "dirty" drug, such as lithium, with its wide range of actions at multiple systems and sites.

This caveat would also appear consistent with new data from molecular biology indicating that, while there is a strong genetic component in bipolar disorder with approximately 50% of patients having a positive family history of the illness, there is no single gene with a large effect. In fact, Craddock and colleagues have suggested that a host of genes, each with small effect, and their combination, is likely to be important in conveying vulnerability for bipolar disorder. In contrast to the huntingtin protein of Huntington's chorea which gives us an important single target for clinical therapeutics, somewhat akin to the deficiency of dopamine in Parkinson's disease, it is highly unlikely that such specific and focused neuropathology will emerge in bipolar disorder, and both multiple targets of therapeutics and multiple systems and their interconnectivity may need to be considered instead in developing novel treatments.

There are already a variety of compounds from many different classes that have shown efficacy in either depression, mania, or as mood stabilizers in the prevention of one or both types of episodes. Thus, a promising path to the next decade would be attempts to bring individualized medicine to fruition in bipolar disorder. Rather than engaging in multiple long-term sequential clinical trials (in an attempt to find which agent may be most effective for a given individual), this process could be focused and accelerated using already available techniques. That is, measuring a substantial array of single nucleotide polymorphisms (SNPs) may provide, by pattern analysis, meaningful hints about the likelihood of clinical response or side effects to a given agent. This approach cited by many investigators, including David Cox of Pergolen, is likely to rapidly yield clinically valuable data based on already available methods and findings of molecular genetics. This promise of pharmacogenetics may come to fruition long before traditional genetics provides strong targets for therapeutics that may have an impact on the illness. Given multiple genes of small effect, altering one neurotransmitter system or signaling pathway may, or not, produce a clinically favorable effect. Instead, the field could rapidly advance if patients were better matched to their most appropriate treatment from the outset and such an approach would even pave the way toward earlier intervention with the possibility of secondary, and even primary, prevention in those at highest risk (Post and Kowatch, 2006). Several studies have begun to explore this possibility and it would appear important to regularly and systematically link SNP profiling to individual outcomes in clinical trials conducted in academia and industry in order to most rapidly usher in the era of personalized medicine. The methodology and technology to achieve this is currently available and is being refined and improved all the time. All that is missing is the motivation, financing, and clinical trials networks to assess individuals response inorder to make this occur in a timely fashion. These obstacles may be as difficult to overcome, as any technical or scientific innovation.

We return to the important notion in the introduction that increasing evidence suggests that the recurrent unipolar and bipolar mood disorders can be associated with a progressive and downhill course if not adequately treated with appropriate and timely interventions. Thus, as a better understanding of the pathophysiology of bipolar illness comes to the fore, it is hoped that this will yield more widespread public knowledge about the potential devastation of the disorder and the need for earlier recognition and treatment. Even when we do find new targets for therapy, it would be important to employ these and currently available treatment options at the earliest possible time in patients' lives. This will help prevent the potential malignant progression of the illness, which can lead to educational, social, and economic dysfunction, and even the possibility of lethality from the illness, either directly from suicide or indirectly by the increased medical mortality associated with bipolar disorder. Therefore, using existing and novel targets of therapeutics in the most expeditious way possible will be an important public health goal of the next several decades, and one that deserves concerted support and new resources for bipolar disorder treatment research in children and adults.

References

Antelman SM, Caggiula AR, Kiss S, Edwards DJ, Kocan D, & Stiller R (1995). Neurochemical and physiological effects of cocaine oscillate with sequential drug treatment: possibly a major factor in drug variability. *Neuropsychopharmacology* 12(4): 297–306.

Bai F, Bergeron M, & Nelson DL (2003). Chronic AMPA receptor potentiator (LY451646) treatment increases cell proliferation in adult rat hippocampus. *Neuropharmacology*, 44(8): 1013–1021.

Bannerman DM, Good MA, Butcher SP, Ramsay M, & Morris RG (1995). Distinct components of spatial learning revealed by prior training and NMDA receptor blockade. *Nature*, 378(6553): 182–186.

Bebchuk JM, Arfken CL, Dolan-Manji S, Murphy J, Hasanat K, & Manji HK (2000). A preliminary investigation of a protein kinase C inhibitor in the treatment of acute mania. *Arch. Gen. Psychiatry*, 57(1): 95–97.

Belanoff JK, Flores BH, Kalezhan M, Sund B, & Schatzberg AF (2001). Rapid reversal of psychotic depression using mifepristone. *J. Clin. Psychopharmacol.*, 21(5): 516–521.

Belanoff JK, Rothschild AJ, Cassidy F, DeBattista C, Baulieu EE, & Schold C, et al. (2002). An open label trial of C-1073 (mifepristone) for psychotic major depression. *Biol. Psychiatry*, 52(5): 386–392.

Belmaker RH, Roitman G, & Birch NJ (1988). A clinical trial of demethylchlortetracycline as a lithium-like agent in excited psychoses. In: *Lithium: Inorganic Pharmacology and Psychiatric Use* (pp 191–193). Oxford: IRL Press Limited.

Bensimon G, Lacomblez L, & Meininger V (1994). A controlled trial of riluzole in amyotrophic lateral sclerosis. ALS/Riluzole Study Group. *N. Engl. J. Med.,* 330(9): 585–591.

Berk M, Copolov DL, Dean O, Lu K, Jeavons S, Schapkaitz I, Anderson-Hunt M, & Bush AI (2008). N-acetyl cysteine for depressive symptoms in bipolar disorder—a double-blind randomized placebo-controlled trial. *Biol. Psychiatry,* 64(6): 468–475.

Berman RM, Cappiello A, Anand A, Oren DA, Heninger GR, & Charney DS, et al. (2000). Antidepressant effects of ketamine in depressed patients. *Biol. Psychiatry,* 47(4): 351–354.

Bertolino A, Crippa D, di Dio S, Fichte K, Musmeci G, & Porro V, et al. (1988). Rolipram versus imipramine in inpatients with major, "minor" or atypical depressive disorder: a double-blind double-dummy study aimed at testing a novel therapeutic approach. *Int. Clin. Psychopharmacol.,* 3(3): 245–253.

Berton O, McClung CA, Dileone RJ, Krishnan V, Renthal W, & Russo SJ, et al. (2006). Essential role of BDNF in the mesolimbic dopamine pathway in social defeat stress. *Science,* 311(5762): 864–868.

Bleakman D, & Lodge D (1998). Neuropharmacology of AMPA and kainate receptors. *Neuropharmacology,* 37(10–11): 1187–1204.

Bloch M, Schmidt P, Danaceau M, & Rubinow D (1999). Dehydroepiandrosterone treatment of midlife dysthymia. *Biol. Psychiatry,* 45(12): 1533–1541.

Bobon D, Breulet M, Gerard-Vandenhove MA, Guiot-Goffioul F, Plomteux G, & Sastre-y-Hernandez M, et al. (1988). Is phosphodiesterase inhibition a new mechanism of antidepressant action? A double blind double-dummy study between rolipram and desipramine in hospitalized major and/or endogenous depressives. *Eur. Arch. Psychiatry Neurol. Sci.,* 238(1): 2–6.

Borges K, & Dingledine R (1998). AMPA receptors: molecular and functional diversity. *Prog. Brain Res.,* 116: 153–170.

Brown GR, McBride L, Bauer MS, & Williford WO (2005). Impact of childhood abuse on the course of bipolar disorder: a replication study in U.S. veterans. *J. Affect. Disord.,* 89(1–3): 57–67.

Callahan AM, Frye MA, Marangell LB, George MS, Ketter TA, & L'Herrou T, et al. (1997). Comparative antidepressant effects of intravenous and intrathecal thyrotropin-releasing hormone: confounding effects of tolerance and implications for therapeutics. *Biol. Psychiatry,* 41(3): 264–272.

Caspi A, Sugden K, Moffitt TE, Taylor A, Craig IW, & Harrington H, et al. (2003). Influence of life stress on depression: moderation by a polymorphism in the 5-HTT gene. *Science,* 301(5631): 386–389.

Chen G, Manji HK, Hawver DB, Wright CB, & Potter WZ (1994). Chronic sodium valproate selectively decreases protein kinase C alpha and epsilon in vitro. *J. Neurochem.,* 63(6): 2361–2364.

Chuang DM, Chen RW, Chalecka-Franaszek E, Ren M, Hashimoto R, & Senatorov V, et al. (2002). Neuroprotective effects of lithium in cultured cells and animal models of diseases. *Bipolar Disord.,* 4(2): 129–136.

Collingridge GL (1994). Long-term potentiation. A question of reliability. *Nature,* 371(6499): 652–653.

Collingridge GL, & Bliss TV (1995). Memories of NMDA receptors and LTP. *Trends Neurosci., 18*(2): 54–56.

DeBattista C, Belanoff J, Glass S, Khan A, Horne RL, & Blasey C, et al. (2006). Mifepristone versus placebo in the treatment of psychosis in patients with psychotic major depression. *Biol. Psychiatry, 60*(12): 1343–1349.

DeBattista C, Posener JA, Kalehzan BM, & Schatzberg AF (2000). Acute antidepressant effects of intravenous hydrocortisone and CRH in depressed patients: a double-blind, placebo-controlled study. *Am. J. Psychiatry, 157*(8): 1334–1337.

Du J, Gould TD, & Manji HK (2003). Neurotrophic signaling in mood disorders. In: Finkel T, & Gutkind JS (Eds). *Signal Transduction and Human Disease* (pp 411–446). Hoboken, NJ: John Wiley & Sons, Inc.

Dubovsky SL, Franks RD, Allen S, & Murphy J (1986). Calcium antagonists in mania: a double-blind study of verapamil. *Psychiatry Res., 18*(4): 309–320.

Ducottet C, Griebel G, & Belzung C (2003). Effects of the selective nonpeptide corticotropin-releasing factor receptor 1 antagonist antalarmin in the chronic mild stress model of depression in mice. *Prog. Neuropsychopharmacol. Biol. Psychiatry, 27*(4): 625–631.

Duman RS (2002). Synaptic plasticity and mood disorders. *Mol. Psychiatry, 7* (Suppl 1): S29–34.

Duman RS, & Monteggia LM (2006). A neurotrophic model for stress-related mood disorders. *Biol. Psychiatry, 59*(12): 1116–1127.

Einat H, & Manji HK (2006). Cellular plasticity cascades: genes-to-behavior pathways in animal models of bipolar disorder. *Biol. Psychiatry, 59*(12): 1160–1171.

Fleischhacker WW, Hinterhuber H, Bauer H, Pflug B, Berner P, & Simhandl C, et al. (1992). A multicenter double-blind study of three different doses of the new cAMP-phosphodiesterase inhibitor rolipram in patients with major depressive disorder. *Neuropsychobiology, 26*(1–2): 59–64.

Flores BH, Kenna H, Keller J, Solvason HB, & Schatzberg AF (2006). Clinical and biological effects of mifepristone treatment for psychotic depression. *Neuropsychopharmacology, 31*(3): 628–636.

Frame S, & Cohen P (2001). GSK3 takes centre stage more than 20 years after its discovery. *Biochem. J., 359*(Pt 1): 1–16.

Friedman E, Hoau Yan W, Levinson D, Connell TA, & Singh H (1993). Altered platelet protein kinase C activity in bipolar affective disorder, manic episode. *Biol. Psychiatry, 33*(7): 520–525.

Frye MA, Gary KA, Marangell LB, George MS, Callahan AM, Little JT, Huggins T, Corá-Locatelli G, Osuch EA, Winokur A, & Post RM (1999). CSF thyrotropin-releasing hormone gender difference: implications for neurobiology and treatment of depression. *J. Neuropsychiatry Clin. Neurosci, 11*(3): 349–353.

Garno JL, Goldberg JF, Ramirez PM, & Ritzler BA (2005). Impact of childhood abuse on the clinical course of bipolar disorder. *Br. J. Psychiatry, 186*: 121–125.

Gary KA, Sevarino KA, Yarbrough GG, Prange AJ, Jr., & Winokur A (2003). The thyrotropin-releasing hormone (TRH) hypothesis of homeostatic regulation: implications for TRH-based therapeutics. *J. Pharmacol. Exp. Ther., 305*(2): 410–416.

Goff DC, Leahy L, Berman I, Posever T, Herz L, & Leon AC, et al. (2001). A placebo-controlled pilot study of the ampakine CX516 added to clozapine in schizophrenia. *J. Clin. Psychopharmacol., 21*(5): 484–487.

Goldberg JF, Burdick KE, & Endick CJ (2004). Preliminary randomized, double-blind, placebo-controlled trial of pramipexole added to mood stabilizers for treatment-resistant bipolar depression. *Am. J. Psychiatry, 161*(3): 564–566.

Goldberg JF, Burdick KE, & Endick CJ (2004). Preliminary randomized, double-blind, placebo controlled trial of pramipede added to mood stabilizers for treatment-resistant bipolar depression. *Am. J. Psychiatry, 161*(3): 564–566.

Gould TD, & Manji HK (2002). The wnt signaling pathway in bipolar disorder. *Neuroscientist, 8*(5): 497–511.

Gould TD, Picchini AM, Einat H, & Manji HK (2006). Targeting glycogen synthase kinase-3 in the CNS: implications for the development of new treatments for mood disorders. *Curr. Drug Targets, 7*(11): 1399–1409.

Gould TD, Quiroz JA, Singh J, Zarate CA, & Manji HK (2004a). Emerging experimental therapeutics for bipolar disorder: insights from the molecular and cellular actions of current mood stabilizers. *Mol. Psychiatry, 9*(8): 734–755.

Gould TD, Zarate CA, & Manji HK (2004b). Glycogen synthase kinase-3: a target for novel bipolar disorder treatments. *J. Clin. Psychiatry, 65*(1): 10–21.

Griebel G, Misslin R, Vogel E, & Bourguignon JJ (1991). Behavioral effects of rolipram and structurally related compounds in mice: behavioral sedation of cAMP phosphodiesterase inhibitors. *Pharmacol. Biochem. Behav., 39*(2): 321–323.

Habib KE, Weld KP, Rice KC, Pushkas J, Champoux M, & Listwak S, et al. (2000). Oral administration of a corticotropin-releasing hormone receptor antagonist significantly attenuates behavioral, neuroendocrine, and autonomic responses to stress in primates. *Proc. Natl. Acad. Sci. USA, 97*(11): 6079–6084.

Hahn CG, & Friedman E (1999). Abnormalities in protein kinase C signaling and the pathophysiology of bipolar disorder. *Bipolar Disord., 1*(2): 81–86.

Hebenstreit GF, Fellerer K, Fichte K, Fischer G, Geyer N, & Meya U, et al. (1989). Rolipram in major depressive disorder: results of a double-blind comparative study with imipramine. *Pharmacopsychiatry, 22*(4): 156–160.

Heim C, Newport DJ, Bonsall R, Miller AH, & Nemeroff CB (2001). Altered pituitary–adrenal axis responses to provocative challenge tests in adult survivors of childhood abuse. *Am. J. Psychiatry, 158*(4): 575–581.

Herrmann LL, & Ebmeier KP (2006). Factors modifying the efficacy of transcranial magnetic stimulation in the treatment of depression: a review. *J. Clin. Psychiatry, 67*(12): 1870–1876.

Holmes A, Heilig M, Rupniak NM, Steckler T, & Griebel G (2003). Neuropeptide system as novel therapeutic targets for depression and anxiety disorders. *Trend. Pharmacol. Sci., 24*(11): 580–588.

Ising M, Horstmann S, Kloiber S, Lucae S, Binder EB, & Kern N, et al. (2007). Combined dexamethasone/corticotropin releasing hormone test predicts treatment response in major depression-a potential biomarker? *Biol. Psychiatry, 62*(1): 47–54.

Jope RS, & Bijur GN (2002). Mood stabilizers, glycogen synthase kinase-3beta and cell survival. *Mol. Psychiatry, 7*(Suppl 1): S35–45.

Kalivas PW (2004). Glutamate systems in cocaine addiction. *Curr. Opin. Pharmacol., 4*(1): 23–29.

Kalivas PW, & Stewart J (1991). Dopamine transmission in the initiation and expression of drug- and stress-induced sensitization of motor activity. *Brain Res. Brain Res. Rev., 16*(3): 223–244.

Kaplan BJ, Simpson JS, Ferre RC, Gorman CP, McMullen DM, & Crawford SG (2001). Effective mood stabilization with a chelated mineral supplement: an open-label trial in bipolar disorder. *J. Clin. Psychiatry, 62*(12): 936–944.

Kitamura Y, Kosaka T, Kakimura JI, Matsuoka Y, Kohno Y, & Nomura Y, et al. (1998). Protective effects of the antiparkinsonian drugs talipexole and pramipexole against 1-methyl-4-phenylpyridinium-induced apoptotic death in human neuroblastoma SH-SY5Y cells. *Mol. Pharmacol., 54*(6): 1046–1054.

Knapp RJ, Goldenberg R, Shuck C, Cecil A, Watkins J, & Miller C, et al. (2002). Antidepressant activity of memory-enhancing drugs in the reduction of submissive behavior model. *Eur. J. Pharmacol., 440*(1): 27–35.

Kraepelin E (1921). *Manic-Depressive Insanity and Paranoia.* Edinburgh: Livingstone.

Kulkarni J, Garland KA, Scaffidi A, Headey B, Anderson R, & de Castella A, et al. (2006). A pilot study of hormone modulation as a new treatment for mania in women with bipolar affective disorder. *Psychoneuroendocrinology, 31*(4): 543–547.

Kunzel HE, Zobel AW, Nickel T, Ackl N, Uhr M, & Sonntag A, et al. (2003). Treatment of depression with the CRH-1-receptor antagonist R121919: endocrine changes and side effects. *J. Psychiatr. Res., 37*: 525–533.

Lauterborn JC, Lynch G, Vanderklish P, Arai A, & Gall CM (2000). Positive modulation of AMPA receptors increases neurotrophin expression by hippocampal and cortical neurons. *J. Neurosci., 20*(1): 8–21.

Leverich GS, McElroy SL, Suppes T, Keck PE, Jr., Denicoff KD, & Nolen WA, et al. (2002). Early physical and sexual abuse associated with an adverse course of bipolar illness. *Biol. Psychiatry, 51*(4): 288–297.

Li X, Tizzano JP, Griffey K, Clay M, Lindstrom T, & Skolnick P (2001). Antidepressant-like actions of an AMPA receptor potentiator (LY392098). *Neuropharmacology, 40*(8): 1028–1033.

Loo CK, & Mitchell PB (2005). A review of the efficacy of transcranial magnetic stimulation (TMS) treatment for depression, and current and future strategies to optimize efficacy. *J. Affect. Disord., 88*(3): 255–267.

Mackin P, Gallagher P, Watson S, Young AH, & Ferrier IN (2007). Changes in brain-derived neurotrophic factor following treatment with mifepristone in bipolar disorder and schizophrenia. *Aust. N Z J. Psychiatry, 41*(4): 321–326.

Malison RT, Anand A, Pelton GH, Kirwin P, Carpenter L, & McDougle CJ, et al. (1999). Limited efficacy of ketoconazole in treatment-refractory major depression. *J. Clin. Psychopharmacol., 19*(5): 466–470.

Manji HK, Etcheberrigaray R, Chen G, & Olds JL (1993). Lithium decreases membrane-associated protein kinase C in hippocampus: selectivity for the alpha isozyme. *J. Neurochem., 61*(6): 2303–2310.

Manji HK, & Lenox RH (1999). Ziskind-Somerfeld Research Award. Protein kinase C signaling in the brain: molecular transduction of mood stabilization in the treatment of manic-depressive illness. *Biol. Psychiatry, 46*(10): 1328–1351.

Manji HK, Quiroz JA, Sporn J, Denicoff K, Gray N, Zarate JA Jr, & Charney DS (2003). Enhancing neuronal plasticity and cellular resilience to develop novel, improved therapeutics for difficult-to-treat depression. *Biol. Psychiatry, 53*(8): 707–742.

McEwen BS (1999). Stress and hippocampal plasticity. *Ann. Rev. Neurosci.,* 22: 105–122.

Meaney MJ, Aitken DH, van Berkel C, Bhatnagar S, & Sapolsky RM (1988). Effect of neonatal handling on age-related impairments associated with the hippocampus. *Science, 239*(4841 Pt 1): 766–768.

Murphy BE, Filipini D, & Ghadirian AM (1993). Possible use of glucocorticoid receptor antagonists in the treatment of major depression: preliminary results using RU 486. *J. Psychiatry Neurosci., 18*(5): 209–213.

Murray SR, Leonard CJ, Lowe DA, & Sachs G (Eds) (2007). MEM1003, a Novel, CNS-Selective L-type Ca2+ Channel Blocker, Versus Placebo in Bipolar Mania. *Seventh International Conference on Bipolar Disorder.* Pittsburgh, PA.

Nahas Z, Burns C, Foust MJ, Short B, Herbsman T, & George MS (2006). Vagus nerve stimulation (VNS) for depression: what do we know now and what should be done next? *Curr. Psychiatry Rep., 8*(6): 445–451.

Nemeroff CB, Mayberg HS, Krahl SE, McNamara J, Frazer A, & Henry TR, et al. (2006). VNS therapy in treatment-resistant depression: clinical evidence and putative neurobiological mechanisms. *Neuropsychopharmacology, 31*(7): 1345–1355.

Nibuya M, Nestler EJ, & Duman RS (1996). Chronic antidepressant administration increases the expression of cAMP response element binding protein (CREB) in rat hippocampus. *J. Neurosci., 16*(7): 2365–2372.

O'Donnell JM (1993). Antidepressant-like effects of rolipram and other inhibitors of cyclic adenosine monophosphate phosphodiesterase on behavior maintained by differential reinforcement of low response rate. *J. Pharmacol. Exp. Ther., 264*(3): 1168–1178.

Ochs G, Penn RD, York M, Giess R, Beck M, & Tonn J, et al. (2000). A phase I/II trial of recombinant methionyl human brain derived neurotrophic factor administered by intrathecal infusion to patients with amyotrophic lateral sclerosis. *Amyotroph. Lateral Scler. Other Motor Neuron Disord., 1*(3): 201–206.

Pazzaglia PJ, Post RM, Ketter TA, Callahan AM, Marangell LB, & Frye MA, et al. (1998). Nimodipine monotherapy and carbamazepine augmentation in patients with refractory recurrent affective illness. *J. Clin. Psychopharmacol., 18*(5): 404–413.

Pazzaglia PJ, Post RM, Ketter TA, George MS, & Marangell LB (1993). Preliminary controlled trial of nimodipine in ultra-rapid cycling affective dysregulation. *Psychiatry Res., 49*(3): 257–272.

Plotsky PM, Owens MJ, & Nemeroff CB (1998). Psychoneuroendocrinology of depression. Hypothalamic-pituitary-adrenal axis. *Psychiatr. Clin. North Am., 21*(2): 293–307.

Post RM (2007a). Animal models of mood disorders: kindling as a model of affective illness progression. In: Schachter S, Holmes G, & Kasteleijn-Nolst Trenite´ D (Eds). *Behavioral Aspects of Epilepsy: Principles and Practice.* Demos Medical Publishing, New York, NY.

Post RM (2007b). Kindling and sensitization as models for affective episode recurrence, cyclicity, and tolerance phenomena. *Neurosci. Biobehav. Rev., 31*(16): 858–873.

Post RM (2007c). Role of BDNF in bipolar and unipolar disorder: clinical and theoretical implications. *J. Psychiatry Res., 41*(12): 979–990.

Post RM, Altshuler LL, Frye MA, Suppes T, McElroy S, & Keck PE, Jr., et al. (2006a). New findings from the Bipolar Collaborative Network: clinical implications for therapeutics. *Curr. Psychiatry Rep., 8*(6): 489–497.

Post RM, Altshuler LL, Leverich GS, Frye MA, Nolen WA, & Kupka RW, et al. (2006b). Mood switch in bipolar depression: comparison of adjunctive venlafaxine, bupropion and sertraline. *Br. J. Psychiatry, 189*: 124–131.

Post RM, Gerner RH, Carman JS, Gillin JC, Jimerson DC, & Goodwin FK, et al. (1978). Effects of a dopamine agonist piribedil in depressed patients: relationship of pretreatment homovanillic acid to antidepressant response. *Arch. Gen. Psychiatry, 35*(5): 609–615.

Post RM, & Kowatch RA (2006). The health care crisis of childhood-onset bipolar illness: some recommendations for its amelioration. *J. Clin. Psychiatry, 67*(1): 115–125.

Post RM, & Speer AM (2007). rTMS and related somatic therapies: prospects for the future. In: Belmaker RH, George MS, Eds. *TMS in Clinical Psychiatry*, Washington DC: Am Psychiatric Press, Inc., 225–255.

Post RM (1992). Transduction of psychosocial stress into the neurobiology of recurrent affective disorder. *Am. J. Psychiatry, 149*(8): 999–1010.

Preskorn S, Baker B, Omo K, Kolluri S, Menniti F, & Landen JA (Eds) (2007). *A Placebo-Controlled Trial of the NR2B Specific NMDA Antagonist CP-101,606 Plus Paroxetine for Treatment Resistant Depression (TRD).* San Diego, CA: APA.

Quiroz JA, Singh J, Gould TD, Denicoff KD, Zarate CA, & Manji HK (2004). Emerging experimental therapeutics for bipolar disorder: clues from the molecular pathophysiology. *Mol. Psychiatry, 9*(8): 756–776.

Riedel G, Platt B, & Micheau J (2003). Glutamate receptor function in learning and memory. *Behav. Brain Res., 140*(1–2): 1–47.

Roceri M, Cirulli F, Pessina C, Peretto P, Racagni G, & Riva MA (2004). Postnatal repeated maternal deprivation produces age-dependent changes of brain-derived neurotrophic factor expression in selected rat brain regions. *Biol. Psychiatry, 55*(7): 708–714.

Sachs GS, Nierenberg AA, Calabrese JR, Marangell LB, Wisniewski SR, & Gyulai L, et al. (2007). Effectiveness of adjunctive antidepressant treatment for bipolar depression. *N. Engl. J. Med., 356*(17): 1711–1722.

Salinska E, & Stafiej A (2003). Metabotropic glutamate receptors (mGluRs) are involved in early phase of memory formation: possible role of modulation of glutamate release. *Neurochem. Int., 43*(4–5): 469–474.

Sapolsky RM (1996). Stress, glucocorticoids, and damage to the nervous system: The current state of confusion. *Stress, 1*(1): 1–19.

Sapolsky RM (2000). Glucocorticoids and hippocampal atrophy in neuropsychiatric disorders. *Arch. Gen. Psychiatry, 57*(10): 925–935.

Sapolsky RM, Romero LM, & Munck AU (2000). How do glucocorticoids influence stress responses? Integrating permissive, suppressive, stimulatory, and preparative actions. *Endocr. Rev., 21*(1): 55–89.

Saunders J, & Williams J (2003). Antagonists of the corticotropin releasing factor receptor. *Prog. Med. Chem., 41*: 195–247.

Scott AI, Perini AF, Shering PA, & Whalley LJ (1991). In-patient major depression: is rolipram as effective as amitriptyline? *Eur. J. Clin. Pharmacol., 40*(2): 127–129.

Simpson GM, El Sheshai A, Loza N, Kingsbury SJ, Fayek M, & Rady A, et al. (2005). An 8-week open-label trial of a 6-day course of mifepristone for the treatment of psychotic depression. *J. Clin. Psychiatry, 66*(5): 598–602.

Sporn J, Ghaemi SN, Sambur MR, Rankin MA, Recht J, & Sachs GS, et al. (2000). Pramipexole augmentation in the treatment of unipolar and bipolar depression: a retrospective chart review. *Ann. Clin. Psychiatry, 12*(3): 137–140.

Szuba MP, Amsterdam JD, Fernando AT, 3rd, Gary KA, Whybrow PC, & Winokur A (2005). Rapid antidepressant response after nocturnal TRH administration in patients with bipolar type I and bipolar type II major depression. *J. Clin. Psychopharmacol., 25*(4): 325–330.

Takahashi M, Terwilliger R, Lane C, Mezes PS, Conti M, & Duman RS (1999). Chronic antidepressant administration increases the expression of cAMP-specific phosphodiesterase 4A and 4B isoforms. *J. Neurosci., 19*(2): 610–618.

Takata K, Kitamura Y, Kakimura J, Kohno Y, & Taniguchi T (2000). Increase of bcl-2 protein in neuronal dendritic processes of cerebral cortex and hippocampus by the antiparkinsonian drugs, talipexole and pramipexole. *Brain Res., 872*(1–2): 236–241.

Tan Y, Hori N, & Carpenter DO (2003). The mechanism of presynaptic long-term depression mediated by group I metabotropic glutamate receptors. *Cell. Mol. Neurobiol., 23*(2): 187–203.

Tsankova NM, Berton O, Renthal W, Kumar A, Neve RL, & Nestler EJ (2006). Sustained hippocampal chromatin regulation in a mouse model of depression and antidepressant action. *Nat. Neurosci., 9*(4): 519–525.

Wachtel H, & Schneider HH (1986). Rolipram, a novel antidepressant drug, reverses the hypothermia and hypokinesia of monoamine-depleted mice by an action beyond postsynaptic monoamine receptors. *Neuropharmacology, 25*(10): 1119–1126.

Watkins J, & Collingridge G (1994). Phenylglycine derivatives as antagonists of metabotropic glutamate receptors. *Trends Pharmacol. Sci., 15*(9): 333–342.

Webster EL, Lewis DB, Torpy DJ, Zachman EK, Rice KC, & Chrousos GP (1996). In vivo and in vitro characterization of antalarmin, a nonpeptide corticotropin-releasing hormone (CRH) receptor antagonist: suppression of pituitary ACTH release and peripheral inflammation. *Endocrinology, 137*(12): 5747–5750.

Winokur A, Amsterdam JD, Oler J, Mendels J, Snyder PJ, Caroff SN, & Brunswick DJ (1983). Multiple hormonal responses to protirelin (TRH) in depressed patients. *Arch. Gen. Psychiatry, 40*(5): 525–531.

Witkin JM, Marek GJ, Johnson BG, & Schoepp DD (2007). Metabotropic glutamate receptors in the control of mood disorders. *CNS Neurol. Disord. Drug Targets, 6*(2): 87–100.

Wolkowitz OM, Reus VI, Chan T, Manfredi F, Raum W, & Johnson R, et al. (1999a). Antiglucocorticoid treatment of depression: double-blind ketoconazole. *Biol. Psychiatry, 45*(8): 1070–1074.

Wolkowitz OM, Reus VI, Keebler A, Nelson N, Friedland M, & Brizendine L, et al. (1999b). Double-blind treatment of major depression with dehydroepiandrosterone. *Am. J. Psychiatry, 156*(4): 646–649.

Yildiz A, Guleryuz S, Ankerst DP, Ongür D, & Renshaw PF (2008). Protein kinase C inhibition in the treatment of mania: a double-blind, placebo-controlled trial of tamoxifen. *Arch. Gen. Psychiatry, 65*(3): 255–263.

Young AH, Gallagher P, Watson S, Del-Estal D, Owen BM, & Ferrier IN (2004). Improvements in neurocognitive function and mood following adjunctive treatment with mifepristone (RU-486) in bipolar disorder. *Neuropsychopharmacology, 29*(8): 1538–1545.

Young LT, Wang JF, Woods CM, & Robb JC (1999). Platelet protein kinase C alpha levels in drug-free and lithium-treated subjects with bipolar disorder. *Neuropsychobiology, 40*(2): 63–66.

Zarate CA Jr, Singh JB, Carlson PJ, Quiroz J, Jolkovsky L, Luckenbaugh DA, & Manji HK (2007). Efficacy of a protein kinase C inhibitor (tamoxifen) in the treatment of acute mania: a pilot study. *Bipolar Disord, 9*(6): 561–570. Erratum in: *Bipolar Disord.*, 2007, *9*(8): 932.

Zarate CA, Jr., Payne JL, Quiroz J, Sporn J, Denicoff KK, & Luckenbaugh D, et al. (2004a). An open-label trial of riluzole in patients with treatment-resistant major depression. *Am. J. Psychiatry, 161*(1): 171–174.

Zarate CA, Jr., Payne JL, Singh J, Quiroz JA, Luckenbaugh DA, & Denicoff KD, et al. (2004b). Pramipexole for bipolar II depression: a placebo-controlled proof of concept study. *Biol. Psychiatry, 56*(1): 54–60.

Zarate CA, Jr., Quiroz JA, Singh JB, Denicoff KD, De Jesus G, & Luckenbaugh DA, et al. (2005). An open-label trial of the glutamate-modulating agent riluzole in combination with lithium for the treatment of bipolar depression. *Biol. Psychiatry, 57*(4): 430–432.

Zarate CA, Jr., Singh JB, Carlson PJ, Brutsche NE, Ameli R, & Luckenbaugh DA, et al. (2006). A randomized trial of an N-methyl-D-aspartate antagonist in treatment-resistant major depression. *Arch. Gen. Psychiatry, 63*(8): 856–864.

Zarate CA, Jr., Quiroz JA, Payne JL, & Manji HK (2002). Modulators of the glutamatergic system: Implications for the development of improved therapeutics in mood disorders. *Psychopharmacol. Bull., 36*(4): 35–83.

Zarate CA Jr, Singh JB, Carlson PJ, Quiroz J, Jolkovsky L, Luckenbaugh DA, & Manji HK (2007). Efficacy of a protein kinase C inhibitor (tamoxifen) in the treatment of acute mania: A pilot study. *Bipolar Disord., 9*(6):561–70.

Zeller E, Stief HJ, Pflug B, & Sastre-y-Hernandez M (1984). Results of a phase II study of the antidepressant effect of rolipram. *Pharmacopsychiatry, 17*(6): 188–190.

Zobel AW, Nickel T, Kunzel HE, Ackl N, Sonntag A, & Ising M, et al. (2000). Effects of the high-affinity corticotropin-releasing hormone receptor 1 antagonist R121919 in major depression: the first 20 patients treated. *J. Psychiatr. Res., 34*(3): 171–181.

Index

A

Agranulocytosis, 474, 485, 487, 508
American Psychiatric Association (APA)
     guidelines, 110
Angiotensin I and II converting enzyme
     inhibitors (ACEIs), 445, 447–448
Anticonvulsants medications, in bipolar
     disorder, 382
   carbamazepine, 383
     antimanic efficacy of, 383–384
     in bipolar depression, 384
     prophylaxis, 384–385
   carbamazepine ER, 385–386
   clonazepam, 399
     acute mania and, 400
     in bipolar depression, 400–401
     prophylaxis, 401
   felbamate, 401–402
   gabapentin
     acute mania/bipolar depression,
        397–398
     prophylaxis, 398
   lamotrigine
     for acute bipolar depression,
        393–395
     in acute mania, 392–393
     prophylaxis, 395–397
   levatiracetam, 402
   oxcarbazepine
     for acute mania, 386
   tiagabine, 401
   topiramate, 398
     in acute bipolar depression, 399
     in acute mania, 399
   valproate/divalproex
     in acute mania, 387–389

in bipolar depression, 389–390
   prophylaxis, 390–392
Antidepressants medications, in bipolar
     disorder, 366
   adverse effects
     (hypo) mania during maintenance
        treatment, 374
     manic switches, 372–374
     rapid cycling, 375–376
   efficacy of
     bupropion, 369
     mirtazapine, 369
     monoamine oxidase inhibitors,
        367–368
     selective serotonin re-uptake
        inhibitors, 368
     tricyclic antidepressants, 367
     venlafaxine, 369
   in maintenance treatment, 372
     imipramine monotherapy, 370–371
     mania during long-term
        monotherapy, 371
   systematic review, 370
   withdrawing of, 376–377
Anxiety disorders, 236–237
Aripiprazole (ARI), 123–124, 500–503
   efficacy and safety, 197
   with placebo double-blind trials, 29
Attention deficit hyperactivity disorder
     (ADHD), 189, 240–241
Atypical antipsychotics, 485
   aripiprazole, 500–503
   clozapine, 485–489
   olanzapine, 492–495
   quetiapine, 495–497
   risperidone, 489–492
   ziprasidone, 497–500

Australian and New Zealand clinical
    practice guidelines, 110
Australian registry of antiepileptic
    drugs, 167

B

Bech-Raefelson mania rating scale
    (BRMS), 386
Beck depression inventory, 66
Beigel–Murphy manic state rating scales,
    268–269
Benzodiazepines (BZs), 511–512
Binge-eating disorder, 240
Bipolar disorder, 2, 366, 592
    and anticonvulsants (see
        Anticonvulsants medications, in
        bipolar disorder)
    antidepressant monotherapy in, 89
    atypical antipsychotics, 91
        BOLDER I and II studies, 92
    chronicity and, 85–86
    clinical and functional sequelae of, 87
    clinical recommendations, 34–37
        for management, 96
    comorbid alcohol and drug use,
        224, 230
        clinical recommendations for,
            245–246
        impact on long-term course and
            clinical features, 232–233
        treatment, 233–234, 236
    conceptualisation and diagnostic
        validity, 83–84
    cross-sectional clinical marker of, 86
    cycling course, 46–47
    and depression, 22–23
        add-on therapies and, 30–33
        antidepressant treatment, 23–24
        early and accurate diagnosis, 20–21
        family history and, 21–22
        first line treatment options, 26–30
        personality disorders, 24–25
        pharmacological treatment
            of, 25–26
        somatic therapies, 33–34
    DSM-IV-TR diagnostic criteria,
        81–83, 186
    epidemiological studies of, 186
        epidemiologic catchment area
            (ECA) study and national
            comorbidity survey, 80

    euthymia and, 87
    gender distribution, 84
    genetic linkage study of, 4
    and hierarchical ordering of
        symptoms, 223
    and illness
        recurrence and adherence, 129–130
        severity, 85
    maintenance treatment, 93–94
        importance of, 108–112
        monitoring of, 128–129
    mood stabilizers
        open-labelled trial of, 91
    mood switching and, 94
    national epidemiologic survey on
        alcohol and related
        conditions, 24
    onset for, 84–85
    peri-pubertal onset of, 189
    pharmacotherapy for (see
        Pharmacotherapy, of bipolar
        disorders)
    physical and psychiatric
        comorbidities, 86
    placebo-controlled data, 90
    prevalence rates of comorbid axis I
        disorders with, 225–229
    psychological therapies, 95
    rapid-cycling subtype, 94–95
    refractory patients, 127–128
    residual/subsyndromal
        symptoms, 109
    risk of relapse, 108
    self-medication hypothesis, 231–232
    somatic treatments, use of (see
        Somatic treatments, for bipolar
        disorder)
    structured clinical interview for
        DSM-III-R (SCID) for
        diagnosis, 4
    subtype and French National EPIDEP
        study, 84
    Zurich cohort study, 80–81
Brain derived neurotrophic factor (BDNF),
    593–597
Brief psychiatric rating scale (BPRS), 265
Bright light therapy, 68
British Association of
        Psychopharmacology (BAP)
        guidelines, 110
Bulimia, 240
Bupropion antidepressant, 32, 369, 506–507

C

Canadian Network for Mood and
 Anxiety Treatment (CANMAT)
 guidelines, 110
Capsulotomy, 425
Carbamazepine, 383–385; *see also*
 Anticonvulsants medications, in
 bipolar disorder
 antimanic efficacy of, 383–384
 in bipolar depression, 384
 prophylaxis of bipolar disorder,
 384–385
Carbamazepine (CBZ), 32, 116–117
 in breast-feeding, 164–165
 as mood stabilizers, 462–463
 adverse events and management,
 474–475
 clinical recommendations, 476–477
 dosing strategies, 475–476
 drug–drug interactions, 465–468,
 473–474
 metabolic pathway of, 463–464
 during pregnancy, 165
 safety and efficacy, 194
Carbamazepine ER, 385–386; *see also*
 Anticonvulsants medications, in
 bipolar disorder
Childhood bipolar disorder, 185
 antidepressant, 198
 atypical antipsychotics, 194–198
 brain imaging, 188–189
 children's clinical global assessment
 scale score, 191
 children's depression rating scale-
 revised (CDRS-R) score, 192–193
 DSM-IV-TR criteria for, 186–187
 electroconvulsive therapy (ECT), 198
 epidemiological studies of, 186
 familial aggregation, 188
 magnetic resonance spectroscopy
 studies, 189
 mood stabilizers, 191–194
 personality symptoms in, 189–190
 placebo-controlled withdrawal trial,
 191–192
 symptoms in, 188
 treatment for, 190–191
Chlorpromazine, 119
Chronotherapeutic interventions, 33
Cingulotomy, 425
Citalopram antidepressant, 32

Clinical global impressions scale (CGI),
 88, 197
 severity and improvement scale,
 393–394
Clinical management package, for
 individual with BP, 551–552
 client's and clinician's goals
 integration, 558–560
 client's "illness" model, understanding
 of, 554–558
 early warning signs, identification of,
 571–572
 engagement, keys to, 554
 enhancing medication adherence,
 561–567
 behavioral interventions for,
 563–564
 cognitive techniques, 564–565
 interventions for, 561
 questions to monitor adherence, 562
 unintentional non-adherence,
 562–563
 guilt and related issues, dealing
 with, 569
 illness awareness, task of improving,
 567–568
 lifestyle regularity, issue of, 569–570
 start of process
 engagement, 553
 therapeutic alliance, development
 of, 552–553
 urgent issue, identification by clinician
 of, 570–571
Clonazepam, 399–401
 acute mania and, 400
 in bipolar depression, 400–401
 prophylaxis, 401
Clozapine (CLZ), 119–120, 485–489
Cognitive behavioral therapy (CBT), 576,
 579–580
Comorbid psychopathology, 222
COMT activity allele, 56; *see also* Rapid-
 cycling (RC) bipolar disorder
Cytochrome P450 isoforms
 as mood stabilizers
 inducers, 472
 inhibitors, 471–472
 substrates, 469–471
Cytochrome P450 monooxygenase (CYP)
 isozymes, 439–440; *see also*
 Pharmacotherapy, of bipolar
 disorders

D

Deep brain stimulation (DBS), 34, 427–428
Dialectical behavior therapy (DBT), 243
Divalproex, 387–392
    divalproex ER versus placebo in acute
        bipolar depression, randomized
        controlled trial, 29
Duloxetine, 506
Dyslipidemia, 215

E

Eating disorders, 240
Efficacy of monotherapy in bipolar
        depression (EMBOLDEN)
        studies, 28–29
Elderly adults and bipolar disorder
    family history of, 205
    national comorbidity survey
        replication study, 205
    neuroimaging studies, 209
    neuropsychological test, 209–210
    onset of, 206–207
        vascular risk factors in, 207–208
    prevalence of, 204
    psychiatric and medical comorbidity,
        205–206
    psychotherapy and psychoeducation in
        patients with, 215
    relapse and rehospitalization, 215–216
    symptoms and diagnosis, 208–209
    treatment of, 210
        antipsychotic agents, 213–215
        carbamazepine, 213
        divalproex sodium, 212
        duration of, 216
        lamotrigine, 212–213
        lithium, 211
Electroconvulsive therapy (ECT), 34–37, 412
    for bipolar disorder, 413
    concomitant medications, use of, 414–415
    double blind controlled data for, 29–30
    euphoria, hypomania, and mania by,
        415–416
    maintenance ECT, 416
Encephalopathic syndrome, 443
Epidemiologic catchment area (ECA)
        survey, 186
Escitalopram antidepressant, 32
Estrogen therapy for depression (MDD)
        during perimenopause, 169–170

F

Family-focused therapy (FFT), 582–584
Felbamate (FBM), 401–402, 513
Female reproductive cycle and bipolar
        disorder
    menarche, 155–156
    menopause, 168–169
        treatment strategies for, 169–170
    menstrual cycle phase and mood,
        156–158
        mood stabilizers, 159–160
        oral contraceptives (OC) and
            hormone therapies (HT),
            158–159
    pregnancy, 160–162
        antidepressant, 168
        carbamazepine, 164–165
        lamotrigine monotherapy, 167–168
        lithium utilization in, 163–164
        treatment strategies during, 162–163
        valproate, 165–167
First-generation antipsychotics (FGAs),
        296–297
    in acute bipolar I mania, 297–299
    in maintenance treatment, 299–300
Fluoxetine antidepressant, 32
Framingham stroke risk score, 208

G

Gabapentin (GBP), 513–515
    acute mania/bipolar depression,
        397–398
    as anxiolytic anticonvulsants, 239
    prophylaxis of bipolar disorder, 398
Generalized anxiety disorder (GAD),
        238–239
Glucuronidation reactions, 440
Glutamatergic neurotransmission,
        603–604
Glycogen synthase kinase-3 (GSK-3),
        lithium action on, 598

H

Haloperidol, 119, 298
Hamilton depression rating scale (HDRS),
        367–368, 389, 393
    Hamilton anxiety scale ratings, 237
    Hamilton rating scale for depression
        (HAM-D), 88

Harvard-McLean first episode mania
    study, 232
Hypomania, 3–5
    management of, 5–6
    treatment strategies in, 15, 87
    topiramate for, 88
Hypothyroidism, and lithium, 450–451

I

Illness model, cognitive representation of,
    555–556
    coping strategies, exploring of,
        557–558
    questions to elicit client's views,
        556–557
Imipramine antidepressant, 32
Inositol, 33, 36
Inpatient multidimension
    psychophathology scale, 386
Integrated family and individual therapy
    (IFIT), 585
Interpersonal and social-rhythm therapy
    (IPSRT), 584–585
Irreversible MAOIs, *see* Monoamine
    oxidase inhibitors (MAOI)

K

Ketamine, 604–605

L

Lamotrigine (LTG), 27, 36, 117–118,
    392–397; *see also* Anticonvulsants
    medications, in bipolar disorder
    for acute bipolar depression, 393–395
    in acute mania, 392–393
    clinical recommendations, 481–482
    International Lamotrigine Pregnancy
        Registry data, 167
    as mood stabilizers, 477–478
        adverse events and management,
            479–480
        clinical recommendations,
            481–482
        dosing strategies, 481
        pharmacokinetic interactions,
            478–479
    prophylaxis, 395–397
    safety and efficacy, 194
LED light device, *see* Litebook

Levetiracetam (LEV), 402, 520–522; *see also*
    Anticonvulsants medications, in
    bipolar disorder
Light therapy, 417–418
    for bipolar disorder, 418–420
Litebook, 417–418
Lithium, 442–443
    antihypertensives and, 447–448
    clinical issues with
        point-of-care (POC) test for levels,
            283–284
    double-blind studies
        anticonvulsants, 268–270
        antipsychotic drugs, 265–268
        placebo, 263–265
    efficacy and age groups, 281–282
    factors affecting clearance of, 446
    history of, 260–262
    lithium/divalproex second mood
        stabilizer, clinical trial, 30–31
    lithium prophylaxis, 46
    maintenance therapy of, 272
        discontinuation trials, 274–279
        prospective trials, 273–274
    as mood stabilizers
        adverse effects and treatment,
            449–453
        and ageing, 448
        analgesics and, 447
        anticonvulsant and, 445
        antidepressants and, 444–445
        antihypertensives and, 447–448
        and antipsychotics interactions,
            443–444
        and benzodiazepines, 445
        calcium channel blockers and, 448
        clinical recommendations, 454–455
        diuretics and, 447
        dosing strategies, 453–454
        encephalopathic syndrome, 443
        factors affecting clearance of, 446
        interactions with carbamazepine, 443
        lamotrigine and, 443
        mania patients and, 448–449
        methylxanthines and, 448
        neuromuscular blocking agents
            and, 448
    predictors of response, 279–281
    pre-DSM era open studies, 263
    in prevention of suicidality, 282–283
    in rapid cycling bipolar disorder, 279
    recommendations for use, 286

treatment
  in acute mania, 262
  as antidepressant, 113
  anti-suicidal properties of, 114
  in breast-feeding, 164
  clinical decision-making and,
      284–286
  in combination with drugs, 114
  efficacy in maintenance treatment
      for bipolar disorder, 113, 270–271
  episodic pattern of mania-
      depressed-euthymia, 113
  FDA indications for, 112
  long-term treatment and, 193
  in mixed and dysphoric manic
      episodes, 272
  in pregnancy, 163–164
  in prevention of manic episodes, 115
  side effects of, 114

M

Maintenance treatment; *see also*
          Antidepressants medications, in
          bipolar disorder
  anticonvulsants, 118–119
  antidepressants, 125–127
  antipsychotics, 119
  aripiprazole, 123–124
  atypical antipsychotics, side effects of,
      124–125
  carbamazepine, 116–117
  clozapine, 119–120
  complex treatment regimens, 111
  episode prevention and treatment
      of sub-syndromal residual
      symptoms, 109–110
  guidlines for, 110
  imipramine monotherapy, 370–371
  importance of, 108
  lamotrigine, 117–118
  lithium, 112–115
  mania during long-term
      monotherapy, 371
  medications for, 110–112
  mood stabilizer, 111–112
  olanzapine, 120–121
  prophylaxis and relapse prevention
      trials, 109
  quetiapine, 121–122
  risperidone monotherapy, 122–123
  side effects, 111

systematic review, 372
topiramate, 118
VPA monotherapy, 115–116
ziprasidone monotherapy, 124
Mania
  Diagnostic and Statistical Manual of
      Mental Disorders (DSM-IV)
      definition of, 1–3
  management of, 5–6
  mania rating scale (MRS), 387, 392
  from schedule for affective
      disorders and schizophrenia,
      307–308
  manic delirium, 414
  treatment algorithm for, 8
  treatment strategies, 12–14
Medical comorbidity, 244–245
Metabotropic glutamate receptors
      (mGluR), 606
Mini mental state examination (MMSE), 208
Mirtazapine, 369, 508
Moclobemide antidepressant, 32, 509
Modafinil, 36
Monoamine oxidase inhibitors (MAOI),
      367–368, 508–510
Montgomery-Åsberg Depression Rating
      Scale (MADRS), 390, 393–395
  with lamotrigine, 27
  score, 89
Mood disorders questionnaire, 4, 208; *see
      also* Bipolar disorder
Mood stabilizers, 111–112, 369–370,
      441–442
  carbamazepine (CBZ), 462–463
      adverse events and management,
          474–475
      clinical recommendations, 476–477
      dosing strategies, 475–476
      drug–drug interactions, 465–468,
          473–474
      metabolic pathway of, 463–464
  cytochrome P450 isoforms
      inducers, 472
      inhibitors, 471–472
      substrates, 469–471
  lamotrigine (LTG), 477–478
      adverse events and management,
          479–480
      clinical recommendations, 481–482
      dosing strategies, 481
      pharmacokinetic interactions,
          478–479

lithium, 442–443
    adverse effects and treatment,
       449–453
    and ageing, 448
    analgesics and, 447
    anticonvulsant and, 445
    antidepressants and, 444–445
    antihypertensives and, 447–448
    and antipsychotics interactions,
       443–444
    and benzodiazepines, 445
    calcium channel blockers and, 448
    clinical recommendations, 454–455
    diuretics and, 447
    dosing strategies, 453–454
    encephalopathic syndrome, 443
    factors affecting clearance of, 446
    interactions with carbamazepine, 443
    lamotrigine and, 443
    mania patients and, 448–449
    methylxanthines and, 448
    neuromuscular blocking agents
       and, 448
  structures of, 441
  valproate (VPA), 455–456
    adverse effects and management,
       449, 459–461
    benzodiazepines and, 458
    clinical recommendations, 462
    dosing strategies, 461–462
    metabolic drug interactions,
       457–459
    metabolic pathways, 456–457
Multidimensional psychiatric scale, 266

N

National comorbidity survey replication
    study, 186
National epidemiologic survey on alcohol
    and related conditions, 224
Nefazodone, 467, 471, 483–486, 507–508
Neuropeptides, stress and HPA axis
    CRF1 receptor antagonists, 601–602
    cytokines and inflammation, 603
    glucocorticoid receptor antagonists,
       600–602
    glutamatergic system, 603–606
    thyrotropin-releasing
       hormone (TRH), 603
NIMH STEP-BD database, 230
Nimodipine, 599

Nonsteroidal anti-inflammatory drugs
    (NSAIDs), 445, 447
Novel therapeutics, in bipolar disorder,
    607–609
  heavy metals, 606–607
  intracellular signaling cascades
    glycogen synthase kinase-3
       (GSK-3), 598
    increased intercellular calcium,
       598–599
    other second messenger targets,
       599–600
    PKC, involvement of, 597–598
  neuropeptides, stress and HPA axis
    CRF1 receptor antagonists, 601–602
    cytokines and inflammation, 603
    glucocorticoid receptor antagonists,
       600–602
    glutamatergic system, 603–606
    thyrotropin-releasing hormone
       (TRH), 603
  neurostimulatory techniques, 607
  neurotrophic cascades
    brain derived neurotrophic factor
       (BDNF), role of, 592–597

O

Obsessive-compulsive disorder (OCD),
    237–238
Olanzapine–fluoxetine combination,
    26–27, 35–36
Olanzapine (OLZ), 120–121, 492–495
    and antidepressant fluoxetine
       (OFC), 333
    and aripipraole studies, 353–354
    efficacy and safety, 196
    in preventing relapse, 354–355
Omega-3 fatty acids, 36
Open-labelled fluoxetine monotherapy, 89
Oppositional defiant disorder (ODD), 189
Organic euphoria, 416
Oxcarbazepine (OXC), 386, 518–520; *see also*
    Anticonvulsants medications, in
    bipolar disorder
    for acute mania, 386

P

Panic disorder, 237
Parkinson's disease, 215
Paroxetine antidepressant, 32

Perphenazine, 119
Personality disorders, 24–25, 241–243
    pharmacotherapy, 243–244
Pharmacodynamic interactions, 439; see
        also Pharmacotherapy, of bipolar
        disorders
Pharmacotherapy, of bipolar disorders,
        438–440
    adjunctive antidepressants, 503–504
        bupropion, 506–507
        mirtazapine, 508
        monoamine oxidase inhibitor,
            508–510
        nefazodone, 507–508
        selective serotonin reuptake
            inhibitors, 504–505
        serotonin-norepinephrine reuptake
            inhibitors, 505–506
        trazodone, 507
        tricyclic antidepressants, 510–511
    antipsychotics, use of, 482 (see also
        Atypical antipsychotics;
        Traditional antipsychotics)
    benzodiazepines, and
        mechanistically related
        drugs, 511–512
    mood stabilizers and (see Mood
        stabilizers)
    newer anticonvulsants, 512–513
        felbamate, 513
        gabapentin, 513–515
        levetiracetam, 520–522
        oxcarbazepine, 518–520
        pregabalin, 523–525
        tiagabine, 517–518
        topiramate, 515–517
        zonisamide, 522–523
Phosphodiesterase (PDE) inhibitors,
        594–596
Phototherapy, see Light therapy
PKC signaling pathways, and lithium
        treatment, 597
Polycystic ovarian syndrome (PCOS),
        157–158, 460
Postpartum psychosis, 161–162
Posttraumatic stress disorder (PTSD),
        239–240
Pramipexole dopamine agonist as mood
        stabilizers, 33, 36, 596
Pregabalin (PGB), 523–525
Premenstrual dysphoric
        disorder (PMDD), 156

Psychosocial interventions, for bipolar
        disorder, 576
    biopsychosocial approaches, 577–578
    cognitive behavioral therapy, 579–580
    design considerations, 578–579
    earlier studies on, 576–577
    family-focused therapy, 582–584
    future research, key issues for
        cost-effectiveness, 587
        moderators and mediators, 586–587
        as preventative intervention,
            587–588
    individual and group
        psychoeducation, 580–582
    interpersonal and social-rhythm
        therapy, 584–585
    STEP-BD program and, 585–586

Q

Quetiapine (QTP), 35–36, 121–122, 495–497
    monotherapy, 28–29

R

Rapid-cycling (RC) bipolar disorder, 46–47
    antidepressants, 58–59
    and antidepressants, 375–376
    and clinical management
            recommendations, 68
        algorithm for, 69
    comparison with non-rapid cycling
            (N-RC) bipolar disorder, 48–51
    DSM-IV and DSM-IV-TR definitions, 47
    follow-Up Studies of, 55
    genetics, 56–57
    illness course, 53–54
    meta-analysis of clinical studies, 58
    mixed episode, 52
    persistence of, 54, 56
    pole-switching pattern, 47, 52
    prevalence of, 54
    risk factors
        hypothyroidism, 57–58
        sex distribution and, 57
        thyroperoxidase (TPO)
            antibodies, 58
    treatment of, 59
        antidepressants, 66
        atypical antipsychotics, 64–65
        combination treatments, 67
        lamotrigine, 63–64

levetiracepam, 64
lithium, 60–62
psychotherapeutic interventions, 67–68
valproate, 62–63
ultra-rapid and ultradian cycling, 52
Refractory bipolar depression
treatment strategies
augmentation, 32–33
combining/adding alternate agents, 31–32
switching agents, 31
Repetitive transcranial magnetic stimulation (rTMS), 34
Reproductive cycle-associated symptoms, 158
Riluzole, 33, 36, 604
Risperidone (RSP), 489–492
as monotherapy, 122–123
safety and efficacy, 195
Rolipram, 596

S

Seasonal affective disorder (SAD), 417–419
Second-generation antipsychotics (SGAs), 297
active comparators in acute bipolar I mania, 310–311
trials, 312–323
in acute bipolar I depression, 333
in bipolar disorder, 300
change in primary outcome measure, 308
combination therapy studies in, 325–331
comparisons with
haloperidol, 311, 324
lithium and divalproex, 324–325
risperidone and olanzapine, 325
dose ranges and, 309
effect on depressive symptoms, 332
efficacy of, 331–332
limitations of, 332
in maintenance treatment of bipolar I disorder, 343, 355–356
meta-analysis, 333
olanzapine-fluoxetine combination and lamotrigine, 341–342
adverse events, 342
onset of action, 308–309

placebo
in acute bipolar I mania, 300, 308
controlled studies, 341
quetiapine studies and, 342
randomized controlled trials of, 307–308, 334–340, 344–352
rates of depressive symptoms, 310
response and remission rates, 309–310
side effects in, 332–333
Selective serotonin reuptake inhibitors (SSRIs), 368, 374, 504–505
in antidepressants medications, in bipolar disorder, 368
for pregnancy, 168
Self-medication hypothesis, 231–232
Serotonin-norepinephrine reuptake inhibitors (SNRIs), 505–506
Sertraline antidepressant, 32
Social phobia, 239
Somatic treatments, for bipolar disorder, 411–412
electroconvulsive therapy, 412–416
light therapy, 417–420
neurosurgical treatments
ablative neurosurgical procedures, 424–425
deep brain stimulation, 427–428
vagus nerve stimulation, 426–427
transcranial magnetic stimulation, 422–424
wake therapy, 420–422
Stanley Foundation Bipolar Network (SFBN), 367, 369
Steven-Johnson's syndrome, 194
Subcaudate tractotomy, 425
Systematic Treatment Enhancement Program for Bipolar Disorder (STEP-BD), 369, 580, 585–586

T

Tamoxifen, 597
Texas Implementation of Medication Algorithms (TIMA), 110
Thioridazine, 119
Thyrotropin-releasing hormone (TRH), 603
Tiagabine (TGB), 401, 517–518; *see also*
Anticonvulsants medications, in bipolar disorder
Topiramate (TPM), 118, 398–399, 515–517, 605–606
in acute bipolar depression, 399

in acute mania, 399
Total sleep deprivation (TSD), *see* Wake
    therapy
Traditional antipsychotics, 482–483
    extrapyramidal symptoms (EPS)
        and, 484
    haloperidol, 483–484
Transcranial magnetic stimulation (TMS),
    422, 607
    repetitive TMS (rTMS), 422–424
Tranylcypromine antidepressant, 32
Trazodone, 469, 479, 507, 512
Tricyclic antidepressants (TCAs), 367,
    510–511

U

University of Cincinnati first-episode
    mania study, 231
Uridine diphosphate glycosyltransferase
    (UGT) isozymes, 440

V

Vagus nerve stimulation (VNS), 34,
    426–427, 607
Valproate (VPA)
    as mood stabilizers, 32, 115, 455–456
        adverse effects and management,
            449, 459–461
        benefit-risk of, 194
        benzodiazepines and, 458
        in breast-feeding, 166
        clinical recommendations, 462
        with combination treatment, 116
        dosing strategies, 461–462
        metabolic drug interactions,
            457–459

metabolic pathways, 456–457
open-label trials of, 193
during pregnancy, 165–166
side effects, 116
valproate/divalproex
    in acute mania, 387–389
    in bipolar depression, 389–390
    prophylaxis of bipolar disorder,
        390–392
Venlafaxine, 369, 505–506
    as antidepressant, 32
    monotherapy trial, 89
Verapamil, 599

W

Wake therapy, 420–422
Weight gain, 452, 493, 496
Winter depression, *see* Seasonal affective
    disorder (SAD)
Wittenborn scale for manic state and
    schizophrenic excitement, 264
World Federation of Societies of Biological
    Psychiatry (WFSBP)
    guidelines, 110

Y

Young mania rating scale (YMRS), 88, 191,
    385, 388, 393

Z

Ziprasidone (ZIP), 497–500
    efficacy and safety, 196–197
    monotherapy, 124
Zonisamide (ZNS), 522–523

Printed and bound by
Baker & Taylor Publisher Services

United States
ior Publisher Services